Gynaecologic Cancer

Gynaecologic Cancer

A Handbook for Students and Practitioners

Rushdan Noor
Eng Hseon Tay
Jeffrey Low

Pan Stanford Publishing

Published by

Pan Stanford Publishing Pte. Ltd.
Penthouse Level, Suntec Tower 3
8 Temasek Boulevard
Singapore 038988

Email: editorial@panstanford.com
Web: www.panstanford.com

British Library Cataloguing-in-Publication Data
A catalogue record for this book is available from the British Library.

Gynaecologic Cancer: A Handbook for Students and Practitioners

ISBN 978-981-4463-06-5 (Hardcover)
ISBN 978-981-4463-07-2 (eBook)

Printed in the USA

Contents

Preface

Gynaecologic oncology is a very challenging field and an important component of gynaecology and oncology. It is one of the most important subjects in gynaecology. The management of patients with gynaecological cancers is complex, as the impact of the outcome of such cancers can be critical. Gynaecologic oncology is always perceived as the most difficult subject in obstetrics and gynaecology. However, this handbook will prove it otherwise. This handbook of gynaecologic oncology is a new addition to the current academic tomes and covers the essential breadth of knowledge ranging from the basics of carcinogenesis to the latest advances in the prevention and management of all gynaecological cancers, including breast cancer. It aims to provide readers with the information and data in a systematic and easy-to-understand format with numerous illustrations and images. It is designed to be handy and compact but with the content equivalent to that of a standard textbook. The book also introduces the readers to the new FIGO staging system, including FIGO staging 2014 for ovarian and fallopian tube carcinoma. It will serve as a useful reference for everyone in the medical field, including researchers, clinicians, house officers, pharmacists, doctors, specialists, postgraduate students, fellows and sub-specialty trainees in gynaecologic, radiation and medical oncology and lecturers in universities.

Rushdan Noor
Eng Hseon Tay
Jeffrey Low

Chapter 1

World Cancer Statistics and Burden of Gynaecological Cancer

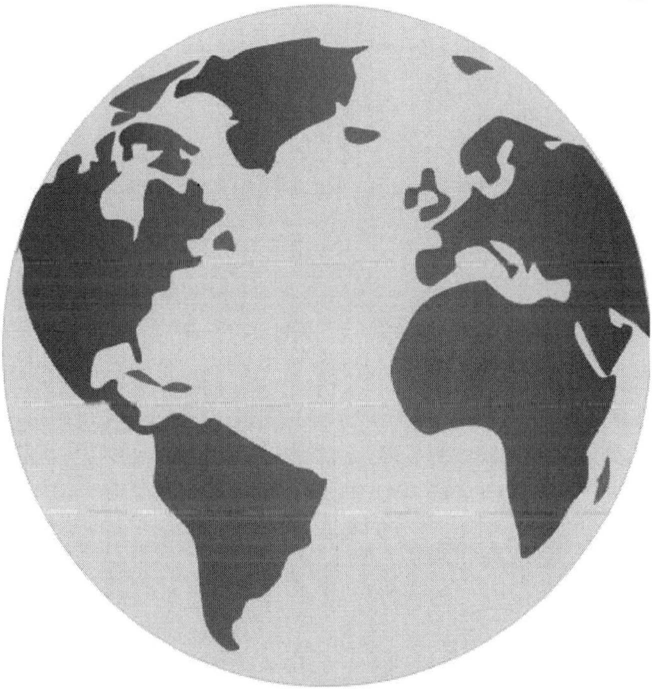

Gynaecologic Cancer: A Handbook for Students and Practitioners
Rushdan Noor, Eng Hseon Tay, and Jeffrey Low

ISBN 978-981-4463-06-5 (Hardcover), 978-981-4463-07-2 (eBook)
www.panstanford.com

Introduction

Cancer is a group of diseases characterized by uncontrolled growth and spread of abnormal cells that can infiltrate to other parts of the body through the blood and lymphatic systems. Unlike normal cells, cancer cells do not undergo programmatic death known as apoptosis and instead continue to grow and divide. There are more than 100 different types of cancer. The aetiology of cancer is multifactorial and involves a very complex process known as carcinogenesis. Cancer carcinogenesis is discussed in Chapter 2.

Cancer kills more people than AIDS, tuberculosis and malaria combined and will soon become the world's single leading cause of death. According to a report by GLOBOCAN 2012, higher proportion of the cancer burden occurs in less developed regions both in terms of cancer incidence (57% new cancers in 2012 occur within less developed regions) and cancer mortality (65% of cancer deaths) (IARC Globocan, 2012).

Smoking, alcohol intake and low fruit and vegetable intake were the leading risk factors for death from cancer worldwide in low- and middle-income countries while in high-income countries, smoking, alcohol use and overweight and obesity were the most important causes of cancer. Smoking alone is estimated to have caused 21% of deaths from cancer worldwide. Low- and middle-income countries accounted for about 50% of all cancers worldwide in 1975; this proportion increased to 56% in 2008 and is projected to reach 61% by 2050 (Bray and Moller, 2006; GLOBOCAN, 2008). A summary of overall cancer statistics in 2008 is shown in Tables 1.1, 1.2 and 1.3 (Globocan, 2008; Ferlay et al., 2010).

Table 1.1 Summary of world cancer statistics 2012

Statistics	Male	Female	Both
Population (million)	3557.717	3496.728	7054.446
Number of new cancer cases (million)	7.4271	6.6630	14.0901
Age-standardized rate*	205.4	165.3	182.3
Risk getting cancer before age 75(%)	21.0	16.4	18.5
Number of cancer death (million)	4.6531	3.5479	8.2010
Risk of dying from cancer before age 75(%)	12.7	8.4	10.4

*per-100,000 population

Source: Globocan, 2012; Ferlay et al., 2010.

Table 1.2 Summary of world cancer statistics in more developed regions in 2012 (GLOBOCAN 2012)

	More developed regions*		
Statistics	**Male**	**Female**	**Both**
Population (million)	605.963	639.750	1245.713
Number of new cancer cases	3.2435 mil	2.8324 mil	6.0759 mil
Age-standardized rate	308.7	240.6	268.3
Risk getting cancer before age 75 (%)	30.9	23.3	26.8
Number of cancer death	1.5912 mil	1.2867 mil	2.8779 mil
Risk of dying from cancer before age 75 (%)	14.3	9.0	11.4
Five most frequent cancers	Prostate, Lung, Colorectum, Bladder, Stomach	Breast, Colorectum, Lung, Corpus uteri, Ovary	Breast, Prostate, Lung Colorectum, Stomach

Source: Globocan, 2012; Ferlay et al., 2010.

*The rates for the more developed regions have been calculated as the population-weighted average of Northern America, Japan, Eastern Europe, Northern Europe, Southern Europe, Western Europe, Australia/New Zealand.

Table 1.3 Summary of world cancer statistics in less developed regions in 2012

	Less developed regions*		
Statistics	**Male**	**Female**	**Both**
Population (million)	2951.754	2856.978	5808.732
Number of new cancer cases	4.1836 mil	3.8306 mil	8.0143 mil
Age-standardized rate#	163.0	135.8	147.7
Risk getting cancer before age 75 (%)	16.6	13.4	14.9
Number of cancer death	3.0619 mil	2.2612 mil	5.3231 mil
Risk of dying from cancer before age 75 (%)	12.0	8.1	9.9
Five most frequent cancers	Lung, Liver, Stomach, Prostate, Colorectum	Breast, Cervix uteri, Lung, Colorectum, Stomach	Lung, Breast, Stomach, Liver, Colorectum

Source: Globocan, 2012; Ferlay et al., 2010.

*The less developed regions: Eastern, Middle, Northern, Southern, Western Africa, Caribbean, Central America, South America, Eastern Asia, South Eastern Asia, Western Asia, Melanesia, Micronesia, Polynesia.

#Age standardized rate: A rate is number of new cases or deaths per 100,000 persons per-year

World Cancer Burden and Contributing Factors

The International Agency for Research on Cancer (IARC) has predicted that by 2030, 27 million new cancer cases and 17 million cancer deaths will occur each year worldwide. This compares to 14.1 million new cancers and 8.2 million cancer death reported by GLOBOCAN 2012. Based on current trends, the rate at which new cancers are diagnosed is expected to grow by 1% annually. China, Russia and India are projected to have the biggest increases in cancers and cancer deaths (Danaei et al., 2005; Globocan, 2008; Ferlay et al., 2010).

The three most important factors that contribute to these trends are

(a) growth and increase in life expectancy of population;
(b) cigarette smoking;
(c) diet, obesity and physical inactivity.

Tobacco use is the single largest preventable cause of cancer and premature death worldwide. Estimated 1.3 billion people in the world currently smoke tobacco. If current trends in smoking and population growth continue, the number of current smokers is expected to be 2 billion worldwide by 2030. Overweight and obesity are also important contributing factors to cancer risk; The WHO estimates that the number of overweight adults in 2005 was approximately 1.6 billion and 300 million were obese (BMI > 30). The number of overweight is expected to increase to 2.3 billion by 2015. The main reasons for this trend are overeating, increased availability of high-calorie food and physical inactivity. Obesity is known to be a risk factor for breast, endometrial, ovarian, colorectal, oesophagus and kidney cancers (Danaei et al., 2005; Globocan, 2008; Ferlay et al., 2010; Sankaranarayanan and Ferlay, 2006).

Chronic infections are known to be primary aetiology for many cancers such as stomach cancer (*Helicobacter pylori*), cervical cancer (human papillomavirus), liver cancer (Hepatitis B and C infections), Kaposi's sarcoma (human herpes virus 8), bladder cancer (*Schistosoma haematobium*), etc. Persistent infections with these various organisms contribute for approximately 18% of cancer worldwide and developing countries have three times the higher percentage of infection-related cancers than developed countries.

Increasing number of elderly population is known contributing factors to increasing rate of cancer incidence worldwide. The life expectancy of the world is 67.2 years: 65 years for males and 69.5 years for female for 2005–2010 according to United Nations World Population Prospects 2006 Revision. Among countries with the highest life expectancy are Japan (82.6), Hong Kong (82.2), Iceland (81.8), Switzerland (81.7) and Australia (81.2) (Ferlay et al., 2010; Globocan, 2008).

According to GLOBOCAN 2012, the total of 14.1 million new cancer cases and 8.2 million cancer deaths have been reported in 2012. Lung cancer remains the most common cancer in the world, both in term of cases (1.8 million cases, 13.0% of total) and deaths (1.6 million deaths, 19.4% of total) (Table 1.4). Breast cancer is the second most common cancer overall with 1.7 million new cases reported in 2012 or 11.9% of total new cancer cases worldwide. While, colorectal cancer is the third most common cancer with 1.4 million new cases reported and 693,881 deaths reported in 2012.

Table 1.4 World's 10 most frequent cancers in men and women in 2012 (GLOBOCAN 2012)

Type of cancer	Number	(%)	ASR (per 100,000)	Mortality (%)
Lung	1,824,701	13.0	23.1	19.4
Breast	1,676,633	11.9	43.3	6.4
Colorectum	1,360,602	9.7	17.2	8.5
Prostate	1,111,689	7.9	31.1	3.7
Stomach	952,594	7.9	12.1	8.8
Liver	782,451	5.6	10.1	9.1
Cervix uteri	527,624	3.7	14.0	3.2
Oesophagus	455,784	3.2	5.9	4.9
Bladder	429,793	3.1	5.3	2.0
Non-Hodgkin lymphoma	385,741	2.5	5.1	2.4

The most common causes of cancer death are lung (1.59 million, 19.4% of total), liver cancers (0.75 million, 9.1%) and stomach (0.72 million, 8.8%). Despite being the second most common cancer, breast cancer ranks fifth as cause of deaths. This is probably due to early detection and more effective treatment; furthermore, breast cancer is more prevalence in developed countries with adequate facilities, finance and human resources for screening and treatment. The world 10 most frequent cancers in men and women are shown in Table 1.5 and 1.6 respectively.

Table 1.5 World's 10 most common cancers in men (GLOBOCAN 2012)

Type of cancer	Number	(%)	ASR (per 100,000)	Mortality (%)
Lung	1,241,601	16.7	34.2	23.6
Prostate	1,111,689	15.0	31.1	6.6
Colorectum	746,298	10.0	20.6	8.0
Stomach	631,293	8.5	17.4	10.1
Liver	554,369	7.5	15.3	11.2
Bladder	330,380	4.4	9.0	2.6
Oesophagus	323,008	4.3	9.0	6.0
Non-Hodgkin lymphoma	217,643	2.5	6.0	2.5
Kidney	213,924	2.9	6.0	2.0
Leukaemia	200,676	2.7	5.6	3.3

Table 1.6 World's 10 most common cancer in women (GLOBOCAN 2012)

Type of cancer	Number	(%)	ASR (per 100,000)	Mortality (%)
Breast	1,676,633	25.2	43.3	14.7
Colorectum	614,304	9.2	14.3	9.0
Lung	583,100	8.8	13.6	13.8
Cervix	527,624	7.9	14.0	7.5
Stomach	320,301	4.8	7.5	7.2
Corpus uteri	319,605	4.8	8.3	2.1
Ovary	238,719	3.6	6.1	4.3
Thyroid	229,923	3.5	6.1	0.8
Liver	228,082	3.4	5.3	6.3
Non-Hodgkin lymphoma	168,098	2.5	4.1	2.4

The regions with the highest cancer incidence rate in females are North America (ASR 274.4 per 100, 000), Australia/New Zealand (ASR 276.4), Northern and Western Europe (ASRs 249.4 and 250.9 respectively) mainly due to the high breast cancer incidence in these regions. The lowest cancer incidence in women is in Middle Africa and Northern Africa (ASR < 100 per 100, 000) (Danaei et al., 2005; Ferlay et al., 2010; Globocan, 2008).

Breast Cancer

Breast cancer is the most common cancer in women and the second most common cancer in both men and women. It was estimated 1.68 million cases or 25.2% of all new women's cancer cases reported in 2012. The incidence rates are highest in developed countries (except Japan). According to GLOBOCAN 2012 reports, breast cancer incidence has increased by more than 20% in 2012 compared to 2008. The mortality rate has also increased by 14%. Incidence rates remains highest in more developed regions, but mortality rate is relatively much higher in less developed countries due to a lack of early detection and access to treatment facilities. The incidence rate in Western Europe is 90 per 100,000 women while in Eastern Africa is 30 per 100,000 women. Breast cancer contributes 12.7% of cancer death in both developing and developed regions (Ferlay et al., 2010; Globocan, 2008; Sankaranarayanan and Ferlay, 2006, GLOBOCAN 2012).

Cervical Cancer

Cervical cancer is the fourth most common cancer in women and the seventh most common overall cancer in 2012. In 2012, cervical cancer is the fourth most common cancers in women worldwide, after breast, colorectal and lung cancers. GLOBOCAN (2012) estimated 527,624 new cases of cervical cancer have been reported in 2012, and this constitutes 7.9% of all female cancer. Regions with high-risk cervical cancer are Eastern Africa (ASR 42.7 per 100,000), Melanesia (ASR 33.3), Southern Africa (ASR 31.5), South Central Asia (ASR 24.6), Middle Africa (ASR

30.6) and South America (ASR 23.9). While, the risk of cervical cancer is lowest in Western Asia (ASR 4.4), Northern America (ASR 5.7), Australia (ASR 5.0) and New Zealand (ASR 5.0). Age-standardized incidence of cervical cancer in South East Asia is 15.8 per 100,000 population. Cervical cancer is responsible for a total of 265,653 deaths in 2012 (mortality:incidence ratio of 0.52), accounting 7.5% of all female cancer deaths. Approximately 88% of cervical cancer death occurs in developing countries; 159,800 deaths (58%) were reported from Asia (Ferlay et al., 2010; Globocan, 2008; Globocan 2012, Sankaranarayanan and Ferlay, 2006). According to GLOBOCAN 2012, cervical cancer is also the fourth most common cause of cancer death in women worldwide (266,000 deaths in 2012) and almost 70% of the global burden falls in areas with lower levels of development. Mortality varies 18-fold between the different regions of the world, with rates ranging from less than 2 per 100,000 in Western Asia, Western Europe and Australia/New Zealand, to more than 20 per 100,000 in Melanesia (20.6), Middle (22.2) and Eastern Africa (27.6) (GLOBOCAN 2012).

Uterine Cancer

According to GLOBOCAN 2012, uterine cancer is the sixth most common women cancer worldwide and a total of 319,605 new cases had been reported with ASR of 8.3 per 100,000 population constituting 4.8% from total women cancers. The highest incidences are observed in United State with ASR of 19.48 per 100,000 women. More than 90% of patients with uterine cancer are more than 50 years old (Ferlay et al., 2010; Globocan, 2008; Sankaranarayanan and Ferlay, 2006, GLOBOCAN 2012).

The incidence of uterine cancer is more common in developed regions (50% of total cases were reported from more developed regions) ranking fourth the most common cancer in women after breast, colorectal and lung. Cancer of the uterine body is also the most common gynaecological cancer in developed regions. A total of 76,155 deaths had been reported in 2012 due to uterine cancer (Globocan 2012). Cancer of the uterus has much more favourable prognosis than ovarian and cervical cancer with 5-year survival rates around 80–90% in developed countries and 70% in the developing countries.

Ovarian Cancer

The cancer of the ovary is one of the most lethal gynaecological malignancies due to late presentation, poor response to treatment and high recurrence rate. Ovarian cancer has a similar geographic distribution to uterine cancer and it is the seventh most common cancer in women and the third most common gynaecological cancer worldwide after cervical and uterine cancer. There was a total of 238,719 new cases of ovarian cancer reported in 2012, which is 3.6% of all women cancer and 151,905 deaths have been reported on the same year (4.3% of all cancer deaths in women). The cumulative risk of developing ovarian cancer is 0.7 (0.7 per 100 lifetime risk). The incidence rates are higher in developed regions (overall ASR of 8–11 per 100,000 compared to 3–5 per 100,000 in less developed regions) and 100,254 new cases (45% from total cases worldwide) of ovarian cancer were reported in more developed regions in 2008 (Ferlay et al., 2010; Globocan, 2008; Globocan 2012, Sankaranarayanan and Ferlay, 2006).

Other Gynaecological Cancers

Vulvar cancer is rare, accounting for 3% of all gynaecological cancers. Approximately, 27,000 cases have been reported annually and 58% of cases are from developed countries. The incidence of vulvar cancer is highest in North America, South America and Europe. The incidence rates are between 1–1.5 per 100,000. Vulvar cancer is rare in developing countries, including Asia.

Vaginal cancer is also rare gynaecological cancer: It is estimated that 13,000–14,000 new cases have been reported annually but the majorities are from developing countries. The incidence rates do not exceed 0.8 per 100,000 women. More than 75% of cases occur in women older than 60 years old.

Glossary of Terms

- **Incidence**: Incidence is the number of new cases that arise in a given period in a specified population. It can be expressed as an absolute number of cases per year or as a rate per 100,000 persons per year. The rate provides an approximation of an average risk of developing cancer.

- **Prevalence**: Prevalence is defined as the total number of cases of the disease in the population at a given time, or the total number of cases in the population, divided by the number of individuals in the population. It is used as an estimate of how common a condition is within a population over a certain period of time.
- **Mortality**: Mortality is the number of deaths that occur in a given period in a specified population. It can be expressed as an absolute number of deaths per year or as a rate per 100,000 persons per year.
- **Crude rate**: Data on incidence or mortality are often presented as rates. For a specific tumour and population, a crude rate is calculated simply by dividing the number of new cancers or cancer deaths observed during a given time period by the corresponding number of person years in the population at risk. For cancer, the result is usually expressed as an annual rate per 100,000 persons at risk.
- **Age-standardized rate (ASR)**: ASR is a summary measure of the rate that a population would have if it had a standard age structure. Standardization is necessary when comparing several populations that differ with respect to age because age has a powerful influence on the risk of cancer. The most frequently used standard population is the world standard population. The calculated incidence or mortality rate is then called age-standardized incidence or mortality rate (world). It is also expressed per 100,000.
- **Cumulative risk**: Cumulative incidence/mortality is the probability or risk of individuals getting/dying from the disease during a specified period. For cancer, it is expressed as the number of new born children (out of 100, or 1000) who would be expected to develop or die from a particular cancer before the age of 75 if they had the rates of cancer observed in the period in the absence of competing causes.

Source: http://globocan.iarc.fr/glossary.htm.

References

Bray F, Moller B. Predicting the future burden of cancer. *Nat Rev Cancer* 2006; **6**(1): 63–74.

Danaei G, Hoorn SV, Lopez AD, et al. Causes of cancer in the world: comparative risk assessment of nine behavioural and environmental risk factors. *Lancet* 2005; **366**: 1784–1793.

Ferlay J, Shin HR, Bray F, et al. Estimates of worldwide burden of cancer in 2008: GLOBOCAN 2008. *Int. J. Cancer* 2010, DOI: 10.1002/ijc.25516.

IARC GLOBOCAN 2008 website: http://globocan.iarc.fr/.

IARC GLOBOCAN 2012: Estimated Cancer Incidence, Mortality and Prevalence Worldwide in 2012. website: http://globocan.iarc.fr/

Sankaranarayanan R, Ferlay J. Worldwide burden of gynaecological cancer: the size of the problem. *Best Pract Res Clin Obstet Gynaecol* 2006; **20**(2): 207–225.

Thun MJ, DeLancey JO, Center MM, et al. The global burden of cancer: priorities for prevention. *Carcinogenesis* 2010; **31**(1): 100–110.

Chapter 2

Genes and Carcinogenesis

Basic Structure of DNA

Deoxyribonucleic acid, or DNA, is a polymer with the basic unit known as nucleotide, which consists of three parts: (1) standard unit of five carbon deoxyribose (sugar) with phosphate and (2) variable unit known as bases known as purine and pyrimidine. Purine comprises adenine (A) and guanine (G), while Pyrimidine comprises cytosine (C) and thiamine (T). Nucleotides are connected to each other through their phosphate group. The bases are free to interact with each other, i.e. Adenine is interacted with Thiamine (A–T), Guanine is interacted with Cytosine (G–C). The DNA molecules are associated with specific proteins to form a chromatics in the nucleus (Figs. 2.1 and 2.2).

Gene

The gene is a fundamental unit of inheritance, and in a normal human cell, DNA contains 30,000 to 100,000 genes. The genes exert their effect through two steps: (1) transcription (DNA to mRNA) and (2) translation of mRNA into protein. Every gene has two main functional units, namely (1) promoter region and (2) coding region. The promoter region determines when and what

Gynaecologic Cancer: A Handbook for Students and Practitioners
Rushdan Noor, Eng Hseon Tay, and Jeffrey Low

ISBN 978-981-4463-06-5 (Hardcover), 978-981-4463-07-2 (eBook)
www.panstanford.com

tissue will be expressed, while the coding region determines the structures of protein produced. Interestingly, gene can be dissected from the DNA using an enzymatic process known as restriction endonucleases. The dissected gene can be captured and replicated by inserting it into a bacterial plasmid or virus. The plasmid is able to replicate independently, and at the same time, the genes that have been inserted to it will also replicate. This process is called cloning and the cloned gene is also known as a probe. Using based pairing on the probes, the cloned gene (DNA sequences) will be identified and this process is called nucleic acid hybridization. Hybridization is the basic concept of many DNA analyses such as Southern blot, microarray analysis and polymerase chain reaction.

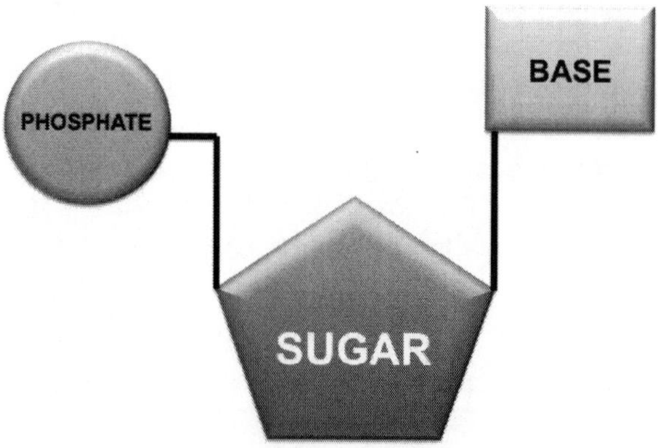

Figure 2.1 Nucleotide is a basic unit of nucleic acids. Each nucleotide has three components: (a) bases belonging to the class of purine or pyrimidine, (b) a five carbon or pentose sugar and (c) a phosphate group.

The DNA will undergo transcription (genetic materials will be copied) to mRNA by mRNA polymerase II enzyme. Subsequently, mRNA will be transported to a cytoplasm. The cytoplasmic mRNA can be detected by northern blotting, nucleus protection assay and modified polymerase chain reaction. It is known that the process of translation to protein is more complex than transcription. After translation, protein has to undergo modification to make it fully functional. The translation from mRNA to protein can be induced in vitro using the cellular extract from animal reticulocytes and wheat germ.

The end result of translation is a functional protein and its acid amino sequences that can be analyzed by various techniques such as electrophoresis, immunoblotting, immunosorbent assay, immune precipitation, mass spectrometry and others. Full process from DNA transcription to RNA and subsequently translation of RNA into protein can be repeated in vivo using the expression system also known as a vector (example of vectors: yeast cell, insect cells and plant cells).

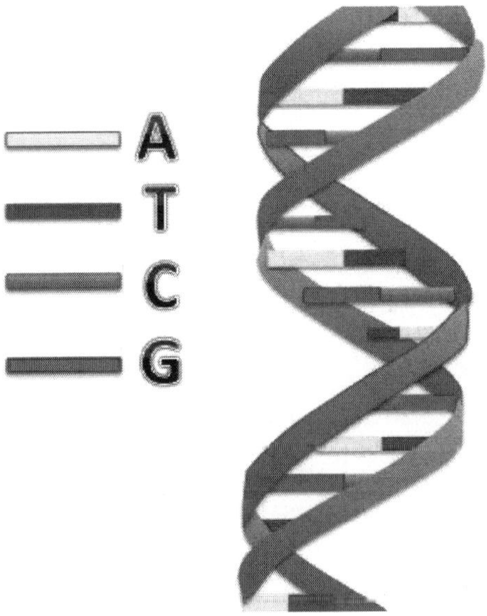

Figure 2.2 DNA molecule. The shape of the DNA is called double helix. The sides of the ladder are a linked chain of alternating sugar and phosphate molecules. Both strands are connected with each other through bases. There are four bases: (a) A: Adenine, (b) T: Thymine, (c) C: Cytosine, and (d) G: Guanine. Adenine is linked to thymine, while cytosine linked to guanine.

Genes and Carcinogenesis

All multicellular organisms have the potential to develop cancer, and the process of cancer development is called carcinogenesis. Carcinogenesis is a highly controversial subject, and it involves many steps and functional processes. Carcinogenesis is built on the foundation of non-lethal genetic changes and these changes may be attributed to acquired factors such as environmental factors (chemical, toxin, radiation, infection, etc.,) and may be inherited from the parent, e.g. defects in repair genes or genes responsible for cell growth and apoptosis.

Phases of Carcinogenesis

Carcinogenesis can be divided into three phases:

(1) initiation phase (irreversible)
(2) promotion phase (reversible)
(3) progression phase

Initiation Phase

The initiation phase follows exposure to carcinogens/mutagens, which are also known as initiators. This phase is an irreversible step cause by DNA damage leading to somatic mutation and mutation to tumour suppressor genes is said to be the first step of carcinogenesis (Fearon–Vogelstein model). During the initiation phase, there will be little or no observable changes in cellular or tissue morphology (Saracin, 2003; Vincent and Gatenby, 2008).

Promotion Phase

The promotion phase consists of changes in tumour suppressor genes and oncogenes, which reduce the tumour cell response to normal tissue proliferation constraints. This phase is a result of prolonged exposure to carcinogens and increased susceptibility of cells to promoters. Promoters are the factors that trigger the promotion phase by promoting the proliferation of mutated cells. The cells have to be first initiated before it can take the effect and enter the promotion phase of carcinogenesis. Therefore, the promoter has no effect on uninitiated cells. In contrast to initiation phase, promotion phase may be reversible. There are two types of promoters: (1) **specific promoters**, which act on the specific receptors, and (2) **non-specific promoters**, which alter gene expression without interaction with receptors. Wound and inflammation are two examples of promoters that promote tumour growth through an increase in local blood flow. In the promotion phase, changes in the cellular or tissue morphology (self-limited tumour growth) may be observed, but it is still reversible (Saracin, 2003; Vincent and Gatenby, 2008).

Progression Phase

The third phase in carcinogenesis is the progression phase. During this phase, the cells that have been promoted are transformed to the malignant cells. One of the most important changes that take place during the progression phase is karyotypic changes leading to aneuploidy. Subsequently, these karyotypic changes will be coupled with an increased growth rate, invasiveness, metastasis and an alteration in biochemistry and morphology.

Stem Cell and Cancer

A stem cell is a special cell type that has both the ability to reproduce exact copies of itself (also called *self-renewal*) and the ability to change (differentiate) into one of the many specialized cell types in the body. An alternative theory of cancer development is the cancer stem cell theory. This theory explained why in some tumours, more than one type of differentiated cell co-exist within a single tumour. The stem cells can also be predisposed to mutagen or carcinogen and undergo mutation. It was also hypothesized that mutated differentiated cells can "reverse backward" and acquire stem cell abilities (Carbone and Pass, 2004; Laconi, 2008).

Cancer stem cells have the ability to produce cells of many different types creating the mixture of cells found in a tumour. Stem cells theory also explained why in many cancers, treatment is difficult, drug resistance is common and recurrence rate is high. Stem cells are more difficult to be killed than normal cell because of their anti-apoptotic properties.

Chronic Inflammation and Cancer

Inflammation has long been associated with the development of cancer. Chronic inflammation due to infection or to conditions such as chronic inflammatory bowel disease is associated with up to 25% of all cancers. Chronic inflammation is an important factor in tumour development due to three main factors (1) It can alter the behaviour of cells, (2) Stimulation of the growth of new blood vessels (angiogenesis) and (3) Tissue remodelling. A recent study done by researchers at Ohio State University found that inflammation stimulates a rise in levels of a molecule called microRNA-155 (miR-155). This, in turn, causes a drop in levels of proteins involved in DNA repair, resulting in a higher rate of spontaneous gene mutations, which can lead to cancer (Laconi et al., 2008).

Infection and Cancer

Infection is an established cause of many cancers in the human being. The *Lancer Oncology* review, which looked at incidence rates for 27 cancers in 184 countries, found four main infections that contribute to cancer development are human papillomaviruses, *Helicobacter pylori* and hepatitis B and C, account for 1.9 million cases of cervical, gut and liver cancers. Some viruses and bacteria have been linked with the initiation and promotion of tumour growth. Viruses such as HPV and hepatitis B can cause cancer from a direct effect on cell division and mutation of gene. Microorganisms such as Schistosoma, *H. Pylori* and Leishmania induce malignant transformation through chronic inflammation.

Genetic Alterations in Cancer

Human Genome and Cancer

A complete constituent of the DNA, all genes and spaces in between them are called genome. A Human Genome Project has identified every chemical base and discovered approximately 25,000 genes in the human genome (Liang et al., 2000; Roest et al., 2000; Sachidanandan et al., 2001). These genes actually contribute to only 3% of total components of genome. Genomics is the study of genes and their functions, while cancer genomics refers to study of human cancer genome. Cancer genomics enable scientists to identify genetic alterations in cancer because all cancer cells have some degree of alteration in gene expression. Formerly, most of the information on genetic alterations in cancer was obtained from the study done in leukaemia and lymphoma because in these cancers, a single malignant cell is easier to be obtained, i.e. peripheral blood or bone marrow.

Types of Genetic Alteration in Cancer

There are two types of genetic alterations in cancer: (a) germ line mutations and (b) somatic mutations. In most cancers,mutation of p53 occurs as a somatic mutation/event but germ line p53 mutations have been identified in some families with rare Li–Fraumeni syndrome. Individuals inheriting the germ line abnormalities are at higher risk of developing malignancy as the penetrance of most of these genes is of the order of 80%. Low penetrance means a relatively small proportion of individuals with the genetic abnormality develop cancer (Elmasry and Gayther, 2006). Malignant transformation is also attributed to epimutation. Epimutation encompasses mechanisms that modify the final outcome of the genetic code without altering the underlying DNA sequence. Three most important epigenetics processes that involved in the normal control of genetic activities are DNA mehylations, histone modification and RNA-mediated silencing. Epimutation is when these processes become deregulated such as hypermethylation or hypomethylation of the DNA.

Germ Line Mutations

The mutations that occur in germ cells are also known as germ line mutations. They may occur de novo (for the first time) or may be inherited from parents. Germ line mutations may involve all cells, including tumour and normal cells, and they can also be passed to descendant and cause cancer family syndromes such as familial adenomatous polyposis and multiple endocrine neoplasia 2B. The occurrences of germ line mutations can be identified in the DNA obtained from normal cells, e.g. peripheral blood sample.

Somatic Mutations

When the mutations occur in non-germ cells line, they are called somatic mutations. Somatic mutations are usually located on the autosomes, and in contrast to germ line mutations, somatic mutations are only found in the tumour cells but not in normal cells. Therefore, they cannot be passed on to the descendants of the patient.

Pathways of Carcinogenesis in Familial and Sporadic Gynaecologic Cancers

Ovarian and endometrial cancer can develop as one of the components of two familiar cancer syndromes, i.e. familial breast/ovarian cancer and Lynch II syndromes.

Persistent infection by high-risk human papillomavirus can initiate genetic alteration involving oncogenes and tumour suppressor genes and subsequently malignant transformation of epithelial cells leading to invasive cancer.

In sporadic ovarian cancer, environmental factors with carcinogenesis operated indirectly by increasing the opportunity of spontaneous mutation.

Specific Genetic Alterations Responsible in Carcinogenesis

In carcinogenesis, the malignant transformation is initiated by various alterations in the genetic make-up of the cells.

Following are specific genetic alterations responsible in carcinogenesis:

(1) **Translocations and inversions**: An example is ovarian adenocarcinoma (t(6;14)(q21;q24)).

(2) **Chromosomal deletions** are most common genetic alterations in solid tumour. Deletion causes loss of function that regulates cell proliferation and differentiation. The p53 tumour suppressor gene-containing region of chromosome 17p is deleted or mutated in a wide variety of human cancers.

(3) **Frameshift mutations** occur as a result of addition or loss of a nucleotide(s).

(4) **Splice-site mutation** occurs within the non-coding regions (introns) resulting in the production of non-functioning proteins.

(5) **Point mutations** involved single base changes in DNA sequences and the most common type of alteration in DNA.

(6) **Gene's amplifications are** manifested as an increase in the number of genes or number of chromosomes. Example:

Amplification of gene her-2/neu in advanced breast and ovarian cancer.

(7) **Aneuploidy**: Gross changes in the number of chromosome occur as tumour progress in the malignant process. In general, tumours that remain localized without metastases have a much lower incidence of aneuploidy.

Genes and Malignant Transformation

The genetic alterations can be acquired either from exposure to exogenous carcinogens or inherited from parents. Three important genes responsible in initiation and progression of cancer are mutated proto-oncogenes, tumour suppressor genes and oncogenes. Proto-oncogenes and tumour suppressor genes exist in normal cells and involved in normal cellular functions. However, genetic alterations to these genes can lead to cellular malfunctions and abnormal proliferation of cells.

Proto-Oncogenes (e.g. c-src, c-abl and c-myc)

The proto-oncogene is a unit of genetic information that encodes a specific protein with specific functions, including cells regulation and differentiation. Actually, proto-oncogene is a normal genetic constituent and it involves in normal cellular functions and growth factors. These genes (growth promoting genes) are responsible in carrying code for proteins that encourage and stimulate cellular replication and control of cell division. Proto-oncogene expression patterns altered (amplification) in malignant tissue as compared to normal tissue; for example, amplification of c-myc was found in small cell carcinoma cell lines.

Tumour Suppressor Genes (e.g. p53, PTEN, BRCA1, BRCA2, APC, RB1)

Tumour suppressor genes are also a normal genes that slow down cell division, repair DNA mistakes and tell cells when to die (apoptosis). Their inactivation and deletion will promote tumour growth. Most of the mutations of tumour suppressor genes are acquired, e.g. mutation of p53 has been found in more than 50% of human cancers. Mutations of tumour suppressor genes can also be inherited, e.g. mutation of APC gene leads to the familial adenomatous polyposis. In some cancers, tumour suppressor genes are normal structurally but not functionally. For example, p53 in cervical cancer is blocked by E6 protein (from HPV).

There are two main categories of tumour suppressor genes: (1) "Gatekeeper genes"; these genes are responsible to stop cell cycle progression when DNA damage is detected. Example of "Gatekeeper genes" is p53, (2) "Caretaker genes", responsible in repairing the damaged DNA during the cell cycle arrest. Example of "Caretaker genes" is BRCA and Mismatch repair genes (MMR genes).

Oncogenes

Oncogenes are mutated proto-oncogenes. In other words, oncogene is a carcinogenic form of proto-oncogene. In contrast to proto-oncogene and tumour suppressor gene, oncogene does not exist in normal cells. Most of the mutations involving oncogenes are acquired, not inherited (e.g. chromosome rearrangement leads to a formation of oncogenes called BCR-ABL that leads to chronic myeloid leukaemia). Some mutations can also be inherited, e.g. inherited mutation of genes called KIT causing hereditary gastrointestinal stromal tumours (GIST). The comparisons between proto-oncogenes and tumour suppressor genes are shown in Table 2.1.

Table 2.1 Comparison between proto-oncogenes and tumour suppressor genes

Properties	Proto-oncogenes	Tumour suppressor gene
Number of mutational event required to initiate cancer	One (one alleles mutated is sufficient) Dominant	Two (both alleles have to be defective) Recessive
Germ line inheritance	No	Frequent
Action of mutated gene	Gain in function	Loss of function
Somatic mutations contribute to cancer	Yes	Yes

Genetic alteration	Point mutation, amplifications, gene rearrangements.	Point mutation, deletion
Effect on growth control	Active cell proliferation	Negatively regulate growth-promoting gene
Tissue specificity of mutation	Not specific to certain tissue (one oncogene may be active in more tissue type)	Commonly tissue-specific

There are six categories of proto-oncogenes: (1) Transcription factors; proteins that bind to DNA regulatory domains to cause transcription of genes, (2) Growth factors; a soluble factors that influence the growth of neighboring cells or the releasing cell itself, (3) Growth factor receptors; a transmembrane proteins that signal intracellular molecules to carry out cell proliferation, (4) Chromatin remodelers; proteins that alter chromatic structure to promote or repress gene transcription, (5) Signal transducer; proteins that carry out receptor signals to initiate gene transcription and (6) Apoptosis regulators; apoptosis contro the net cell production. Mutated proto-oncogenes will become oncogenes and this mutation could be inherited or acquired from exposure to carcinogen. There are many types of mutation involving proto-oncogenes such as point mutation, deletions, insertion and chromosomal translocation.

Other Genes Responsible in Carcinogenesis

Carcinogenesis involves very complex processes and poorly understood. Studies have shown that there are actually more genes involved in this process and alterations of one or more of these genes can potentially lead to malignant transformation. Following is the list of genes that have been linked with carcinogenesis:

(1) DNA repair genes
(2) carcinogen-activating genes
(3) carcinogen-deactivating genes
(4) cell cycle genes

(5) cell cycle checkpoint genes
(6) cell death genes
(7) cell signalling genes
(8) cellular differentiation genes
(9) cellular senescence genes
(10) metastasis/invasion genes

Additional Facts about Oncogenes and Tumour Suppressor Genes

- Studies have shown that the genes implicated in malignant diseases were often **altered forms of human genes** (not a virus genes) that were picked up by viruses during their travels. Or in other occasions, this virus activated the "rest" gene. This is so in "virus-induced" cancer.
- Majority of cancer is not virus-related and the only explanation for this is a spontaneous mutation of proto-oncogene into carcinogenic forms called **oncogenes.**
- Some viruses carry a specific gene that is capable of transforming the infected cell to become a malignant cell. This type of transforming gene is termed as the **viral oncogene.** Viral oncogene can cause alteration to proto-oncogene and transforming it to become oncogene.
- Mutation of proto-oncogene can also be due to certain chemical or physical elements.
- Knowledge about tumour suppressor genes and oncogenes can assist researchers and clinicians in preventing and treating cancers. Knowing about these genes can also assist in predicting the risk of cancer recurrence and prognosis.
- Detection of inherited form of mutated tumour suppressor genes and oncogenes can also be useful information for calculating the risk of developing a certain type of cancer.
- Genetic testing can be done to identify such mutation.
- Studies have shown that oncogene activation, resulting in increased gene expression (amplification) or the synthesis of an altered gene product (mutation), plays an important role in the process of malignant transformation.

- Women whose tumours contained amplification or overexpression of certain genes were more likely to develop recurrence and had shortened overall survival. (1) Women with breast cancer who produce too much of HER2/neu proteins had the worse prognosis. Drugs such as trastuzumab are designed to attack cells with too much HER2/neu. (2) *HER-2/neu oncogene* has also been studied in ovarian carcinoma. More aggressive lesions were more likely to have Her-2/neu amplification. Therefore, some oncogene alteration can be used as a prognostic factor. (3) Expression of ***c-myc proto-oncogene*** correlates with the proliferative capacity of a number of malignant and non-malignant cell types.
- Following are the examples how laboratory testing can demonstrate the effect on tumour suppressor gene:
  (a) Injection of anti p53 monoclonal antibody to the mouse cell line with wild type p53 will result in cell growth being arrested.
  (b) Rat embryonic fibroblast injected with p53 cDNA will cause cell immortalization while if the same cell injected with p53cDNA and activated Ha-ras will lead to the transformation of the cell.

Proposed Mechanism How Oncogenes Can Transform Normal Cells to Malignant Cells

The growth and division of normal cell within the normal tissue is controlled largely by its surrounding. The normal cells listen to and obey messages that originate from its neighbours in the tissue. These messages may carry growth-stimulatory or growth-inhibitory information/signal, which is conveyed largely by growth factors that are released by some cells. This growth factor will attach to the receptor in the surface of recipient cell. Each recipient cell possesses complex machinery that enables it to receive these signals, process and launch a growth program.

Proto-oncogene encodes many of the proteins in this process that enables a normal cell to respond to exogenous growth factors. However, when proto-oncogene becomes an oncogene, it required no external stimuli to activate this process. The oncogene forces a cell to grow; even its surroundings contain none of the clues normally required to provoke growth. However, in many occasions, the oncogene cannot act alone. It needs other factors to be present before it can be effective. The other factor that equally important is **tumour suppressor genes**.

Cancer Spread (Invasion and Metastases)

Malignant cells are defined by their ability to invade adjacent normal structures and be disseminated or metastasize. Metastasis is a process whereby there is spread of malignant cells from a primary origin to a distant site. It can occur through a direct mechanism or transfers of malignant cells via the blood streams or the lymphatics. For metastases to take place, sequential process must take place, which includes proliferation, angiogenesis, invasion, embolisation, circulation and transport, adherence to vessel walls and organs of distant site and extravasation of malignant cells at the new site.

At the molecular level, interactions between the malignant cells and host cells are an integral part of cancer growth created by more stimulatory signals being produced as opposed to the inhibitory signals. An example of stimulatory signals is vascular endothelial growth factor A (VEGF-A), which induces angiogenesis by increasing vascular permeability, stimulates endothelial cells proliferation and migration thus enhancing cancer cells survival. Metastasis is induced by activation of EGFR and through complex chain of events eventually it produce enzyme metalloproteinases (MMP). MMP degrade the collagen to allow cancer cell migrate towards vessels. MMP also causes enzymatic action of the basement membranes of the vessel to allow cancer cell enter into the blood stream or lymphatic channels.

Apoptosis

Apoptosis or programmed cell death is one of mechanism by which organism limits the growth and replication of the cellls. Apoptosis occur in normal cell allows to removed the damaged cells and maintain the balance between cell death and cell proliferation. In average human adult, there are 50–70 billion cells undergo apoptosis everyday. Apoptosis is activated by two pathways: (1) Death receptor or extrinsic pathway, by activation of tumour necrosis factor receptor and (2) Mitochondrial or Intrinsic pathway triggered by DNA damage. Both of these pathways ultimately stimulated the set of enzymes called Caspases enzymes which interact with inhibitor of apoptosis protein i.e., IAP and Bcl-2 family proteins. Overexpressed of these anti-apoptotic proteins and loss of function of pro-apoptotic proteins contributed to malignant transformation.

Telomerase and Cancer

Telomere is a region of repetitive nucleotide sequences at each end of a chromatid which protects the end of the chromosome from deteriorating or fusion with neighboring chromosome. Telomere control the number of DNA replication and cell division or it act as "division counter". The telomeres are consumed during cell division and when it become shortened, this will blocks cell division, therefore it acts as protective mechanism against uncontrolled cell division. It has also been linked to the mechanism of human cellular ageing. With this mechanism, cell is said to have their own biological clock and it will programmed to die after 50–60 reproductions. Natural loss of telomere can be replenish by an enzyme known as telomerase. Activation of telomerase enzyme allows addition of new repeats at the end of chromosomes or telomere. Therefore, telomerase prevents shortening of the DNA during each cell reproduction. Telomerase is almost undetectable in most normal somatic cells and increase telomerase expression produces vulnerability of uncontrolled cell division and malignant transformation. In contrast, inhibition of telomerase may limits the growth of human cancer celis. Research on anti-telomerase or telomerase inhibitor as one of the anti-cancer therapy is ongoing.

Genetic Studies in Gynaecologic Malignancies

Ovarian Cancer

In ovarian cancer, there are two types of genetic alterations either inheritance (familial) or somatic mutation (sporadic) and approximately, 90% of ovarian cancers are sporadic.

Inherited genetic alterations are related to BRCA1 and BRCA2 genes. Altered BRCA1 (BRCA: breast cancer) may be passed from one generation to another. BRCA1 mutant is associated with breast and/or ovarian cancer.

Studies on families with breast–ovarian cancer syndrome indicate that 52% are due to BRCA1, 32% due to BRCA2 and 16% due to neither. Studies have suggested a lifetime risk of ovarian cancer in BRCA1 carriers is 39% compared with 11% in BRCA2 carriers.

In sporadic ovarian cancer, BRCA1 mutation is detected in 7% of cases. Some ovarian cancer is also associated with over-expression of oncogene erb B-2 (her-2neu). Amplification of erb B-2 oncogene is observed in approximately 26% of primary ovarian malignancies, and it correlates with a poor clinical outcome (Elmasry and Gayther, 2006; Hogdall et al., 2003).

Beside BRCA 1 and BRCA 2 mutation, the other genetic alterations discovered in ovarian cancer are amplification of C-myc (oncogene) observed in 30–50% of ovarian carcinoma and p53 mutations, found in 36–50% of cases. Overexpression of p53 is noted in 50% of advanced ovarian cancer.

The other genetic mutations found are Ki-ras mutation occurs in 48% of borderline tumour and 57% mucinous cystadeno-carcinoma. PTEN (tumour suppressor gene) mutation has been identified in about 20% of endometrioid ovarian cancers but rare in other histotype (Elmasry and Gayther, 2006).

Cervical Cancer

In cervical cancer, genetic alterations not associated with HPV are possible such as loss of function of PTEN tumour suppressor gene (mainly in adenocarcinoma and HPV negative tumour) and reduced expression of p14 and p16. Human papillomavirus DNA sequences have been found integrated near cellular oncogene c-myc and n-myc in at least a few cervical cancer cell lines. The molecular basis for differences in the oncogenic potential between various strains of HPV remains unclear. Overexpressions of proteins E6 and E7 are observed in cervical cancer cell lines. Overexpression of proteins E6 and E7 is due to the deletion of E2 and E4, which control the function of former oncogenes/oncoproteins. E6 and E7 proteins will bind to p53 and Rb protein leading to inactivation and subsequently cell transformation. Despite powerful association between HPV infection and cervical cancer, the genetics of cervical cancer remains poorly understood. For details on carcinogenesis in cervical cancer, see Chapter 6.

Vulvar Cancer

Human papillomavirus types 16 and 18 have been identified in vulvar intraepithelial neoplasm and invasive squamous carcinoma of the vulvar (mainly in younger and baseloid subtype). P53 inactivation (with or without HPV) is observed in 50–80% of cases of squamous cell carcinoma of the vulva. Loss of functions on PTEN and CDKN2A genes are also identified in 60% and 68% of vulvar carcinoma respectively.

Endometrial Cancer

Approximately, 10% of endometrial cancers have a hereditary basis as part of Hereditary Non-polyposis Coli Syndrome (HNPCC) or Lynch II syndrome. Endometrial cancer has it pre-invasive stage (hyperplasia); however, compared with other gynaecological cancers, particularly cervical and ovarian cancer, the knowledge related to carcinogenesis and genetic alterations in endometrial cancer is still limited. Small proportion of endometrial cancers occurred as part of the *Lynch II syndrome (HNPCC)*. Defective MMR genes were identified in 85% of HNPCC-associated endometrial carcinoma. Individual with germ line MSH6 mutations are more likely to develop endometrial cancer than patients with MLH1 mutations.

Majority of endometrial cancers are sporadic, i.e. due to somatic mutations. Somatic mutations demonstrated in sporadic endometrial cancer include microsatellite instability in 17–32%, mutations of tumour suppressor genes such as PTEN (37–61%) and p53 and mutations of proto-oncogene KRAS. PTEN mutation/deletion is more common in endometrioid type. Loss of expression of oestrogen and progesterone receptors correlates with poor prognosis (Elmasry and Gayther, 2006).

The other genetic alterations noted in endometrial cancer is mutations of P53 tumour suppressor gene demonstrated in 10–20% of endometrial cancers, mainly in advanced stage and in

Type 2 endometrial cancers such as clear cell and serous carcinoma. Mutations of Ki-ras genes are detected in 19% of endometrial cancers and overexpression and amplification of ErbB2 oncogenes were reported in 10–30% of cases mainly in serous papillary tumour.

Clinical Implications of Molecular Genetics in Gynaecological Cancer

The knowledge about molecular genetics and genetic alterations in cancers, including gynaecological cancers will benefit patients in many ways. Genetic analysis will allow accurate assessment of familial cancer risk. Molecular genetic can provides a basis for design cancer preventative techniques such as (a) genetic analysis may help to identify pre-malignant conditions amenable to conventional therapy, tb) in familial cancer syndromes, it may be possible to transfer normal copies of the abnormal gene (e.g. p53, BRCA 1) to the tissue at risk using tissue specific viral vectors, (c) development of Vaccine, e.g. HPV vaccine and (d) possible to generate an immune response to viral transforming proteins, i.e. E6, E7 using either a protein vaccine or presentation of these antigens in a viral or bacterial vector.

The knowledge can also assist in the detection of cancer at an early stage, example (a) screening of ovarian cancer based upon genetic markers via identification of gene products in peripheral blood, (b) protein products of abnormal genes involved in carcinogenesis can be detected in the serum, e.g. protein product of M-CSF gene increase in ovarian cancer and (c) endometrial sampling can be used for genetic analysis to detect mutation of gene associated with endometrial cancer.

The genetic markers can also be valuable as prognostic indicators. The behaviour of a malignancy is a consequence of the complex interaction of all of the genetic alterations, which have accumulated during the process of carcinogenesis, e.g. erbB2 amplification is associated with reduce survival in ovarian cancer. Genetic study has also found that p53 mutation does not correlate with prognosis. Studies have shown that loss of heterozygosity (LOH) on chromosome 3 or 11 results in high-grade malignancy, while LOH on chromosome 6 is consistent with a well-differentiated phenotype (ovarian cancer). Interestingly, pattern of LOH is an independent prognostic indicator for ovarian cancer.

Molecular genetics are also important in the research of gene therapy. There are two types of gene therapy namely **ex vivo approaches of gene therapy** and **in situ approaches of gene therapy**. In ex vivo approaches, the cells from an individual are removed and manipulated in vitro, the altered cells are then re-injected into the body to trigger an immune response. Example of this approach is removing tumour cells from patients with cancer and inserting genes encoding cytokines or MHC clonal Ag in vitro to enhance their immunogenicity then re-injecting it into cancer patients to stimulate an immune response. Immune system will then acts against respective tumour antigens and destroy cancer cells. In situ approaches of gene therapy involves replacing a normal copy of tumour suppressor gene, e.g. p53 or suppression expression of the product of an oncogene, e.g. K-ras. This is based on evidence inserting a wild type p53 and anti sense K-ras into the tumour cells with abnormalities of these genes, which had shown to suppress a tumourigenicity.

Proteomics and Cancer

There are four causes of genetic message alterations in cancer:

(1) DNA mutation
(2) chromosomal aberrations
(3) epigenetic modification
(4) protein–protein interaction

Generally, 2% of diseases are monogenic (caused by mutation of single gene) and 98% of major diseases involve multiple genes (polygenic). The proteins are the end product of genes and proteomics is the analysis of the protein complement of the genome. Proteomics encompasses knowledge of the structure, function and expression of all proteins as a function of time, age, state and external factors (Baak, 2003; Li et al., 2002).

There are approximately 100,000–10 millions proteins, but only a small percentage of it had been studied. The study of these proteins is a step forward and will provide new molecular-biological insights, tumour markers and drugs.

There are various methods of proteomics techniques (method to analyze protein) such as 2D poly-acrylamide gel electrophoresis (2D-PAGE), high-performance liquid chromatography (HPLC), capillary array (CA), yeast two-hybrid system (Y2HS), protein microarrays, fluorescence resonance energy transfer (FRET) and others (Baak et al., 2003; Li et al., 2002).

Potential role of proteomics in cancer are for detection, diagnosing, monitoring (including identification of new biomarkers) and treatment. An example of the application of proteomic in detection of cancer is the study by Li and colleagues in which they used a proteomic and bioinformatic approach to identify biomarkers for breast cancer with SELDI-TOF-MS; they discovered three discriminatory biomarkers with sensitivity of 93% and specificity of 91%.

Researchers hope that proteomics research will help find new ways to diagnose cancer early, identify the best screening and treatment method for specific type of cancer and determine the best way to monitor patients during and after treatment.

References

Alberts B, Johnson A, Lewis J, et al. *Molecular Biology of the Cell*. 4th ed. New York: Garland Press, 2002.

Baak JPA, Path FRC, Hermsen MAJA, Meijer G, Schmidt J, Janssen EAM. Review genomics and proteomics in cancer. *Eur J Cancer* 2003; **39**: 1199–1215.

Bookman MA, Darcy KM, Clarke-Pearson D, et al. Evaluation of monoclonal humanized anti-HER2 antibody, trastuzumab, in patients with recurrent or refractory ovarian or primary peritoneal carcinoma with overexpression of HER2: a phase II trial of the Gynecologic Oncology group. *J Clin Oncol* 2003; **21**: 283–290.

Carbone M, Pass HI. Multistep and multifactorial carcinogenesis: when does contributing factor become a carcinogen? *Semin Cancer Biol* 2004; **14**: 399–405.

Elmasry K, Gayther SA. Genetic mutations in gynaecological cancers. *Rev Gynaecol Perinat Pract* 2006; **6**: 115–125.

Hogdall EV, Christensen L, Kjaer SK, et al. Distribution of HER-2 overexpression in ovarian carcinoma tissue and its prognostic value in patients with ovarian carcinoma: from the Danish MALOVA Ovarian Cancer Study. *Cancer* 2003; **98**: 66–73.

Laconi E, Doratiotto S, Vineis P. The microenvironments of multistage carcinogenesis. *Semin Cancer Biol* 2008; **18**: 322–329.

Li J, Zhang Z, Rosenzweig J, Wang YY, Chan DW. Proteomics and bioinformatics approaches for identification of serum biomarkers to detect breast cancer. *Clin Chem* 2002; **48**: 1296–1304.

Liang F, Holt I, Pertea G, et al. Gene index analysis of the human genome estimates approximately 120,000 genes. *Nat Genet* 2000; **25**: 239–240.

Roest CH, Jaillon O, Bernot A, et al. Estimate of human gene number provided by genome-wide analysis using *Tetraodon nigroviridis* DNA sequence. *Nat Genet* 2000; 25: 235–238.

Sachidanandan R, Weissman D, Schmidt SC, et al. A map of human genome sequence variation containing 1.42 million single nucleotide polymorphisms. *Nature* 2001; **409**: 928–933.

Saracin A. An overview of mechanisms of mutagenesis and carcinogenesis. *Mutat Res* 2003; **544**: 99–106.

Slamon DJ, Leyland-Jones B, Shak S, et al. Use of chemotherapy plus a monoclonal antibody against HER2 for metastatic breast cancer that overexpresses HER2. *N Engl J Med* 2001; **344**: 783–792.

Sonnenschein C, Soto AM. Review: Theories of carcinogenesis: an emerging perspective. *Semin Cancer Biol* 2008; **18**: 372–377.

Tili E, Michaille J-J, Wernicke D, Alder H, Costinean S, Volinia S, Croce CM. Mutator activity induced by microRNA-155 (miR-155) links inflammation and cancer. *Proc Natl Acad Sci* 2011; **108** (12): 4908 DOI: 10.1073/pnas.1101795108.

Vincent TL, Gatenby RA. An Evolutionary model for initiation, promotion and progression in Carcinogenesis. International. *J Oncol* 2008; **32**: 729–737.

Chapter 3

Cancer of Vulva

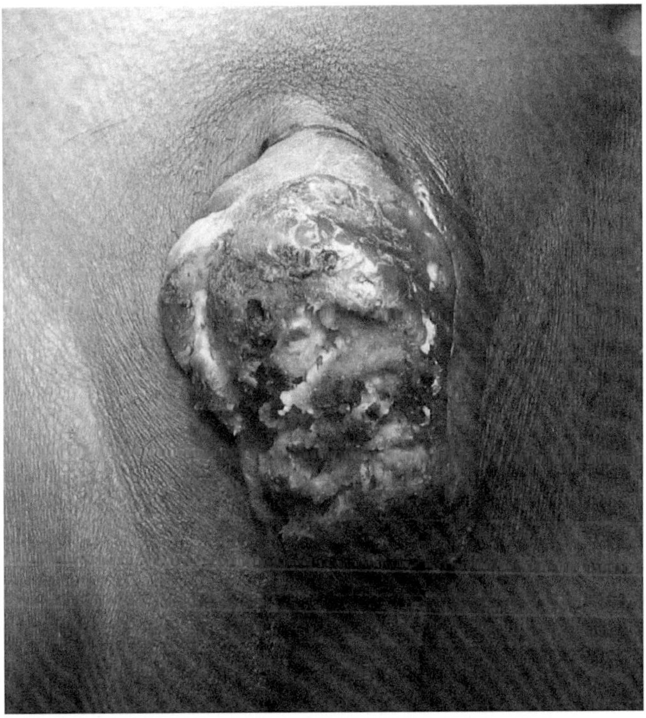

Gynaecologic Cancer: A Handbook for Students and Practitioners
Rushdan Noor, Eng Hseon Tay, and Jeffrey Low

ISBN 978-981-4463-06-5 (Hardcover), 978-981-4463-07-2 (eBook)
www.panstanford.com

Introduction to Anatomy of Vulva

Vulva

The vulva includes mon pubis, labia minora, labia majora, clitoris, vestibule, glands (Bartholin's glands, skene glands and minor vestibular glands) and perineal body. The other term for vulva is pudendum. Vulva is bounded by anterior abdominal wall and mon pubis superioly, labia-crural fold at a medial thigh laterally and anus posteriorly (Fig. 3.1).

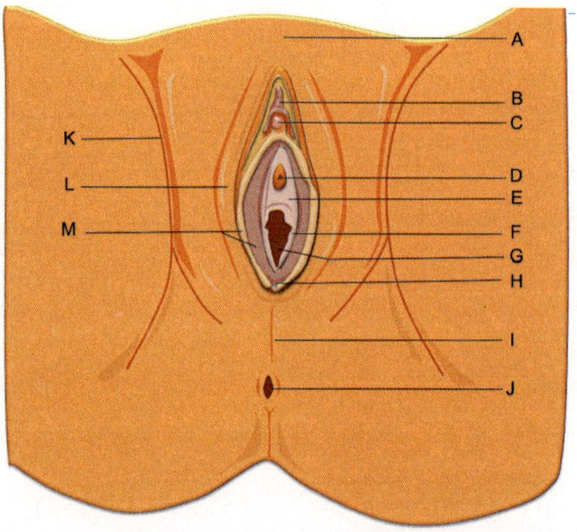

Figure 3.1 The female external genitalia. A: mons pubis, B: prepuce of clitoris, C: glans of clitoris, D: urethral meatus, E: vestibule, F: hymen, G: vagina opening, H: fourchet, I: perineum, J: anus, K: labia-crural fold, L: labia majora, M: labia minora.

The mons pubis is the superior border of the vulva described as directly anterosuperior to the pubic symphysis. This area is covered by skin where sexual hair development occurs at the time of puberty.

The labia majora form the lateral boundaries of the vulva. They are composed of folds of adipose and fibrous tissue. The labia majora correspond to the scrotum in male. Labia majora fuse anteriorly into the mons pubis and posteriorly they terminate 3–4 cm in front of the anus where they are united by the posterior commissure or fourchette. The labia majora is covered by skin contains of stratified squamous epithelium.

The labia minora or nymphae consists of two folds of connective tissue which has little or no adipose tissue. Labia minora is situated between the labia majora and extending from the clitoris to the fourchette. Labia minora is divided into two parts anteriorly, one part passes over the clitoris to form the prepuce, while the other part joins beneath the clitoris to form a frenulum. Posteriorly, labia minora blend with the medial surfaces of the labia majora. The skin and mucosa covering the labia minora are rich in sebaceous glands.

The clitoris is situated at the middle and upper part of the labia minora. The clitoris is an erective structure, homologous with the penis. The clitoris is made up of two crura, which attach to the periosteum of the ischiopubic rami. It has two small muscles called ischiocarvernosa, which are inserted into the crura of the clitoris. The average length of the clitoris is 1.5–2.0 cm and about 1 cm width in adult female. Clitoris is innervated by the terminal branch of the pudendal nerve known as dorsal nerve of the clitoris.

The vestibule is the area (triangular shape) between the labia minora and behind the gland of clitoris and extends to the fourchette posteriorly. The vestibule is where the urethral meatus and vaginal orifices are found. It also gives rise to the opening of the glands, i.e. Skene glands and Bartholin's glands bilaterally. It is lined by non-keratinized squamous epithelium. The squamous cells in the epithelium are well glycogenated and resemble the vaginal or cervical squamous cells. The structures found in the vestibule include the Bartholin's glands (Major vestibular glands), the minor vestibular glands, Skene's glands (periurethral gland), the opening of the urethra and vaginal orifice. The external urethral orifice is a sagittal cleft situated about 2.5 cm behind the clitoris. The total length of female urethra is from 3.5 to 5.0 cm.

The hymen is a thin mucous membrane partially covered the vaginal orifice. In other words, the opening of the vaginal orifice is actually a cleft between the hymen. The hymen has many shapes and when stretched, the posterior part is the broadest. It can be absent or form a complete septum across the vaginal opening and this condition is known as imperforate hymen. When the hymen is ruptured, the remaining part will form rounded elevations known as carunculae hymenales. The shallow depression between the hymen and the frenulum of the labia is called navicular fossa.

The other structure found in the vulva is the vestibular bulbs or bulbus vestibuli. The vestibular bulbs are two masses of erectile tissue that lie deep to the bulbocavernosus muscles bilaterally, on each side of the vagina orifice. Each mass measures approximately 2.5 cm in length and united to each other anteriorly by a median band known as pars intermedia. Their posterior end is in contact with the Bartholin's gland. The deeper surface of vestibular bulb is in contact with fascia of pelvic diaphragm, while superficially they are covered by the bulbocavernosus.

Skene's glands or periurethral glands are glands that secrete the mucous for lubrication at the opening of the urethra. The duct of this gland is about 0.5 to 1.5 cm long and located in the floor of the terminal end of the urethra and open just within or external to the meatus.

Batholin glands (or greater vestibular glands) are two small mucus secreting glands situated within a subcutaneous tissue of the posterior labia majora, have ducts that open onto the posterolateral portion of the vestibule. Batholin glands are homologous of bulbo-urethral glands in male. There are two Bartholin's glands, one on each side of the vaginal orifice in contact with the posterior end of each lateral mass of the bulb of the vestibule. It has a 2 cm duct opening immediately lateral to the hymen and medial to the posterior part of labia minora. It secretes mucus for lubrication of the vagina.

The minor vestibular glands are small glands corresponding to the penile glands of Littre in male. These glands are located within the vestibule and lined by a single layer of columnar cells secreting a mucin.

The other glands located in the vulva are apocrine glands, sebaceous glands and sweat glands. Sweat glands are primarily involved in heat regulation.

Blood Supply and Innervation of the Vulva

The main blood supply to a vulva is from the **internal pudendal artery** (terminal branch of anterior division of internal iliac artery) and **external pudendal artery** from a femoral artery. Internal pudendal artery supply ischiocavernosus, bulbocavercosus muscle, perineal body, urethra and clitoris. External pudendal artery supplies labia majora and their deep structures.

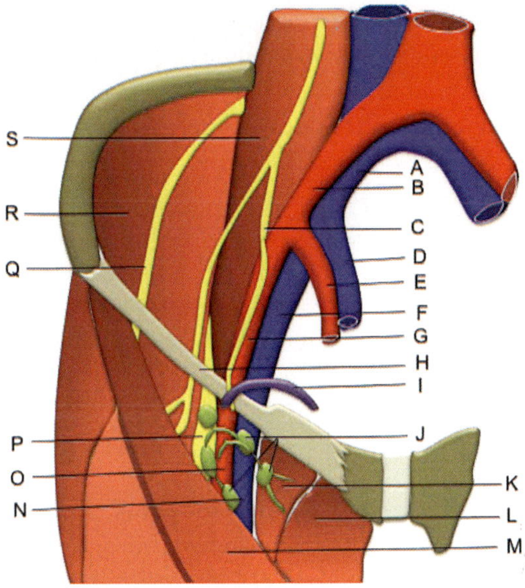

Figure 3.2 Anatomy of the right hemipelvis and groin. A: common iliac vein, B: common iliac artery, C: genito-femoral nerve, D: internal iliac vein, E: internal iliac artery, F: external iliac vein, G: external iliac artery, H: inguinal ligament, I: round ligament, J: right inguina-femoral lymph nodes K: pectineus muscle, K. femoral artery, L: adductor longus muscle, M: sartorius muscle, N: femoral vein, O: femoral artery, P: femoral nerve, Q: right lateral cutaneous nerve of thigh, R: iliacus muscle, S: psoas major muscle.

The mons pubis and upper labia majora are supplied by **ilioinguinal nerve (L1)** and **genitofemoral nerve (L1-2)**, while lower vagina, labia, clitoris, perineal body and their supporting structures are supplied by **pudendal nerve (S2-3)**.

Lymphatic Supply of the Vulva

Lymphatic drainage of the vulva is mainly to superficial inguinal lymph nodes (10 nodes in a triangle below, along the saphenous vein). Some part of clitoris and middle structures drain to the pelvic lymph nodes (obturator and iliac nodes). Generally, the lymphatic drainage of one side of the vulva does not cross the midline. The midline is defined as 1 cm within an imaginary line from the clitoris to the anus.

There are two groups of inguinal lymph nodes: (a) superficial inguinal lymph nodes (subcutaneous lymph nodes situated between Camper's fascia and cribriform fascia) and they are further subdivided into oblique and vertical groups; (b) deep inguinal lymph nodes (within the cribriform fascia and medial to the femoral vein and runs towards the femoral canal).

Superficial inguinal lymph nodes drain into the deep inguinal lymph nodes and subsequently into the external iliac lymph nodes. Direct spread of the cancer to the deep inguinal nodes without metastasis to the superficial group has been documented, although it is uncommon, representing in less than 5% of cases. Furthermore, 10–20% of lymphatic flow from the superficial inguinal group travels directly to the pelvis without passage through the deep inguinal group.

The lymphatic vessels draining the midline structures of the vulva decussate and drain to the bilateral groin nodes. The lymphatic vessels of the anterior vulva also drain directly into the deep nodes—accounting for the direct metastasis of cancer to the deep nodes without involving the superficial nodes in less than 5% of patients.

Some part of clitoris and middle structures drain to pelvic lymph node (obturator, iliac nodes). Approximately 10–20% of lymphatic flow from the superficial inguinal group travels directly to the pelvis without passing through the deep inguinal group.

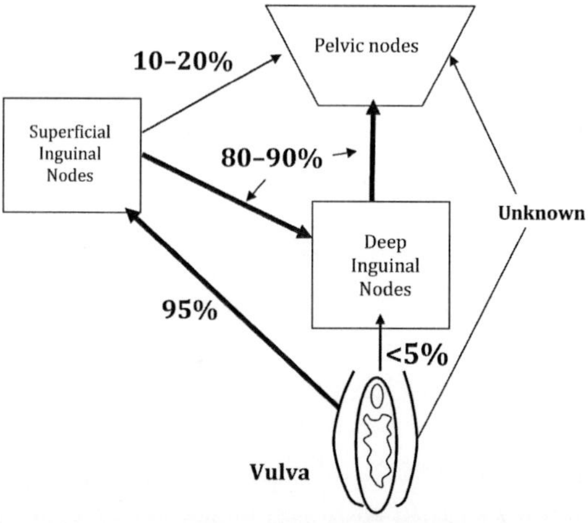

Figure 3.3 Lymphatic drainage of the each side of vulva.

Premalignant Vulvar Lesions

Squamous cell carcinoma is the most common vulvar carcinoma. There are two types of squamous cell carcinoma of the vulva: (a) HPV-related squamous cell carcinoma and (b) non-HPV-related squamous cell carcinoma (Lyengar and Acheson, 2008; Zeaps et al., 1990).

In some textbooks, pre-malignant squamous cell carcinoma of vulva is also classified into HPV related and non-HPV related. Pre-malignant condition of the vulva is also known as vulva intra-epithelial neoplasm (VIN). The non-HPV related VIN is more common and often affects older women with histology of differentiated keratinizing squamous cell carcinoma. HPV-related VIN is a pre-malignant condition of HPV-related squamous cell carcinoma of the vulva. This type of lesions is caused by high-risk HPV, predominantly HPV 16 and 18 and often it is also seen adjacent to approximately 30% of squamous cell carcinoma of the vulva (Lyengar and Acheson, 2008; Zeaps et al., 1990). Twenty-two percent of patients with HPV-related VIN have concurrent cervical intraepithelial neoplasia (CIN). HPV-related squamous cell carcinoma of vulvar occurs in the younger age group of less than 50 years old. The diagnosis of VIN must be made by biopsy preferably using keyhole biopsy or punch biopsy from the edge of the lesion, including a small piece of normal tissue.

Lichen Sclerosus

Lichen sclerosus (LS) is a non-HPV-related premalignant condition of the vulva. The majority of women with this condition are aged 50–70 years old; however, lichen sclerosis can occur at all ages. Studies have shown that 7–13% of women with chronic vulvar symptoms were found to have lichen sclerosis (Carli et al., 1995).

The exact aetiology of lichen sclerosis is unknown. Hormonal factors have been suggested as a possible aetiology of lichen sclerosis because the highest incidence of this condition was observed in patients with a low oestrogen level (prepubertal girls and postmenopausal women) (Carli, et al., 1995). There was also a strong association between lichen sclerosis and autoimmune disorders, e.g. vitiligo, alopecia areata, pernicious anaemia and others. One third of women with LC are asymptomatic while others may be presented with chronic itchiness, pain, burning sensation, dyspareunia, bleeding and blistering (Carli et al., 1995). The lesions are white plaques and papules with areas of erythema, ecchymosis, hyperkeratosis, pallor, excoriation and ulceration. In extreme lesions, the skin became scarring, labia minora disappeared and vaginal introitus became narrower. The classical histological features of LS are thinned epidermis, loss of a normal rete pegs, oedema of the dermis, basal layer vacuolor changes and paucity of melanocytes. Long term followed up of women with lichen sclerosis revealed 2–6% risk of malignant change to squamous cell carcinoma of the vulva. Some postulated that LS would progress to VIN and subsequently squamous cell carcinoma of the vulva.

Treatment for Lichen Sclerosus

Generally, there is no cure for lichen sclerosus. In some cases, spontaneous resolution is possible. Medical treatment is the first line treatment and the most effective medical treatment is topical superpotent corticosteroid ointment (Carli et al., 1995). The other medical treatments are topical testosterone (controversial), retinoids (may be indicated in refractory LS even with steroid treatment), tacrolimus, pimecrolimus, calcipotriol, oxitomide and others. Surgical treatment can be offered to patients with lichen sclerosis. Local excision, laser ablation, cryotherapy and even vulvectomy are acceptable in selected patients. It is also important to provide supportive care by treating problems related to LS such as bacterial infection (antibiotic), fungal infection (anti-fungal), vulvodynia (topical xylocaine), vulvar atropy (local oetrogen cream) and itchiness (anti-histamine).

Extramammary Paget's Disease of Vulva

Paget's disease is a rare neoplasm of apocrine-bearing skin. Paget's disease of the nipple was first described by James Paget in 1874 and 15 years later extramammary Paget's disease affecting the scrotum and penis was reported by H. Radchliffe Crocker (Crocker, 1889; Paget, 1874). First case of extramammary Paget's disease involving the vulva was reported by Dubreuith in 1901 (Chanda, 1985; Chang et al., 1996). The most common site of extramammary Paget's disease is a vulva, scrotum and perianal region.Extramammary Paget's disease has also been described in other apocrine gland-bearing areas such as axilla, groin, thigh, eyelid, external ear and nose. Some described this condition as an epidermal adenocarcinoma extending into the contiguous epithelium of the hair follicles and eccrine sweat ducts. It may also be described as an adenocarcinoma in situ of the vulvar skin.

Paget's disease involving nipple always associated with underlying malignancy of the breast. Extramammary Paget's disease in contrast may or may not be associated with underlying malignancy.

Table 3.1 Comparison between Paget's disease, Melanoma and VIN III based on immunostaining.

Staining	Paget's disease	Melanoma	VIN III
PAS with diastase	+	–	–
Mucicarmine	+	–	–
CAM 5.2	+	–	–
Pankeratin	I		+
S-100	–	+	-
Vimentin	–	+	–

Extramammary Paget's disease of the vulva is a rare condition, affecting mainly white women aged 50–80 years with the peak incidence of 65 years (Chanda, 1985; Chang et al., 1996; Levy et al., 2010). Most common symptoms are pruritus, burning, irritation, pain and swelling. Clinically, the lesion appeared well-demarcated erythematous or leukoplakic plaques. Typical appearance is "cake-icing" effect (whitish top and hyperaemic below). There may be crusting, scaling and ulceration. Histologically, Paget's cells are large intraepithelial cells with abundant cytoplasm and large vesicular nuclei. There may also present with hyperkeratosis, parakeratosis and acanthosis. Histochemistry study can differentiate Paget's disease from malignant melanoma, VIN III and Bowen's disease (Table 3.1). Paget's cells stain positively with periodic acid Schiff reaction and mucicarmine. If this failed, immunohistochemical staining for CAM 5.2, EMA, Cytokeratin 7 and GCDFP-15 are all positive in Paget cells (Black et al., 2007; Goldblum and Hart, 1998). Ten to fifteen percent of women with Paget's disease of the vulva have underlying primary adenocarcinoma and 30% of patients will later have adenocarcinoma at other site such as breast, colon, rectum and upper female genital *tract* (Black et al., 2007; Chanda, 1985).

Treatment for Non-mammary Paget's Disease

The most acceptable mode of treatment is surgery. Excision of the lesions must be complete and with adequate margin, during surgery, the margin must be sent for frozen section to ensure free from disease because recurrence rate is high. Recurrence rate after surgical treatment is up to 32–38% despite negative surgical margin. Patients with positive margin will have higher risk of recurrence (up to 70% in the study done by Black, et al.). Radiotherapy is reserved for selected patients who are unfit for surgery, with persistent disease despite surgery and those who refuse surgical intervention (Luk et al., 2003). Topical 5-Fluorouracil may be useful for symptomatic relief or as a cytoreductive measure prior to surgery. Topical 5-FU is not curative because it cannot penetrate deep enough.

Vulva Intraepithelial Neoplasm

Vulva intraepithelial neoplasm or VIN is characterized histologically by an abnormal proliferation of cells with an increased nuclear: cytoplasmic ratio, nuclear hyperchromasia, pleomorphism and mitosis involving the epithelium of the vulva. The incidence of VIN is increasing and 20% of affected women are younger than 50 years old.

The International Society for Study of Vulval Disease (ISSVD) 2004 has classified VIN into two groups namely (a) Usual type (HPV-related) VIN, which is subdivided into warty type, basaloid type and mixed type and (b) Differentiated type VIN (Non-HPV related).

Usual Vulvar Intraepithelial Neoplasia

Usual type vulvar intraepithelial neoplasia or HPV-related VIN was formerly known as Bowen's disease. This lesion is closely related to human papillomavirus infection. Formerly, ISSVD classified VIN into VIN 1, VIN 2 and VIN 3 similar to classification of preinvasive lesions of the cervix (CIN) (Sideri et al., 2005). In 2003, ISSVD decided to abolish the three grades system (VIN 1, 2, 3) because the behaviour of VIN is not similar to CIN. Vulva intraepithelial neoplasm 1 is not considered as premalignant lesions. Vulva intraepithelial neoplasm 2 and VIN 3 are grouped under usual VIN, which is further subdivided into warty VIN, Basaloid VIN and Mixed VIN. According to ISSVD 2004 classification, the lesion previously known as VIN simplex is now classified as differentiated VIN (Sideri et al., 2005).

The incidence of usual VIN is approximately 5 per 100,000 women per-year and increasing worldwide due to Human Papillomavirus Infection. Usual VIN relatively more common in the younger age group as compared to differentiated VIN (Jones et al., 2005; Joura, 2002; Lara, 2004). Almost 100% of usual VIN is due to HPV infection, mainly HPV 16 and 18. The most common sites of usual VIN are labia majora, labia minora and posterior fourchette. Pruritus is the most common presenting complaint (60%). Other symptoms are pain, ulceration and dysuria. Approximately, 20% of patients do not have any specific symptoms.

Clinically, the lesions are either whitish, erythematous plaques or pigmented. Coexisting preinvasive lesions of vagina, cervix and anus are seen in 25–66% of cases. Histologically the epidermis is thickened and accompanied by a hyperkeratosis and/or parakeratosis. The epithelial cells appeared enlarged, high nuclear:cytoplasmic ratio, nuclear hyperchromasia and numerous mitotic figures. There is also koilocytes, which represent HPV-infected epithelial cells. Warty type of usual VIN presented with warty lesions or condylomatous appearance while basaloid type presented with flat and non-papillamatous lesions (Jones et al., 2005; Joura, 2002). The malignant potential for usual VIN is lower than differentiated VIN. Metanalysis by (van Seters et al., 2005) and study by Jones et al. have found that the risk of progression to invasive cancer was 3.3% and 4.2%, respectively.

Treatment of Vulva Intraepithelial Neoplasm

The treatment of VIN is not always easy. The diagnosis of VIN must be performing with biopsy preferably using keyhole punch biopsy, with correct procedure the diagnosis of VIN can be made accurately and invasive lesions can be ruled out. The aims of treating the VIN are (a) to obtain a full tissue biopsy and exclude co-existing invasive disease, (b) to relief the symptoms, (c) to restore of normal epithelial architecture, (d) to reduce the risk of malignant progression and (e) to cure the disease. Treatment of VIN can be divided into surgical and medical treatment.

Surgical Treatment for Vulva Intraepithelial Neoplasm

Wide local excision is the treatment of choice; in extensive disease, vulvectomy may be indicated. Excision can also be done using laser or loop electrosurgical excision procedure (LEEP). Laser vaporization is a local destructive technique indicated in a patient with extensive or multifocal lesions not amenable to excisional treatment. Laser vaporization, however, will not provide tissue for histological diagnosis. Prior to laser vaporization, invasive disease of vulvar must first be excluded by thorough colposcopic examination and biopsy of suspicious areas (Joura, 2002).

Medical Treatment for Vulva Intraepithelial Neoplasm

Topical **5-fluorouracil** is effective only in small proportion of patients. The response rate is low (30%) and high failure rate (58%). **Imuiquimod** act indirectly to inhibit HPV replication through up-regulation of cell mediated immunity (Mathiesen et al., 2007). Data on imuiquimod is limited, complete response rate was reported in 47–80% of patients. Interferon therapy has been tried in patients with VIN but due to limited evidence and high cost, its use is not widely accepted. The side-effects of imuiquimod include burning, irritation and erythema. Antiviral drug such as **Cidofovir** may be potentially useful in the treatment of VIN but the data is still very limited (Joura, 2002).

Photodynamic Therapy for Cervical Intraepithelial Neoplasia

Photodynamic therapy is a treatment that uses a drug, called photosensitizer or photosensitizing agent and a particular type of light (Martin, 2002). When photosensitizers are exposed to a specific wavelength or light (3–4 hours after application of photosensitizing agent), they produce a form of oxygen that kills nearby cells. In VIN, topical 5-aminolaevulinic acid was used as photosensitizer agent. Studies involving 100 patients have shown a response rate of 40%, best in small unifocal lesions. The type of lesions and the optimum dose of light will determine the success of treatment. PDT did not induce ulcers or scar formation; however, pain over the treatment site is a known problem (Joura, 2002; Martin, 2002).

Differentiated Vulva Intraepithelial Neoplasm

Differentiated vulval intraepithelial neoplasm (Differentiated VIN) was formerly known as intraepithelial carcinoma of simplex type. Differentiated VIN is not related to HPV infection and occurs mainly in postmenopausal women with mean age of 67 years (Jones et al., 2005; Sideri et al., 2005). It may be associated with lichen sclerosis and has close relation with squamous cell hyperplasia. Differentiated VIN is more commonly seen adjacent to lichen sclerosis or invasive vulvar carcinoma and it rarely exists alone. On histology, cellular abnormalities seen in differentiated VIN are less prominent as compared to usual VIN, and it can be mistaken

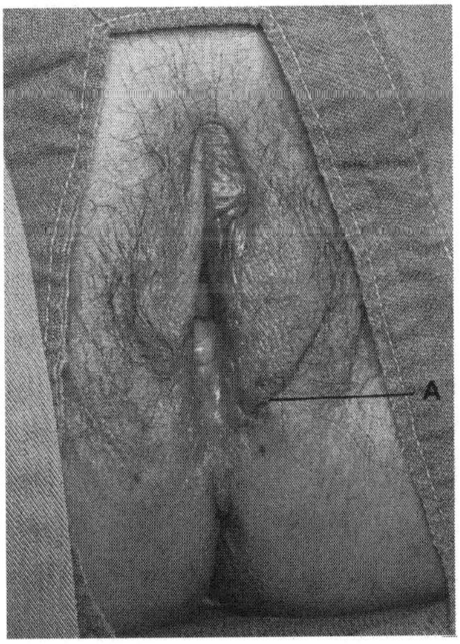

Figure 3.4 Vulva intraepithelial neoplasm 3. VIN can be presented as hyperpigmented skin lesion as shown in A.

easily with a benign dermatosis or epithelial hyperplasia (Sideri et al., 2005). Clinically, it can be presented as an area of red lesions (ulcerative or erythematous) or white-grey discoloration of the skin. Differentiated VIN is characterized by an increased amount of eosinophilic cytoplasm in dysplastic cells immediately above the basal cell layer and is said to be more likely to progress to invasive cancer as compared to lichen sclerosis and usual VIN (Sideri et al., 2005). Treatment for differentiated VIN is mainly by radical excision and medical treatment is generally ineffective (Jones et al., 2005; Sideri et al., 2005).

Vulvar Cancer

Vulvar cancer accounts for about 3–5% of all female genital cancers and 1% of all malignancies in women. In Western countries, the average annual age-adjusted incidence is 1.2 cases per 100,000 women-years (Ghurani and Penalver, 2001; Mutch, 2009). Approximately, 75% of women with vulvar cancer are older than 60 years old. The incidence is increasing due to increase in life expectancy and increase in prevalence of HPV infection. Since vulvar cancer is rare and is not monitored by the World Health Organization, the global incidence of this disease in not precisely known. The American Cancer Society has reported a total of 3460 cases of vulvar cancer in 2008 (Mutch, 2009).

Squamous cell carcinoma of vulvar is the most common type accounting 90% of all vulvar cancer. There are five variants of squamous cell carcinoma of the vulva:

(1) adenoid squamous cell carcinoma
(2) squamous cell carcinoma of giant cells
(3) sebaceous cell carcinoma
(4) spindle-cell squamous cell carcinoma
(5) squamous cell carcinoma with sarcoma like stroma

Second most common vulvar cancer is malignant melanoma. Other histological type of vulvar cancer is adenocarcinoma of Bartholin's gland, adenocarcinoma related to Paget's disease and sarcoma. Squamous cell carcinoma of vulvar can be divided into two groups, i.e. HPV-related and non-HPV-related vulvar cancer. Younger age women tend to be diagnosed as HPV-related vulvar cancer. In older women with non-HPV-related vulvar cancer, the aetiology of this carcinoma is attributed to chronic irritation; immunological problems or other poorly understood co-factors.

Following are the factors associated with risks of developing squamous cell carcinoma of vulvar:

(a) smoking; increases the risk four- to fivefold
(b) HPV infection, recent or past infection
(c) women with genital warts; relative risk of 14.5 for vulvar cancer
(d) women with multiple sexual partners
(e) immunosuppression, HPT, DM and obesity

Approximately, 40% of patients with vulvar cancer were diagnosed at advanced stage (3, 4) and 70% of vulvar cancers occur in labia while, 15–20% involved clitoris and perineal body.

Presentations and Diagnosis

The most common presentation is lump or mass on the vulva and the lesion is frequently itchy and may bleed. Other presenting symptoms include pain, ulceration, dysuria and vaginal discharge. The diagnosis must be made by biopsy. Punch biopsy is taken via keyhole biopsy or Keyes dermal punch size 4–6 mm, under local anaesthesia. Evaluation of entire vulvar, vagina and cervix should also be done to rule out any co-existing preinvasive and invasive lesions of other genital tracts.

Patterns of Spread in Vulvar Cancer

Direct extension is common, spread to adjacent organs, e.g. urethra, anus, vagina and even deep to the pelvic bone. **Lymphatic spread** occurs when the tumour invasion is more than 1 mm depth. Lymphatic spread is the most common method of spread and may occur with apparently small lesions, initially to the superficial inguino-femoral nodes, then up to femoral nodes and into the pelvis. Direct spread to the deep inguinal nodes without metastasis to the superficial group has been documented although it is uncommon representing in <5% of cases. Approximately, 20% of patients with positive groin nodes will have involvement of pelvic nodes. Lateralized lesions more than 1 cm from the midline will spread to ipsilateral lymph nodes while centralized lesions may spread to both sides of lymph nodes. The risk of contralateral lymph node metastasis in lateralized lesion is 0.9% if the lesion is <2 cm (Ghurani and Penalver, 2001; Hampl et al., 2008; Robison et al., 2006). **Haematogenous spread** is usually a late manifestation of vulvar cancer. Cancer can spread to solid organs, e.g. liver, lung, bone, brain, and others.

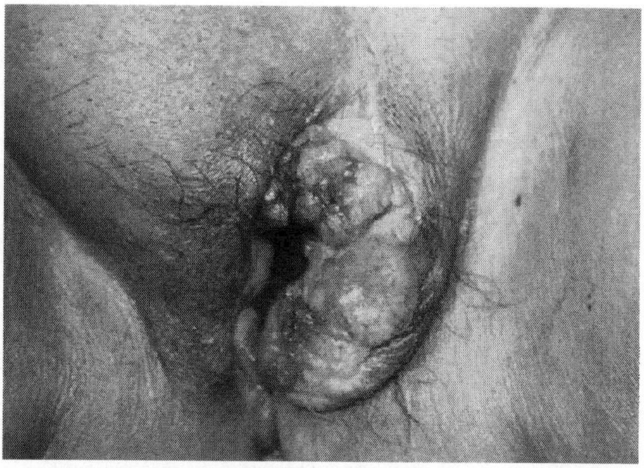

Figure 3.5 Squamous cell carcinoma of the vulva.

Staging of Vulvar Cancer

Radiological assessment is one of the most important investigations. Radiological examination is performed after the diagnosis of vulvar carcinoma is confirmed and it includes chest x-ray, CT scan or MRI of the pelvis. If suspected bone metastasis, bone scan may be helpful. Prior to 1988, the staging for vulvar cancers was clinical but now the staging of vulvar cancer is by surgico-pathological. Any spread beyond inguinal lymph nodes is considered as distant metastasis. See Tables 3.2 and 3.3 for old and new FIGO staging for vulvar cancer (Mutch, 2009).

Table 3.2 Staging system for vulvar cancer by the International Federation of Gynecology and Obstetrics (FIGO) Montreal 1994

Stage	Descriptions
Stage 1	Lesions 2 cm or less in size confined to the vulva or perineum; no nodal metastasis
Stage 1A	Lesions 2 cm or less in size confined to the vulva or perineum and with stromal invasion no greater than 1.0 mm*; no nodal metastasis
Stage 1B	Lesions 2 cm or less in size confined to the vulva or perineum and with stromal invasion greater than 1.0 mm; no nodal metastasis
Stage 2	Tumour confined to the vulva and/or perineum of more than 2 cm in the greatest dimension; no nodal metastasis
Stage 3	Tumour of any size with (1) adjacent spread of the lower urethra and/or the vagina or anus and/or (2) unilateral regional lymph node metastasis
Stage 4A	Tumour invades any of the following: upper urethra, bladder mucosa, rectal mucosa, pelvic bone and/or bilateral regional node metastasis
Stage 4B	Any distant metastasis including pelvic lymph nodes

*The depth of invasion is defined as the measurement of the tumour from the epithelial-stromal junction of the adjacent most superficial dermal papilla to the deepest point of invasion.

Table 3.3 New FIGO staging of vulva cancer (2009)

Stage	Descriptions
Stage 1	Tumour confined to the vulva; no nodal metastasis
Stage 1A	Lesions 2 cm or less in size confined to the vulva or perineum and with stromal invasion no greater than 1.0 mm*; no nodal metastasis
Stage 1B	Lesions >2 cm in size or with stromal invasion >1.0 mm, confined to the vulva or perineum; no nodal metastasis
Stage 2	Tumour of any size with extension to adjacent perineal structures (1/3 lower urethra, 1/3 lower vagina, anus); no nodal metastasis

(*Comtinued*)

Table 3.3 (*Comtinued*)

Stage	Descriptions
Stage 3	Tumour of any size with or without extension to adjacent perineal structures (1/3 lower urethra, 1/3 lower vagina, anus) with positive inguino-femoral lymph nodes
Stage 3A	(a) With 1 lymph node metastasis (≥5 mm), or (b) 1–2 lymph nodes metastasis (es) (<5 mm)
Stage 3B	(a) with two or more lymph node metastases (≥5 mm), or (b) three or more lymph node metastases (<5 mm).
Stage 3C	Positive nodes with extracapsular spread
Stage 4	Tumour invades other regional (2/3 upper urethra, 2/3 upper vagina), or distant structures.
Stage 4A	(a) Tumour invades any of the following: upper urethra and/or vaginal mucosa, bladder mucosa, rectal mucosa or fixed to pelvic bone, or (b) Fixed or ulcerated inguino-femoral lymph nodes
Stage 4B	Any distant metastasis including pelvic lymph nodes

*The depth of invasion is defined as the measurement of the tumour from the epithelial-stromal junction of the adjacent most superficial dermal papilla to the deepest point of invasion.

Reference: (Mutch DG, 2009).

Prognostic Factors in Squamous Cell Carcinoma of Vulvar

Nodal status is the most significant independent prognostic factor for survival (Hazard ratio 3.47 (CI 95% 1.85, 7.85). The risk of nodal metastasis is correlating with few other important factors such as (a) Size of tumour (23% if tumour size less than 2 cm, 37% when the diameter 2–4 cm) and (b) Depth of invasion (5% risk of nodal metastasis if depth of invasion ≤3 mm) (Ghurani and Penalver, 2001; Leibowitch et al., 1990; Origoni et al., 1992; Paladini et al., 1994).

The other factors that determine the prognosis of vulvar cancer are listed below:

(a) Presence of lymphvascular space invasion (HR 2.06, CI95% 1.57–12.07)

(b) Stage of the disease

(c) Presence of extracapsular spread in the lymph node correlates with survival. Patients with an intracapsular spread have 10-year survivals of 71% as compared to 30% in patients with the extracapsular spread (Raspagliesi et al., 2006). Another study done by Paladini et al. based on multivariate analysis had concluded that extracapsular spread was the most important independent prognostic factor, 5-year survivals dropped from 51% in patients with intracapsular metastasis to 15% if one node showed extracapsular involvement (Paladini et al., 1994).

(d) Number of lymph nodes was found to correlate with survival in some study but others suggested that the prognostic value of the number of positive nodes is dependent upon the other lymph node variables.

(e) Size of involved lymph node. Paladini et al. reported when only one lymph node involved, the most important prognostic factor was the greatest dimension of metastasis within the lymph node (5-year survivals were 86% in patients with nodal metastasis <5 mm and 40% if larger than 5 mm) (Paladini et al., 1994).

The diameter of involved lymph node was also found to correlate with survival. Origoni et al. reported that survival rate varied from 90.9% for diameter of less than 5 mm and 20% when the diameter is more than 15 mm) (Origoni et al., 1992).

Management of Squamous Cell Carcinoma of Vulva

Surgical Treatment

Surgery is the most important primary treatment for a patient with squamous cell carcinoma of the vulva. Traditionally, surgery for vulvar cancer was very radical (radical vulvectomy with "en bloc" bilateral inguino-femoral and pelvic lymphadenectomy), although the cure rate was good but morbidity associated with this surgery was very significant. The inguino-femoral lymphadenectomy or groin node dissection is often performed together with excision of the primary tumour. However, pelvic lymphadenectomy is not recommended even in a patient with positive groin lymph node. Routine pelvic lymphadenectomy was found to be inferior to adjuvant pelvic irradiation in patients with groin node metastasis. Routine pelvic lymphadenectomy may lead to unnecessary procedures, as the risk of pelvic lymph node metastasis is low if groin nodes are negative. Recently, the surgery for patients with squamous cell carcinoma of the vulva has become more conservative and individualized with the intention to reduce morbidity without compromising the prognosis.

Surgery for Early Stage

Patients with tumour size less than 2 cm and stromal invasion <1 mm (stage 1A) can be managed by wide local excision alone (with margin of at least 10 mm). Lymphadenectomy can be omitted because the risk of groin lymph node metastases is <1%. The tumour free margins are the most important predictive factor for local recurrences. Study had shown that the rate of local recurrence is 50% if the histopathological margin is less than 8 mm (Heaps, et al.) and in another study by de Hullu et al., no patients with tumour free margins of >8 mm developed local recurrence. Free surgical margin of 1 cm is safe but 2 cm margin is better if feasible (Ve Hullu et al., 2002; Zeaps et al., 1990).

Patients with early-stage disease but with invasion more than 1 mm and/or tumour size more than 2 cm required groin node assessment. If sentinel node mapping is not available, inguino-femoral lymphadenectomy is indicated either unilaterally or bilaterally depending on the location of the primary tumour. The surgery is done via a separate incision. Separate incision technique is defined as when inguino-femoral lymphadenectomy and excision of primary tumour are done via separate incision. The rationale of this technique (as compared to traditional en bloc butterfly shape incision) is based on the fact that the dissemination of cancer to inguino-femoral lymph nodes is by embolization and does not have continuity with the primary lesions. The risks of wound breakdown and lymphoedema are lower in separate incision technique. Large prospective randomized trial is not yet available to address this concept; however, Cochrane's review has reported that the risk of skin bridge recurrence was only 1% and therefore, separate skin incision is considered as a safe technique (Van Doorn et al., 2006).

Patients with lateralized lesions and the tumour size less than 2 cm have only 0.9% risk of contralateral groin node metastasis and therefore, unilateral inguino-femoral lymphadenectomy is sufficient. However, controversy remains whether contralateral groin requires treatment (irradiation or inguino-femoral lymphadenectomy) when ipsilateral lymph node metastases have been identified. While, patients with centralized lesions, invasion >1 mm and/or tumour size >2 cm required bilateral inguino-femoral lymphadenectomy.

Surgical Tips during Vulvectomy and Inguino-Femoral Lymphadenectomy

Following are some important tips for surgeons who perform vulvectomy and inguino-femoral lymphadenectomy:

(1) In wide local excision, surgical margin should be 1–2 cm and depth of incision is down to the fascia lata. Primary closure is preferable.

(2) A position of neurovascular bundles in the femoral triangle from lateral to medial is femoral nerve, femoral artery and femoral vein.

(3) In inguino-femoral lymphadenectomy, the skin incision can either be parallel and 2 cm above the inguinal ligament or vertical incision. The saphenous vein is preferably preserved although it has not been proven to reduce morbidity mainly lymphoedema. Femoral lymph nodes are only 1–3 in number and always situated medial to the femoral vein within the opening of the fossa ovalis.

(4) The perforated membrane contiguous with fascia lata is called the cribriform fascia.

(5) In superficial inguinal lymphadenectomy, the cribriform fascia is left intact and none of the nodes below this landmark is removed.

(6) There is no need to remove the fascia lata lateral to the femoral vessels.

(7) Superficial inguinal lymphadenectomy with medial femoral lymphadenectomy are probably the most commonly performed procedure.

Lymphatic Mapping and Sentinel Node Biopsy

Lymphatic is one of the most important modes of spread in carcinoma of the vulva and lymph node metastasis is the most important prognostic factor for survival in squamous cell carcinoma of the vulva. Information regarding the status of inguino-femoral lymph nodes is also vital in the planning of treatment and adjuvant therapy. It is known that clinical palpation of groin nodes is unreliable with the sensitivity and specificity of 57% and 62%, respectively. While, fine needle aspiration cytology (FNAC) can be used to assess enlarged lymph nodes but there is a high false-negative rate, mainly due to sampling error. Imaging techniques such as ultrasound, CT scan, MRI and positron emission tomography has yet to show any promise in the detection of groin node metastases in vulvar cancer. Lack of sensitivity is the main problem with these imaging techniques. New technique such as MR lymphography using ultra-small-iron-oxide-particles (USIOP) is still investigational but promising in differentiating benign and metastatic lymph nodes.

Lymphatic Mapping and Sentinel Node Biopsy in Vulva Cancer

Sentinel lymph node technology has become the standard of care in penile cancer, melanoma and breast cancer. Sentinel node is defined as the first lymph node in the lymphatic chain to receive lymphatic flow from the malignant lesion. If the sentinel lymph node is free from metastatic disease, the rest of the nodes in the lymphatic chain should theoretically be free of tumour as well (Hampl et al., 2008; Moore et al., 2003, 2008; Robison et al., 2006).

Identification of a sentinel node is done by injection of a tracer around the primary tumour and to follow the course of the tracer to the first lymph node in the region. The tracer can be a radioactive tracer (injection pre-operatively, ^{99m}Tc-labelled nanocolloid) or blue dye (injection done during operation under anaesthesia). Using hand-held gamma probe and gamma camera, accumulation of radioactive tracer in the sentinel node will be identified. Sentinel node biopsy will subsequently perform and sent for histological examination to determine the presence of metastasis. Combined technique (radioactive tracer and blue dye) was found to be more effective in detection of a sentinel node with the detection rate of 99.5% and negative predictive value of >95% (Moore et al., 2008; Moore et al., 2003). In patients with clinically normal nodes, complete lymphadenectomy should be omitted if the sentinel node biopsy (frozen section) did not show metastasis.

Not all patients with operable vulvar cancer are suitable for sentinel node mapping. Following are the selection criteria for lymphatic mapping in vulvar cancer:

(a) squamous cell carcinoma with depth of invasion >1 mm
(b) patient who is a candidate for primary surgical treatment
(c) technically possible to inject around the tumour
(d) no fixed lymph nodes in the groins
(e) no enlarged lymph nodes on preoperative CT scan
(f) tumour located in or close to the midline seem to be less suitable for sentinel lymph node mapping due to higher false negative rate (Hampl et al., 2008)

Despite the advantages and potential role in the management of vulvar cancer, there are a number of concern arises from the practice of lymph node mapping and sentinel node biopsy in vulvar cancer. Some of the concerns are (a) the procedures require training, quality control and radioactive handling, (b) the possibility of failure to detect sentinel node, (c) false negative rate, (d) sensitivity and specificity of frozen section, (e) presence of skip lesions because in small proportion of patients, femoral lymph nodes metastases were detected despite negative inguinal lymph nodes and (f) failure to detect micrometastases.

Moore, et al. had shown that when sentinel nodes are found to be negative for metastatic disease the negative predictive value is near 100% for predicting the status of the remaining inguinal nodes (Moore et al., 2003, 2008). Robison K, et al. had also discovered that when a sentinel node harbour only micrometastasis (<2 mm focus of metastatic cells), remaining inguinal nodes in the same basin will be negative to metastatic disease (Robison et al., 2006). A multicenter prospective study on safety of the sentinel node mapping in vulvar cancer known as Groningen International Study on Sentinel nodes in vulvar cancer (GROINSS-V I) had completed and following are the outcome of this trial (Van der Zee et al., 2008); (a) the study involves 15 hospitals from year 2000 until

2006, (b) total number of patients recruited were 403 patients with early carcinoma of vulva stage T1–T2 (<4 cm), (c) sentinel node mapping (combined technique) and biopsy were done in all patients, (d) approximately, 33% has positive sentinel nodes and had full inguinal-femoral lymphadenectomy, (e) patients with negative sentinel node did not undergo any further lymphadenectomy, (f) women with negative sentinel node had significantly fewer short and long-term complications. The 3-year disease-specific survival rate was 97%. Their rate of recurrence was 3%, which was comparable to patients with early stage treated with excision and full inguino-femoral lymphadenectomy and (g) the authors concluded that sentinel node mapping is safe and should be part of the standard treatment in patients with early-stage vulvar cancer (Van Der Zee et al., 2008).

Method of Sentinel Node Detection

Two intradermal peritumoral injections on both the medial and lateral edge of the tumour with a total of 2 mCi of unfiltered technetium-99m sulphur colloid (Tc-99m) in a volume of 1 cm^3 90 to 180 minutes prior to surgery. Lymphoscintigraphy was obtained to illustrate the presence of a sentinel node. Intraoperatively, 5–10 min prior to the groin dissection, 3 cm^3 of methylene blue was injected at the peritumoral edge in a manner and location similar to the Tc-99m above (Moore, et al., 2003, 2008).

Prior to groin node dissection, a hand held collimated gamma counter is used to identify the location of the sentinel node, and this area is marked with ink on the skin. Inguinal sentinel node dissection is performed through 2–3 cm groin incision prior to excision of the vulvar tumour. The inguinal nodal beds are gently dissected to identify blue lymphatic tracts leading to sentinel node or blue stained sentinel nodes. An intraoperative hand held gamma counter is also used to identify any lymph nodes labelled with Tc-99m sulphur colloid. Each sentinel node that had taken up blue dyes only is labelled as cold sentinel nodes. Sentinel nodes that had taken up Tc-99m sulphur colloid alone were labelled as hot sentinel nodes, while sentinel nodes that had taken up both were labelled as hot and blue sentinel nodes. A 10s gamma count was taken for each hot sentinel node and recorded. Radiolabelled lymph nodes with a 10 s gamma count of at least 10% of the hottest sentinel node are considered as hot sentinel nodes.

Upon completion of the sentinel node dissection, the lymphatic beds were re-examined with the gamma probe to ensure that all sentinel nodes had been removed and that the background count of the lymphatic basin is less than 10% of the gamma count of the hottest sentinel node. The groin incisions are closed with a subcuticular suture or staples.

A sentinel node ultra-staging protocol was used to evaluate each sentinel node as described in publication by Moore RG, et al. Each sentinel node is cut at 2 mm intervals parallel to the long axis of the node. These 2 mm-thick sections are submitted for histologic evaluation in one or more blocks. From each block, five levels were cut at 100 micrometer interval with a 5 micrometer section cut at each level and stained with hematoxylin and eosin.

Wide local excision or radical vulvectomy is performed for the primary tumour and patients with sentinel node metastasis will subsequently undergo a complete groin node dissection. Patients with negative sentinel nodes for metastatic disease do not undergo a complete groin node dissection and are followed up in the postoperative period. If the sentinel nodes are undetected, complete groin node dissection will be performed (unilateral groin node dissection for lateralized lesions and bilateral dissection for centralized lesions).

Radiotherapy in Early-Stage Vulvar Cancer

Patients with early-stage vulvar cancer can be treated with primary radiotherapy if they are not fit for surgical treatment. The main role of radiotherapy in early vulvar cancer is an adjuvant treatment given to patients with high-risk of recurrence (Faul, 1997; Moore, 2009; Van Doorn et al., 2006). Patients with early vulvar cancer who undergo wide excision and inguino-femoral lymphadenectomy do not require adjuvant treatment if the microscopic margin is free (at least 10 mm) and no lymph node involvement. In some institution, radiotherapy was not given if only one lymph node involved (micrometastasis).

The indications for postoperative adjuvant radiotherapy in an early-stage vulvar cancer are (a) positive surgical margin, (b) narrow microscopic surgical margin of less than 10 mm and not amenable to repeat surgical resection, (c) extracapsular spread of any lymph node and (d) more than one lymph node with micrometastasis.

Radiotherapy has at least three major roles in vulvar cancer (Faul, 1997; Moore, 2009): (a) postoperative adjuvant pelvic radiotherapy (to pelvis and groin), indicated in a patient with lymph node metastasis, (b) in a patient with narrow resection margin, repeat excision can be performed but if, for some reason, repeat excision is not feasible or patient refuses, radiotherapy (brachytherapy) to the primary site is acceptable and (c) as a primary radiotherapy to groins and pelvis, indicated in a patient who is not fit for surgical treatment or the tumour is located closed to vital structures such as clitoris and urethra. Primary radiotherapy consists of external beam radiotherapy followed by interstitial brachytherapy. Complete response rates are ranging from 53% to 89%.

Objectives of Radiotherapy in Vulvar Cancer

Generally there are four possible main objectives of radiotherapy in the treatment of patients with vulvar carcinoma: (1) to decrease the incidence of locoregional failures after wide local excision in patients with early-stage disease, (2) to reduce the incidence of post-surgical failure in patients with locally advanced disease, (3) to serve as an alternative to inguinal or pelvic lymph node dissection in patients with clinically negative nodes and (4) to treat patients before surgery for locally advanced tumours that may be considered inoperable initially. Type and indications of radiotherapy in vulvar cancer is shown in Table 3.4.

Table 3.4 Type and indications of radiotherapy in vulvar cancer

Type of radiotherapy	Indication
Local vulvar RT	Resection margin involved; surgical margin less than 1 cm; perineural tumour involvement
Groin and Pelvic Radiotherapy (Standard vulvar EBRT* and inguinal nodal radiotherapy)	Macroscopically involved lymph node; more than one lymph node involved; extracapsular spread of tumour in lymph node

*Superior margin: Mid sacro-iliac join, Inferior: 1 cm beyond the vulva, Lateral: Anterior superior iliac crest (encompass both inguinal regions).

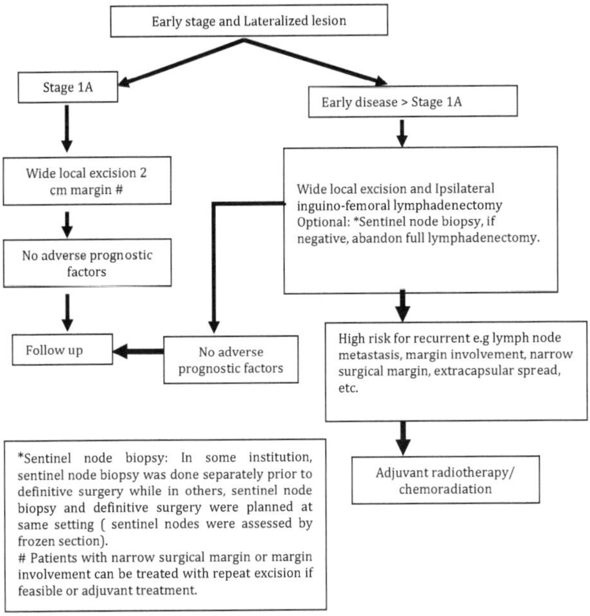

Figure 3.6 Summary of treatment for early vulvar cancer (lateralized lesions, >1 cm away from the midline).

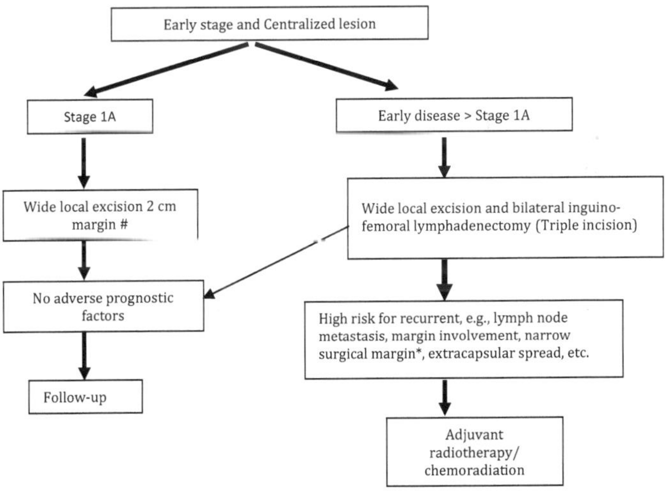

* For narrow surgical margin (microscopically <10 mm), recommended treatment is repeat surgical resection.
# Patients with narrow surgical margin or margin involvement can be treated with repeat excision if feasible or adjuvant treatment.

Figure 3.7 Summary of treatment for early vulvar cancer (centralized lesion).

Treatment for Advanced-Stage Carcinoma of Vulva

Advanced-stage carcinoma of the vulva can be classified into locally advanced disease and metastatic disease. Locally advanced disease is when the primary tumour is large involving important local structures and tumour with obvious groin node involvement. Approximately, one third of patients with vulvar cancer present with locally advanced disease. Surgery in patients with locally advanced disease will carry high morbidity not only because of the radicality of the surgery but also related to patient's age, physical status and co-morbidity.

Treatment for Locally Advanced Disease

Surgery in locally advanced disease involves ultraradical surgery consists of radical excision or radical vulvectomy followed by plastic reconstruction. In some cases, exenterative procedure has been undertaken. Postoperative mortality rate in patients with locally advanced disease is ranging from 0 to 20% with a mean of 4% and 5-year survivals are <50%. The other alternative to primary surgery is neoadjuvant radiotherapy/chemotherapy to shrink the tumour and subsequently followed with less radical surgery (Van Doorn et al., 2006). Radiotherapy followed by surgical excision carries a higher rate of surgical complications due to radiation effect to the tissue and poor vascularization (Moore, 2009). Neoadjuvant chemoradiation followed by surgery was associated with significant more morbidity than either treatment given on its own (Moore, 2009). An acceptable regime for neoadjuvant chemotherapy prior to surgical treatment for vulvar carcinoma is platinum-based such as platinum-5-Fluorouracil or platinum-taxane given in 2–4 cycles (Moore, 2009; Thomas et al., 1989). Patients with enlarged groin node do not require complete groin node dissection. Nodal debulking is sufficient because full groin node dissection followed by radiotherapy carry higher risk of severe lymphoedema. Chemoradiation (cisplatin-5-FU or Mitomycin C-5FU) in locally advanced squamous cell carcinoma of the vulva either as primary treatment or in neoadjuvant setting was found to be a promising approach with mean complete response rate of 60%. Large phase II prospective trial conducted by GOG (Protocol 101) was conducted to evaluate the role of chemoradiation in patients with unresectable locally advanced vulvar cancer. Two cycles of 5-FU and cisplatin were given to shrink the tumour size prior to surgery, complete response rate was 48%. Only 3% had an unresectable disease following neoadjuvant chemoradiation. Despite lower dose of radiation therapy, the result of this GOG trial was encouraging. Subsequently, GOG conducted the trial using a higher dose of radiation (GOG 205). The main concern about neoadjuvant chemoradiation is toxicity and surgical morbidity. Therefore, van Doorn, et al. in their critical review had concluded that (1) Patients with an inoperable primary tumour or lymph nodes benefit from chemoradiation if an operation of lesser scope can ultimately be performed (2) Neoadjuvant therapy is not justified in patients with tumours that can be adequately treated with radical vulvectomy and bilateral groin node dissection (Van Doorn et al., 2006).

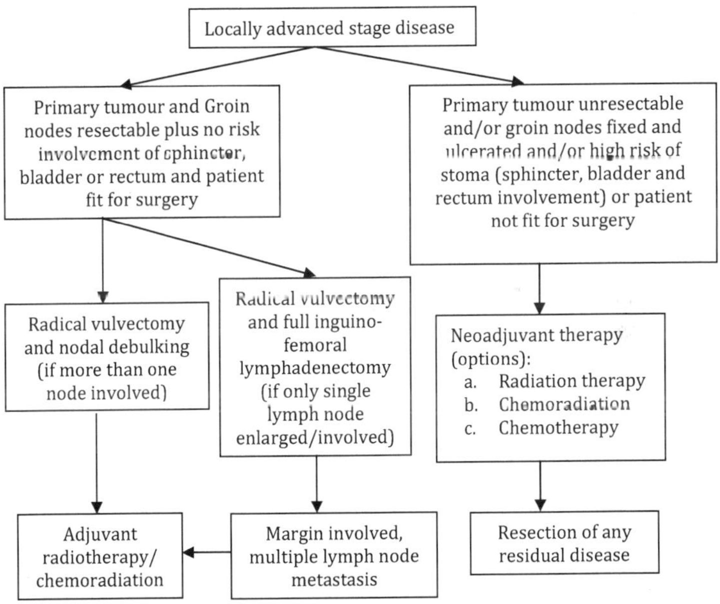

Figure 3.8 Summary of treatment for locally advanced vulvar carcinoma.

Treatment for Metastatic and Recurrent Disease

The intention of treatment in metastatic vulvar cancer is palliative. Metastatic squamous cell carcinoma can be treated with palliative chemotherapy. In general, one third of patients with vulvar cancer will develop recurrent disease and approximately 80% of recurrences occur within first 2 years of treatment. The treatment for patients with recurrent vulvar cancer depends on the several factors such as (a) the extend of recurrence disease, (b) the extend and the nature of primary surgery, (c) previous use of radiotherapy/chemoradiation, (d) previous regimen of chemotherapy, (e) current medical status and performance status of patients and (f) patient's wishes.

Approximately, 50% of patients with recurrent vulvar cancer have isolated local recurrence and 14% have multiple site recurrence including distance metastases. A five-year survival rate for patients with recurrent vulvar cancer is 25–35%. Patients with negative groin nodes are more likely to developed local recurrence as compared to patients with positive groin nodes at initial presentation. The risk of recurrence in patients with positive groin nodes is 52% as compared to 31% in patients with negative nodes. Treatment for isolated local recurrence is radical excision with good surgical margin. Wider free surgical margin of 2 cm and more is recommended and this surgery may require flap reconstruction. Five-year survivals are ranging from 50–70%. Inguino-femoral lymphadenectomy can also be performed if it was not done before. The type and extend of lymphadenectomy follows the same principles, e.g. bilateral lymphadenectomy in centralized lesions. In radiation naïve patients, post-operative radiation therapy is indicated if the surgical margin is involved or groin node metastasis is presence.

In some patients with operable localized but extensive recurrence, they may be recommended for exenterative procedure if surgery is the only option for a cure and at the same time, radiotherapy is not suitable for some reasons such as patients with prior radiotherapy.

Nodal recurrence carries poorer prognosis as compared to local recurrence. There is no standard treatment for nodal recurrence. Nodal debulking followed by chemoradiation may be indicated in some cases; however, if the involved lymph nodes are unresectable, prior chemotherapy/chemoradation followed by nodal resection may be the only option available.

Patients with distance solid organ metastasis or with multiple paraaortic lymph node metastases, palliative chemotherapy may be useful for symptom control. The most common chemotherapy regimen used in squamous cell carcinoma of the vulva is platinum (mainly cisplatin) and 5-Fluorouracil (5-FU). Combination of 5-FU and Mitomycin C was also found to be useful (Moore, 2009).

Post-Operative Care for Vulvectomy

Vulvectomy and groin node dissection potentially carries high morbidity because the patient tends to be an elderly and has co-morbidities. Furthermore, the surgery involves genitalia and groins, which are easily contaminated, and prevents early ambulation. The priorities in post-op management are analgesia, antibiotics, perineal care, prevention of deep vein thrombosis and lymphoedema, as well as specific measures if reconstruction has been performed.

General measures

Provision of adequate analgesia to avoid chest complications. Administering DVT prophylaxis according to protocol including TED stocking and calf compressors especially for the first 3 days.

Urinary catheter

Left for free drainage for about 5–7 days until the patient is ambulating well and there is no significant periurethral oedema.

Drain

Radivac drains are usually placed in the inguinal lymphadenectomy sites for about 10–14 days to prevent early formation of lymphocysts.

Perineal care

An ice pack may be left at the vulvar area immediately post-operatively to reduce the pain and swelling and this can be removed when it is no longer cold. Nurse patient in the circumcision frame. Perineal washing can commence on day 3 POD with the shower or cotton swabs with normal saline three times/day. This must be followed by drying of the area with a hair dryer on low setting. Sitz baths are NOT recommended as this may promote tissue maceration and wound breakdown. Ring cushions are also not recommended as they can increase oedema to the central area.

Bowel

If involve anal canal sphincter, bower function will have to be delayed with low residue diet and antispasmodic.

Mobilization

Important to prevent atelectasis and DVT but should be delayed depending on the extent of vulvar reconstruction performed. Excessive movement may disrupt healing of any graft.

Complications of Surgery in Vulva Cancer

Groin lymph node dissection is associated with the risk of lymphocyst (7–19%) and chronic lymphoedema (10–20%) (Ghurani and Penalver, 2001; Simcock, 2008). Lymphocyst usually presented with asymptomatic mass at the groin. Treatment for lymphocyst is conservative, including aspiration, pressure bandage and antibiotic treatment. The other complications of groin node dissections are infection (cellulitis, lymphangitis), wound breakdown, seroma, and venous thromboembolism. The incidence of wound breakdown and infection is approximately 15% (Simcock, 2008). Rare complications include femoral nerve injury, femoral hernia, vaginal fistula and osteitis pubis. Chronic lymphoedema is an important complication and more commonly experienced by patients who were treated with a combination of surgery and radiotherapy. The other important complications related to vulvectomy or radical excisions of vulvar cancer are micturition problems, coital difficulties and psychosexual problems.

Following measures can minimize the risk of complications; (a) adequate preoperative preparation, including thromboprophylaxis and administration of prophylactic antibiotic, (b) good surgical techniques, e.g. good haemostasis, tension-free wound closure, avoiding dead space, and others, (c) adequate wound drainage, (d) preservation of saphenous vein can reduce the risk of lymphoedema and (e) risk of lymphoedema is higher if groin nodes are involved and complete inguino-femoral lymphadenectomy is performed (instead of nodal debulking).

Follow-Up of Patients with Vulvar Cancer

Close monitoring and regular follow up is very important, especially within 2 years after treatment as 80% of recurrence occurs during this period. The common follow up schedules are three monthly follow up for the first year, four monthly on the second year, six monthly from third to fifth year and yearly from sixth year onwards. During each visit, history and thorough physical examination must be performed to detect any sign of early recurrence.

Prognosis

The most important prognostic factors for survival are staging and nodal status (Homesley et al., 1991; Origoni et al., 1992). Patients with groin node negative have 5-year survivals of 90% but may fall to 50% if they have nodal metastases (Ghurani and Penalver, 2001). The other important prognostic factors are the number of lymph node involved, size of involved lymph nodes and presence extracapsular spread of tumour (Origoni et al., 1992). Patients with pelvic node involvement have 5-year survivals of only 10–15% (Homesley et al., 1991). Based on FIGO staging 1994, corrected 5-year survivals rate were 90% for stage 1, 77% (stage 2), 51% (stage 3) and 18% (stage 4).

Other Carcinoma of Vulvar Carcinoma

Verrucous carcinoma

Verrucous carcinoma is the variant of squamous cell carcinoma. It appears as an exophytic and locally destructive tumour. This tumour carries an excellent prognosis, rarely metastasize and majority of cases occur in postmenopausal women. Cytogenetic study showed diploid cells instead of eneuploid in other variants of squamous cell carcinoma. Usually the lesions are large cauliflower-like, condylomatous lesion. It is important that diagnosis of this tumour needs multiple biopsies to establish a correct diagnosis. Human papilloma virus has been implicated as a causative factor and may be detected in verrucous carcinoma in approximately 25% of cases. Radiotherapy can transform it into anaplastic and therefore, radiotherapy is contraindicated in verrucous carcinoma. Surgery is the mainstay of treatment for verrucous carcinoma of the vulva.

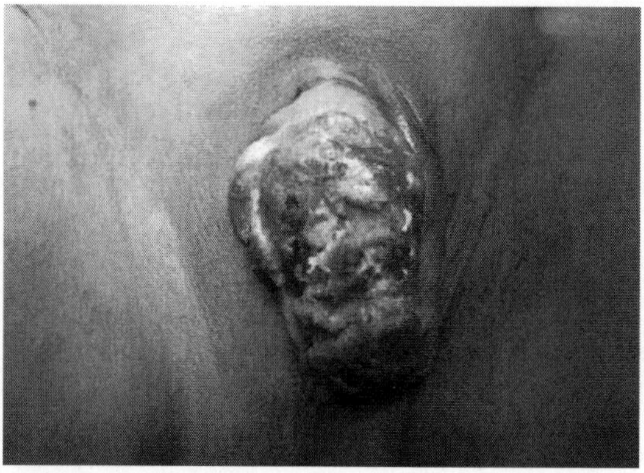

Figure 3.9 Verrucous carcinoma of the vulva.

Basal cell carcinoma

Basal cell carcinoma of the vulvar is rare, accounts for 2–4% of vulvar cancer and occurs more commonly in post-menopausal women. This cancer is most commonly arises from the labia majora and usually a locally invasive disease. The treatment is surgery and if the margin is free (1 cm margin is adequate), most patients will achieve a cure and no further treatment required.

Merkel-cell tumours

Merkel-cell tumour is a neuroendocrine tumour of skin and 95% occurs in the head and neck. Merkel-cell carcinoma has similar histological features with poorly differentiated neuroendocrine carcinoma of the lung (oat-call carcinoma). Merkel-cell carcinoma involving the vulva is extremely rare and it resembles small cell carcinoma and an aggressive tumour carries poor prognosis. It can be classified into three types: (a) Carcinoid type, (b) Intermediate type and (c) Oat cell (small cell) type. Treatment for this cancer is surgery for an early disease and adjuvant treatment similar to small-cell carcinoma of the lungs.

Transitional cell carcinoma

Transitional cell carcinoma of the vulvar is also very rare tumour and it can be divided into primary or secondary. Secondary tumour is more common and primary transitional cell carcinoma is arising from Batholin's gland.

Carcinoma of Batholin's gland

Most of primary adenocarcinoma of the vulva is arising from Batholin's gland. Majority of the women is more than 50 years of age. Therefore, it is advisable to excise an enlarged Batholin's gland in women above 50 years ago. The presenting symptoms are painless lump in the posterior half of the vulva, abnormal bleeding, pruritus and rarely vulvar pain. Carcinoembryonic antigen (CEA) may be elevated. The diagnostic criteria for Batholin's gland carcinoma are shown in Table 3.5 (Copeland et al., 1986; Finan and Barre, 2003).

Table 3.5 Diagnostic criteria of Batholin's gland carcinoma (Copeland, 1986)

(1) Anatomical position consistent with Batholin's gland
(2) Intact overlying skin
(3) Tumour located deep in the labia majora
(4) Normal glandular elements present on histology
(5) Areas of transition from normal to cancerous epithelium
(6) Histology tumour type consistent with a Batholin's gland origin
(7) No evidence of a coexisting primary tumour elsewhere

Approximately, 20% of women with Batholin's gland carcinoma already have lymph node metastasis at first presentation. Other variants of carcinoma of Batholin's gland are adenosquamous, adenoid cystic carcinoma and squamous cell carcinoma (Copeland et al., 1986; Finan and Barre, 2003). The treatment is similar to squamous cell carcinoma of the vulva.

Other Malignant Tumour of Vulva

Malignant melanoma of the vulva

Malignant melanoma of the vulva accounts in 5–10% of all vulvar cancer and second most common vulvar cancers. The median age is approximately 67 years old (range from 18–92) (Irvin Jr et al., 2001; Gungor et al., 2009). It can be subclassified into three groups; (a) Superficial spreading malignant melanoma (most frequent), (b) Nodular melanoma (poorer prognosis) and (c) Mucosal lentiginous melanoma. Malignant melanoma carries poor prognosis, spread predominantly via lymphatic and metastasize early. One of the most important differences between vulvar and cutaneous melanomas is the recurrence rate. Vulva melanoma carries a higher risk of recurrence and reported lower 5-year survivals rate (27–60% versus 88%) as compared to cutaneous melanomas (Irvin Jr, 2001; Gungor et al., 2009). Malignant melanoma of the vulva most commonly arises in labia minora and clitoris with a tendency for superficial spread toward urethra and vagina. Lymph node status is the most important independent prognostic factor in melanoma of the vulva. For node negative patients, 5-year survivals were 65% while for node positive patients, the survival dropped to <37% (Raspagliesi et al., 2000).

There are two staging systems in malignant melanoma, i.e. (1) Clark's staging system and (2) Breslow staging system (see Table 3.6). Breslow staging system is more widely used than Clark's system. The comparison between Clark's staging system and Breslow system is shown in Table 3.6.

Table 3.6 Staging of melanoma

	Clark's staging (level)	**Breslow system (thickness)**
Level 1	In situ melanoma: all demonstrable tumour is above the basement membrane in the epidermis	Thickness < 0.76 mm
Level 2	Melanoma extends through the basement membrane into the papillary dermis	Thickness 0.76–1.5 mm
Level 3	The tumour fills the papillary dermis and extends to the reticular dermis but does not invade it.	Thickness 1.51–2.25 mm
Level 4	The tumour extend into the reticular dermis	Thickness 2.26–3 mm
Level 5	The tumour extends into the subcutaneous fat	Thickness >3 mm

The Clark system is applicable to vulvar melanoma where there are skin appendages (cutaneous melanoma) and hence, it cannot be used where the melanoma involves or arises in the mucosal membrane of the vulva. Chung's staging system is the combination of Clark and Breslow systems. In the melanoma of the vulva, poor prognosis is correlated to Clark's level 5, thickness of more than 2 mm, nodal metastasis and mitotic count of more than $10/\text{mm}^2$.

Radical vulvectomy and bilateral inguino-femoral lymphadenectomy is a treatment of choice, especially when the invasion is more than 2 mm. If Breslow's thickness is less than 0.76 mm, nodal metastasis is very rare and a radical local excision is an adequate treatment. Early stage could be treated with wide local excision and sentinel node biopsy is useful to avoid unnecessary routine groin node dissection. The actual role and appropriate type of adjuvant therapy in malignant melanoma of the vulva are still unknown.

Dacarbazine is probably the most active chemotherapeutic agent, which can produce response rate of 15–25% (Irvin Jr et al., 2001). The other systemic therapy for vulva melanoma is interferon alpha-2b (20 MIU/m^2/day, 3–5 days a week for 12 weeks) (Gungor et al., 2009). Apart from dacarbazine and interferon alpha, FDA also approves interleukin 2 for the treatment of melanoma. There was also a report of successful treatment with the combination of chemotherapy and biological therapy (cisplatin, vinblastin, dacarbazine, interferon alfa or interleukin 2) (Harting and Kim, 2004).

Radiotherapy might be offered in patients who are not fit or refuse surgery and in patients with inoperable tumour to facilitate surgical treatment. Radiotherapy is ineffective to treat gross disease. Radiotherapy was also used as adjuvant treatment for nodal metastases.

Vulvar sarcoma

Sarcoma of the vulvar is rare and there is no large prospective series' reporting experience with management of vulvar sarcoma. Leiomyosarcoma is the most common primary vulvar sarcoma and often presented with painful tender mass, which may arise in the arrector pili muscle of the skin, vascular smooth muscle or the origin of the round ligament. Other types of sarcomas are (a) malignant fibrous histiocytoma, (b) epithelioid sarcoma, (c) malignant rhabdoid tumour, (d) rhabdomyosarcoma (sarcoma botryoides is its variant), (e) others such as angiosarcoma, Kaposi's sarcoma, haemangiopericytoma and liposarcoma.

Other vulvar malignancies

Vulvar lymphoma is extremely rare and chemotherapy and/or radiation therapy regimens similar to those used for cutaneous lymphoma. Malignant schwannoma is often associated with neurofibromatosis. Yolk-Sac Tumour is primarily arising from the labia and clitoris, young age. Metastatic disease to the vulva had been reported from the primary site in endometrium, ovary, cervix, breast, kidney, urethra and lymphoma.

Appendix

Tips on Surgical Techniques in Vulvar Cancer Surgery

(1) Traditional Radical vulvectomy and Bilateral Inguino-femoral lymphadenectomy.

(a) Butterfly incision

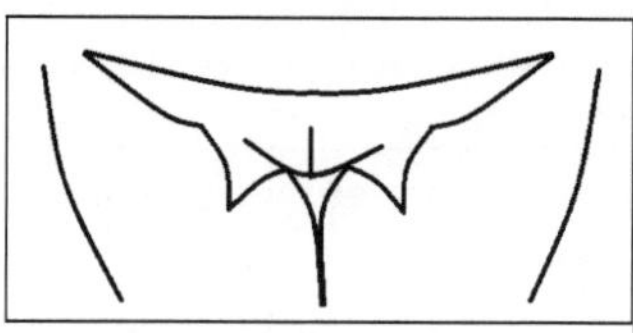

Butterfly incision was practised previously based on the traditionally belief that the vulvar cancer is a diffuse disease that spread by permeation to regional lymphatics.

(b) Longhorn incision

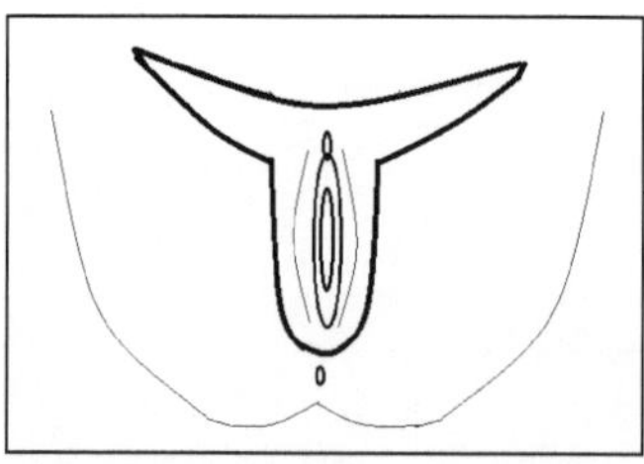

Give long-term survival of 70% with 5-year survivals 90% in stage 1 disease. Mortality rate 2% and lymphoedema rate 30-70%. 70% loss of sexual function.

(2) Radical Wide Excision and skin flap

(a) Margin should be 1–2 cm, 1 cm may be adequate

(b) May have to do rhomboid flap repair if difficult to close the incision.

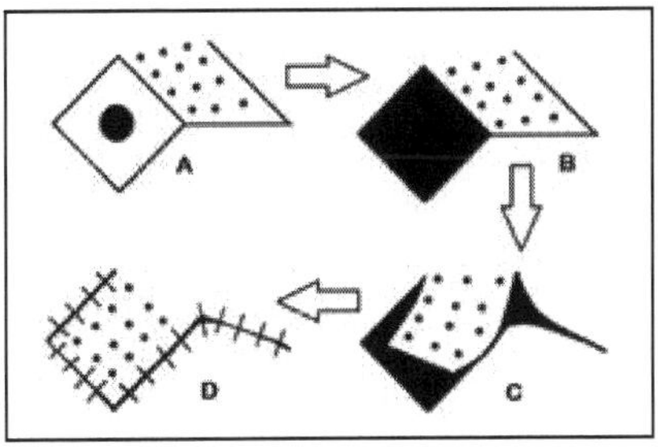

The thickness of rhomboid flap is 1–1.5 cm, practical size is 4 × 4 cm

(c) Myocutaneous flaps for large vulvar and groin defect, can use gracilis, gluteus muscle and rectus abdominis.

(3) Triple incision technique

(a) Alternative to butterfly or longhorn incision is triple incision. Triple incision technique can still preserve the radicality of vulvar resection while retaining skin over the groin.

(b) Incidence of wound breakdown reduced to 15–20%.

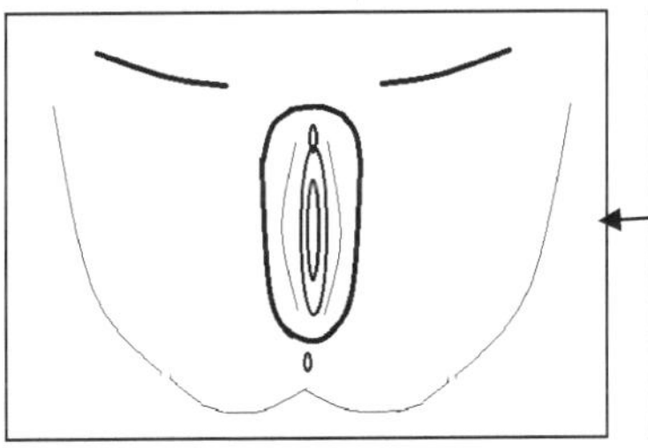

The rationale of triple incision is based on a clear understanding of the regional anatomy, the mechanism of lymphatic spread (embolization and not permeation) and incidence of nodal metastases.

Contraindications for separated groin incision (triple incision) are (a) clinically positive groin node (b) clitorial lesion and (c) lesion in the mons pubis. Surgical margin of resection is the best predictor of local recurrence (it should be clear of tumour by 1 cm in all direction).

(4) Inguinal lymphadenectomy

(a) Fine needle aspiration cytology (FNAC) can be done to assess the status of lymph node

(b) Excised enlarged lymph node because bulky lymph nodes do not respond well to radiation.

(c) Superficial lymphadenectomy should involved removing 8–10 superficial inguinal lymph nodes along the saphenous vein and branches.

(d) Deep inguinal (femoral) lymphadenectomy
- Nodes within the cribriform fascia (3–5 nodes)
- Medial to femoral vein
- Most superficial deep nodes known as Cloquet's node

(5) Surgical resection of recurrence

- Radical wide resection for resectable local recurrence can be curative. Resection is done with 2 cm margin.
- Pelvic exenteration
  (a) In a selected patient
  (b) Distant metastasis should be ruled out
  (c) Similar like in cervical cancer
- Resection of groin recurrence
  (a) In selected patient
  (b) Combined with radiation in a patient with no previous radiation
  (c) The aim is to reduce the tumour bulk to achieve better local control by subsequent radiation.

Anatomical Landmarks for Inguinal Lymphadenectomy

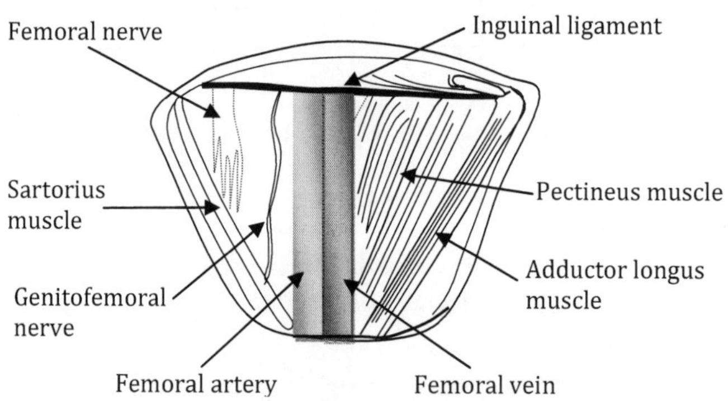

The above illustration shows the anatomy of the femoral triangle after complete inguinal lymphadenectomy. Femoral nerve lies beneath the fascia covering iliopsoas muscle. Iliopsoas muscle lies beneath the Sartorius muscle.

Modified Radical Vulvectomy

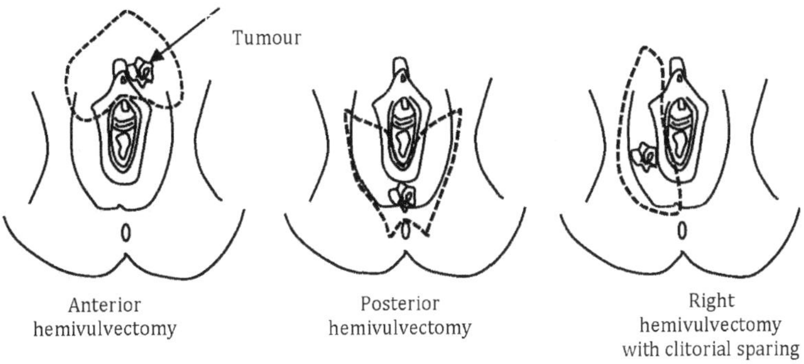

References

Abdel-Hady ES, Martin-Hirsch P, Duggan-Keen M, et al. Immunological and viral factors associated with the response of vulval intraepithelial neoplasia to photodynamic therapy. *Cancer Res* 2001; **61**: 192–196.

Black D, Tornos C, Soslow RA, et al. The outcomes of patients with positive margins after excision for intraepithelial Paget's disease of the vulva. *Gynecol Oncol* 2007; **104**: 547–550.

Booth S, Poole D, Moghissi K. Initial experience of the use of photodynamic therapy (PDT) in recurrent malignant and pre-malignant lesions of the vulva. *Photodiagn Photodyn Ther* 2006; **3**: 156–161.

Carli P, Cattaneo A, De MA, Biggeri A, Taddei G, Giannotti B. Squamous cell carcinoma arising in vulval lichen sclerosus: a longitudinal cohort study. *Eur J Cancer Prev* 1995; **4**(6): 491–495.

Chanda JJ. Extramammary Paget's disease: prognosis and relationship to internal malignancy. *J Am Acad Dermatol* 1985; **13**: 1009–1014.

Chang YT, Liu HN, Wong CK. Extramammary Paget's disease: a report of 22 cases in Chinese males. *J Dermatol* 1996; **23**: 320–324.

Chung AF, Woodruff JM, Lewis Jr. JL. Malignant melanoma of the vulva: a report of 44 cases. *Obstet Gynecol* 1975; **45**: 638–646.

Copeland LJ, Sneige N, Gershenson DM, et al. Adenoid cystic carcinoma of Batholin's gland. *Obstet Gynecol* 1986; **67**: 115–120.

Crocker HR. Paget's disease affecting the scrotum and the penis. *Trans Pathol Soc (London)* 1888–1889; **40**: 187–191.

Crosbie EJ, Slade RJ, Ahmed AS. Anti-Tumour Treatmen. The management of vulval cancer. *Cancer Treat Rev* 2009; **35**: 533–539.

Darier J, Couillaud P. Sur un cas de maladie de Paget de la region perinea-annale et scrotale. Ann Dermatol Syphiligr 1893; **4**: 25–31.

Faul CM, Mirmow D, Huang Q, Gerszten K, Day R, Jones MW. Adjuvant radiation for vulvar carcinoma: improved local control. *Int J Radiat Oncol Biol Phys* 1997; **38**(2): 381–389.

Fehr MK, Hornung R, Degen A, et al. Photodynamic therapy of vulvar and vaginal condyloma and intraepithelial neoplasia using topically applied 5-aminolevulinic acid. *Lasers Surg Med* 2002; **30**(4): 273–279.

Finan MA, Barre G. Bartholin's gland carcinoma, malignant melanoma and other rare tumours of the vulva. *Best Pract Res Clin Obstet Gynaecol* 2003; **17**(4): 609–633.

Fischer GO. The commonest causes of symptomatic vulvar disease: a dermatologist's perspective. Australas *J Dermatol* 1996; **37**(1): 12–18.

Fischer GO, Spurrett B, Fischer A. The chronically symptomatic vulva: aetiology and management. *Br J Obstet Gynaecol* 1995; **102**(10): 773–779.

Ghurani GB, Penalver MA. An update on vulvar cancer. *Am J Obstet Gynecol* 2001; **185**(2): 294–299.

Goldblum JR, Hart WR. Perianal Paget's disease: a histologic and immunohistochemical study of 11 cases with and without associated rectal adenocarcinoma. *Am J Surg Pathol* 1998; **22**: 170–179.

Gungor T, Altinkaya SO, Ozat M, et al. Primary malignant melanoma of the female genital tract. *Taiwan J Obstet Gynecol* 2009; **48**(2): 169–175.

Hampl M, Hantschmann P, Michels W, Hillemanns P. Validation of the accuracy of the sentinel node procedure in patients with vulvar cancer: Results of a multicenter study in Germany. *Gynecol Oncol* 2008; **111**: 282–288.

Hart WR. Vulvar intraepithelial neoplasia: historical aspects and current status. *Int J Gynecol Pathol* 2001; **20**: 16–30.

Harting MS, Kim KB. Biochemotherapy in patients with advanced vulvovaginal mucosal melanoma. *Melanoma Res* 2004; **14**: 517–5120.

Homesley HD, Bundy BN, Sedlis A, et al. Assessment of current International Federation of Gynecology and Obstetrics staging of vulvar carcinoma relative to prognostic factors for survival (a Gynecologic Oncology Group Study). *Am J Obstet Gynecol* 1991; **164**(4): 997–1003.

Irvin WP Jr, Legallo RL, Stoler MH, et al. Vulvar melanoma: a retrospective analysis and literature review. *Gynecol Oncol* 2001; **83**: 457–465.

Jabbar AS. Perianal extramammary Paget's disease. *Eur J Surg Oncol* 2000; **26**: 612–614.

Jones RW, Rowan DM, Stewart AW. Vulvar intraepithelial neoplasia: aspects of the natural history and outcome in 405 women. *Obstet Gynecol* 2005; **106**: 1319–1326.

Joura EA. Epidemiology, diagnosis and treatment of vulvar intraepithelial neoplasia. *Curr Opin Obstet Gynecol* 2002; **14**: 39–43.

Lara-Torre E, Perlman SE. Vulvar intraepithelial neoplasia in adolescents with abnormal pap smear results: a series report. *J Pediatr Adolesc Gynecol* 2004; **17**: 45–48.

Leibowitch M, Neill S, Pelisse M, Moyal-Baracco M. The epithelial changes associated with squamous cell carcinoma of the vulva: a review of the clinical, histological and viral findings in 78 women. *Br J Obstet Gynaecol* 1990; **97**(12): 1135–1139.

Levy RS, Bean SM, Vollmer RT, et al. Paget disease of the vulva: a study of 56 cases. *Eur J Obstet Gynecol Reprod Biol* 2010; **149**: 86–91.

Luk NM, Yu KH, Yeung WK, Choi CL, Teo ML. Extramammary Paget's disease: outcome of radiotherapy with curative intent. *Clin Exp Dermatol* 2003; **28**: 360–363.

Lyengar S, Acheson N. Review: Premalignant vulvar conditions. *Obstet, Gynaecol Reprod Med* 2008; 60–63.

Martin-Hirsch P, Kitchener HC, Hampson IN. Photodynamic therapy of lower genital tract neoplasia. *Gynecol Oncol* 2002; **84**:187–189

Mathiesen O, Buus SK, Cramers M. Topical imiquimod can reverse vulvar intraepithelial neoplasia: a randomized, double-blinded study. *Gynecol Oncol* 2007; **107**: 219–222.

Medeiros F, Nascimento AF, Crum CP. Early vulvar squamous neoplasia: advances in classification, diagnosis, and differential diagnosis. *Adv Anat Pathol* 2005; **12**: 20–26.

Minsky B, Hoffman J, Kelsedeir D. Cancer of the anal region. In DeVita V Jr, Hellman S, Rosenberg SA, eds. *Cancer: Principles and Practice of Oncology*. 6th ed. Philadelphia, Pa: JB Lippincott Co; Chapter 33, 2001: 1319–1342.

Monk BJ, Burger RA, Lin F, Parham G, Vasilev SA, Wilczynski SP. Prognostic significance of human papillomavirus DNA in vulvar carcinoma. *Obstet Gynecol* 1995; **85**: 709–15.

Moore DH. Review: Chemotherapy and radiation therapy in the treatment of squamous cell carcinoma of the vulva: Are two therapies better than one? *Gynecol Oncol* 2009; **113**: 379–383.

Moore DH, Thomas GM, Montana GS, Saxer A, Gallup DG. Preoperative chemoradiation for advanced vulvar cancer: a phase II study of the Gynecologic Oncology Group. *Int J Radiat Oncol Biol Phys* 1998; **42**: 79–85.

Moore RG, Robison K, Brown AK, et al. Isolated sentinel lymph node dissection with conservative management in patients with squamous cell carcinoma of the vulva: a prospective trial. *Gynecol Oncol* 2008; **109**: 65–70.

Moore RG, DePasquale S, Steinhoff MM, Gajewski W, Steller MA, Falkenberry S. Sentinel node identification and the ability to detect metastatic tumour to inguinal lymph nodes in vulvar malignancies. *Gynecol Oncol* 2003; **89**(3): 475–479.

Moore RG, Granai CO, Gajewski W, Steinhoff MM. Pathologic evaluation of inguinal sentinel nodes in vulvar cancer patients: a comparison of immunohistochemical staining versus ultra-staging with hematoxylin and eosin staining. *Gynecol Oncol* 2003; **88**(2): 190.

Mutch DG. Meeting Report: the new FIGO staging system for cancers of the vulva, cervix, endometrium and sarcomas. *Gynecol Oncol* 2009; **115**: 325–328.

Origoni M, Sideri M, Garsia S, Carinelli SG, Ferrari AG. Prognostic value of pathological patterns of lymph node positivity in squamous cell carcinoma of the vulva stage III and IVA FIGO. *Gynecol Oncol* 1992; **45**: 313–316.

Paget J. On disease of the mammary areola preceding cancer of the mammary gland. *St. Bartholomew Hosp Res* (*London*) 1874; **10**: 87–89.

Paladini D, Cross P, Lopes A, Monaghan JM. Prognostic significance of lymph node variables in squamous cell carcinoma of the vulva. *Cancer* 1994; **74**: 2491–2496.

Piura B, Rabinovich A, Cohen Y, Friger M, Glezerman M. Squamous cell carcinoma of the vulva in the south of Israel: a study of 50 cases. *J Surg Oncol* 1998; **67**(3): 174–181.

Piura B. Management of primary melanoma of the female urogenital tract. *Lancet Oncol* 2008; **9**: 973–981.

Preti M, van Seters M, Sideri M, van Beurden M. Squamous culvar intraepithelial neoplasia. *Clin Obstet Gynecol* 2005; **48**: 845–861.

Raspagliesi F, Hanozet F, Ditto A, et al. Clinical and pathological prognostic factors in squamous cell carcinoma of the vulva. *Gynecol Oncol* 2006; **102**: 333–337.

Raspagliesi F, Ditto A, Paladini D, et al. Prognostic indicators in melanoma of the vulva. *Ann Surg Oncol* 2000; **7**(10): 738–742.

Robison K, Steinhoff MM, Granai CO, et al. Inguinal sentinel node dissection versus standard inguinal node dissection in patients with vulvar cancer: a comparison of the size of metastasis detected in inguinal lymph nodes. *Gynecol Oncol* 2006; **101**(1): 24–27.

Shutze WP, Gleysteen JJ. Perianal Paget's disease: classification and review of management. Report of two cases. *Dis Colon Rectum* 1990; **33**: 502–507.

Sideri M, Jones RW, Wilkinson EJ, et al. Squamous vulvar intraepithelial neoplasia: 2004 modified terminology, ISSVD Vulvar Oncology Subcommittee. *J Reprod Med* 2005; **50**(11): 807–810.

Sillman FH, Sedlis B, Boyce JG. A review of lower genital intraepithelial neoplasia and the use of topical 5-fluorouracil. *Obstet Gynecol Surv* 1985; **40**: 190–220.

Simcock B. Review: Invasive vulval cancer. *Obstet, Gynaecol Reprod Med* 2008; **18**(3): 64–68.

Tabatabaei S, Harisinghani M, McDougal WS. Regional lymph node staging using lymphotropic nanoparticle enhanced magnetic resonance imaging with ferumotran-10 in patients with penile cancer. *J Urol* 2005; **174**(3): 923–927.

Thirlby RC, Hammer CJ, Galagan KA, et al. Perianal Paget's disease: successful treatment with combined chemoradiotherapy. Report of a case. *Dis Colon Rectum* 1990; **33**: 150–152.

Thomas G, Dembo A, DePetrillo A, et al. Concurrent radiation and chemotherapy in vulvar carcinoma. *Gynecol Oncol* 1989; **34**(3): 263–267.

Van de Nieuwenhof HP, van der Avoort IAM, de Hullu JA. Review of squamous premalignant vulvar lesions. *Crit Rev Oncol/Hematol* 2008; **68**: 131–156.

van der Avoort I, Shirango H, Hoevenaars BM, et al. Vulvar squamous cell carcinoma is a multifoctorial disease following two separate and independent pathways. *Int J Gynecol Pathol* 2006; **25**(1): 22–29.

Van der Zee AG, Oonk MH, De Hullu JA, et al. Sentinel node dissection is safe in the treatment of early-stage vulvar cancer. *J Clin Oncol* 2008; **26**: 884–889.

Van Doorn HC, Ansink A, Verhaar-Langereis M, Stalpers I. Neoadjuvant chemoradiation for advanced primary vulvar cancer. *Cochrane Database Syst Rev* 2006; **3**: CD003752.

van Seters M, van Beurden M, de Craen AJ. Is the assumed natural history of vulvar intraepithelial neoplasia III based on enough evidence? A systematic review of 3322 published patients. *Gynecol Oncol* 2005; **97**: 645–651.

Ve Hullu JA, Hollema H, Lolkema S, et al. Vulvar carcinoma, the price of less radical surgery. *Cancer* 2002; **95**: 2331.

Zeaps JM, Fu YS, Montz FZ, et al. Surgical-pathologic variables predictive of local recurrence in squamous cell carcinoma of the vulva. *Gynecol Oncol* 1990; **38**: 309.

Chapter 4

Carcinoma of Vagina

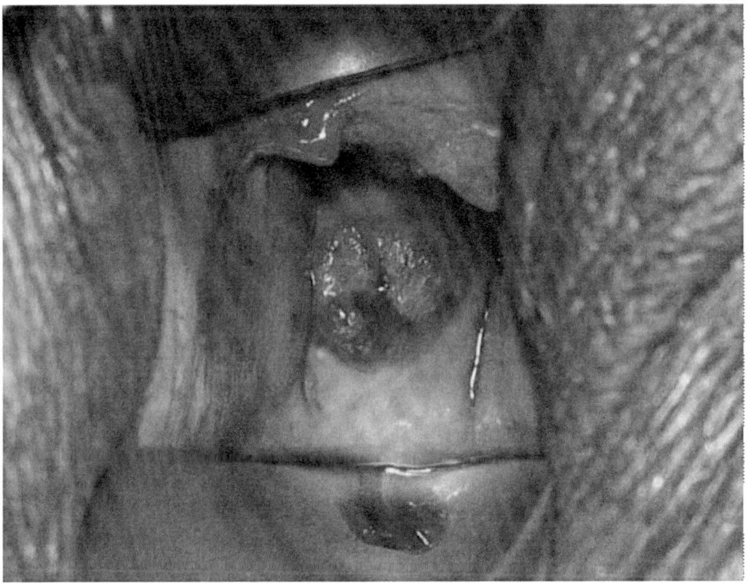

Gynaecologic Cancer: A Handbook for Students and Practitioners
Rushdan Noor, Eng Hseon Tay, and Jeffrey Low

ISBN 978-981-4463-06-5 (Hardcover), 978-981-4463-07-2 (eBook)
www.panstanford.com

Basic Anatomy of the Vagina

Vagina is a muscular tube extends from the cervix to hymenal ring. Inner mucosal layer of the vagina is formed by a thick, non-keratinizing, stratified, squamous epithelium overlying a basement membrane containing many papillae. Levator ani muscle and urogenital diaphragm support the vagina. Vagina is attached to the rectum posteriorly via rectal pillar and anteriorly attached to the bladder via bladder pillar. The upper vagina receives its blood supply from uterine and internal pudendal arteries. The lower part of the vagina receives its blood supply from inferior rectal artery and other branches from internal pudendal artery. Vaginal venous plexus mainly drains into the pelvic wall through a parametrial vein, and lesser degree to vesical and rectal plexuses. Lymphatic drainage from the vagina is as follows: (a) lower third to inguinal femoral then to external iliac lymph nodes, (b) middle third to mainly internal iliac and external iliac lymph nodes and (c) upper third to common iliac, internal iliac and pre-sacral lymph nodes. Basic anatomy of the vagina is shown in Fig. 4.1.

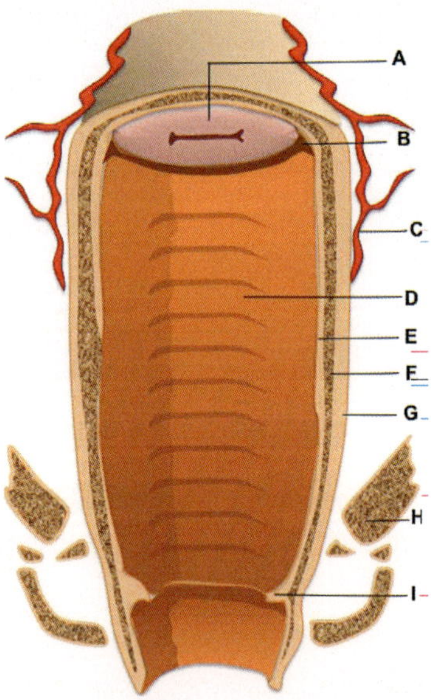

Figure 4.1 Anatomy of the vagina. A: cervix, B: vagina fornix, C: vaginal branch of uterine artery, D: vagina cavity/canal, E: vagina mucosa, F: muscular layers of vaginal wall, G: adventitia, H: levator ani muscle, I: hymen.

Carcinoma of Vagina

Carcinoma of the vagina is very rare, with primary vaginal carcinoma representing only 2–3% of all gynaecological malignancies. The incidence of vagina carcinoma is about 0.7 per 100,000 women (Grigsby, 2002; Kirkbride et al., 1995). The most common site is the upper third of the posterior vaginal wall because it is believed that the upper posterior wall of the vagina is more predisposed to irritating substances such as vaginal secretions and semen, which pool in the posterior fornix.

The diagnosis of primary carcinoma of vagina is not always easy to make; it cannot be considered a primary vaginal cancer if the portio and external os of the cervix or vulva are also involved in the tumour at presentation. About 80–90% of carcinomas of the vagina are metastatic and 60% of patients with vaginal cancer have had a prior hysterectomy. The mean age at presentation is approximately 67 years, and 20% of vaginal cancers are diagnosed in women younger than 50 years. More than 90% are epithelial cancers, mainly squamous cell carcinoma (about 80%), while adenocarcinoma of the vagina accounts for about 10% of cases (Frank et al., 2007; Grigsby, 2002). Figure 4.2 showed primary vaginal carcinoma diagnosed several years following hysterectomy for benign gynaecological condition.

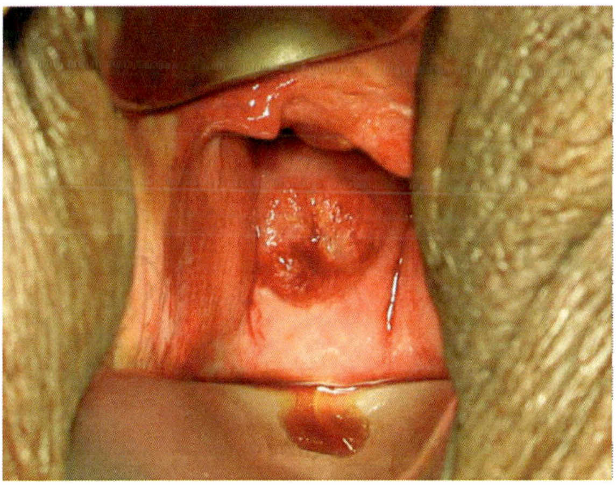

Figure 4.2 Primary vaginal cancer. Patient had hysterectomy for benign uterine pathology. Later she presented with postmenopausal bleeding, speculum examination showed raised, friable lesions with contact bleeding at the posterior vaginal wall.

Aetiology of Vaginal Cancer

The actual aetiology of primary vaginal cancer has not been identified. A single aetiologic factor is unlikely. The strongest aetiologic factor for vaginal cancer is the human papilloma virus, especially types 16 and 18. In utero exposure to DES accounts for 10% of patients with vaginal cancer (Frank et al., 2007; Herbst et al., 1971). The number of cases is declining. Up to 30% of patients with primary vaginal cancer have a previous history of in situ or invasive carcinoma of the cervix treated at least 5 years before the diagnosis. Prior pelvic irradiation or chronic irritation from vaginal ring pessaries may also be possible causes. There is also some association with HIV infection, smoking and alcohol consumption.

Histological Types of Primary Vaginal Cancer

The most common histotype for primary vaginal cancer is squamous cell carcinoma accounting 80–90% of cases and the peak age is 60 years old. Adenocarcinoma is the second most common accounting 10% of cases; however, it occurs in a younger age group between 7 and 34 years old (Frank et al., 2007). The other rare variant of primary vaginal cancer are verrucous carcinoma (rare) with peak age of 60 years old, vaginal melanoma (0.5–2%), peak age 60 years and carries poor prognosis and leiomyosarcoma (<2%) which can occur secondary to pelvic irradiation. Sarcoma botryoides or embryonal rhabdomyosarcom of vagina is also a rare cancer with a peak age of 3 years. Sarcoma botryoides is the most common vaginal cancer in children. The other type of vaginal cancer is endodermal sinus tumour (yolk sac tumour) which is rare and occurs in the young age group with peak age of, this tumour is very aggressive and is associated with raised alpha fetoprotein (Grigsby, 2002; Kirkbride et al., 1995).

Adenocarcinoma of the Vagina

Adenocarcinoma of vagina accounts for 14% of cases and occurs exclusively in young women under 20 years of age (Herbst et al.,

1971; Frank et al., 2007). There are four types of adenocarcinoma of vagina: (a) clear cell carcinoma, (b) papillary adenocarcinoma, (c) mucinous adenocarcinoma and (d) adenosquamous carcinoma.

Clear Cell Adenocarcinoma of the Vagina

The association of in utero exposure to diethylstilbestrol is well known. The incidence of clear cell adenocarcinoma (CCA) of the vagina in relation to diethylstilbestrol exposure is 1 in 1,000 exposures. Diethylstilbestrol (DES) is a synthetic oestrogen and it was used in the first trimester (from 1941 to 1971) to prevent pregnancy loss; however, the FDA withdrew DES in 1971. Approximately, 75% of patients with CCA of vagina had a history of DES exposure, and unfortunately DES-related adenocarcinoma of the vagina carries poorer prognosis (Frank et al., 2007; Hellman et al., 2004).

Almost 50% of women who had in utero exposure to DES have vaginal adenosis. Vaginal adenosis is a glandular epithelial similar with endocervical gland in the vagina it appears red, velvety and grapelike clusters lesions. Not all vaginal adenoses are DES-related; congenital adenosis has been reported in patients as young as 6 years of age. Vaginal adenosis may also develop after destruction or denudation of the overlying vagina squamous epithelium, examples following treatment with 5-fluorouracil and carbon dioxide laser. Vaginal adenosis is usually asymptomatic; however, some presented with vaginal bleeding and vaginal discharge. Rare complications of vaginal adenosis are atypical adenosis and vaginal CCA.

In the reproductive tract, clear cell carcinoma of the vagina is more common than clear cell carcinoma of cervix with a ratio of 60%:40%. The age group of patients with this cancer is between 7 and 34 years old 70% diagnosed at stage 1 disease. The cancer occurs mainly in the upper third of anterior vaginal wall. The risk of clear cell carcinoma of vagina is higher if the exposure occurs before 16-week gestation. About 60% of patients with this cancer had an exposure during the first trimester (Frank et al., 2007; Herbst et al., 1971; Robboy et al., 1981).

Vaginal Intraepithelial Neoplasia

The preinvasive lesion of the vagina is known as vaginal intraepithelial neoplasm (VAIN). Graham and Meigs did the first report of VAIN in 1952. Unlike cervical intraepithelial neoplasm, VAIN is uncommon and does arise from a transformation zone.

The actual aetiology has not been identified and single aetiologic factor is unlikely. Similar to invasive carcinoma of the vagina, the strongest aetiologic factor for VAIN is a human papilloma virus infection, especially types 16 and 18. Vaginal intraepithelial neoplasm is extremely rare condition, accounting for approximately 0.4% of lower genital tract intraepithelial neoplasm. The incidence of VAIN in United State is found to be 0.2–0.4 per 100,000 women. VAIN can be divided into VAIN 1, VAIN 2 and VAIN 3 (Kirkbride et al., 1995). In contrast to CIN, there is very limited knowledge about the rate of progression from VAIN to invasive cancer. VAIN 1 is characterized by slight nuclear and cellular atypia with preservation of stratification. While VAIN 3 demonstrated by gross nuclear atypia involving and complete loss of stratification. In VAIN, only VAIN 3 is considered as high-grade lesion while VAIN 1 and 2 are low-grade lesions.

VAIN is more common among 50–60-year-old patients. A history of tobacco use is frequent among women diagnosed with VAIN. The other risk factors for VAIN are pelvic radiotherapy and patient with chronic immunocompromised state such as AIDs.

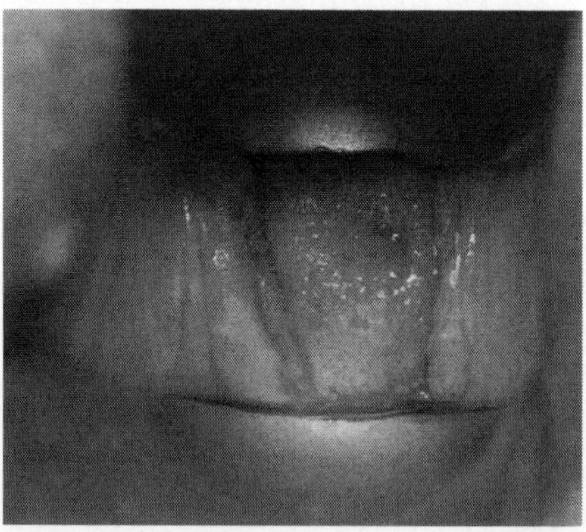

Figure 4.3 Colposcopic view of VAIN lesion on the vaginal vault. Observe the raised, irregular lesions; on further magnification, atypical vessels were seen, representing the high-grade lesions.

Most of patients with VAIN are asymptomatic. Some of them may present with vaginal discharge or abnormal vaginal bleeding. VAIN is also often diagnosed incidentally, following assessment of patient who had been treated for CIN or cervical carcinoma in the past. The diagnosis of VAIN is made through colposcopic examination and vaginal wall biopsy. Colposopic features of VAIN are flat warty lesions with multicentric foci of dense and white epithelium after application of acetic acid (Figs. 4.3 and 4.4). The colposcopic directed biopsy is important for the diagnosis of VAIN and to exclude the pre-existing invasive cancer.

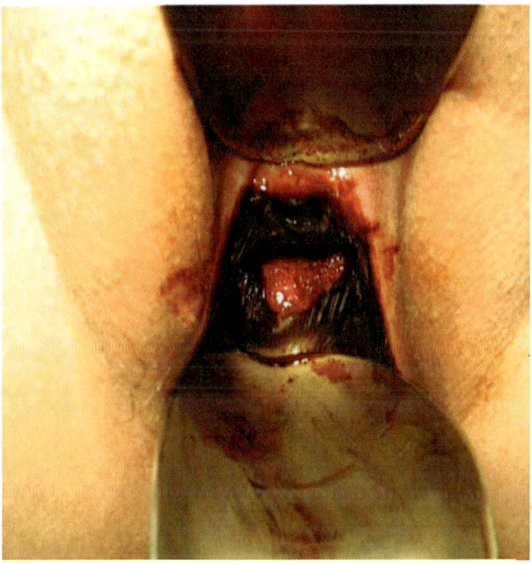

Figure 4.4 Same lesions as seen in Fig. 4.2 but following the application of Lugol's iodine. The abnormal lesion lacks of iodine uptake.

Treatment of Vaginal Intraepithelial Neoplasm

Before treating VAIN, patient must be thoroughly evaluated to rule out the pre-existing pre-invasive disease of the vulva and the cervix. It is also important to rule out the invasive carcinoma of the vagina. If the lesion is unifocal and small, local excision is the treatment of choice and the depth of treatment must be at least 1 mm (Fig. 4.5). Local ablative therapy is indicated in large and multifocal lesions. Local ablative therapy can be performed by electrocoagulation, cryotherapy or laser vaporization in superpulse or ultrapulse mode (to the depth of 2–3 mm). The other option for local treatment is application of topical 5-Fluorouracil 20% 1.5 gm weekly for 10 weeks or 1 gm nightly for one week with the response rate of 75–90%. The other option is application of 5% imiquimoid cream especially for extensive and multifocal lesions. In some patients who failed to respond to local ablative treatment, radical surgical excision such as partial or total vaginectomy may be indicated with reconstructive surgery of the vagina in sexually active women. Radiation therapy is the last choice and not recommended in majority of patient due to high recurrence rate and the risk of complications such as vaginal stenosis and other radiation toxicities. Radiotherapy in form of low dose intracavitary radiotherapy 65–80 Gy for in situ lesion and the whole vagina need to be irradiated using 50–60 Gy to the entire vagina for multifocal lesions. Radiotherapy and vaginectomy should be avoided in young patients as this treatment may compromise their sexual function.

Patients with VAIN must be followed up once in three to six months for few years because these women are at increased risk of recurrence. Cervical and vaginal wall smear should be done during each follow-up visit and if necessary, and repeated colposcopic evaluation must be performed if recurrent disease is suspected.

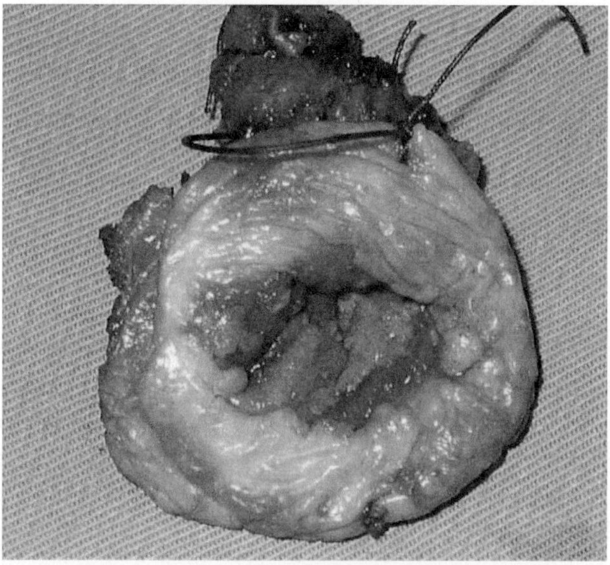

Figure 4.5 Upper vaginectomy specimen in patient with VAIN 3.

Clinical Presentation of Vaginal Carcinoma

Approximately, 10–27% of patients with vaginal carcinoma are asymptomatic. Painless vaginal bleeding is the most presenting symptom accounting for 65–80% of the symptomatic patients. Thirty percent of patients presented with vaginal discharge and 20% with urinary symptoms such as bladder pain, dysuria and haematuria (Hellman et al., 2004; Kirkbride et al., 1995). The other presenting symptoms are postmenopausal bleeding, postcoital bleeding and intermenstrual bleeding. Pelvic pain, tenesmus and vaginal ulceration with utero-vaginal prolapse are rare presentation.

Staging of Vaginal Carcinoma

The staging of vaginal cancer is clinical, similar to cervical cancer. The latest FIGO staging 2009 is shown in Table 4.1. There are no changes in this latest staging as compared to the earlier FIGO staging.

Table 4.1 FIGO staging (cancer of vagina)

Stage	Descriptions
Stage 1	The carcinoma is limited to the vaginal wall
Stage 2	The carcinoma has involved the subvaginal tissue but has not extended to the pelvic wall
Stage 3	The carcinoma has extended to the pelvic wall
Stage 4	The carcinoma has extended beyond the true pelvis or has involved the mucosa of the bladder or rectum; bullous oedema as such does not permit a case to be allotted to stage IV
Stage 4A	Tumour invades bladder and/or rectal mucosa and/or direct extension beyond the true pelvis
Stage 4B	Spread to distant organs

During staging procedures, multiple cervical biopsies are strongly recommended; if the cervical biopsy is positive, vagina cancer is considered secondary from cervical carcinoma. In vaginal cancer, risk of nodal metastasis is difficult to determine because of the rarity of this disease and patients were mostly treated with radiotherapy. The risk of pelvic recurrence depends on the stage (stage I, 10–20%; stage II, 35%; stage III, 25–37%; stage V, 58%).

Management of Vaginal Cancer

Radiation therapy is a preferred modality of treatment because it provides an excellent tumour control and good functional results (Chyle et al., 1996; Samant et al., 2005; Lian et al., 2008). Surgery is indicated in the following patients: (a) small localized stage 1 lesions, (b) stage 1 CCA in young women, (c) in young women who want to preserve fertility and ovarian function, (d) in selected stage 4A disease, particularly in the presence of rectovaginal or vesicovaginal fistula, (e) failed radiation therapy, (f) recurrence after irradiation (usually requiring exenteration), (g) verrucous carcinoma (radiation therapy is contraindicated) and (h) non-epithelial tumours (Cutillo et al., 2006).

Surgery in Stage 1 Disease

The type of surgical treatment depends on the site of the tumour. If the tumour is located in the middle and upper third of the vagina, radical hystero-vaginectomy and pelvic lymph nodes dissection is the treatment of choice. For localized lesion, partial colpectomy may be performed instead of total vaginectomy. Tumour in the lower third of the vagina is best treated with radical vulvovaginectomy (or hemivulvectomy and lower vaginectomy) and bilateral groin lymph node dissection. Radical vaginectomy usually requires a combined abdominal-perineal approach. An omental graft can be used to cover the upper vagina, while the lower vagina requires a split-thickness skin graft or a myocutaneous flap. In selected young patients who wanted to preserve their fertility, a radical wide local excision with surgical margin of at least 1 cm (radical tumorectomy) and pelvic lymphadenectomy (laparotomy or laparoscopically) can be considered (Cutillo et al., 2006).

Treatment of Stage 2–4 Vaginal Cancer

The treatment of choice for stage 2 and 3 vaginal cancer is radiation therapy. In premenopausal patients, pre-treatment ovarian transposition and resection of enlarged nodes can be performed. Ovarian transposition will minimize the risk of radiation-induced premature menopause. Stage 4A can be treated with either radiotherapy or pelvic exenteration, whereas patients with stage 4B disease are treated with palliative intent.

Radiation Therapy in Vaginal Cancer (Stage by Stage)

There are two types of radiation therapy: (a) external beam radiotherapy and (b) brachytherapy (intracavitary/interstitial therapy).

Radiation Therapy for Stage 1

The majority of cases of stage 1 vaginal cancer require brachytherapy alone. For superficial tumours, intracavitary cylinder covering the entire vagina (60 to 70 Gy mucosal dose) and additional 20–30 Gy mucosal dose to the tumour area are given. In larger and deeper lesions (>1 cm, some defined as >5 mm), the above treatment is given plus single plane interstitial implants to increase the depth dose. Some have suggested using interstitial implants for lesions involving the lateral and anterior wall of the lower two-thirds of the vagina, while intracavitary BRT is favoured for posterior wall lesions and lesions in the upper 1/3 of the vagina. More invasive, aggressive and poorly differentiated tumours require an additional dose to the parametrium and whole pelvis (Chyle et al., 1996; Samant et al., 2005; Lian et al., 2008).

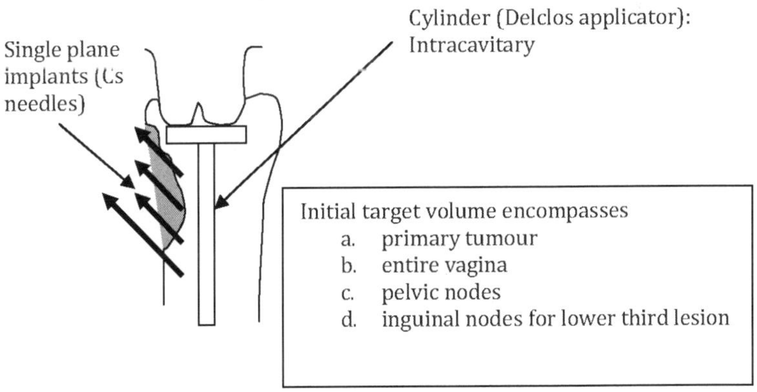

Figure 4.6 Example of radiation therapy technique for vaginal cancer (different institutions may have a different technique).

Radiation Therapy for Stage 2A

Stage 2A vaginal cancer is treated with interstitial (double-plane or volume plane) and intracavitary irradiation with greater external irradiation to the whole pelvis with 20 Gys and additional parametrial dose (total 45–50 Gys).

Radiation Therapy for Stage 2B, Stage 3 and Stage 4A

In more advanced stage 2B, 3 and 4A, higher dose of radiation (40 Gy whole pelvis, 55–60 Gys additional parametrial dose) using a similar method are given. Para-aortic irradiation may be indicated if bulky pelvic or para-aortic nodes are present.

There is lack of good prospective data to substantiate the use of concurrent chemotherapy with radiation in locally advanced vaginal cancer. However, with the frequent local failure in these high-risk patients, the use of concurrent 5-fluorouracil and/or cisplatin appears appropriate (Dalrymple et al., 2004). Lesions involving lower part of the vagina may require additional inguinal nodes irradiation (if node positive), i.e. a further 15–20 Gy in 7–10 fractions given in 10–14 days.

Survival

Five-year overall survival rate for vaginal cancer is 55.6%. Overall survival is influenced by (a) the stage (stage I and II are early disease and have a better prognosis), (b) dose of radiotherapy (poorer prognosis if the total dose < 70 Gy and BRT < 20 Gy) and (c) size of tumour (>4–5 cm tumour has significantly lower overall survival) (Chyle et al., 1996; Lian et al., 2008; Tabata et al., 2002). Some study showed tumour located at the upper third of the vagina has a better prognosis. The most important prognostic factor is the stage. The 5-year survival rates are 70–90% for stage 1, 45% for stage 2, 30% for stage 3 and 15% for stage 4 (Anderson et al., 2003; Emberger et al., 2006).

Vaginal Melanoma

Primary vaginal melanoma is extremely poor prognosis and the 5-year survival rates are only 9.1%. It has a high incidence of distant metastases and the best treatment for vaginal melanoma remains controversial. Radical surgery has been the main treatment modality. The treatment options for vaginal melanoma are (a) local excision/partial vaginectomy, (b) radical surgery, (c) radiotherapy using high dose fraction and (d) surgery plus irradiation. Small lesions in the upper vagina are treated by radical hysterectomy, upper vaginectomy and pelvic lymphadenectomy. Lesions in the lower vagina are treated by partial vaginectomy, total or partial vulvectomy and bilateral inguinal lymphadenectomy. The recurrence rate of vaginal melanoma is high: local recurrence rate of 40.7%, regional failures in 20% and distant metastases in 35%.

Small Cell Carcinoma of Vagina

As in small cell carcinoma of the lung, these tumours have a great propensity for distant dissemination and can be rapidly fatal. The usual chemotherapeutic agents used in small cell carcinoma arecyclophosphamide, doxorubicin (Adriamycin), and vincristine sulfate (CAV), with administration of 8–12 cycles, some before initiation of irradiation. Cisplatin and etoposide (VP-16) are also frequently used.

In some patients, radiotherapy is the only option and the dose of irradiation is similar to those administered for squamous cell carcinoma.

Clear Cell Adenocarcinoma of Vagina

Most young women with CCA of the vagina have a history of prenatal exposure to diethylstilbestrol; however, some develop vaginal CCA without this history. Surgery for stage I CCA may have the advantage of ovarian preservation and better vaginal function after skin graft; however, surgery for vaginal CCA requires removal of most of the vagina and reconstructive procedures. A radical hysterectomy and lymph node dissection are necessary to encompass the area from the parametria and paracolpium to the sidewalls of the pelvis. The periaortic nodes should be sampled before the procedure to determine if there is a lymphatic disease beyond the pelvis.

Fletcher and Wharton (1980) advocate intracavitary or transvaginal irradiation for treatment of small tumours because it may yield excellent tumour control with a functional vagina and preservation of ovarian function. For more extensive lesions, external radiation therapy is essential. Techniques are similar to those described earlier.

Vaginal Recurrences

Post-irradiation local failures can sometimes be effectively treated with surgery. Surgical procedures range from wide local excision or partial vaginectomy to exenterative procedures. Meticulous and regular follow-up examinations are important to detect recurrences early.

Other Vaginal Cancers

- **Leiomyosarcoma:** For low-grade tumour, local excision may be sufficient, but for high-grade lesion, the patient should receive radiotherapy.
- **Rhabdomyosarcoma** of the vagina generally is treated with a combination of surgical resection, irradiation, and systemic chemotherapy. **Sarcoma botryoides** is treated with a combination of chemotherapy, surgery and radiotherapy. In small-localized lesion, local excision followed by either chemotherapy or radiotherapy is effective. In large tumour, preoperative chemotherapy or radiotherapy can be administered to facilitate surgical resection. Chemo-therapy regimen is VAC (vincristine, actinomycin D and cyclophosphamide) regimen.
- **Lymphomas:** Radical surgery occasionally has been used for treatment of localized malignant of the vagina. Satisfactory results with a combination of external irradiation and intravaginal brachytherapy combined with chemotherapy have been reported. Six cycles of chemotherapy usually are given; most frequently, chemotherapy consists of cyclophosphamide, doxorubicin, vincristine, and prednisone (CHOP), or CHOP plus bleomycin sulfate (BACOP).

- **Endodermal sinus tumour** of the vagina is preferentially are treated with surgery and chemotherapy (VAC regimen), because this lesion often occurs in young women and preservation of the ovarian function is desired. Brachytherapy may occasionally be used.

References

Anderson ES, Hanselaar AG, Paavonen J, et al. Tumors of the vagina. In: Tavassoli FA, Devilee P, eds. *Tumors of the Breast and Female Genital Organs*. Lyon: IARC Press, 2003: 292–311.

Chyle V, Zagar GK, Wheeler JA, Wharton JT, Delsclos L. Definitive radiotherapy for carcinoma of vagina: outcome and prognostic factors. *Int J Radiat Oncol Biol Phys* 1996; **35**: 891–905.

Cutillo G, Cignini P, Pizzi G et al. Conservative treatment of reproductive and sexual function in young woman with squamous carcinoma of vagina. *Gynecol Oncol* 2006; **103**: 234–237.

Dalrymple JL, Russell AH, Lee SW, et al. Chemoradiation for primary invasive squamous carcinoma of the vagina. *Int J Gynecol Cancer* 2004; **14**: 110–117.

Davies M, Mount S. Premalignant and malignant lesions of the vagina. *Diagn Histopathol* 2010; **16**(11): 508–516.

Emberger M, Lanschuetzer CM, Laimer M, Hawranek, Staudach A. Vaginal adenosis induced by Stevens–Johnson syndrome. *J Eur Acad Dermatol Venercol* 2006; **20**: 896–898.

Fletcher GH, Wharton JT. Tumour of the vagina and female urethra. In: Fletcher GH, ed. *Textbook of Radiotherapy*, 3rd ed. Philadelphia: Lea & Febiger, 1980: 821–824.

Frank SJ, Deavers MT, Jhingran A, Bodurka DC, Eifel PJ. Primary adenocarcinoma of vagina not associated with DES exposure. *Gynecol Oncol* 2007; **105**: 470–474.

Grigsby PW. Vaginal cancer. *Curr Treat Options Oncol* 2002; **3**: 125–130.

Hellman K, Lundell M, Silfversward C, Nilsson B, Hellstrom AC, Frankendal B. Clinical and histopathologic factors related to prognosis in primary squamous cell carcinoma of the vagina. *Int J Gynecol Cancer* 2006; **16**(3): 1201–1211.

Hellman K, Silfversward C, Nilsson B, Hellstrom AC, Frankendal B, Pettersson F. Primary carcinoma of the vagina: factors influencing the age at diagnosis. The Radiumhemmet series 1956–96. *Int J Gynecol Cancer* 2004; **14**: 491–501.

Herbst A, Ulfelder H, Poskanzer D. Adenocarcinoma of the vagina: an association of maternal stilbestrol therapy with tumor appearance in young women. *N Engl J Med* 1971; **284**: 878–881.

Kirkbride P, Fyles A, Rawlings GA, Manchul L, Levin W, Murphy KJ, Simm J. Carcinoma of vagina: experience at the Princess Margaret Hospital (1974–1989). *Gynecol Oncol* 1995; **56**(3): 435–443.

Lian J, Dundas G, Carlone M, Ghosh S, Pearcey R. Twenty-year review of radiotherapy for vaginal cancer: an institutional experience. *Gynecol Oncol* 2008; **111**: 298–306.

Martino MA, Nevadunsky NS, Magliaro TJ, Golberg MI. The DES year: bridging the past to the future. Prim Care Update Ob/Gyns 2002; 9: 7–12.

Robboy S, Szyfelbein W, Goellner J, et al. Dysplasia and cytologic findings in 4,589 young women enrolled in Diethystilbestrol-Adenosis (DESAD) Project. *Am J Obstet Gynecol* 1981; **140**: 579–586.

Samant R, Tam T, Dahrouge S. Radiotherapy for treatment of primary vaginal cancer. *Radiother Oncol* 2005; **77**: 133–136.

Tabata T, Taheshima N, Nishida H, et al. Treatment failure in vaginal cancer. *Gynecol Oncol* 2002; **84**: 309–314.

Chapter 5

Screening for Cervical Cancer

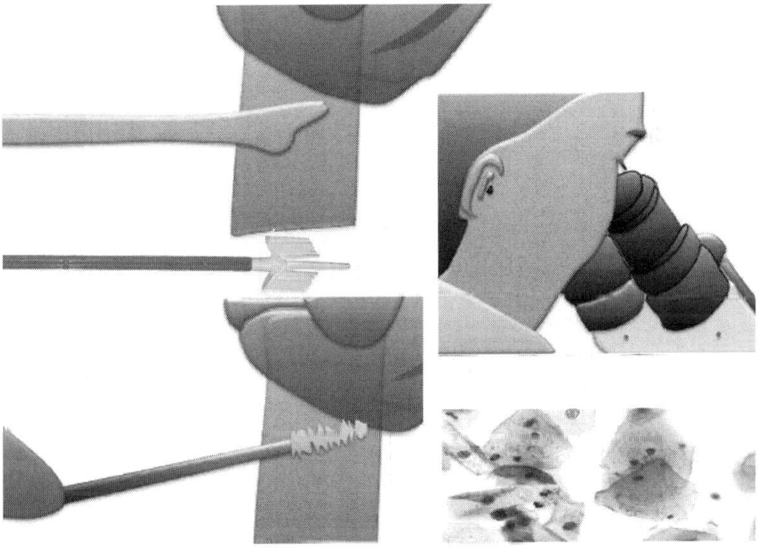

Gynaecologic Cancer: A Handbook for Students and Practitioners
Rushdan Noor, Eng Hseon Tay, and Jeffrey Low

ISBN 978-981-4463-06-5 (Hardcover), 978-981-4463-07-2 (eBook)
www.panstanford.com

Basics in Cancer Screening

The purpose of cancer screening is to identify asymptomatic individuals who have a significant risk of acquiring cancer, which warrants further diagnostic procedures.

Following are the criteria for an effective cancer-screening program:

- The cancer is a major health problem.
- The cancer is treatable at an early stage.
- The screening test is acceptable.
- The screening test is inexpensive.
- The screening test has high sensitivity (the bulk of subjects with the cancer should test positive).
- The screening test has a high specificity (the vast majority of subjects without the cancer should test negative).
- Screening has been shown to reduce mortality in randomized controlled trials.
- Screening has been shown to be a cost-effective means of controlling this cancer.

How to Calculate Sensitivity and Specificity

In any cancer-screening test, sensitivity and specificity of the test are the most important statistical measures to evaluate the efficacy of the test. The definition of and how to calculate the sensitivity and specificity are shown in Table 5.1.

The ideal screening test must have high sensitivity and specificity. There are four main criteria for a good screening test: (a) high sensitivity so the tests do not miss the cases with the disease, (b) high specificity to reduce the number of people with false-positive results who require diagnostic evaluation, (c) high positive predictive value and (d) simplicity and low cost.

Screening for any health problems is not without risk. The possible adverse effects from screening are

(a) discomfort from the test
(b) anxiety
(c) potential side effects related to test, e.g. radiation exposure in mammography

(d) false positive test

(e) risk of overdiagnosis (pseudodisease) (screening can lead to the detection of the early stage of cancer and this will accompanied by a temporary increase in the cancer incidence; in slow-growing tumour with excellent prognosis, screening might lead to "overdiagnosis"; some of these tumours may even regress spontaneously, e.g. neuroblastoma).

Table 5.1 Sensitivity and specificity

	Screen result	
Cancer present	**Negative**	**Positive**
No	A	B
Yes	C	D

A: Number of persons who do not have cancer and screen negative

B: Number of persons who do not have cancer but screen positive

C: Number of persons who do have cancer but screen negative

D: Number of persons who have cancer and screen positive

Sensitivity = D ÷ (C + D): The proportion of disease that test positive

Specificity = A ÷ (A + B): The proportion without disease and test negative

Positive Predictive Value = D ÷ (B + D): The proportion testing positive who will have disease.

Cervical Cancer Prevention

Cervical cancer is preventable disease because it has the most effective screening test. There are three modalities of cervical cancer prevention:

(a) **Primary prevention:** prevention of HPV infection through sexual abstinence, healthy lifestyle and HPV vaccination;

(b) **Secondary prevention:** detection and treatment of precancerous state through screening;

(c) **Tertiary prevention:** detection and treatment of an early stage of cancer.

Screening of Cervical Cancer

Screening of precancerous lesions and invasive cervical cancer is considered secondary prevention. Secondary prevention stops the progression of disease once it has already started. There has been lack of the number of randomized trials to evaluate the impact of screening on cervical cancer incidence and mortality. Majority of data on the effectiveness of screening were from cohort and case-control studies.

A comprehensive analysis of data by International Agency for Research on Cancer (IARC) showed the following:

(a) Well-organized screening programs were effective in reducing cervical cancer incidence and mortality.
(b) In Nordic countries, the greatest fall in a cumulative mortality rates was in Iceland (84% from 1965 to 1982).
(c) The greatest reduction in the cervical cancer incidence was in women aged between 30 and 49 years, for whom the focus of screening was the most intense.
(d) Target age range of a screening program was a more important determinant of risk reduction than frequency of screening within the defined age range.
(e) Screening interval every 2–3 years have been found to be as effective as annual screening (Table 5.2).
(f) The protective effect of 5 years' screening interval in the organized screening program was still high, i.e. more than 80%.
(g) Screening every 2 years is approximately 50% more expensive than screening every 3 years.
(h) Risk of developing invasive cervical cancer is 3–10 times greater in women who have not been screened. Risk also increases with long duration following the last normal screening test.

Table 5.2 Effectiveness (reduction in cervical cancer incidence) of the cervical cancer screening program based on the target age group and screening interval (Sasieni et al., 2003)

	20–39 years	40–54 years	55–69 years
3 yearly screening	41%	69%	73%
5 yearly screening	30%	63%	73%

There are four main modalities of screening tests for cervical cancer: (a) cytology, (b) visual inspection, (c) HPV testing and (d) combination.

Screening Population

One of the most important factors to determine the success of any cancer-screening program is the target population and age groups. In cervical cancer screening program worldwide, there are slight variations in the target age group and interval of screening between countries and institutions. In United Kingdom under NHS (UK), 2004 guideline, the age group for screening is all women between ages of 25–64, Interval: 3 yearly (age 25–49), 5 yearly (age 50–64), and for women age above 64 years old, only screen those who have not been screened since age 50 or have had recent abnormal tests. In United States, according to revised ACOG guidelines, the target age group is 21–65 years old, begins at the age of 21 years, regardless of sexual history, end at 65–70 years old. The recommended interval of screening is 2 yearly (age 21–29) and for women age more than 30 years old; the recommended testing is cytology and HPV testing. If both tests are normal, re-screening should be performed no sooner than 3 years later. The screening is stopped at the age of 65–70 if three consecutive smears are normal or no abnormal smears in last 10 years. Cervical Screen program of Singapore (CSS) recommended screening at the age of 25–64 year old (who had sexual exposure) with the interval of 3 years; women age 35–64 years old will receive a letter of invitation.

Based on the guidelines from US Preventive Services Task Force (USPSTF), the target group for screening is women aged 21–65 years old, begins the screening within 3 years of onset of sexual activity or age 21 (whichever comes first) with the interval of at least 3 yearly. Finally, in Australia; National Cervical Screening Program (NCSP Australia) recommended screening at the age of 18–70 year old (sexually active women begin to screen at the age of 18–20 or 1–2 years after first sexual exposure, whichever is later). National Cervical Screening Program suggested stopping screening after age of 70 when two consecutive smears are normal within last 5 years. The interval of screening is 2 years.

Women with high risk factors such as smokers, multiple sexual partners, sex workers, history of in utero exposure to DES, history of CIN and immunosuppresion (HIV, renal transplant, chronic steroid treatment, etc.) should have yearly screening.

Cytologic Screening for Cervical Cancer and Its Precursors

Dr. George Papanicolaou first proposed the cytologic evaluation of cells taken from the cervix and vagina in the 1940s, and in 1947 Ayre's introduced wooden spatula. Pap smear screening program significantly reduced the incidence and mortality of cervical cancer (see screening of cervical cancer above). In the United Kingdom, since the introduction of the organized Pap smear screening program in 1988, the incidence and mortality rate of cervical cancer have fallen by more than 50%.

Studies have shown that pap smear is highly specific in detecting invasive cervical cancer and high-grade squamous intraepithelial lesions, although it is less specific in low-grade lesion. Unfortunately, Pap smear is not very sensitive. Meta-analyses suggested that the sensitivity of single conventional Pap test for CIN 2/3 or higher is 50–60% (Wright, 2007; Nanda et al., 2000). In other cross-sectional studies evaluating the accuracy of cytologic testing from developing countries, the sensitivity of this testing was between 44–78% (Sankaranarayanan et al., 2009).

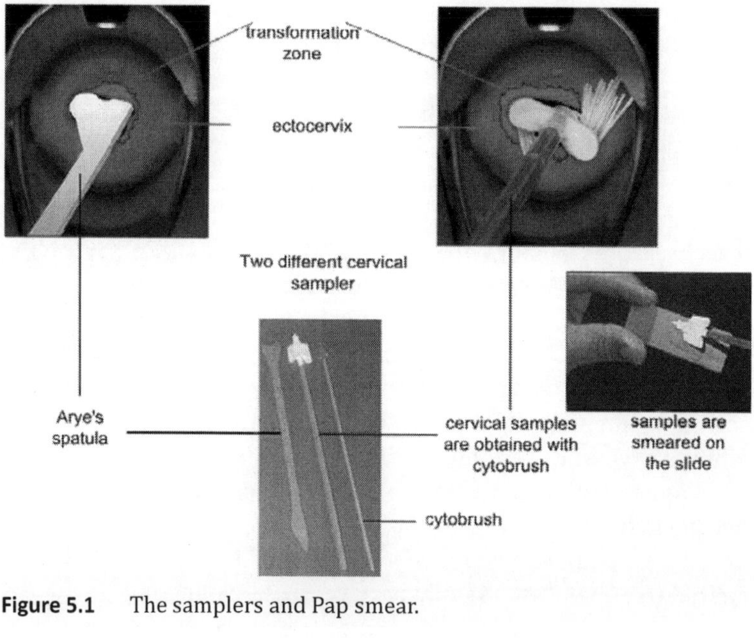

Figure 5.1 The samplers and Pap smear.

In general, cytologic testing has a wider range of sensitivity but high specificity ranging from 60–96% (Sankaranarayanan et al., 2004; Denny et al., 2006; Nanda et al., 2000) and low sensitivity of Pap smear was attributed to poor sample collection, incorrect slide preparation and laboratory interpretation errors. False negative rate of Pap smear is ranging from 8–50%. In order to reduce the false negative rate, sample from the endocervix has to be taken. Many have recommended using cytobrush to sample the cervix because it can obtain more cells than Ayre's spatula and cotton tipped applicator (Figs. 5.1 and 5.2).

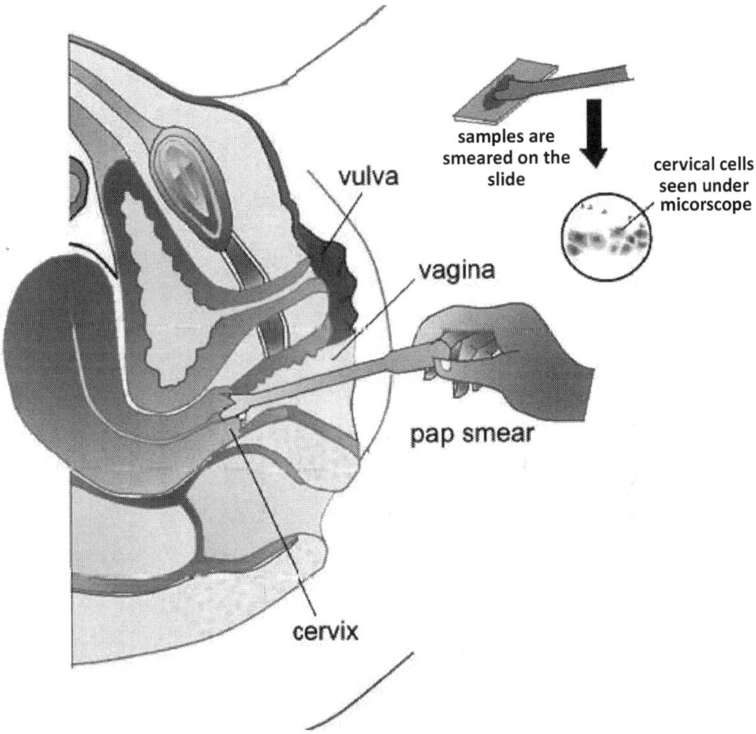

Figure 5.2 Pap smear, how the sampling is performed.

Timing and methods of taking Pap smear are very important and there are several tips on how to obtain optimum Pap smear:

(a) Before smear, there should be no douching and vaginal washing, and the last sexual intercourse must have happened more than 24 hours earlier.

(b) Pap smear should not be done during menses and within 1 week after discontinuation of antimicrobs.
(c) Smear is taken before a bimanual examination and no lubricant.
(d) No acetic acid should be used before Pap smear.
(e) Ayre's spatula rotated 360° twice or by cytobrush rotated 180° and place in same slide: Spread smear on slide and roll brush over the same slide.
(f) Immediate fixation in alcohol: Either use spray fixative, at a right angle to, and a distance of 20 cm from the slide or immerse the slide in a container of 95% alcohol (ethanol) for at least 5 minutes.

Currently, there are two types of cytologic testing: (1) conventional cytology and (2) liquid-based cytology.

Liquid-Based Cytology

Liquid-based cytology (LBC) was introduced in the mid-1990s to increase the sensitivity and specificity of cervical screening. In conventional Pap test, 80% of patient's cell sample containing important diagnostic information is discarded with the sample devices. In LBC, sampling technique is similar with a conventional method. The samples are washed in a medium (ethanol-based) and a monolayer of cervical cells is spread on a slide. Because the cells are not "smeared", they do not clump together and all the samples are preserved. The remaining samples can also be used for HPV DNA testing.

Numerous studies have compared the accuracy of LBC and conventional cytology; however, results have been inconsistent. Cluster randomized controlled trial involving 89,784 women aged 30 to 60 years indicates that LBC does not perform better than conventional Pap tests in terms of relative sensitivity and PPV for detection of cervical cancer precursors (Siebers et al., 2009). A randomized controlled trial by Ronco, involving 45,000 participants, has shown that (a) liquid-based cytology showed no statistically significant difference in sensitivity to conventional cytology for detection of cervical intraepithelial neoplasia of grade 2 or more, (b) there were more positive results with LBC and

(c) there was large reduction in unsatisfactory smear in the LBC group (from 4.1% to 2.6%). The per test cost of LBC is higher than the conventional Pap smear but this is compensated for by reduction in inadequate samples, repeat tests and screening time together with the ability to perform additional tests from the same cervical specimen. The principle of pap smear test is shown in Fig. 5.3.

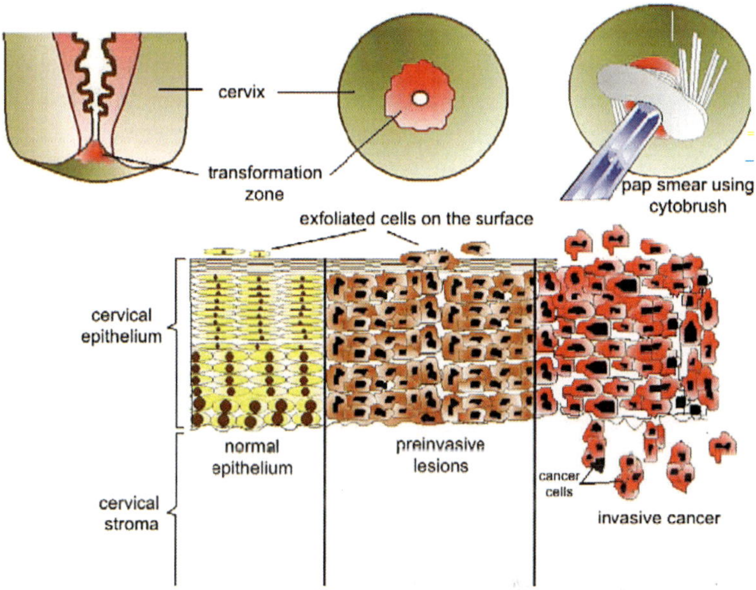

Figure 5.3 During Pap smear, the cells exfoliated on the surface of the cervical epithelium are obtained. These cells are the representatives of the underlying cervical pathology.

Technologies Related to Liquid-Based Cytology

ThinPrep Pap Test

ThinPrep Pap Test is approved by the FDA in 1996. This technique uses the filter method and the detection rate is better than conventional method. It separates cells from the background material, results in uniform layers of cells and improves the detection rate. The method is 65% more effective than conventional Pap test in detecting pre-cancerous lesions. However, some argue that this test is no better than the conventional one and that it would result in too many false warnings, unnecessary alarming the patient. The end result is a circular layer cells of 20 mm size and same sample can be used to test for HPV using Digene Hybrid Capture HPV DNA assay.

AutoCyte PREP

The other sample preparation system is AutoCyte PREP, approved by the FDA in 1999. In this method, brush pad used to collect cells is "disconnected" and dropped into the vial (contain ethanol-based preservation). The end result is a circular layer cell of size 13 mm.

PapNet

PapNet is based on computerized re-screening, utilizing LBC technology. PAPNET is an automated interactive system for the analysis of Pap smears, which has been shown to detect abnormalities that were repeatedly missed on manual screening.

AutoPap

AutoPap system scanned slides of Pap smears and ranked specimens according to their degree of abnormality. The system will identify 25% of slides that have the lowest risk and excluding it from rescreening, thus reducing the screener's workload by 25%. The FDA has approved AutoPap in May 1998. AutoPap rescreening identified 3–5 times more false-negative cases than traditional quality control measures.

ThinPrep Imaging System

The ThinPrep imaging system (TIS) consists of three components: an image processor, a PC-based computer that runs on Windows NT and a review microscope. The TIS uses algorithms to select 22 fields of view (FOV), which include the cells most likely to be dysplastic according to computer imaging characteristics. The TIS has been shown to provide increased sensitivity and specificity over manually reviewed ThinPrep Pap Test slides. In one study, the TIS was found to have a 50% reduction in a false negative fraction when compared to manually reviewed ThinPrep Pap Test slides.

Bethesda System of Reporting Pap Smear Results

Terminology of Cytologic Reports

Cervical cytology became the standard screening test for cervical cancer and premalignant cervical lesions with the introduction of the Papanicolaou smear in 1941. The terminology and reporting system was first introduced by Papanicolaou, who devised the Class 1–5 systems. In 1973, the WHO proposed mild, moderate and severe dysplasia, CIS, invasive Ca and adenocarcinoma. Since then, the terminology and reporting system had gone through various stages and changes to suit with the current technology and understanding of preinvasive disease of the cervix. In 1988, National Institutes of Health consensus panel formed a new terminology known as Bethesda System. Bethesda system has been revised in 1991 and currently been widely used worldwide. The major features of Bethesda Systems are: (a) estimation of the adequacy of a specimen, (b) general categorization into normal and benign cellular changes due to inflammation and epithelial abnormality and (c) descriptive diagnosis in details. The latest Bethesda system is Bethesda System 2001, shown in Table 5.3.

Bethesda 2001 Reporting System

Table 5.3 Bethesda System 2001

Category	Reporting
Specimen adequacy	(a) Satisfactory for evaluation (*note presence/absence of endocervical/transformation zone component*) (b) Unsatisfactory for evaluation . . . (*specify reason*) (c) Specimen rejected/not processed (*specify reason*) (d) Specimenprocessedandexamined,butunsatisfactory for evaluation of epithelial abnormality because of (*specify reason*)

(*Continued*)

Table 5.3 (*Continued*)

General categorization (optional)	(a) Negative for intraepithelial lesion or malignancy (b) Epithelial cell abnormality (c) Others
Interpretation/results	
Negative for Intraepithelial lesion or malignancy	(a) Organisms (*Trichomonas vaginalis*, fungal organisms morphologically consistent with Candida species, shift in flora suggestive of bacterial vaginosis, bacteria morphologically consistent with Actinomyces species, cellular changes consistent with herpes simplex virus) (b) Other non-neoplastic findings (optional to report; list not comprehensive): Reactive cellular changes associated with inflammation (includes typical repair), radiation, intrauterine contraceptive device, glandular cells status post-hysterectomy, atrophy
Epithelial cell abnormalities	(a) Squamous cell (atypical squamous cells (ASC), atypical squamous cell of undetermined significance (ASC-US), atypical squamous cell cannot exclude HSIL (ASC-H), low-grade squamous intraepithelial lesion (LSIL) encompassing HPV/mild dysplasia/CIN 1, high-grade squamous intraepithelial lesion (HSIL) encompassing moderate and severe dysplasia, CIS, CIN2 and CIN3, squamous cell carcinoma) (b) Glandular cell (atypical glandular cells (AGC): specify endocervical, endometrial, or not otherwise specified, atypical glandular cells, favour neoplastic: specify endocervical or not otherwise specified, Endocervical adenocarcinoma in situ (AIS), adenocarcinoma) (c) Others (list not comprehensive): Endometrial cells in a woman ≥40 years old

Non-Cytologic Method of Screening

Cytologic screening test is the most widely used primary screening tool for cervical cancer worldwide. Besides cytology, there are two non-cytologic methods that have been recommended for the screening of cervical cancer: (a) visual inspection and (b) HPV testing.

Visual Inspection

Visual inspection is the direct visualization of the cervix after application of a solution of either acetic acid 3–5% (**VIA**) or Lugol's iodine (**VILI**). A result is obtained immediately and treatment can be performed at the same setting (see and treat approach). Visual inspection is a potential screening method in countries with low-resource setting. In visual inspection with acetic acid (VIA), CIN lesions will turn white for a few minutes after application of acetic acid. The effect of acetic acid is thought to depend on the amount of nuclear proteins, and cytokeratins present in the cervical epithelium, which increases in CIN.

The alternative to VIA is VILI or visual inspection with Lugol's iodine. Instead of acetic acid, VILI uses Lugol's iodine, which is taken up by the normal columnar cells, glycogen containing cervical cells, while an abnormal epithelium remains unstained or iodine negative. The large cross-sectional studies evaluating VIA and VILI (detection of HSIL) involving more than 56,000 women have reported the following results (Sankaranarayanan et al., 2003, 2004): (a) VIA (pooled data), sensitivity: 76.8% (95% Cl: 74.2–79.4%), specificity: 85.5% (95% Cl: 85.2–85.8%), positive predictive value: 9.4% (95% Cl: 8.8–10.8%) and negative predictive values: 99.5% (95% Cl: 99.4–99.6%), (b) range sensitivity for VIA: 56.1–93.9%, range of specificity: 74.2–93.8%, (c) VILI (pooled data), Sensitivity: 91.7% (95% Cl: 89.7–93.4%), specificity: 85.4% (95% Cl: 85.1–85.7%), positive predictive value: 10.9% (95% Cl: 10.2–11.6%), negative predictive values: 99.8% (95% Cl: 99.7–99.9%) and (d) range sensitivity for VILI: 56.1–93.9%, range specificity: 74.2–93.8%.

Compared with Pap smear, a meta-analysis shows that screening with VIA or VILI allows detection of cervical cancer and its precursors with an accuracy as good or even better than the standard Pap smear test, although VIA and VILI is less specific in comparison to the Pap smear test; however, they are more sensitive in detecting pre-invasive lesions (Arbyn et al., 2008; Qureshi et al., 2010). There is evidence that VILI is at least as specific as but more sensitive than VIA. Similar to cytology, VIA and VILI may be less effective for older women in their 50s or 60s because of the tendency of the transformation zone together with any lesions within it to recede into the endocervical canal.

Visual inspection was also evaluated in screening and treat approach (single visit "see and treats" approach). Patients with a positive screening test were offered an immediate treatment at the same setting. The treatment was a cryotherapy. The evidence from published studies indicates that cryotherapy is an effective, safe and acceptable treatment with cure rates exceeds 86% if performed by trained staff. Sankaranayanan and colleagues had evaluated the effectiveness, safety and acceptability of "see and treat" with VIA and cryotherapy by nurses in a cervical screening study in India (N = 2513). The nurses were trained in performing VIA, colposcopy and cryotherapy. Women with a colposcopic impression of low- or high-grade lesions were advised immediate cryotherapy after a directed biopsy (see Table 5.4). The acceptability rate was approximately 75%. The cure rate for CIN 1 and CIN 2–3 was 81.4% and 70.6%, respectively. In this study, "see and treat" with cryotherapy resulted in 40% of the women being unnecessarily treated.

Steps to Perform VIA/VILI

(a) counselling
(b) visual technique not recommended in postmenopausal women
(c) speculum examination
(d) adjusting the light source to get the best view of the cervix
(e) use of a cotton swab to remove any discharge, blood or mucus
(f) identification of the squamo-columnar junction and area around it
(g) application of acetic acid 3–5% or Lugol's iodine solution to the cervix and then waiting for 1–2 minutes (VIA is positive if the epithelium change to white, while VILI is positive if there is no iodine uptake; iodine uptake is manifested as dark brown epithelium)
(h) documentation
(i) use of fresh swab to remove any remaining acetic acid or iodine solution from the cervix and vagina

Table 5.4 Criteria for immediate cryotherapy in see and treat approach

Criteria for immediate cryotherapy
(1) The lesion involved less than three quadrants of the transformation zone.
(2) No extension of the lesion into the endocervical canal
(3) No extension of the lesion onto the vaginal walls
(4) Entire lesion could be covered by the cryoprobe
(5) Squamo-columnar junction was visible in its entirety
(6) No clinical or colposcopic suspicion of invasive cancer

Source: Sankaranarayanan et al., 2007, *Br J Cancer*; **96**: 738–743.

HPV Testing

Human papillomavirus DNA is identified in almost all (99.7%) verified cases of cervical cancer worldwide (Walboomers et al., 1999). The FDA approved HPV testing using Hybrid Capture 2 in April 2003 as a primary screening test for women age more than 30, and currently it has been incorporated into the National Screening Program in the United States. The specificity of HPV testing was found to be higher in women older than 30 years.

The recognition that cervical cancer is caused by HR-HPV led to the development of several NTCC prevention measures:

(a) HPV DNA testing
(b) HPV RNA testing
(c) molecular markers related to HPV infection
(d) HPV vaccine

Role of HPV Testing

There are at least four potential roles of HPV testing in the prevention of cervical cancer:

(1) triage of women with equivocal cytology
(2) follow-up of the patient after treatment of CIN
(3) HPV testing by the "see and treat" approach
(4) HPV testing as primary screening test

Triage of Women with Equivocal Cytology (ASCUS)

The HPV testing can be used to triage women with equivocal cytology result. **ALTS** or ASCUS-LSIL Triage Study is a randomized multicenter trial (3488 women recruited) to determine the best way to manage women with ASCUS and LSIL. The trial was organized by the US National Cancer Institute, and recruitment began in 1996. Women with ASCUS and low-grade squamous intraepithelial lesions (LSIL) on Pap smear were assigned into three study arms: immediate colposcopy, conservative management or HPV testing (Hybrid capture 2). Following were the results:

(a) HPV testing had high sensitivity (96%) in the detection of CIN in women with ASCUS (9–10% had CIN2; 4–5% had CIN 3).
(b) HPV testing is not useful for LSIL because 82.9% have a positive test.
(c) HPV triage was found to be at least as sensitive as immediate colposcopy for detecting CIN3 but accomplished this with referring only about 50% as many women to colposcopy.
(d) Single enrolment HPV test identified 92.4% of the women diagnosed with CIN3+ over 2 years. In this study, the term "ASCUS" was based on earlier Bethesda system. In Bethesda 2001, ASCUS is divided into two groups, i.e. ASC-US (Atypical squamous cell of undetermined significance) and ASC-H (Atypical squamous cell, cannot rule out high grade).

Arbyn and colleagues conducted meta-analyses of all valid studies reported on the comparative accuracy of repeat cervical cytology and HPV testing to detect CIN2+ in women with ASC-US or LSIL. HPV testing using Hybrid Capture 2 (HC2) was found to be more sensitive and equally specific in comparison to cytology for the triage of patients with ASC-US Pap results. The meta-analysis also confirmed the high rate of HPV positivity in LSIL and therefore, HPV testing for LSIL is not cost effective.

The Italian Multicentric Study (Mistro et al., 2010) evaluated the role of HPV testing in the triage of ASC-US. Patients with ASC-US were randomized into immediate colposcopy, conventional Pap test and HPV testing using Hybrid Capture 2. The results were

(a) Total samples: 749 (age 25–64).
(b) Abnormal colposcopy was reported in 34.2%.

(c) Positive high-risk HPV in 24.2%, (43.4% in women age less than 35, 17.2% in age more than 35).
(d) HPV testing gave the highest sensitivity and specificity in detecting CIN2+, especially in women older than 35 years (sensitivity 100%, specificity 84.8% and PPV 13.7%).

Follow-Up of Patient after Treatment for CIN 2–3

Studies and meta-analyses have shown that women who test HPV negative 6–18 months after their treatment can be safely returned to routine screening, while those who test positive should be followed up more closely. Meta-analysis by Arbyn and colleagues (2005) also reported that HPV testing performed better than follow-up cytology to predict success or failure of treatment (higher sensitivity). In the follow-up analysis of ALTS trial, 610 women were treated with LEEP for CIN and follow-up either with PCR HPV testing or cytology. During follow-up, 40% of patients were found positive to HPV. The sensitivity and specificity of PCR HPV testing in detecting CIN2+ was 96.9% and 69.1%, respectively, better than cytology (HPV testing is more sensitive (96.9% versus 78.1%) but with same specificity). Meanwhile, Hybrid Capture 2 was found to have sensitivity of 90.6% and specificity of 63.8% as compared to PCR HPV testing. Therefore, women treated for CIN2+ could be followed up with either cytology or combination of cytology and colposcopy 4–6 months until three normal cytologic tests are obtained. With HPV testing, initial follow-up can be done at longer interval, e.g. 6 months. If three consecutive cytologies are normal or negative to HPV DNA testing, they can continue routine screening at a yearly interval.

HPV Testing in Screening and Treat Approach

The role of a screen/see-and-treat approach has been evaluated in various studies using a cytologic test or visual technique, and the results were encouraging. The treatment (either LEEP/LLETZ or cryotherapy) is offered during the same setting following a thorough colposcopic evaluation. In low-resource setting, VIA followed by cryotherapy was evaluated and was found to be safe, feasible and acceptable. Trained nurses can perform the procedure, and no anaesthesia was required. High cure rate of up to 89% was reported with this approach (Sankaranarayanan et al., 2007; Blumenthal et al.). The concern about this approach is overtreatment (up to 40%) due to false positive test or spontaneous regression, especially, in low-grade lesions.

HPV testing may play an important role either as a single test or in combinations with others in identifying a patient who required treatment. With combination test, false positive rate can be reduced and therefore, reducing the overtreatment rate. Further, large randomized control trial is needed to evaluate this approach.

HPV Testing as Primary Screening Test for Cervical Cancer

The role of HPV testing as a potential primary screening for cervical cancer has been evaluated in various studies. Sherman and colleagues evaluating almost 21,000 women, followed up for 10 years from 1992, they had found that the risk of developing CIN3+ from initial Pap smear > ASCUS or positive HPV testing or both were nearly 7% as compared to 0.79% for women with negative test (Sherman et al., 2003). Therefore, the combination of both negative cytology and negative HPV test provides strong reassurance that the women will free from the disease for many years.

In HART (HPV in Addition to Routine Testing) study, 11,085 women age 30–60 were recruited. Women with borderline cytology and positive to high-risk HPV (using Hybrid Capture 2) were selected and randomized to immediate colposcopy or to surveillance by repeat HPV testing with cytology at 12 months. HPV testing was found to be more sensitive (97.1% versus 76.6%) in detecting CIN2+ than Pap smear without increasing colposcopy referral rate.

The randomized study known as Canadian Cervical Cancer Screening Trial (CCCaST) had recruited more than 10,000 women aged 30–69 years old to compare conventional Pap smear with Hybrid Capture 2 HPV DNA testing in screening of cervical cancer. All trial participants were randomized to receive either cytologic test or HPV test first and followed by second test with the primary end-point of CIN2+. The sensitivity and specificity of HPV test alone was 97.4% and 94.3%, respectively. The sensitivity of HPV test alone was more superior to Pap smear alone (56.4%), Pap with reflex HPV (53.8%) and HPV with reflex Pap (53.8%). HPV test with reflex Pap smear was found to have highest specificity of 99.1%. The approach that has the highest sensitivity (100%) was HPV test plus Pap smear although the specificity was lower (92.5%) with higher rate of colposcopy referral (7.9%) (Mayrand et al., 2006, 2007). See Table 5.4 for full results.

New Technologies for Cervical Cancer (NTCC) study (Italian multicentre RCT) was designed to compare the effectiveness, acceptability and cost of HPV testing (HC2) compared with the Pap smear or LBC as a primary screening test. Cytologic test was compared to HPV testing using HC2. Women with ASCUS+ or HPV positive were referred for colposcopy. The study showed that HPV testing and/or liquid-based cytology had higher sensitivity than conventional Pap smear. Conventional Pap smear, however, had higher positive predictive value. By using the 2pg/ml threshold for positive test, HPV testing alone was found to have similar relative sensitivity but higher relative positive predictive value. Therefore, 2 pg/ml threshold may be appropriate for HPV testing as a primary screening for cervical cancer (Ronco et al., 2006).

A study known as ARTISTIC (Randomized Trial in Screening to Improve Cytology) was conducted to evaluate the effectiveness of HPV testing (HC2) as compared to LBC for primary cervical screening, involving more than 24,000 women. Results: (i) 87% of women < 30 years old with mild dyskaryosis have positive HR-HPV, the proportion decreased with age (ii) 96% of severe dyskaryosis have positive HR-HPV (iii) Prevalence of HR-HPV in women above 30 was ranging from 6–18.5%, (iv) Prevalence of moderate dyskaryosis was found to be 20–30-times higher and severe dyskaryosis was over 100 times higher in HPV-positive women compared with those who were HPV-negative (v) HPV testing is more practical in women age above 30.

Systematic Review and Meta-analysis of Non-Randomized Studies by Koliopoulos et al., 2007 involving 25 studies found that pooled sensitivity of Hybrid Capture 2 (HC2) was higher than cytology (ASCUS or worse), i.e. 90% versus 72.7%. However, cytology was found to be more specific than HC2 (91.9% versus 86.5%).

Nauclear and colleagues (Swedescreen trial) evaluated the role of HPV test (HC2) in the cervical screening strategy and reported that the most effective screening combinations were screening first with a HPV test and if positive, followed by Pap test (HPV test with reflex Pap smear). This approach increased the number of screening tests by 12% but improved the sensitivity by 30%.

Table 5.5 Results from randomized trial comparing different screening tests either alone or in combinations

Randomized Canadian Cervical Cancer Screening Trial[a] (final endpoint: CIN2+)					
Test	**Sensitivity (%)**	**Specificity (%)**	**PPP (%)**	**NPV (%)**	**Colposcopy rate (%)**
HPV alone	97.4	94.3	7.0	100	6.1
Pap alone	56.4	97.3	8.5	99.8	2.9
Pap with reflex HPV	53.8	98.7	14.9	99.8	1.6
HPV with reflex Pap	53.8	99.1	21.4	99.8	1.6
HPV plus Pap	100	92.5	5.5	100	7.9

[a]Mayrand et al. *N Engl J Med* 2007; **357**: 1579–1588.

In 2005, the IARC/WHO recommended that HPV-DNA testing can be used for primary screening. The first FDA approved method of HPV DNA testing is a Digene Hybrid Capture 2 assay, which is tested for 13 oncogenic HPV types. This test was, however, expensive and needs high-quality laboratory support and maintenances and therefore may not be suitable in low-resource setting.

Cuzick et al. (2006) have reported that negative HPV test (HC2) offered about twice the protection of a negative Pap for at least 5 years. They found that a positive HPV test was far more predictive of increased risk in the follow-up period than a positive Pap smear. Women with positive HPV test but negative cytology were found to have 10% risk of cumulative incidence of CIN3+ by 6 years while the risk in women with negative HPV test was only 0.27%. (Dillner et al., 2009).

In general, the sensitivity of HC2 for CIN2+ in primary screening was 33% higher than cytology at an ASC-US threshold for referral to colposcopy; however, the specificity was slightly lower (Cuzick et al., 2008). Combining HPV testing and Pap smear increased sensitivity marginally but compromise the specificity by 5%. Castle et al. (2009) reported that only 4% of more than 800,000 women age 30 and above have cytology negative but HPV positive results (highest among women age 30–34 (6.76%) and lowest for women age 60–64 (2.56%). These figures are important for cost-analysis purposes if co-testing of Pap smear and HPV test is to be implemented as a screening test.

A cluster-randomized trial by Sankaranarayanan, et al. in 52 clusters of villages in rural India involving more than 131,000 healthy women were conducted to evaluate the efficacy of three cervical screening methods, i.e. HPV testing (HC2 assay), VIA and cytologic testing. The screened group was compared to unscreened population. The primary outcomes measured were the incidence of cervical cancer and associated rates of death. The results were as follows: (a) Total recruitment was 131,806 women. (b) The positivity rate for HPV test, cytology and VIA was 10%, 7%, and 13.9%, respectively. (c) Positive predictive value for HPV test, cytology and VIA was 11.3%, 19.3% and 7.4%, respectively (with endpoint of detecting CIN2+). (d) After 8-year follow-up, the age-standardized incidence of cervical cancer in women with negative HPV test, cytology and VIA was 3.7, 15.5 and 16.0 per 100,000 person-years, respectively. There was no reduction in the rate of cervical cancer in VIA group. (e) HPV testing was associated with significant reduction in the number of advanced cervical cancers and death from cervical cancer. No significant reduction in number of advanced cancer or deaths was observed in the cytology and VIA groups. (f) HPV testing was found to be most objective and reproducible of all cervical screening tests and was less demanding in term of training and quality assurance. (g) The drawback of HPV testing with HC2 was that it is more expensive and time consuming and requires a sophisticated laboratory infrastructure.

Two new methods of HPV testing, Digene FastHPV and Arbo Vita E6 Strip test, were subsequently introduced specially design for the country with low-resource setting. Digene FastHPV (careHPV) was being tested in the demonstration project in China and India, careHPV was developed by Digene Corporation (now known as QIAGEN). This method is more rapid, simpler, portable and affordable. The test needs no mains electricity or running water, and can be done by technical support staff in roughly 2.5 hours. CareHPV uses a signal amplification assay that detects a target HPV-DNA from 14 different oncogenic HPV types. A cross-sectional study of the accuracy of careHPV as rapid primary screening test was done in rural China (comparison between care HPV, Hybrid Capture 2, VIA and liquid-based cytology). The sensitivity and specificity of this new rapid test were 90.0% and 84.2%, respectively. The sensitivity and specificity of Hybrid Capture 2 were 97.1% and 85.6%, respectively. Liquid-based cytology and VIA had higher specificity (97.0%, 94.5%, respectively) but lower sensitivity (85.3% for LBC and 41.4% for VIA) (Qiao et al., 2008).

Arbo Vita E6 Strip test is also a rapid HPV testing developed by Arbo Vita Corporation (AVC) in 2008; the result can be obtained in less than 20 minutes, and the test is against E6 oncoprotein of HPV. Arbo Vita E6 strip test is expected to be cheaper.

Testing against HPV 16 and 18 (type-specific HPV test) was evaluated as an alternative test to HC2 (testing against 13 types). Narrowing the testing to 16 and 18 was found to improve the predictive value of detecting CIN2+ as both of these HPV are responsible in at least 70% of cervical cancer. Women with positive HPV 16 have 17.2% cumulative incidence rate of ≥ CIN3 in 10 years while if they were positive to HPV 18, the incidence was 13.6%. Detection of these oncogenic viruses may reduce the unnecessary intervention in women with other high risks HPV because it is known that HPV 16 and 18 carry a higher risk of CIN3+ (Khan et al., 2005). With this new HPV test, it will now be possible to separate Pap negative/HPV positive women into higher risk of CIN3+ from those at lesser risk. In March 2009, FDA announced approval two new HPV DNA diagnostic test (HPV DNA genotyping test) that is Cervista™ HPV HR Test (testing 14 types high-risk HPV similar to HC2 plus type 66 in three probes, i.e. A5/6, A7, A9) and type specific HPV 16/18 test (Cervista™ HPV 16/18). Study comparing Cervista™ HPV 16/18 versus HC2 demonstrated better specificity and PPV of the former test (Ginocchio et al., 2008). ASCCP has included this test into their guidelines and the indications of Cervista™ HPV HR are similar to Hybrid Capture 2 HPV DNA Assay.

In the era of HPV vaccination, it is expected that the number of cervical lesions will decrease and so the colposcopic referral perhaps by 40–60%. The positive predictive value of these tests/procedures will gradually reduce especially Pap smear and colposcopy because these tests are more subjective as compared to HPV testing. Being more objective, HPV testing will perhaps become a better screening test. A cost-effective analysis of the cervical screening program during HPV vaccination era have indicated that for both vaccinated and unvaccinated women, the following recommendation may be logical: (a) HPV testing as a triage test for equivocal results in younger women, (b) HPV testing as a primary screening test in older women. Figure 5.4 is a proposed algorithm of screening test incorporating type specific HPV test. This is only a recommendation and may not be applicable certain countries.

The other alternative to the screening test shown in Fig. 5.4 is primary HPV testing with reflex Pap smear for women with positive HR HPV. The second Pap smear test is to reduce the false positive HPV testing and therefore reduce the rate of unnecessary colposcopy (Fig. 5.5).

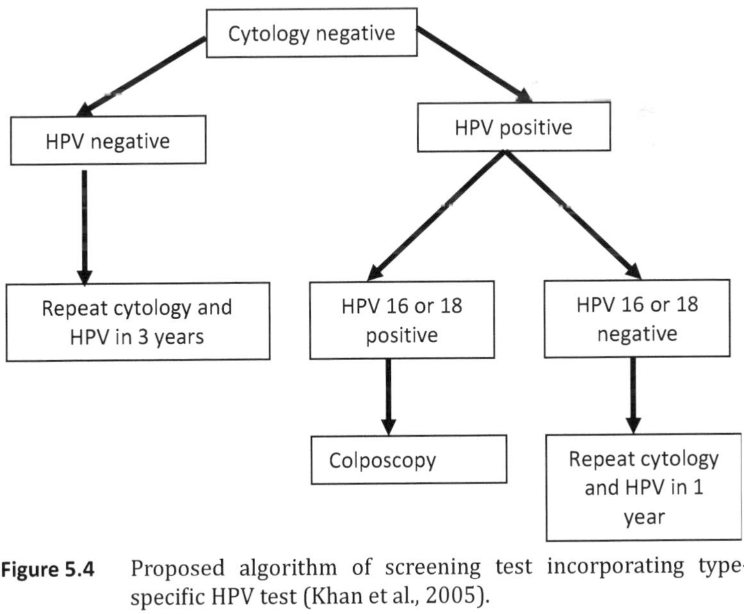

Figure 5.4 Proposed algorithm of screening test incorporating type-specific HPV test (Khan et al., 2005).

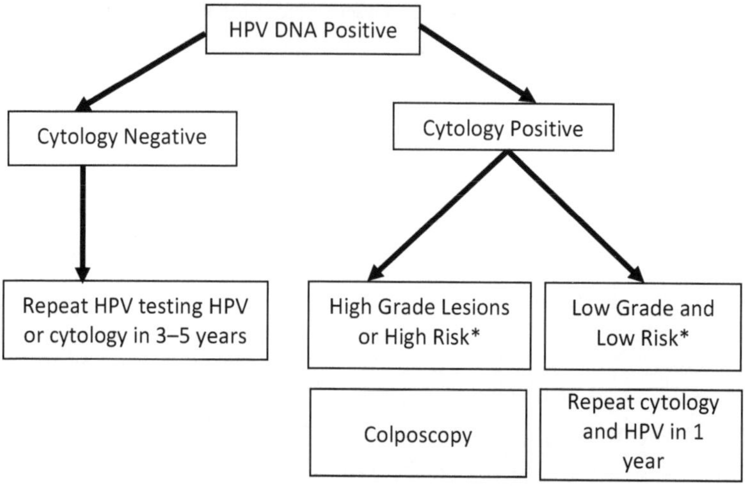

Figure 5.5 The alternative pathway for cervical cancer screening with HPV DNA testing (*risk factors are smoking, multiple sexual partners, immunosuppression, and poor compliance).

Optoelectronic Device for Cervical Cancer Screening

Optical and electrical assessment of the cervix can be used to detect any abnormal epithelium. To date, there are at least three devices have been developed, i.e. TruScreen, Polaprobe and TruScan; TruScreen was developed by Polartechnics, Sydney, Australia. The device consists of a probe and a console, which are connected to each other by a cable. The electrical and optical assessment of the cervix detected by the probe is sent to a microcomputer in the console and compared with the data of 14 tissues types studied previously. The type of cervical tissue is diagnosed and the results are expressed as "normal" or "abnormal" on the printed paper. This procedure is done immediately after cytologic testing. It is used as an adjunctive test to improve the accuracy of cytologic testing. Women with abnormal test will be subjected for colposcopic examination without need to wait for cytology reports. In multicentre evaluation by Singer A et al. (2003), the sensitivities for histologically confirmed CIN 2/3 lesions by TruScreen, Pap and TruScreen/Pap combined were 70%, 69% and 93%, respectively.

New Technologies in Cervical Cancer Screening

With the introduction of the HPV vaccination program, cervical cancer prevention will become increasingly costly. Positive predictive value of current screening strategies will be diminished in a vaccinated population. New screening technologies should have higher positive predictive value, able to reduce overtreatment of low-grade lesions and have higher specificity. Therefore, most likely solution to the goals of improving existing screening program is to incorporate molecular approaches into existing screening program. Following are some of the promising new technologies for cervical cancer screening: (a) **HPV genotyping**. (b) **HPV mRNA**. Problem with HPV genotyping is that in a significant proportion of women without disease, HR-HPV DNA can also be detected. Detection and quantitation of mRNA from E6 and E7 genes of high-risk genotypes could be a more specific marker of the presence of high-grade lesion and cancer. (c) **HPV viral load**. High viral load had been associated with CIN2+ and with progression of disease. Viral load can be quantitated using both conventional and real-time PCR. (d) **HPV integration**. HPV-16 integration is commonly detected in high-grade CIN and invasive cervical cancer. However, the limitation of this technology is that, in many women, both HPV DNA integration and episomal DNA often co-exist and therefore can lead to misinterpretation and misclassification. (e) **p16 enzyme linked immunosorbent assay**. p16(INK4a) is a cell cycle regulation protein which accumulates in abnormal epithelial cells infected with HR-HPVs. p16(INK4a) can be a potential immunohistochemical biomarker in both histopathology and LBC specimens. Recently, detection of p16 by immunostaining of high-risk HPV-positive women was strongly associated with CIN2+, suggesting that p16 may serve as a triage to high-risk HPV positive results to increase specificity. (f) **Methylation markers**. DNA methylation is absent in disease-free women. Study in Senegal have confirmed a high specificity for detection of CIN3/cancer (95–97%) using a panel of 1–3 methylated gene targets (DAPK1, RARB and TWIST1).

References

Arbyn M, Buntinx F, Van Ranst M, Paraskevaidis E, Martin-Hirsh P, Dillner J. Virologic versus cytologic triage of women with equivocal Pap smears: a meta-analysis of the accuracy to detect high-grade intraepithelial neoplasia. *J Natl Cancer Inst* 2004; **96**: 280–293.

Arbyn M, Paraskevaidis E, Martin-Hirsch P, Prendiville W, Dillner J. Clinical utility of HPV-DNA detection: triage of minor cervical lesions, follow-up of women treated for high-grade CIN: an update of pooled evidence. *Gynecol Oncol* 2005; **99**(3 Suppl 1): S7–S11.

Arbyn M, Sankaranarayanan R, Muwonge R, et al. Pooled analysis of the accuracy of five cervical cancer screening tests assessed in eleven studies in Africa and India. *Int J Cancer* 2008; **123**: 153–160.

Bray F, Carstensen B, Moller H, et al. Incidence trends of adenocarcinoma of the cervix in 13 European countries. *Cancer Epidemiol Biomarkers Prev* 2005; **14**: 2191–2199.

Castle PE, Fetterman B, Poitras N, Lorey T, Shaber R, Kinney W. Five-year experience of human papillomavirus DNA and Papanicolaou test cotesting. *Obstet Gynecol* 2009; **113**: 595–600.

Colposcopy and Programme Management. Guidelines for the NHS Cervical Screening Programme. NHSCSP Publication No 20, April 2004.

Coppleson M, Reid BL, Skladnev VN, et al. An electronic approach to the detection of pre-cancer and cancer of the uterine cervix: a preliminary evaluation of Polarprobe. *Int J Gynecol Cancer* 1994; **4**: 79–83.

Cox JT. Review: history of the use of HPV testing in cervical screening and in the management of abnormal cervical screening results. *J Clin Virol* 2009; **45**: S3–S12.

Cuzick J, Clavel C, Petry KU, et al. Overview of the European and North American studies on HPV testing in primary cervical cancer screening. *Int J Cancer* 2006; **119**(5): 1095–1101.

Cuzick J, Szarewski A, Cubie H, et al. Management of women who test positive for high-risk types of human papillomavirus: the HART study. *Lancet* 2003; **362**(9399): 1871–1876.

Cuzick J, Szarewski A, Mesher D, Cadman L, Austin J, Perryman K, et al. Long-term follow-up of cervical abnormalities among women screened by HPV testing and cytology Results from the Hammersmith study. *Int J Cancer* 2008; **122**: 2294–300.

Cuzick J, Arbyn M, Sankaranarayanan R, Tsu V, Ronco G, Mayrand MH, et al. Overview of human papillomavirus-based and other novel options for cervical cancer screening in developed and developing countries. *Vaccine* 2008; **26**(Suppl 10): K29–K41.

Denny L, Sankaranarayanan R. Secondary prevention of cervical cancer. *Int J Gynecol Obstet* 2006; **94**: 565–570.

Dillner J, Rebolj M, Birembaut P, Petry K, Szarewski A, Munk C, et al. Long term predictive values of cytology and human papillomavirus testing in cervical cancer screening: joint European cohort study. *BMJ* 2009.

Dray M, Russel P, Dairymple C, et al. P16(INK4a) as a complementary marker of hgh-grade intraepithelial lesions of the uterine cervix: experience with squamous lesions in 189 consecutive cervical biopsies. *Pathology* 2005; **37**(2): 112–124.

Gravitt PE, Coutlee F, Iftner T, et al. ICO Monograph series on HPV and Cervical Cancer: General Overview. New technologies in cervical cancer screening. *Vaccine* 2008; **26S**: K42–K52.

Ginocchio CC, Barth D, Zhang F. Comparison of the Third Wave Invader human papillomavirus (HPV) assay and the Digene HPV Hybrid Capture 2 assay for detection of high-risk HPV DNA. *J Clin Microbiol* 2008; **46**: 1641–1646.

Goldhaber-Fiebert JD, Stout NK, Salomon JA, Kuntz KM, Goldie SJ. Costeffectiveness of cervical cancer screening with human papillomavirus DNA testing and HPV-16, 18 vaccination. *J Natl Cancer Inst* 2008; **100**: 308–320.

Hakama M, Miller AB, Day Ne, eds. *Screening for Cancer of the Uterine Cervix*. Lyon, France: IARC Press; 1986. iaRC Scientific Publication No. 76.

IARC Working Group on Evaluation of Cervical Cancer Screening Programmes. Screening for squamous cervical cancer: the duration of low risk after negative result of cervical cytology and its implication for screening policies. *Br Med J* 1986; **293**: 659–664.

IARC, WHO. *IARC Handbooks of Cancer Prevention: Cervical Cancer Screening*. Vol. 10. IARC Press; 2005.

Khan MJ, Castle PE, Lorincz AT, Wacholder S, Sherman M, Scott DR, et al. The elevated 10-year risk of cervical precancer and cancer in women with human papillomavirus (HPV) type 16 or 18 and the possible utility of type-specific HPV testing in clinical practice. *J Natl Cancer Inst* 2005; **97**: 1072–1079.

Kitchener HC, Almonte M, Wheeler P, et al. HPV testing in routine cervical screening: cross sectional data from the ARTISTIC trial. *Br J Cancer* 2006; **95**(1): 56–61.

Koliopoulos G, Arbyn M, Hirsch PM, et al. Diagnostic accuracy of human papillomavirus testing in primary cervical screening: A systematic review and meta-analysis of non-randomized studies. *Gynecol Oncol* 2007; **104**: 232–246.

Kreimer AR, Guido RS, Solomon D, Schiffman M, Wacholder S, Jeronimo J, et al. Human papillomavirus testing following loop electrosurgical excision procedure identifies women at risk for posttreatment cervical intraepithelial neoplasia grade 2 or 3 disease. *Cancer Epidemiol Biomarkers Prev* 2006; **15**: 908–914.

Kyrgiou M, Koliopoulos G, Martin Hirsch P, et al. Management of minor cervical cytological abnormalities: a systematic review and a meta-analysis of the literature. *Cancer Treat Rev* 2007; **33**(6): 514–520.

Lee SJ, Bae JH, Kim JH, et al. A real-time optoelectronic device in screening of cervical intraepithelial neoplasia. *J Women's Med* 2009; **1**(2): 23–28.

Mayrand MH, Duarte-Franco E, Rodrigues I, et al. Human papillomavirus DNA versus Papanicolaou screening tests for cervical cancer. *N Engl J Med* 2007; **357**: 1579–1588.

Mayrand MH, Duarte-Franco E, Coutlée F, et al. Randomized controlled trial of human papillomavirus testing versus Pap cytology in the primary screening for cervical cancer precursors: design, methods and preliminary accrual results of the Canadian cervical cancer screening trial (CCCaST). *Int J Cancer* 2006; **119**(3): 615–623.

Mayrand MH, Duarte-Franco E, Rodrigues I, et al. Human papillomavirus DNA versus Papanicolaou screening tests for cervical cancer. *N Engl J Med* 2007; **357**(16): 1579–1588.

Miller FS, Nagel LE, Kenny-Moynihan MB. Implementation of the ThinPrep imaging system in a high volume metropolitan laboratory. *Diag Cytopath* 2007; **35**: 213–217.

Mistro AD, Salamanca HF, Trevisan R, et al. Triage of women with atypical squamous cells of undetermined significance (ASC-US): Results of an Italian multicentric study. *Gynecol Oncol* 2010; **117**: 77–81.

Myers E, Huh WK, Wright JD, Smith JS. The current and future role of screening in the era of HPV vaccination. *Gynecol Oncol* 2008; **109**: S31–S39.

Nanda K, McCrory DC, Myers ER, et al. Accuracy of the Papanicolaou test in screening for and follow-up of cervical cytologic abnormalities: a systematic review. *Ann Int Med* 2000; **132**(10): 810–819.

Naucler P, Ryd W, Tornberg S, Strand A, Wadell G, Elfgren K, et al. Efficacy of HPV DNA testing with cytology triage and/or repeat HPV DNA testing in primary cervical cancer screening. *J Natl Cancer Inst* 2009; **101**: 88–99.

Nobbenhuis MA, Meijer CJ, van den Brule AJ, et al. Addition of high-risk HPV testing improves the current guidelines on follow-up after treatment for cervical intraepithelial neoplasia. *Br J Cancer* 2001; **84**(6): 796–801.

Peto J, Gilman C, Deacon J, et al. Cervical HPV infection and neoplasia in a large population-based prospective study: the Manchester cohort. *Br J Cancer* 2004; **91**: 942–953.

Qiao YL, Sellors JW, Eder PS, et al. A new HPV-DNA test for cervical-cancer screening in developing regions: a cross-sectional study of clinical accuracy in rural China. *Lancet oncol* 2008; **9**: 929–936.

Qureshi S, Das V, Zahra F. Evaluation of visual inspection with acetic acid and Lugol's iodine as cervical cancer screening tools in a low-resource setting. *Trop Doct* 2010; **40**: 9–12.

Ronco G, Cuzick J, Pierotti P, et al. Accuracy of liquid based versus conventional cytology: overall results of new technologies for cervical cancer screening: randomised controlled trial. *BMJ* 2007; **335**: 28 (7 July).

Ronco G, Segnan N, Giorgi-Rossi P, et al. Human papillomavirus testing and liquid-based cytology: results at recruitment from the new technologies for cervical cancer randomized controlled trial. *J Natl Cancer Inst* 2006; **98**(11): 765–774.

Ronco G, Giorgi-Rossi P, Carozzi F, et al. Results at recruitment from a randomized controlled trial comparing human papillomavirus testing alone with conventional cytology as the primary cervical cancer screening test. *J Natl Cancer Inst* 2008; **100**(7): 492–501.

Sankaranarayanan R, Gaffikin L, Jacob M, Sellors J, Robles S. A critical assessment of screening methods for cervical neoplasia. *Int J Gynaecol Obstet* 2005; **89** (Suppl 2): S4–S12.

Sankaranarayanan R, Rajkumar R, Esmy PO, et al. Effectiveness, safety and acceptability of "see and treat" with cryotherapy by nurses in a cervical screening study in India. *Br J Cancer* 2007; **96**: 738–743.

Sankaranarayanan R, Basu P, Wesley RS, et al. Accuracy of visual screening for cervical neoplasia: results from an IARC multicentre study in India and Africa. *Intl J Cancer* 2004; **110**: 907–913.

Sankaranarayanan R, Wesley R, Thara S, Dhakad N, Chandralekha B, Sebastian P, et al. Test characteristics of visual inspection with

4% acetic acid (VIA) and Lugol's iodine (VILI) in cervical cancer screening in Kerala, India. *Int J Cancer* 2003; **105**(3): 404–408.

Sankaranarayanan R, Nene BM, Shastri SS, et al. HPV screening for cervical cancer in rural India. *New Eng J Med* 2009; **360**(14): 1385–1394.

Sasieni P, Adam J, Cuzick J. Benefits of cervical screening at different ages: evidence from the UK audit of screening histories. *Br J Cancer* 2003; **89**(1): 88–93.

Schiffman M, Soloman D. Findings to date from the ASCUS-LSIL Triage Study (ALTS). *Arch Pathol Lab Med* 2003; **127**(8): 946–949.

Sherman ME, Lorinzc AT, Scott DR, Wacholder S, Castle PR, Glass AG, et al. Baseline cytology, human papillomavirus testing, and risk for cervical neoplasia: a ten year cohort analysis. *J Natl Cancer Inst* 2003; **95**: 46–52.

Siebers AG, Klinkhamer PJJM, Grefte JMM, et al. Comparison of liquid-based cytology with conventional cytology for detection of cervical cancer precursors. a randomized controlled trial. *JAMA* 2009; **302**(16): 1757–1764.

Singer A, Coppleson M, Canfell K, et al. A real time optoelectronic device as an adjunct to the Pap smear for cervical screening: a multicenter evaluation. *Int J Gynecol Cancer* 2003; **13**: 804–811.

Solomon D, et al. The 2001 Bethesda System: terminology for reporting results of cervical cytology, *J Am Med Assoc* 2002; **287**(16): 2114–2119.

Stoler MH Schiffman M. Interobserver reproducibility of cervical cytologic and histologic interpretations: realistic estimates. From the ASCUS-LSIL Triage Study, *J Am Med Assoc* 2001; **285**(11): 1500–1505.

The ASCUS LSIL Triage Study (ALTS) Group. Results of a randomized trial on the management of cytology interpretations of atypical squamous cells of undetermined significance. *Am J Obstet Gynecol* 2003; **188**: 1383–1392.

Walboomers JM, Jacobs MV, Manos MM, et al. Human papillomavirus is a necessary cause of invasive cervical cancer worldwide. *J Pathol* 1999; **189**(1): 12–19.

Wright TC. Cervical Cervical cancer screening in the 21th century: is it time to retire the PAP smear? *Clin Obstet Gynecol* 2007; **50**(2): 313–323.

Wright Jr TC, Massad LS, Dunton CJ, Spitzer M, Wilkinson EJ. Solomon D. 2006 consensus guidelines for the management of women with abnormal cervical cancer screening tests. *Am J Obstet Gynecol* 2007; **197**: 346–355.

Yeoh KG, Chew L, Wang SC. Cancer screening in Singapore, with particular reference to breast, cervical and colorectal cancer screening. *J Med Screen* 2006; **13** (Suppl 1): S14–S19.

Chapter 6

Human Papillomavirus and HPV Vaccination

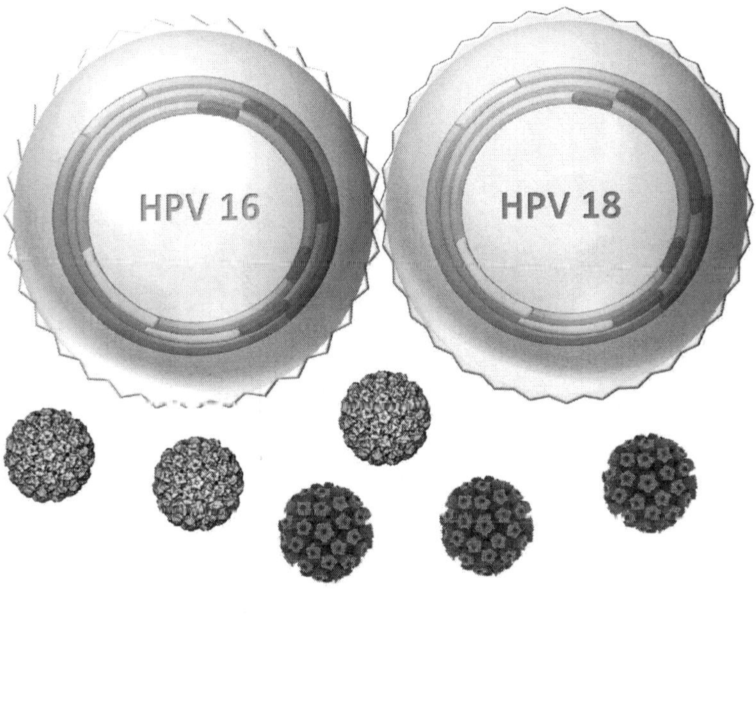

Gynaecologic Cancer: A Handbook for Students and Practitioners
Rushdan Noor, Eng Hseon Tay, and Jeffrey Low

ISBN 978-981-4463-06-5 (Hardcover), 978-981-4463-07-2 (eBook)
www.panstanford.com

HPV Infection in Lower Genital Tracts

Human Papillomavirus

The link between human papillomavirus (HPV) and cervical cancer was first proposed by Harald zur Hausen, Professor Emeritus at the German Cancer Research Centre. He suggested the link between HPV and cervical cancer since 1976 but only in 1980s, his opinion was proven by laboratory evidence. He was awarded the 2008 Nobel Prize in Medicine.

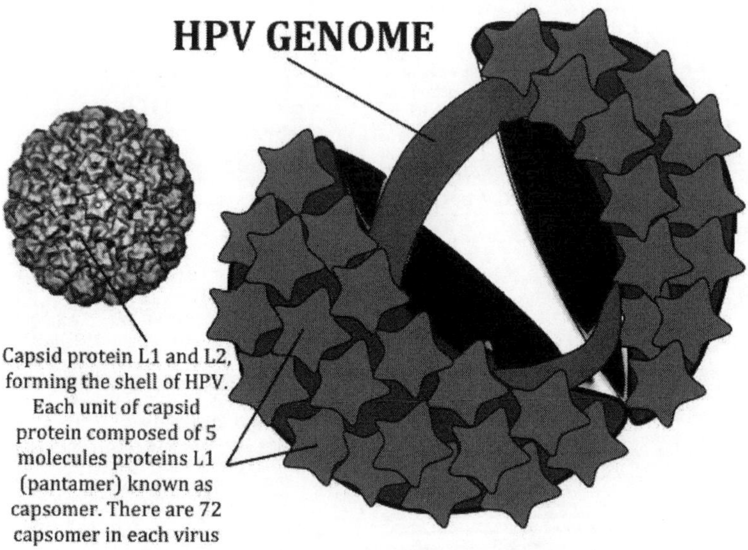

Figure 6.1 Human papillomavirus. The DNA is circular in shape within the shell of the virus. The shell is formed by capsid proteins. L2 capsid proteins are located at the central point of each capsomer.

Human papillomavirus is a member of family Papovaviridae, double stranded DNA virus with the diameter from 52–55 nm (Fig. 6.1). The HPV genome comprises 8000 base-pair long circular DNA molecules and encodes a maximum of eight proteins, six of which are known as early proteins (E1, E2, E4, E5, E6, and E7) and two late proteins known as L1 and L2 (Fig. 6.2). The DNA molecules are wrapped into a protein shell (capsid) that is composed of two molecules L1 (major capsid protein) and L2 (minor capsid protein). L1, the major capsid protein constitutes 80% of the virion while L2 minor capsid protein makes up the remaining 20%. The other region in HPV genome is known as a long control region (LCR), which has no coding potential. Early proteins are necessary for the replication of the viral DNA and for the assembly of newly produced virus particles within the infected cells. E6 and E7 are oncoproteins.

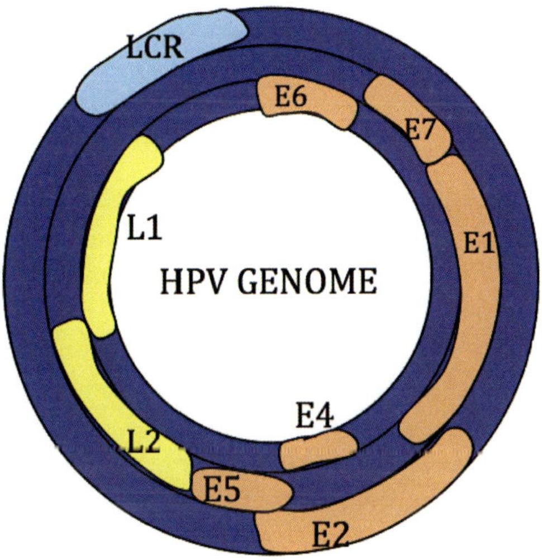

Figure 6.2 Genome of Human Papillomavirus. The HPV genome comprises 8000 base-pair long circular DNA molecules and encodes a maximum of eight proteins, six of which are known as early proteins (E1, E2, E4, E5, E6 and E7) and two late proteins known as L1 and L2. LCR: long control region; E: early region; L: late region.

HPV is epitheliotropic, it infect the skin and mucous membranes and produce local epithelial proliferation or warts. Papillomaviruses are absolutely species-specific; thus HPVs only infect humans, rabbit papillomaviruses only infect rabbits, and so forth.

In contrast to other viral infections, human papillomavirus can evade from the body immune system; antibody levels following natural infection are low and not reliably protective. Following are the sophisticated immune evasion mechanisms by HPV:

(a) Infection is exclusively intraepithelial.
(b) There is no viraemia following infection.
(c) Local immunosuppression.
(d) HPV uses the natural life cycle of epithelial cells to release new viruses and does not cause cell death.
(e) HPV infection does not induce inflammation and therefore, no attraction of immune cells. No pro-inflammatory signals mean no activation of dendritic cells.
(f) Production of high immunogenic capsid protein is limited to the well-differentiated outer layers that are well away from the basal cell and subepithelial region.
(g) Factors (a)–(f) lead to poor exposure to antigen presenting cells.

There is a suggestive of natural protection, mainly by cell-mediated immunity, however, antibody levels after natural infections are low and have not been shown to be consistently protective against re-infection with the same type.

In human, there are more than 150 genotypes of HPV identified by sequence of genes encoding major capsid protein L1 and early proteins E6 and E7. The incidence of HPV positive in women with normal smear is very variable from 4% to 43% and different subtype has different site of epithelial and different type of lesions produced. More than 40 types of HPVs were recognized to infect anogenital tract of human. In women 15–25 years of age, almost 80% of HPV infections are transient.

HPV-related diseases can be divided into three categories: (1) skin lesions, (2) genital lesions and (3) non-genital lesions (see Table 6.1). Human papillomavirus has a predilection for either cutaneous or mucosal surfaces. Within the groups of skin or mucosal viruses, they can be separated into high-risk HPV (HR HPV) and low risk HPV (LR HPV) depending upon their oncogenic potential. Most important high-risk HPVs associated with cervical cancer are HPV 16 and 18. The WHO has recognized HPV 16 and HPV 18 as carcinogenic agents for humans. Persistent infection is a prerequisite for malignant transformation of cervical epithelial cells. Evidence shows HR HPV infections tend to persist longer than LR HPV infections. Among HR HPV, HPV 16 and 18 infections are more likely to persist than other types.

Table 6.1 Clinical manifestations and type of HPV

Clinical manifestations	Type of HPV
Skin lesions	
Plantar warts	1, 2, 4
Common warts	2, 4, 26, 27, 29, 57
Butcher's warts	7
Epidermodysplasia verruciformis	2, 3, 5, 8, 9, 10, 12, 14, 15, 17, 19, 20–25, 36, 37, 46, 47, 50
Genital lesions	
Condyloma acuminata	6, 11, 16, 30, 40, 41, 42, 44, 45, 54, 55, 61
SIL, VIN, VAIN, PAIN, PIN	6, 11, 16, 18, 30, 31, 33, 35, 39, 40, 42, 45, 51, 52, 55, 59, 61, 62, 64, 66–70
Cervical cancer	16, 18, 31, 33, 35, 39, 45, 51, 52, 54, 55, 56, 58, 59, 66, 68
Non-cervical anogenital cancers	6, 11, 16, 18, 30, 31, 33
Non-genital mucosal lesions	
Mouth (local epith. Hyperplasia)	13, 32
Recurrent resp. papillovatosis	6, 11, 30
Carcinoma (head/neck/lung)	2, 6, 11, 16, 18, 30

Source: Modified from Koutsky LA, Kiviat NB. Genital HPV. In Holmes KK, Mardh PA, Sparling PF, et al., eds. *STD* (3rd ed.). New York McGraw-Hill, 1999; 347–359.

Almost 100% of cervical cancers contain HPV DNA sequences from a high-risk HPV and the most important HPV related to cervical cancer is HPV 16 responsible in 50–70% of cases and HPV 18, found in 7–20% of cases. Molecular and epidemiological data suggest that each HPV type has variants or subtypes; variants of the same type are biologically distinct and may confer differential pathogenic risk (e.g. HPV 16 has five distinct phylogenetic branches, i.e. European (E), Asian (As), Asian American (AA) and two African (Af-1, Af-2). A clinical and epidemiological study done in Mexico had indicated that HPV 16 variants in Asian American (AA) might be more oncogenic than European (E) variants. Existence of HPV subtypes or intratype distributions suggest that these viruses evolved with humans over a period of time (Berumen, 2001). Based on the accumulation of molecular and epidemiologic evidence supporting a causal association, the International Agency for Research on Cancer (IARC) has concluded that there is sufficient evidence to classify HPV infection as a Group I carcinogen for cancers of the anus, cervix, oropharynx, penis, vagina, and vulva.

Transmission of HPV

HPV infection is the most common sexually transmitted disease. Based on 78 studies worldwide, the world prevalence of age-adjusted HPV infection is 10%, highest in Africa (23%) and lowest in Asia and Europe (8%) (Burchell, et al. 2006).

Following are the mechanisms of HPV transmissions and acquisitions:

(1) **Sexual contact**

- (a) Sexual intercourse
- (b) Genital-genital, manual-genital, oral-genital contacts
- (c) Genital HPV infection in virgin is rare, but may result from non-penetrative sexual contact
- (d) Condom use may reduce the risk of transmission but not fully protective. Regular and consistent use of condom can provides 60% protection against HPV infection; HPV can still be transmitted through contact with areas of unprotected genital skin such as the vulva or scrotal sacs.

(2) **Non-sexual routes**

- (a) Vertical transmission from mother to newborn resulting in respiratory papillomatosis
- (b) Possibly through fomites such as undergarments, surgical glove, and biopsy forceps, would be very rare.

At least 85% of transmission is through sexual contact while remaining 15% is through non-sexual routes. Up to 75% of sexually active women acquired HPV infection at least once in their lifetime. However, 80% of infections are cleared after 12 months.

The prevalence of HPV infection in women without cervical abnormalities varies from one continental to others; estimated prevalence of high-risk HPV infection in Asian women without cervical abnormalities was 5.4%. Following are the risk factors for HPV infection in women: (a) young age (peak age at 20–24 years old), (b) lifetime and recent number of sex partners, (c) male partner's sexual behaviour, (d) uncircumcised male partners, (e) smoking, (f) oral contraceptive use and (g) early age of first sexual intercourse. In men, three important risk factors for HPV infections are (a) young age (peak age from 25–29 years old), (b) lifetime number of sex partners and (c) being uncircumcised.

Burden of HPV Infections

The burdens of HPV infections are tremendous; it can be divided into two categories (applicable to males and females):

(a) HPV-related precancerous and cancerous lesions
(b) HPV-related benign lesions

Human papillomavirus is attributable in 5% of human cancers, 10% of cancers in women and 15% of female cancers in developing countries. Human papillomavirus is responsible in more than 500,000 new cases of cervical cancer worldwide in 2008. If current incidence trends continue, incidence of cervical cancer will rise to estimate 1 million cases per year by 2050. In 2005, more than 260,000 cervical cancer deaths occurred, resulting in 2.7 million years of life lost. If current trends persist, cervical cancer deaths are expected to rise by nearly 25% in the next 10 years. About 80% of cervical cancer deaths occur in developing countries. The incidence rates are highest in parts of Latin America and the Caribbean, sub-Saharan Africa, Melanesia and parts of south Asia.

The burden of non-cervical cancers among men and women are more than 95,000 cases annually worldwide, including approximately 50,000 cancers among men (anal cancer (26%), oropharyngeal cancer (52%) and penile cancers (22%)) and 46,000 cancers among women (anal cancers (32%), oropharyngeal cancers (13%), vulvar/vaginal cancers (55%)) (Chaturvedi, 2010).

The worldwide burden of cervical compared to non-cervical HPV-related cancers has demonstrated that the cervix is uniquely most susceptible to HPV-induced carcinogenesis when compared to other anatomic sites. In fact, when the causal relationship between HPV infection and cervical cancer was compared to other non-HPV–related cancers; the relative risk of cervical cancer from HPV infection was found to be the highest (see Table 6.3).

Table 6.2 HPV types in anogenital malignancies (both males and females)

Lesion	HPV types involved	% cases HPV
Cervical carcinoma	16, 18, 31, 33, 35, 39, 45, 51, 52, 66, 58, 59, 66 (26, 68, 73, 82[a])	>95%
Vulval carcinoma		
Basaloid	16, 18	>50%
Warty	16, 18	>50%
Keratinizing	16	<10%
Vaginal carcinoma	16, 18	>50%
Penile carcinoma		
Basaloid	16, 18	>50%
Warty	16, 18	>50%
Keratinizing	16	<10%
Carcinoma of the anus	16, 18	>70%

[a]Rare type of HPV.

Reference: Stanley M. HPV vaccines. *Best Pract Res Clin Obstet Gynaecol* 2006; **20**(2): 279–293.

Table 6.3 The causal relationship between causative agent and cancer

Cancer and causative agent	Relative risk
Cervical cancer from HPV	300–500
Liver cancer from Hepatitis B virus (Taiwan)	100
Liver cancer from Hepatitis C virus (Italy)	20
Lung cancer and smoking	10

Currently, organized cytologic screening is still implemented in many developed countries to prevent cervical cancer; today, it is estimated that 50 million pap tests are performed annually in the United States alone. Although, screening program reduces the incidence and mortality rate, the cost of implementing organized screening program is very huge. Out of 50 million pap tests, 2–3 million women were diagnosed with atypical squamous cells (ASC),

1.25 million with low-grade squamous intraepithelial lesions (LSIL), 300,000 with high-grade squamous intraepithelial lesions (HSIL) and more than 10,000 with cervical cancer; many of these cases required repeat testing, treatment and follow-up. Therefore, the economic and psychological burden associated with screening program is substantial. Furthermore, despite an organized screening program, there are still many women die of cervical cancer annually.

Apart from HPV-related cancer, HPV infection is also attributed to pre-cancerous lesions and benign genital warts. Worldwide, approximately 10 million cases of high-grade cervical lesions and 30 million cases of low-grade cervical lesions were reported; all were associated to HPV infections. Low risk HPV has also contributed to tremendous numbers of genital wart lesions with the estimation of 30 million cases annually. Anogenital warts or condylomata acuminata are the most commonly diagnosed viral sexually transmitted disease (STD) in the United States and United Kingdom. More than 90% of anogenital warts are due to HPV type 6 and 11. Majority of anogenital warts are not clinically visible. It is estimated that 1% of US adult population has visible anogenital warts and estimated lifetime risk of developing genital warts is approximately 10%. Treatment modalities are often painful, costly, required follow-up and repeat treatment. Furthermore, the recurrence rate is high up to 75% after 6 months, despite treatment.

Human papillomavirus can also be transmitted from mother to a newborn through vertical transmission during delivery. Infection to newborn may lead to recurrent respiratory papillomatosis (RRP). More than 90% of RRP is associated with infection by HPV type 6 and 11. RRP is a rare disease characterized by the formation of wart-like lesions on the respiratory tract, most frequently at the larynx. The incidence of RRP is estimated to be 4.3 per 100,000 in children and 1.8 per 100,000 in adults. Both males and females have a similar incidence. RRP is the most common benign neoplasm of the larynx among children and the second most common cause of chronic hoarseness. The disease is more aggressive in children, and it can cause hoarseness of voice, stridor and airway obstruction requiring multiple surgeries. In US, 1500 new cases have been reported every year; 15,000 surgical procedures were involved to treat this condition costing approximately US$ 100 million/year.

Pathogenesis of HPV Infections

Human papillomavirus has a very unique process of infection. The earlier understanding of HPV infection was based on in vitro studies mostly involving either non-infectious virus-like particles, virions generated in organotypic raft culture or infectious pseudoviruses. Currently, in order to obtain better and more accurate understanding, the study of pathogenesis of HPV infection has shifted to in vivo investigations. The first step in HPV infection is called attachment. Major capsid protein L1 contains the major determinant for initial attachment. The most critical attachment factors on the epithelial cell are called heparan sulfate proteoglycans (HSPGs). The viruses enter the epithelium through microabrasion straight to the cells in the basement membrane. Several hours after initial binding on the basement membrane, the capsids were detected on the surfaces of epithelial cells. After attachment, the viral genome makes its way to the nucleus through ways not yet completely defined. After some time, the virus then uses the host cell DNA replication machinery to begin its own replication process, and increasing the number of viral to around 50–100 copies per-cell. The infected cells are then moved toward the surface of epithelium, and now the number of viral copies increase to 1000 per-cell. The time taken for infected cells at basal layers to move upward until to the superficial layers are said to be from 2–3 weeks.

Most of the infections are subclinical and transient (80–90%); infection or any low-grade lesions developed from the infectious processes will resolve as a consequence of the development of the host cell- mediated immunity (CMI). In minority of women, perhaps 10–15% of them fail to eradicate the infection, and the infection persists. These groups of women are those at risk of developing high-grade lesions and invasive carcinoma.

The incubation period is the time from initial infection until to the appearance of clinical lesions; the duration of the incubation period is from 3 weeks to 8 months or even more (Fig. 6.3). Majority of the clinical lesions are seen after 2–3 months of infection, however, up to 30% of the infection will regress within 3 months by CMI. The time of clearance is longer for HR HPV (12–18 months) as compared to LR HPV (4–9 months). Persistent infection by HR HPV; with the presence of co-factors eventually transform the epithelial cells into neoplastic cells either as high-grade lesions such as CIN 2/3 or as invasive cervical cancer. During this event, viral DNA may be integrated into the host genome, and subsequently E6/E7 oncoproteins are overexpressed throughout the epithelium. E6 oncoprotein can inactivate p53 (tumour suppressor/DNA repair) while E7 protein binds to pRb protein (gene transcription inhibitor). Normally, Rb protein is responsible in preventing the cell to enter S-phase (acting like a "brake"). When the Rb proteins are degraded by E7 proteins, the "brake" mechanism will be eliminated and the cell enters S-phase and continue to replicate. Protein E6 is also said to eliminate proteins involved in regulating the shape and polarity of the epithelial cells, therefore preventing apoptosis (anti-apoptotic affect). The epithelial cells become genetically unstable; acquiring further mutation and have the capability of progression from CIN 2, CIN 3 and subsequently invasive cancer. The time taken from HRHPV infection to the development of CIN 3 is 3–5 years; progression to invasive cancer takes much longer, i.e. 10–20 years.

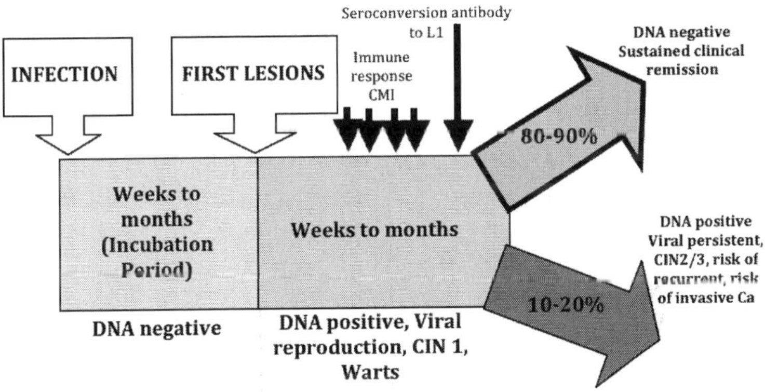

Figure 6.3 Natural history of genital HPV infection. Adapted from Stanley. *Gynecol Oncol* 2010; **117**: S5–S10.

In general, there are two important growth characters of malignant cells: (a) Immortalization, the cancer cells replicate indefinitely and (b) Anchorage-independent growth; cancer cells are able to grow when suspended in fluid or semisolid agar gel and this is a transformation character. When oncogenic HPV such as HPV 16 and 18 are introduced into already immortalized cell lines, the cells become transformed and developed capacity of anchorage-independent growth. These transformed cells are tumorigenic. Immortalization is a prerequisite for cell transformation, i.e.

tumorigenic by HPV 16 and 18. Non-immortalize cervical cells when exposed to oncogenic viruses will be immortalized but will not be transformed and therefore non-tumorigenic. The HPV DNA has two separate effects on cell growth that is (a) able to immortalize (without transforming) human cells and (b) able to transform immortalized human cells. Both effects are determined by specific gene in HPV genome, i.e. E6/E7 oncogenes. These genes encode specific proteins. E7 protein is the major transforming and immortalizing protein of HPV. These genes, through a very complex processes act with oncogenes (activate) and tumour suppressor gene (inhibit, e.g., p53). HPV E6 enhanced the activity of HPV E7 oncoprotein. The binding capacity E7 and E6 protein to oncoprotein (Rb) and tumour supressor protein (p53) respectively, determine the level of oncogenic potential of specific type of HPV, e.g. HPV 16 has higher oncogenic potential than HPV 6 because E6/E7 oncoprotein from HPV 16 has higher binding capacity than that in HPV 6.

Majority of HPVs cause benign lesions. In benign HPV-related lesions, majorities are asymptomatic and few clinical lesions are manifested. In clinically visible HPV-infected lesions or condylomata acuminata, there are four typical histologic features suggestive of HPV infection: (a) thickening of the superficial cell layers (keratosis), (b) presence of koilocytosis (layer of cells with enlarged nuclei, irregular chromatin, perinuclear clearing (halo) and thickening or thinning of the cytoplasmic border), (c) proliferation of the prickle cell layer (acanthosis) and (d) localized hyperplasia of basal cells (basal cell hyperplasia). Majority of HPV infections are cleared spontaneously without treatment and study had shown that the clearance of HPV infections likely involve both innate immunity (non-specific, the first-line defence against infection, e.g. anatomic barrier, physiologic barrier, phagocytic barrier endocytosis, etc.) and adaptive immunity (specific, it reacts against a specific microorganism; adaptive immunity has two components, i.e., humoral and cell-mediated immunity).

HPV Infection in Man

The prevalence of genital warts is highest among men aged 25–29 years; and similar to women, the prevalence decreases with age. In general, the prevalence of HPV infection in males is almost similar or even higher than female. In some report, HPV DNA of both oncogenic and non-oncogenic type was noted in 50.5% of men (Giuliano and Palefsky and Giuliano 2008). Approximately, 4% of sexually active male ages between 18 and 59 years old have been diagnosed as genital warts at least once. The most common sites of infection (>95% of cases) are penile shaft, coronal sulcus, glan penis and scrotum. HPV infections may be less likely to persist in men than in women (6% versus 20%) (Van Doornum, 1994). Approximately, 75% of infections clearing within 12 months and reduced risk of persistent infection has been observed among circumcised men (Lu et al., 2009). Many studies have reported that prevalence of HPV infection and HPV detection rate were lower in circumcised men (Dunne et al., 2006; Giuliano et al., 2010; Nielson et al., 2009). More than 90% of genital warts are due to HPV type 6 and 11. One third of genital warts are due to multiple infections, including with co-existing oncogenic HPV infections. Similar to women, apart from genital warts, man can also develop recurrent respiratory papillomatosis. The incidence of RRP in man is similar to women. Approximately, 85% of anal canal cancer cases worldwide are attributable to HPV and the incidence of anal cancer in men in the United States was 1.3 per 100,000. The American Cancer Society has estimated that 2000 new cases of anal cancer will be reported in 2010. The DNA of HPV was found in 47% of penile squamous cell carcinoma; HPV 16 and 18 were found in 60% and 13% respectively. The prevalence of HPV DNA in penile tumours varies with histological subtype—most common in basaloid and warty subtypes.

Subsets of head and neck squamous cell carcinoma (HNSCC) originating in the oropharynx, tonsil, base of the tongue, soft palate and pharyngeal wall are found to be increasingly associated with human papillomavirus infection. The prevalence of HPV infection in oropharygeal carcinoma varies widely between studies from 18–82%. HNSCC is more common in males; American Cancer Society has estimated that in 2010, there will be a total of 25,420 cases of oral cavity and pharyngeal cancer in males as compared to 11,120 cases in females (US data). Most cases (90–95%) of HPV positive oropharyngeal carcinoma is associated with HPV type 16. Case control studies have demonstrated an association between HPV positive oropharyngeal carcinoma and certain sexual behaviours, including a high lifetime number of oral sex or vaginal sex partners, early age of first intercourse and infrequent use of condoms. Patients with HPV-positive head and neck squamous carcinoma (HNSCC) has a better prognosis with 50–80% reduction in the risk of cancer-related death as compared to HPV-negative HNSCC (Evan and Powell 2010).

Methods of HPV Detection

There are various methods of HPV detection and each of this method has their advantage and disadvantages (Table 6.4). Newest methods of HPV detection are generally more sensitive but require higher maintenance cost. In general, HPV detection can be classified into three broad categories:

(1) **Culture methods**: This method is currently not widely available, very cumbersome and restricted to only few types of HPV. The examples of culture methods are (a) *nude-mouse transplantation system* (human epithelial tissues are exposed to the HPV-infected tissues and transplant beneath the renal capsule of mice; a specific cytopathic effect will be observed after several months) and (b) *Collagen-raft culture system* (culturing the human HPV-infected keratinocytes in collagen-raft culture and treated with substances that can increase the expression of keratinocyte differentiation accompanied with production of HPV virion).

(2) **Immunologic methods**: The limitation of immunologic methods is that HPV lack of appropriate antigen targets for immunologic assays. HPV 16 E7 protein expressed by bacteria has been used to produce an antibody against HPV. Only 50% patient with cervical cancer (HPV 16 related) will have an antibody to HPV 16 E7. None of patients with HGSIL has antibody to E7. Antibody to E7 therefore, only useful in the advanced stage. Antibody to HPV capsid proteins is currently being studied. This protein is also a candidate for future HPV vaccines.

(3) **Molecular detection methods**: There are various molecular detection methods to detect HPV DNA: (a) *filter hybridization method* (Southern blot Dot blot), (b) *polymerase chain reaction (PCR)*, (c) *ligase chain reaction* and (c) *solution hybridization method*. Southern blots are the gold standard for detection of

specific type of HPV. PCR is more sensitive than Southern blots for detecting specifics DNA sequence. Both PCR and Southern blots are labour intensive and difficult. Hybrid Capture HPV DNA assay (solution hybridization methods) is the most widely used HPV DNA assay for clinical used, approved by FDA. This method is using chemiluminescence principle. The detection rate is higher when the specimen is obtained from cervico-vaginal lavage rather than swab or spatula.

HPV Vaccine

The fact that human papillomavirus is the primary aetiology of cervical cancer is undeniable. Persistent infection by oncogenic HPV and presence of co-factors are prerequisites for malignant transformation of cervical epithelial cells. Persistent cervical infection causes cellular changes in the epithelium that can be detected through cytologic screening. This is the basis of Pap smear, which is currently the most common method of secondary prevention for cervical cancer. HPV detection and genotyping are also increasingly used as screening method either together with cytologic screening or as a primary screening modality. Oncogenic types of HPV are estimated to cause almost 100% of cervical cancer, 90% of anal cancers, 40% of cancers of the vulva, vagina and penis, and at least 12% of head and neck cancers. HPV 16 is the most common cause of cervical cancer, causing 52–58% of cases in all regions and HPV 16 is also the most common cause of non-cervical anogenital cancers. Overall, the top ranked HPV types responsible in cervical cancer are 16, 18, 31, 58 and 52. Apart from precancerous and cancerous lesions, HPVs are also responsible in large number of benign lesions involving mucosal and non-mucosal surfaces. HPV type 6 and 11 are non-oncogenic HPV (low-risk HPV), however, are responsible in 90–100% cases of external anogenital warts and recurrent respiratory papillomatosis.

Secondary prevention via cytologic testing is successful in preventing cervical cancer in developed countries where organized screening program and high coverage of screening population are feasible. However, secondary prevention in developing countries and underdeveloped countries is less successful due to poor coverage, lack in infrastructures, inadequate facilities for treatment and inadequate number of human resources. Cytologic screening is more effective in detecting precancers and cancers of squamous cell type than adenocarcinoma in situ and adenocarcinoma because of sampling difficulties. Therefore, screening with cytology has a limitation in prevention of endocervical lesions.

Table 6.4 Comparison of various methods of HPV detection

Method	Sensitivity	Specificity	Comments
Cytology	Low	Low	Easy, relatively inexpensive, but subjective, insensitive and non-specific
Dot blot	Moderate	Moderate	Radioactive, commercially available, labour intensive
Filter in situ hybridization	Moderate		Detect HPV in paraffin-embedded tissue
Southern blot hybridization	High	High	Not feasible for large scale clinical use
Hybrid capture	High	High	Approved by FDA and for commercial use, non-radioactive, easier to use and less expensive than dot blot
PCR	Very high	High	Uses amplification and so is prone to contamination errors

Following are the limitations of secondary prevention (cytologic test, HPV testing and visual inspection):

(a) Secondary prevention does not prevent HPV infection or pre-invasive lesions of the cervix,

(b) Lesion that has rapid progression rate may not be detected in time,

(c) There is a higher chance of missing the lesions in the cervical canal,

(d) It has limited sensitivity and specificity,

(e) It involves high cost and is labour intensive,

(f) Early stages of adenocarcinoma can be difficult to detect due to lesion within endocervical canal,

(g) Many lesions will regress and are thus "overtreated" and

(h) Adverse pregnancy outcomes are associated with treatment of precancerous lesions.

Due to the limitations of secondary prevention, there has been a shift in paradigm to primary prevention. Primary prevention of cervical cancer can be achieved through prevention and control of genital HPV infection. Primary prevention includes health promotion strategies geared at a change in sexual behaviour, i.e. promoting healthy sexual life, avoiding or minimizing exposure to co-factors such as stop smoking, promoting healthy lifestyles and perhaps the most promising effort is through HPV vaccination. Historically, vaccination has proven to be an effective means to reduce infectious disease and mortality related to it, for example, prophylactic Hepatitis B vaccine had reduced the incidence of infection by 72%. Study in Taiwan shows that vaccination of newborns with hepatitis B immunoglobulin at birth (if the mother is infected with Hepatitis B) was associated with a reduction in the average annual incidence of hepatocellular cancer from 0.70 per 100,000 children in 1981 to 0.36 per 100,000 in year 1990–1994 (Chang et al., 1997).

The HPV vaccine was discovered by Professor Ian Frazer and his co-researcher Dr. Jian Zhou. Ian Frazer was born in Glasgow in 1953. He met Jan Zhou in 1989 while he was working in the Department of Immunology, University of Queensland, Australia. They decided to work together and began to use molecular biology to synthesize particles in vitro that could mimic the virus. They discovered that the L1 capsid protein could be expressed in eukaryotic cells and could self-assemble into virus-liked particles (VLPs). VLPs contain reassembled capsid proteins without viral genome; therefore, VLP is non-infectious (see Figs. 6.4 and 6.5). When injected, they generate high levels of systemic anti-HPV L1 IgG antibodies and provide type-specific protection. Studies have found that, they also confer some degree of protection against phylogenetically-related HPV types.

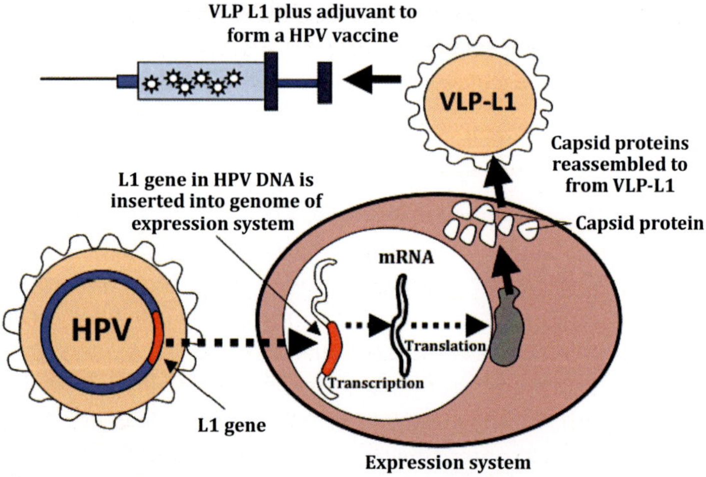

Figure 6.4 Illustration of how HPV vaccine is manufactured using recombinant technology. Expression system in quadrivalent vaccine is the yeast cell while in Bivalent vaccine, using Baculovirus. VLP L1: Viral-liked particle L1.

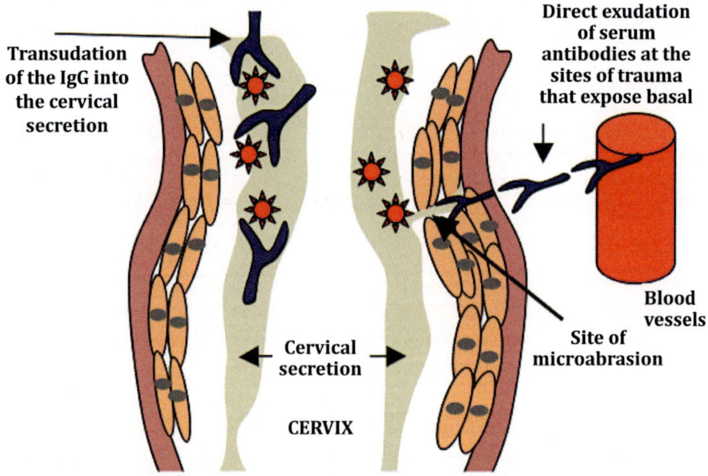

Figure 6.5 Theoretical mechanism of local protection by IgG after HPV vaccination. Adapted from Schiller and Davies. *Nat Rev Microbiol* 2004; **2**: 343–347.

There are two potential benefits of HPV vaccination: (a) Prevention of HPV-related precancerous and cancerous lesions and (b) Prevention of HPV-related benign lesions. At present, there are two types of prophylactic HPV vaccines available in the market: quadrivalent HPV vaccine against HPV 16, 18, 6, 11 and bivalent HPV vaccine against HPV 16 and 18. The differences between quadrivalent and bivalent vaccine are shown in Table 6.5. Both Quadrivalent and Bivalent vaccines were found to be highly immunogenic in clinical trials, resulting in essentially 100% seroconversion. The antibody titres reach peak at month 7, decline over the next year and then remained relatively stable for at least 5–6 years. Both vaccines were also shown to induce production of memory B cells. Human studies have shown that high titres of specific antibodies are also present in cervical secretions of women receiving HPV 16 VLP L1. The most likely mechanism of these findings is transudation from the cervical secretion and exudation from the blood stream at the site of microtrauma or microabrasion. These antibodies are said to provide local protection against HPV infection (see Fig. 6.5). Natural HPV infection induces type-specific immunity to HPV infections. Individuals who are infected with one HPV type may seroconvert and show some level of protection against future infection with that HPV type but will remain immunologically naïve to other HPV types.

Table 6.5 Characteristics of quadrivalent and bivalent HPV vaccine

	Quadrivalent vaccine	Bivalent vaccine
Manufacturer and trade name	Merck, Gardasil®, Silgard®	GlaxoSmithKline, Cervarix®
HPV Genotypes	16, 18, 6, 11	16, 18
Manufacturing and Expression system	Yeast cells (Saccharomyces cerevisiae) with recombinant plasmid	*Trichoplusia ni* insect cell line infected with L1 encoding recombinant baculovirus
Adjuvant	Amorphous aluminium hydroxyphosphate sulphate (AAHS), dose: 225 ug	Aluminium hydroxide and monophosphoryl lipid A (ASO4); dose: 500 ug + 50 ug
Other content	Sodium chloride, L-histidine, polysorbate 80, sodium borate, and water for injection	Sodium chloride and sodium dihydrogen phosphate dehydrate, and water for inject.

(*Continued*)

Table 6.5 *(Continued)*

	Quadrivalent vaccine	Bivalent vaccine
Dose (0.5 mL per injection)	20 ug anti HPV 6, 18 and 40 ug anti HPV 11, 16	20 ug anti HPV 16 and 18
Administration	Intramuscular	Intramuscular
Schedule (3 intramuscular inj. within 6 months)	0, 2, 6 months	0, 1, 6 months
Initial study age group	16–26 years old	15–25 years old
Approval (age group)	FDA, European Medicines Agency (FDA: females 9–26 years old, male aged 9–26 years old. EMA: females 9 years or older, males 9–15 years old, M'sian DCA: females 9–26)	FDA, European Medicine Agency (EMA) (FDA: females 10–25 years old, EMA: females 10 years or older, Malaysia DCA: females 10–45 years old)
Indications	Prevention of HPV 6/11/16/18-related cervical cancer, adenocarcinoma in situ, CIN1-3, VAIN 2/3, VIN2/3, vulvar cancer, vaginal cancer and genital warts. Prevention of genital warts in males (approved by FDA for use in females age 9–26 and males age 9–21. ACIP has given a permissive recommendation for male age 22–26 years old and routine catch-up vaccination for MSM (men who has sex with men) and HIV positive male in same age group.)	Prevention of HPV 16, 18-related cervical cancer, denocarcinoma in situ, CIN1-3 (approved by FDA for use in female age 9–25)
Require for storage and cold-chain system	Yes	Yes
Preservative	None	None
Temperature storage	Store refrigerated at 36°–46°F (2°–8°); do not freeze	Store refrigerated at 36°–46°F (2°–8°C). Do not freeze

Table 6.6 Conditions associated with HPV type 16, 18, 6 and 11 and potential benefits of HPV vaccination

Type of HPV	Lesions	Estimated attributable
HPV 16 and 18	Cervical cancer	70%
	High-grade cervical abnormalities	50%
	Low-grade cervical abnormalities	30%
	Anal cancer	70%
	Vulva/Vagina/Penile	40–50%
	Head and neck cancers	3–12%
HPV 6 and 11	Low-grade cervical abnormalities	10%
	Genital warts	90%
	Recurrent respiratory papillomatosis	90%

HPV Vaccine Trial

The process of the development of any vaccine involves four phases or stages of trials:

(a) proof of principles (animal model)
(b) toxicity studies (phase I)
(c) induction of immunity; immunogenicity study (phase II)
(d) prevention of mucosal infection (phase III)

In HPV vaccine development, the first proof-of-principle study to test the safety and immunogenicity of VLP L1 was done, and it was found to be safe and inducing a significant immune response. Subsequently, both Quadrivalent and Bivalent HPV vaccines have been evaluated in large double blind randomized control trial.

Quadrivalent Vaccine Trials

The results of first double blind efficacy trial using HPV VLPs were published in November 2002 (Koutsky et al., 2002). In this first proof-of-principle trial, HPV 16 VLP (plus adjuvant) was given to women age 16–23 years old in three doses (0, 2 and 6 months); the vaccine was found to be 100% efficacious in preventing persistent HPV infection and 99.7% of women received the vaccine was seroconverted and the level of the immune response was >50-fold higher than natural infection.

The results of first double blind randomized placebo control trial (phase II) evaluating the efficacy of quadrivalent HPV vaccine (involving 552 women age 16–23 years old) was published in 2005 and the primary endpoints were persistent HPV infection and vaccine-type HPV-related diseases (Protocol 007). The vaccine was found to be very efficacious in preventing persistent infection and clinical diseases related to HPV 6, 11, 16 and 18. Quadrivalent HPV vaccine was also found to be well tolerated and safe (Villa et al., 2005). The extended follow-up for 5 years was done and the high efficacy of this vaccine was found to be sustained. At 5 years, the quadrivalent vaccine prevented 96% and 100% of HPV 6, 11, 16, 18 infections and cervical and genital diseases, respectively (Villa et al., 2006). All women receiving the quadrivalent vaccine developed neutralizing antibodies to HPV 6, 11, 16 and 18 at completion of the vaccine regimen at month 7; the geometric mean titers decline after month 7 until month 24 when the level was plateauing. Immune memory was also observed among vaccinees who received an antigen challenge after 5 years (anamnestic response) (Olsson et al., 2007).

Quadrivalent vaccine was initially licensed and approved by FDA for use in females aged 9–26 years old in October 2006. The Advisory Committee on Immunization Practices (ACIP) recommended routine quadrivalent vaccination of females aged 11 or 12 years, and catch-up vaccination for females aged 13 through 26 years. Phase II trials were not only important in evaluating the efficacy and safety of the vaccine but also in guiding the appropriate dose of vaccine for subsequent phase III trial. Phase III trial for quadrivalent HPV vaccine is also known as FUTURE trial (Female United to Unilaterally Reduce Endo/ectocervical disease). The aim of FUTURE trial is to further define the efficacy and safety of quadrivalent vaccine against HPV-6, 11, 18, 18–related infections and diseases including external genital lesions. There are two FUTURE trials, i.e. FUTURE I and FUTURE

II. The study designs of FUTURE I and FUTURE II trials are shown in Table 6.7. Combined analysis of phase II trial (Protocol 007) and phase III trials (FUTURE I and FUTURE II trials) showed that the quadrivalent vaccine prevented 100% of HPV 16, 18–related high-grade cervical lesions. Vaccine also showed 100% efficacy in preventing HPV 16, 18–related VAIN 2/3 and VIN 2/3; more than 95% efficacy in preventing HPV6, 11, 16, 18–related CIN 1/2/3, AIS, genital warts, vulvar and vaginal neoplasias. In summary, Quadrivalent vaccine was very effective in reducing the incidence of HPV 6/11/16/18–related disease in HPV naïve women (seronegative and HPV DNA negative by PCR). Interestingly, vaccine also beneficial to women who had been previously exposed to at least one vaccine HPV type at enrolment, but had no ongoing HPV infection (seropositive but HPV DNA negative by PCR) (Joura et al., 2007; Ault, 2007). Quadrivalent vaccine also demonstrated vaccine efficacy against CIN2+ associated with 10 other oncogenic types, which were 32.5% (Brown et al., 2009). The other completed and ongoing studies related to quadrivalent HPV vaccine are phase III adolescent immunogenicity study for males and females aged 9–15, efficacy study in mid-adult women (age 24–45), men safety and efficacy study (male age 16–26) and safety and immunogenicity in HIV-infected children (protocol 021).

The results of randomized double blind trial on the safety, immunogenicity and efficacy of quadrivalent HPV vaccine in women aged 24–45 years old have been published in Lancet 2009. The efficacy against the HPV 6, 11, 16 and 18–related disease or infection in per-protocol population was 90.5% while the efficacy against second coprimary endpoint that is disease or infection related to HPV 16 and 18 alone was 83.1%. The efficacy of quadrivalent HPV vaccine in intention-to-treat population (including women who had been infected) was approximately 22–30%. The authors concluded that quadrivalent HPV vaccine is efficacious in women aged 24–45 years not infected with the relevant type at enrolment (Munoz et al., 2009).

Men safety and efficacy study (protocol 020) is a randomized double blind placebo control trial involving more than 4000 male subjects (age 16–26 males including heterosexual and gays). Preliminary analysis (after 30 months) of this study reported the efficacy in per-protocol population of 100% for prevention of PIN

1/2/3, 89% for prevention of condyloma and 90% for external genital lesions (EGLs). Based on immunogenicity bridging study among boys age 9–15 (protocol 016 and 018), FDA has agreed that immune responses to quadrivalent vaccine in 9–15 years old boys and girls are non-inferior to those in 16–26 years old and it is also well tolerated. On October 2009, ACIP provided guidance that quadrivalent HPV vaccine may be given to males age 9 through 26 years to reduce their risk of acquiring genital warts.

Table 6.7 Characteristics of trials evaluating efficacy and safety of quadrivalent HPV vaccine

Study design	Protocol 007[a] (phase II trial)	FUTURE I[b] (phase III trial)	FUTURE II[c] (phase III trial)
Sample size	550	5455	12, 167
Study sites	International, multicenter, double blind	International, multicenter, double blind	International, multicenter, double blind
Study vaccine	Quadrivalent	Quadrivalent	Quadrivalent
Schedule	0, 2, 6 months	0, 2, 6 months	0, 2, 6 months
Age	16–23	16–24	15–26
Previous history of HPV-related disease	Not allowed	Not allowed	Not allowed
Sexual exposure	Allowed	Allowed	Allowed
Requirement for biopsy	All abnormal areas	All abnormal areas	All abnormal areas
HPV detection	PCR assay on frozen specimens	PCR assay on frozen specimens	PCR assay on frozen specimens

Note: More than 20,000 women involved in the trials from Europe, North America, Latin America and Asia Pacific region.

[a]Villa LL, et al. *Lancet Oncol* 2005; **6**: 271–278.

[b]Garland et al. *N Engl J Med* 2007; **356**: 1928–1943.

[c]FUTURE II study group. *N Engl J Med* 2007; **356**: 1915–1927.

For quadrivalent HPV vaccine, titres of anti-HPV remained substantially higher than those obtained after natural infection for type 16 and 6, while as for type 18 and 11, the titres were approaching close to that of natural infection after 5-year follow-up. Despite this observation, no breakthrough disease occurred in all subjects, including HPV 16 and 6–related conditions.

Bivalent HPV Vaccine Trials

The bivalent HPV vaccine was first evaluated in double blind randomized placebo control trial (phase II) involving more than 1000 women age 15–25 years old and was published in 2004. This study is also known as HPV-001 trial. Bivalent HPV vaccine was found to be very efficacious, well tolerated and safe (Harper et al., 2004). Extended follow-up study from HPV-001 trial is known as HPV-007 trial. Both HPV-001 and HPV-007 trials are phase II trials to evaluate the efficacy and safety of bivalent HPV vaccine. The efficacy endpoints for HPV-007 trial were HPV 16, 18–related incident of infection, persistent infection, abnormal cytology and CIN lesions. Final analysis of HPV-007 (after 6.4 years) indicates that bivalent HPV vaccine remains efficacious (97–100%) in prevention of persistent infection (for 12 months) and HPV 16/18–related abnormal cytology and CIN. The combined HPV-001 and 007 analyses have also shown evidence of cross protection against HPV 45 and 31. HPV-001 and HPV-007 trials have justified the currently used dose of bivalent HPV vaccine for clinical use and phase III trial (PATRICIA). Long term followed up study from HPV-001/007 trial is continued in Brazil and is expected to be completed at 9.5 years; this trial is known as HPV-023 trial. De Carvalho N and colleagues have reported the analysis of HPV-023 trial up to 7.3 years, and they have reported that vaccine efficacy up to 7.3 years was 94.5% for incident of infection, 100% for 12 months persistent infection and 100% for CIN2+. Antibody titres for total IgG and neutralizing antibodies remained several folds above natural infection levels and more than 96% of women were seropositive. Almost similar findings were elicited at 8.4 years of HPV023 trial. The vaccine also remains safe.

Phase III double blind randomized control trial evaluating the efficacy and safety of bivalent HPV vaccine is known as PATRICIA trial or HPV-008 trial. PATRICIA or Papilloma Trial against Cancer In young Adults is multinational randomized control trial, assessing the efficacy and safety of bivalent HPV vaccine against persistent infection, CIN2+, CIN3+ associated with HPV 16/18 and infection as well as lesions caused by the non-vaccine oncogenic HPV types. Participants in this trial were healthy women age 15–25 years at the time of first vaccination; participants were recruited from 135 centres in 14 countries in Asia Pacific, Europe, Latin America and North America (from May 2004). Women who had sexual exposure were also included. Women were enrolled irrespective of their HPV DNA status, HPV serostatus or cytology at baseline. The results of PATRICIA were published in July 2009. Vaccine efficacy against CIN2+ associated with HPV 16/18 was 98.4% in HPV naïve women. Vaccine efficacy against CIN2+ irrespective of HPV DNA in lesions was 30.4% in a total vaccinated cohort (included all women receiving at least one dose, regardless of their baseline HPV status; representing general population). In HPV naïve women, the efficacy of bivalent HPV vaccine against HPV 16/18-related CIN3+ was 100%. The vaccine also showed significant efficacy (54%) against CIN2+ not associated with HPV 16 and 18 indicating cross protection, especially with HPV 31, 33 and 45 (Paavonen et al., 2009). This additional efficacy could translate into approximately 11–16% extra protection against cervical cancer over and above the protection afforded by efficacy against HPV 16 and 18 alone.

Bivalent HPV vaccine was first licensed and approved by FDA for use in females aged 10–25 years old in October 2009. Vaccination with bivalent HPV vaccine induced a strong immune response with the average level of antibodies for both HPV 16 and 18 remains 11 times greater than antibody levels associated with natural HPV infection over a period of up to at least 8.3 years. Einstein HM and colleagues compared the immunogenicity between bivalent and quadrivalent HPV vaccine given to healthy women age 18–45; bivalent HPV vaccine induced higher neutralizing antibody level for both HPV 16 and 18. Although the bivalent vaccine induces higher antibody titres, it is unclear if this will translate into a more durable response. Currently bivalent HPV vaccine has been selected for national cervical cancer immunization programs in many countries such as United Kingdom, Netherlands, Sweden, Latvia, Gibraltar, Italy, Spain, Mexico and

Malaysia. Safety and immunogenicity of bivalent HPV vaccine in adolescent girls were evaluated in randomized controlled trial involving over 2000 girls with the means age of 12. This study shows that Bivalent HPV vaccine has a favourable safety profile and stimulates high anti HPV 16 and 18 antibody levels ; higher than in young women (Medina et al., 2010).

Table 6.8 Characteristics of clinical trials for Bivalent HPV vaccine (Cervarix)

Study design	HPV-001/007/023[a]	PATRICIA[b]	NCI/COSTA RICA[c]
Sample size	1113 (for HPV 001/007)	18,644	7466
Study sites	USA, Canada, Brazil (HPV-023 trial is an extended trial but participants are only from Brazil)	North America, Latin America, Europe, Asia Pacific and Australia	Costa Rica
Phase of study	Phase II	Phase III	Phase III
Control arm	500 ug Aluminium hydroxide	Hepatitis A Vaccine	Hepatitis A Vaccine
Age	15–25	15–25	18–25
Frequency of monitoring	6 months	12 months	12 months
Primary end point	Incidence of type 16/18 infections	HPV 16, 18-related CIN2+	HPV 16, 18-related persistent infection and CIN2+
Secondary endpoints	Persistent infection, CIN1+; adverse effects	Persistent infection or CIN1+ by any type of HPV; adverse effects	Adverse effects

[a]Harper et al., *Lancet* 2004; **364**: 1757–1765; Carvalho et al., *Vaccine* 2010; **28**: 6247–6255; HPV-023 is still ongoing.

[b]Paavonen et al., *Lancet* 2007; **369**: 2161–2170, Paavonen et al., *Lancet* 2009; **374**: 301–314.

[c]Costa Rica Vaccine trial sponsored by NCI (Herrero et al., *Vaccine* 2008; **26**: 4795–808).

Table 6.9 Efficacy of bivalent and quadrivalent HPV vaccine in female

Vaccine/endpoint/HPV type	Vaccine efficacy (%, 95% CI)
Bivalent HPV vaccine	
1. CIN 2/3 or adenocarcinoma in situ	
HPV 16 and/or 18	92.9% (79.9–98.3)
HPV 16	95.7% (82.8–99.6)
HPV 18	86.7 % (39.7–98.7)
Quadrivalent HPV vaccine	
1. CIN 2/3 or adenocarcinoma in situ	
HPV 6, 11, 16 and/or 18	98.2% (93.3–99.8)
HPV 16	97.6% (91.1–99.7)w
HPV 18	100% (86.6–100.0)
2. VIN2/3 or VAIN 2/3	
HPV 6, 11, 16 and/or 18	100% (82.6–100.0)
HPV 16	100% (76.5–100.0)
HPV 18	100% (<0–100.0)
3. Genital warts	
HPV 6 and/or 11	99% (96.2–99.9)

Source: Adapted from Centers for Disease Control and Prevention, Morbidity and Mortality weekly reports, Volume 59, No 20, May 2010.
CIN: Cervical intraepithelial neoplasm.
VIN: Vulvar intraepithelial neoplasm.
VAIN: Vaginal intraepithelial neoplasm.

Safety of Quadrivalent HPV Vaccine

Pain, erythema and swelling at the injection sites were the most common side effects but same problems were also found in the placebo arm (87% versus 77%). Serious vaccine-related adverse events were very rare, less than 2%. There was no adverse pregnancy outcome to women who had accidentally vaccinated while pregnant (66% of vaccine recipients and 63% in placebo recipients who became pregnant had a live birth). HPV vaccination did not increase the risk of the miscarriage and abnormal foetus. Among women who received the quadrivalent vaccine while lactating, the few adverse events among infants were judged not to be related to vaccine.

The 3-year post-licensure surveillance has reported that as of June 2009, more than 25 million doses of quadrivalent HPV vaccine had been distributed in the United States with more than 50 million doses globally. The rate of treatment-related serious adverse effect was 0.05% in the vaccine group as compared to 0.02% in the placebo group. A total of 18 deaths were reported but all were considered unrelated to study treatment. There was no difference in the rate of new autoimmune phenomena. The vaccine adverse events reporting system has received approximately 14,000 reports for the quadrivalent vaccine since licensure, with only 7% being serious adverse events, about half the average reported for licensed vaccines in general. The authors concluded that based on review of post-licensure safety information, the benefits of vaccination to prevent the majority of genital tract precancers and cancers continue to far outweigh its risks (Block et al., 2010). Based on the official statements of national and international agencies and expert immunization groups (WHO, CDC, FDA, PHAC, ATAGI, EMEA, STIKO, PEI, etc.) to date, as well as the review of the reports presented herein, HPV vaccine seems to be safe and effective vaccines. However, it is vital that continued and careful monitoring is undertaken.

Safety of Bivalent Vaccine

Pooled analysis on the safety of bivalent HPV vaccine showed almost similar findings with quadrivalent HPV vaccine. Rate of adverse events, including serious adverse effects were generally similar between the bivalent vaccine and control groups and there was no increased in the risk of the autoimmune condition. Similar to quadrivalent vaccine, injection site symptoms such as pain, swelling and redness were reported more frequently; however, these were transient, easily managed and did not affect compliance.

The pooled safety analysis included >29,000 females aged 10 through 25 years; approximately, 16,000 females received at least one dose of bivalent vaccine. In the bivalent vaccine group, 92% reported injection-site pain, 48% redness, and 44% swelling compared with 64–87%, 24–28% and 17–21% in the control group. Fatigue, headache and myalgia were the most common general symptoms (Descamps et al., 2009; Verstraeten el al., 2008).

Proportions of persons reporting a serious adverse event were similar in vaccine and control group (5.3% and 5.9% respectively). Medically significant adverse events occurred in 8.1% of women in the vaccine group and 6.2% of women in the placebo group, no women experienced new onset chronic disease and new onset autoimmune disease (Carvalho et al., 2010).

The outcome of pregnant women receiving bivalent HPV vaccine was similar to placebo; there was no increase in the rate of premature delivery, elective termination and spontaneous miscarriage. Bivalent HPV vaccine has been classified as category B on the basis of animal studies that revealed no evidence of impaired fertility or harm to the foetus. No data are available on use of bivalent HPV vaccine in lactating women.

Overall, both bivalent and quadrivalent vaccines are well tolerated, safe and so far there was no report on death directly related to the content of the vaccines. In June 2013, the WHO Global Advisory Committee on vaccine safety concluded that both HPV vaccines are generally safe and well tolerated.

WHO Global Advisory Commitee (GAC) Statement on the Update of HPV Vaccine Safety by 2013

At its meeting on 13 June 2013, WHO GAC reviewed updated information about safety of HPV vaccines. There was a approximately 175 million doses of HPV vaccines have been distributed worldwide. Although there were reported of new side-effects such as syncope, venous thromboembolism, stroke, Guillain-Barre syndrome and complex regional pain syndrome, their occurrence were very low and none have been found to have direct causal relationship to HPV vaccine. Surveillance of pregnancy outcomes among women inadvertently vaccinated during pregnancy through spontaneous reports and registries have not detected any adverse outcomes above expected rates. Therefore the Committee continues to reassure that both vaccines are generally safe and well tolerated. This statements is also endorsed by FIGO (International Federation of Gynecology and Obstetrics) and their Gynaecologic Oncology Committee as well as FIGO subcommittee for Cervical Cancer Prevention supports the continued administration of the HPV vaccines in appropriate population.

HPV Vaccination in Males

HPV vaccination is not only effective in females but recently, evidence has shown that HPV vaccine is also safe and efficacious against HPV infection and external genital lesions in young men (Palefsky, 2010; Giuliano et al., 2008). US Food and Drug Administration (FDA) had approved the use of Quadrivalent HPV vaccine in males (age 9–26 years old) in October 2009 for the prevention of genital warts. The new indication for Quadrivalent HPV vaccine is based on two trials. The first included 4055 males ages 16 through 26 that measured the vaccine's effectiveness in preventing genital warts. Overall, the study found a 90% reduction in genital warts and pre-cancerous lesions (PIN) caused by HPV (Giuliano et al., 2009; Palefsky 2008). The second trial studied immune response in boys ages 9 to 15, and the study suggested that the vaccine should have similar effectiveness in younger boys as the first study found for older males (Reisinger et al., 2007).

In 2011 the US Advisory Committee on Immunisation Practices approved and recommended routine use of Quadrivalent HPV vaccine for boys aged 11–21 years, with approval for administration up to age 26 years, in order to prevent genital warts and anal cancer (Palefsky et al., 2011). HPV vaccine has been approved for use in males by local health authority in Australia, Mexico and several other countries, including in some Asian countries such as Malaysia.

At present, HPV vaccination to males is still not a priority and we are still awaiting a conclusive data regarding the role of HPV vaccination in prevention of HPV-related cancers in males and HPV transmission to female. Following are the arguments of why HPV vaccination in males should be considered (Zimet and Rosenthal Rosenthal SL, 2010):

(a) The fastest way to achieve the greatest protection for females from cervical cancer and its precursors is to vaccinate males as well (through herd immunity).
(b) HPV vaccination to males will protect men who have sex with men from HPV and HPV-related diseases.
(c) Vaccination of males may be more acceptable to some cultural groups than vaccinating females.

(d) Implementations of risk-based (or gender-based) vaccination policies have been less effective and more confusing to the public.

(e) HPV vaccination in males will also reduce the burden of HPV-related precancerous, cancerous lesions as well as benign lesions accounted by male.

The main argument against the HPV vaccination to males is cost-effectiveness. Several studies have shown that vaccinating both males and females is less cost-effective than vaccinating females alone especially in young males and in countries with limited financial support (Kim, 2009). This cost-effective analysis study is still inconclusive as the study had assumed that 75% of eligible women would be vaccinated (lower than current coverage in US). If the coverage of female HPV vaccination is low, adding male vaccination may have clear health benefits for both genders. Furthermore, cost-effective analysis should also include prevention of HPV-associated diseases in men.

HPV Vaccine: Policy and Administration Guidelines

(1) HPV vaccine is most effective when given before exposure to HPV infection.

(2) Both HPV vaccines are given intramuscularly in three doses.

(3) Second dose is administered 1–2 months after the first dose and the minimum interval between the first and second dose is 4 weeks while the minimum interval between the second and third dose is 12 weeks.

(4) If the dose is given at the shorter minimum interval should be readministered.

(5) Coadministration of a different vaccine (either inactivated or live vaccine) is permitted because HPV vaccine is not a live vaccine.

(6) HPV vaccine can be administered to persons with immunocompromised state; however, the immune response may be less in the immunocompromised patient compared with a healthy individual.

(7) Person with mild acute illness (e.g. diarrhoea, mild upper respiratory tract infection) can receive the HPV vaccine. Vaccination of people with moderate or severe acute illnesses should be deferred until after the illness improves.

(8) Patient who received HPV vaccine is recommended to be observed for about 15 minutes after vaccination as syncopal attach is common.

(9) Whenever feasible, the same HPV vaccine should be used for the entire vaccination series, however, if the previous vaccine is not available, either vaccine can be used to complete the series to provide protection against HPV 16 and 18.

(10) Testing for HPV is currently not recommended before vaccination.

(11) HPV vaccines are not recommended for use in pregnant women; if women are found to be pregnant after initiating the vaccination series, the remainder of the three-dose series should be delayed until completion of pregnancy. If the vaccine dose has been administered during pregnancy, no intervention is needed.

(12) It is not known whether the vaccine antigens or antibodies are excreted in human milk. Lactating women can receive the HPV vaccine such as this, because it is an inactivated vaccine without live viral DNA.

(13) Women with previous abnormal cervical cytology or genital warts can receive the HPV vaccine but it may be less effective in women who have been infected with HPV before vaccination than in women who have not.

(14) Women with previous HPV infection will benefit from protection against infection of HPV genotypes with which they have not been infected.

(15) HPV vaccine can be given to patients with previous cervical intraepithelial neoplasia, but the benefits may be limited to protection against infection of HPV genotypes with which they have not been infected.

(16) HPV vaccines are contraindicated for persons with a history of immediate hypersensitivity to any vaccine component. A person who is allergic to yeast is contraindicated from quadrivalent HPV vaccine. While a person who is allergic

to latex should not be given vaccine which has latex in the rubber stopper of their prefilled syringes (in bivalent HPV vaccine).

(17) HPV vaccines should be introduced as part of a coordinated cervical cancer and other HPV-related diseases prevention strategy, including education on risk reducing behaviours, diagnosis and treatment of precancerous lesions and cancer.

(18) HPV vaccine introduction should not undermine or divert funding from effective cervical cancer screening programmes and it should not replace cervical cancer screening.

Table 6.10 Advantages and disadvantages of current prophylactic HPV vaccines

Advantages	Disadvantages
Highly immunogenic	Expensive (for low-income countries, the per dose cost would need to be less than US$ 5 for vaccination to be affordable.
High efficacy	Protection only against 2 oncogenic types and 6, 11 for quadrivalent vaccine. Cross protection only provided extra 11–16% reduction in cervical cancer incidence (prediction). Furthermore, the duration of cross protection is still unknown.
Induce memory B cells	Unsure duration of protection, decay of antibody response
Cross protection	Unsure the need for booster
Benefited in older age group up to 45 years old	Cost-effective analysis still unclear, perhaps cost-effective if the cost per-dose is much cheaper and when use in children & adolescents
Safe and well tolerated	Safety concerns and public perception
Potential effective in reducing the incidence and mortality of HPV 16, 18–related precancerous and cancerous lesions	Require 3 injections, proper storage and cold chain
Potential reduction in the burden of HPV 6, 11–related lesions with quadrivalent vaccine	A result on final endpoint (incidence and mortality rate of cervical cancer) can only be obtained after many years of vaccination.

Future Direction

Current HPV vaccine is very costly; the price will drop with time. However, using basic structural units of the HPV capsid known as L1 capsomer instead of whole VLPs was found to be much cheaper; besides L1 capsomer is more thermostable. L1 capsomers can be produced in Escherichia coli and expression of L1 in recombinant Salmonella enteric serovars. Inventing needle free administration route such as oral drop or nasal spray can also lower the cost of vaccine. The spectrum of coverage by HPV vaccine can be broadening by manufacturing multivalent HPV vaccine comprising more oncogenic HPV types. Merck also known as MSD outside the United State and Canada had conducted phase III clinical trials on nine-valent vaccine, V503. In this phase III trial (Protocol 001), V503 was compared to Quadrivalent vaccine (Gardasil) in term of efficacy, safety and immunogenicity. V503 consists of vaccine against 9 HPV types i.e 6, 11, 16, 18, 31, 33, 45, 52, 58 and was given to 7,099 females age between 16–26 years old. The results were:

(a) 96.7% reduction in the combined incidence of high grade lesions of cervical,vulvar and vagina, caused by HPV types 31, 33, 45, 52, 58,
(b) 97.1% reduction in the combined incidence of any grade of CIN/VIN/VaIN,
(c) 96.0% efficacy against 6-months persistent HPV infection with HPV types 31, 33, 45, 52 and 58,
(d) Similar immunogenicity against HPV 6, 11, 16 and 18 in V503 compared to Gardasil,
(e) similar safety profiles and frequencies of adverse event between V503 and Gardasil.

In Protocol 002 trial, immonogenicity "bridging data" of V503 administered to younger male and female age 9–15 years old were evaluated. Results from this study showed non-inferior immunogenicity of V503 in adolescent males and females compared with females 16–26 years old for all nine vaccine HPV type. The safety and tolerability were also comparable. Both of these trials were presented at the European Research Organisation on Genital Infection and Neoplasia (EUROGIN) Congress in November 2013. An effort must be made to manufacture a cheaper Multivalent HPV vaccine, which is more suitable for low-income countries. This can be achieved by reducing the cost of production, producing longer shelf life vaccine, vaccine that does not require cold chain and producing the vaccine that is effective even with a single dose. The other promising method to broaden the protection of HPV vaccine is by using L2 minor capsid protein instead of L1 major capsid protein. Study has shown that L2 minor capsid protein has broader cross protection across HPV genotypes. However, L2 protein is less immunogenic than L1 protein. Upon successfully finding an appropriate adjuvant, this approach may be explored in clinical trials. There is an urgent need for therapeutic HPV vaccine. The current HPV vaccines are prophylactic, and it would take many years through a well-organized vaccination program before it can reduce the incidence of cervical cancer. With therapeutic HPV vaccine, cell-mediated immunity will be employed (instead of humoral immunity in prophylactic vaccine) to immediately destroy the HPV-infected cells and therefore the outcome of this vaccine will be observed in the shorter period of time. Long overlapping peptides have stirred enthusiasm for therapeutic HPV E6/E7 peptide-based vaccines because they could limit the obstacle of major histocompatibility complex restriction by broadening the range of antigenic epitopes. Long overlapping peptides that represent E6 and E7 of HPV 16 was evaluated in phase II trial by Kenter GG in patients with vulvar intraepithelial neoplasia; the outcome from this trial was promising. The potency of therapeutic vaccine can be enhanced by using DNA vaccine, which has undergone microencapsulation to avoid degradation by enzyme nucleases. The example of this type of vaccine is Amolimogene bepiplasmid (ZYC101A); this vaccine comprised plasmid DNA that encodes E6/E7 proteins of HPV16/18 and encapsulated in biopolymer has been evaluated in the phase II/III trial for patients with CIN2/3.

The latest morbidity and mortality weekly report from the Centers for Disease Control and Prevention on vaccination coverage indicates that in 2012, only 53.8% of girls between 13 and 17 years old initiated HPV vaccination, and only 33.4% of them received all three doses. NCI-funded phase III trial had evaluated the efficacy of less than 3 doses of HPV vaccine (Bivalent) received by a group of women from Costa Rica. In this study, 78, 192 and 120 women received one, two and three doses of the vaccine respectively. The immune response was evaluated in all of these women and compared to 113 women who did not received the vaccine but had antibodies against the viruses because they were infected with HPV in the past. All vaccinated groups were found to have significant levels of antibody for at least 4 years, although the lesser dose was associated with lower antibody levels. The antibody levels in women received one and two doses were 5–24 times higher than the levels of antibodies in women who did not receive vaccination. Results from this study raise the possibility that even a single dose of HPV VLPs will induce long-term protection (Safaeian et al., 2013).

References

Agorastos T, Chatzigeorgiou K, Brotherton JML, Garland SM. Safety of human papillomavirus (HPV) vaccines: A review of the international experience so far. *Vaccine* 2009; **27**: 7270–7281.

Ault KA. Effect of prophylactic human papillomavirus L1 virus-like-particle vaccine on risk of cervical intraepithelial neoplasia grade 2, grade 3, and adenocarcinoma in situ: a combined analysis of four randomised clinical trials. *Lancet* 2007; **369**: 1861–1868.

Berumen J, Ordonez RM, Lazcano E, et al. Asian-American variants of human papillomavirus 16 and risk for cervical cancer. *J Natl Can Inst* 2001; **93**: 1325–1330.

Bonanni P, Boccalini S, Bechini A. Efficacy, duration of immunity and cross protection after HPV vaccination: A review of the evidence. *Vaccine* 2009; **27**: A46–A53.

Block SL, Brown DR, Chatterjee A, et al. Clinical trial and post-licensure safety profile of a prophylactic human papillomavirus (type 6, 11, 16 and 18) L1 virus-like particle vaccine. *Pediatr Infect Dis J* 2010; **29**: 95–101.

Brown et al. The impact of quadrivalent human papillomavirus (HPV; type 6, 11, 16 and 18) L1 virus-liked particle vaccine on infection and disease due to oncogenic nonvaccine HPV types in generally HPV-naïve women aged 16–26 years. *J Infect Dis* 2009; **199**: 926–35.

Carvalho ND, Teixeira J, Roteli-Martin CM, et al. Sustained efficacy and immunogenicity of the HPV 16/18 AS04 adjvanted vaccine up to 7.3 years in young women. *Vaccine* 2010; **28**: 6247–6255.

Castellsague X, Bosch FX, Munoz N, et al. Male circumcision, penile human papillomavurus infection, and cervical cancer in female partners. *N Engl J Med* 2002; **346**: 1105–1112.

Chang MH, Chen CJ, Lai MS, et al. Universal hepatitis B vaccination in Taiwan and the incidence of hepatocellular carcinoma in children. Taiwan Childhood Hepatoma Study Group. *N Engl J Med* 1997; **336**(26): 1855–1859.

Chaturvedi AK. Beyond cervical cancer: burden of other HPV-related cancers among men and women. *J Adolesc Health* 2010; **46**: S20–S26.

Chaturvedi AK. Beyond Cervical Cancer: burden of other HPV related cancers among men and women. *J Adolesc Health* 2010; **46**: S20–S26.

Descamps D, Hardt K, Spiessens B, et al. Safety of human papillomavirus (HPV)-16/18 AS04-adjuvanted vaccine for cervical cancer prevention: a pooled analysis of 11 clinical trials. *Hum Vaccin* 2009; **5**: 332–340.

Division of STD Prevention. Prevention of genital HPV infection and sequelae: Report of an External Consultants Meeting, December 1999. Atlanta, GA: department of Health and Human Services, Centers for Disease Control and Prevention: 1999.

Dunne EF, Nielson CM, Stone KM, Markowitz LE, Giuliano AR. Prevalence of HPV infection among men: a systematic review of the literature. *J Infect Dis* 2006; **194**: 1044–1057.

Einstein MH, Baron M, Levin MJ, et al. Comparison of the immunogenicity and safety of Cervarix and Gardasil human papillomavirus (HPV) cervical cancer vaccine in healthy women aged 18–45 years. *Hum Vaccin* 2009; **5**(10): 1–15.

Evans M, Powell NG. The changing aetiology of Head and Neck Cancer: the role of human papillomavirus. *Clin Oncol* 2010; **22**: 538–546.

Food and Drug Administration. Product approval-prescribing information [package insert]. Cervarix [human papillomavirus bivalent (types 16 and 18) vaccine, recombinant], Glaxo Smith Kline Biologicals: Food and Drug Administration 2009. Available at http://www.fda.gov/biologicsbloodvaccines/vaccines/approvedproducts/ucm186957.htm. Accessed May 25, 2010.

Frazer IH, Cox JT, Mayeaux EJ, et al. Advances in prevention of cervical cancer and other human papillomavirus-related diseases. *Pediat Infect Dis J* 2006; **25**(2): S65–S81.

Future II Study Group. Quadrivalent vaccine against human papillomavirus to prevent high-grade cervical lesions. *N Engl J Med* 2007; **356**: 1915–1927.

Garland SM, Hernandez-Avila M, Wheeler CM, Perez G, Harper DM, Leodolter S, et al. Quadrivalent vaccine against human papillomavirus to prevent anogenital diseases. *N Engl J Med* 2007; **356**: 1928–1943.

Gillison ML, Chaturvedi AK, Lowy DR. HPV prophylactic vaccines and the potential prevention of noncervical cancers in both men and women. *Cancer* 2008; **113**(S10): 3036–3046.

Gissmann L. Review Artcle: HPV vaccine: Preclinical Development. *Arch Med Res* 2009; **40**: 466–470.

Giuliano AR, Anic G, Nyitray AG. Epidemiology and pathology of HPV disease in males. *Gynecol Oncol* 2010; **117**: S15–S19.

Giuliano AR, Lazcano Ponce E, Villa LL, et al. The human papillomavirus infection in men study: human papillomavirus prevalence and type distribution among men residing in Brazil, Mexico, and the United States. *Cancer Epidemiol Biomarker Prev* 2008; **17**: 2036–2043.

Giuliano AR, Lazcano E, Villa LL, Flores R, et al. Circumcision and sexual behavior: factors independently associated with human papillomavirus detection among men in the HIM study. *Int J Cancer* 2009; **124**: 1251–1257.

Giuliano AR, Palefsky J. The efficacy of quadrivalent HPV (type 6/11/16/18) vaccine in reducing the incidence of HPV-related genital disease in young men. EUROGIN 2008; France: Abstract SS 19-7a.

Giuliano AR, Palefsky J. The efficacy of quadrivalent HPV (type 6/11/16/18) vaccine in reducing the incidence of HPV-related genital disease in young men. Presented in 25th International Papillomavirus Congress, May 8–14, 2009, Malmo, Sweden. Presentation O-01.07.

Harper DM, Franco EL, Wheeler C, et al. Efficacy of a bivalent L1 virus-like particle vaccine in prevention of infection with human papillomavirus type 16 and 18 in young women: a randomized controlled trial. *Lancet* 2004; **364**: 1757–1765.

Herrero R, Hildesheim A, Bratti C, et al. Population-based study of human papillomavirus infection and cervical neoplasia in rural Costa Rica. *J Natl Cancer Inst* 2000; **92**: 464–74.

Herrero R, Hildesheim A, Rodriguez AC, Wacholder S, Bratti C, Solomon D, et al. Rationale and design of a community-based double-blind randomized clinical trial of an HPV 16 and 18 vaccine in Guanacaste, Costa Rica. *Vaccine* 2008; **26**: 4795–808.

IARC. *IARC Monographs on the Evaluation of Carcinogenic Risk to Humans*. Human Papillomaviruses, vol. 90. Lyon, France: IARC Press, 2007.

Joura EA, Leodolter S, Hernandez-Avila M, Wheeler CM, Perez G, Koutsky LA, et al. Efficacy of a quadrivalent prophylactic human papillomavirus (types 6, 11, 16, and 18) L1 virus-likeparticle vaccine against high-grade vulval and vaginal lesions: a combined analysis of three randomised clinical trials. *Lancet* 2007; **369**: 1693–1702.

Kenter GG, Welters MJ, Valentijin AR, et al. Vaccination against HPV 16 oncoproteins for vulvar intraepithelial neoplasia. *N Eng J Med* 2009; **361**: 1838–1847.

Kim JJ, Brisson M, Edmunds WJ, Goldie SJ. Modeling cervical cancer prevention in developed countries. *Vaccine* 2008; **26** (Suppl 10): K76–K86.

Kim JJ, Goldie SJ. Cost effectiveness analysis of including boys in a human papillomavirus vaccination program in the United State. *BMJ* 2009; b3884: 339 doi: http://dx.doi.org/10.1136/bmj.b3884.

Koutsky LA, Ault KA, Wheeler CM, et al. A controlled trial of a human papillomavirus type 16 vaccine. *N Engl J Med* 2002; **347**: 1645–1651.

Koutsky L. The epidemiology behind the HPV vaccine discovery. *Ann Epidemiol* 2009; **19**: 239–244.

Lizano M, Berumen J, Garcia-Carranca A. Review Article: HPV-related carcinogenesis: Basic concepts, viral types and variants. *Arch Med Res* 2009; **40**: 428–434.

Lu B, Wu Y, Nielson CM, et al. Factors associated with acquisition and clearance of human papillomavirus infection in a cohort of US men: a prospective study. *J Infect Dis* 2009; **199**: 362–371.

Marina VM, Poveda KT, Toledo GL, Caranca AG. Advantages and disadvantages of current prophylactic vaccines against HPV. *Arch Med Res* 2009; **40**: 471–477.

Medina DMR, Valencia A, de Velsquez A, et al. Safety and immunogenicity of the HPV 16/18 adjuvanted vaccine: A randomized, controlled trial in adolescent girls. *J Adolesc Health* 2010; **46**: 414–421.

McCredie MR, Sharples KJ, Paul C, et al. Natural history of cervical neoplasia and risk of invasive cancer in women with cervical intraepithelial neoplasia 3: a retrospective cohort study. *Lancer Oncol* 2008; **9**: 425–434.

Moscicki AB. Review article. HPV vaccines: today and in the future. *J Adolesc Health* 2008; **43**: S26–S40.

Munoz N, Castellsaque X, de Gonzalez AB, Gissmann L. Chapter 1: HPV in the etiology of human cancer. *Vaccine* 2006; **24** (Suppl 3) S3/1–10.

Munoz N, Manalastas Jr R, Pitisuttithum P, et al. Safety, immunogenicity and efficacy of quadrivalent human papillomavirus (type 6, 11, 16, 18) recombinant vaccine in women aged 24–45 years: a randomized, double blind trial. *Lancet* 2009; **373**: 1949–1957.

Nielson CM, Schiaffino MK, Dunne EF, Salemi JL, Giuliano AR. Associations between male anogenital human papillomavirus infection and circumcision by anatomic site sampled and lifetime number of female sex partners. *J Infect Dis* 2009; **199**: 7–13.

Olsson SE, Villa LL, Costa RL, Petta CA, Andrade RP, Malm C, et al. Induction of immune memory following administration of a prophylactic quadrivalent human papillomavirus (HPV) types 6/11/16/18 L1 virus-like particle (VLP) vaccine. *Vaccine* 2007; **25**(26): 4931–4939.

Paavonen J, Naud P, Salmeron J, et al. Efficacy of human papillomavirus (HPV)16/18 AS04-adjuvanted vaccine against cervical infection and precancer caused by oncogenic HPV types (PATRICIA): final analysis of a double-blind, randomized study in young women. *Lancet* 2009; **374**: 301–314.

Palefsky JM. Human Papillomavirus-related disease in men: not just a women's issue. *J Adolesc Health* 2010; **46**: S12–S19.

Palefsky J, Giuliano A. Efficacy of the quadrivalent HPV vaccine against HPV 6/11/16/18-related genital infection in young men. Presented at the 2008 conference of the European research organization on genital infection and neoplasia (EUROGIN); 2008 November 12–15; Nice, France. Abstract PS 1–3a.

Palefsky JM, Giuliano AR, Goldstone S, et al. HPV vaccine against anal HPV infection and anal intraepithelial neoplasia. *N Eng J Med* 2011; **365**: 1576–1585.

Reisinger KS, Block SL, Lazcano-Ponce E, et al. Safety and persistent immunogenicity of a quadrivalent human papillomavirus types 6, 11, 16, 18 L1 virus-like particle vaccine in preadolescents and adolescents: a randomized controlled trial. *Pediatr Infect Dis J* 2007; **26**(3): 201–209.

Safaeian M, Porras C, Pan Y, et al. Durable Antibody Responses Following One Dose of the Bivalent Human Papillomavirus L1 Virus-Like Particle Vaccine in the Costa Rica Vaccine Trial. *Cancer Prev Res*, November 2013; **6**(11): 1242–50. doi:10.1158/1940-6207.CAPR-13-0203.

Schiffman M, Castle PE, Jeronimo J, et al. Human papillomavirus and cervical cancer. *Lancet* 2007; **370**: 890–907.

Stanley M. Pathology and epidemiology of HPV infection in female. *Gynecol Oncol* 2010; **117**: S5–S10.

The Future II Study Group. Prophylactic efficacy of a quadrivalent HPV vaccine in women with virologic evidence of HPV infection. *J Infect Dis* (in press) 2007; **196**(10): 1438–1446.

The GlaxoSmithKline Vaccine HPV 007 study. Sustained efficacy and immunogenicity of the HPV 16/18 AS04 adjuvanted vaccine: analysis of a randomized placebo-controlled trial up to 6.4 years. *Lancet* 2009; **374**: 1975–1985.

Van Doornum GJ, Prins M, Juffermans LH, et al. Regional distribution and incidence of human papillomavirus infection among heterosexual men and women with multiple sexual partners: a prospective study. *Genitourin Med* 1994; **70**: 240–246.

Verstraeten T, Descamps D, David MP, et al. Analysis of adverse events of potential autoimmune aetiology in a large integrated safety database of AS04 adjuvanted vaccines. *Vaccine* 2008; **26**: 6630–6638.

Villa LL, Costa RL, Petta CA, Andrade RP, Ault KA, Giuliano AR, et al. Prophylactic quadrivalent human papillomavirus (types 6, 11, 16, and 18) L1 virus-like particle vaccine in young women: a randomised double-blind placebo-controlled multicentre phase II efficacy trial. *Lancet Oncol* 2005; **6**: 271–278.

Villa LL, Costa RL, Petta CA, Andrade RP, Paavonen J, Iversen OE, et al. High sustained efficacy of a prophylactic quadrivalent human papillomavirus types 6/11/16/18 L1 virus-like particle vaccine through 5 years of follow-up. *Br J Cancer* 2006; **95**: 1459–1466.

Villa LL. Overview of the clinical development and results of a quadrivalent HPV (type 6, 11, 16, 18) vaccine. International *J Infect Dis* 2007; **11**(Suppl 2): S17–S25.

Winer RL, Hughes JP, Feng Q, et al. Condom use and the risk of genital human papillomavirus infection in young women. *N Engl J Med* 2006; **354**: 2645–2654.

Zimet GD, Rosenthal SL. HPV vaccine and males: issues and challenges. *Gynecol Oncol* 2010; **117**: S26–S31.

Chapter 7

Management of Preinvasive Disease of the Cervix

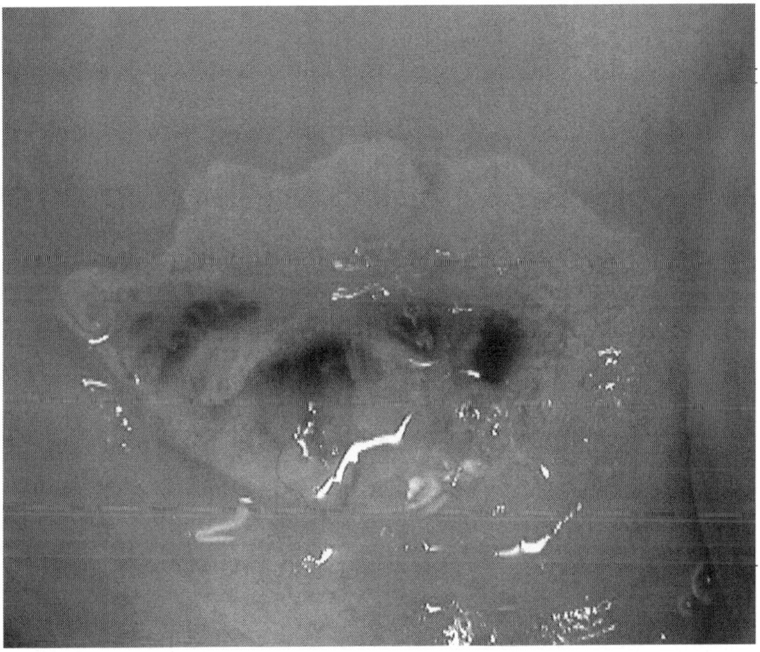

Gynaecologic Cancer: A Handbook for Students and Practitioners
Rushdan Noor, Eng Hseon Tay, and Jeffrey Low

ISBN 978-981-4463-06-5 (Hardcover), 978-981-4463-07-2 (eBook)
www.panstanford.com

Introduction

Cytology, visual inspection and HPV testing are screening tests for preinvasive and invasive cervical cancer. They are not diagnostic and, therefore, their results must not be used as an indication for treatment. Patients with a positive screening test must be referred for diagnostic test/procedure. Colposcopy and biopsy are diagnostic procedures for preinvasive disease of the cervix. Diagnosis of preinvasive disease of the cervix must be made based on histology reports from cervical biopsy. Treatment of preinvasive disease reduces the incidence of invasive carcinoma of the cervix. In selected patients and with the presence of well-trained colposcopist, "screen and treat" approach may be acceptable. This is, however, a relatively new approach and the long-term impact on the cancer incidence has yet to be evaluated.

Descriptive histologic term for preinvasive lesion of the cervix is called cervical intraepithelial neoplasm (CIN). CIN is subdivided into CIN 1 (mild), CIN 2 (moderate) and CIN 3 (severe dysplasia). The CIN subdivision is based on the degree of penetration of cellular abnormalities from the basal membrane to the surface of the cervical epithelium. The CIN 1 is referred to when one third of the epithelium is involved in the dysplastic changes, two-third involvement in CIN 2 and full-thickness involvement in CIN 3. Many CIN lesions regress spontaneously over time even without treatment. CIN can also progress from mild to moderate and then to severe lesions. Progression rate is depending on the grade of lesions and age of patients. Low-grade and younger age group (<30 years old) are more likely to regress. Rate of progression in biopsy-proven CIN is shown in Table 7.1.

Table 7.1 Rate of progression for biopsy-proven CIN (Ostor, 1993)

	Regression	Persistent	Progression
CIN 1	57%	32%	11%
CIN 2	43%	35%	22%
CIN 3	32%	56%	12%

Some studies have shown that the spontaneous regression rate for CIN 1 was actually much higher in younger women, i.e.

>90% within 24–36 months' follow-up (Schlecht et al., 2003; Nobbenhuis et al., 2001; Moscicki et al., 2004).

Management of Abnormal PAP Smear

If the Pap smear is reported as unsatisfactory, identify the cause, treat and repeat the smear in 3 months; treat the infection if it exist, and give a course of local oestrogen therapy if the cytology reported as atrophic changes. Refer for colposcopy if a same finding in three consecutive smears. If the Pap smear is reported as inflammatory, identify the cause and source of infections, treat inflammatory smears with antifungal, antibiotic or antiviral according to the organisms involved. Refer for colposcopy if three consecutive inflammatory changes persist on smear.

Management of atypical squamous cells is as follows: (a) ASCUS-H (Atypical squamous cell of unknown significant, cannot exclude high-grade lesion: Refer for colposcopy, (b) ASCUS: Repeat smear in 6 months, refer for colposcopy if ASCUS persist and (c) ASCUS and positive to high-risk HPV: Refer for colposcopy.

Patients with low-grade squamous intraepithelial lesions (LSIL) should be referred for colposcopy if they have the following criteria: (a) age > 30 years old, (b) poor compliance, (c) immuno-compromised patient, (d) positive to high-risk HPV and (e) had CIN in the past. Other low-risk patients should be managed expectantly; repeat Pap smear in 6 months and refer for colposcopy if persistent LSIL for more than 12 months.

Patients with following Pap smear abnormalities require urgent colposcopy referral: (a) high-grade squamous intraepithelial lesion (HSIL), (b) atypical glandular cells (AGUS), (c) adenocarcinoma in situ, (d) squamous cell carcinoma and (e) adenocarcinoma.

Colposcopy

Colposcopy was first introduced by Hinselman in 1925. A colposcope is a low-power, stereoscopic, binocular field microscope with a powerful light source (Fig. 7.1). Colposcopy is the direct inspection of magnified areas of vulva, vagina and cervix using the colposcope. During colposcopy, biopsy will be performed from abnormal area. Colposcopy is also done to guide the colposcopist in the treatment for preinvasive disease of vulva, vagina and cervix. See Table 7.2 for the preparation and step-by-step colposcopic procedures.

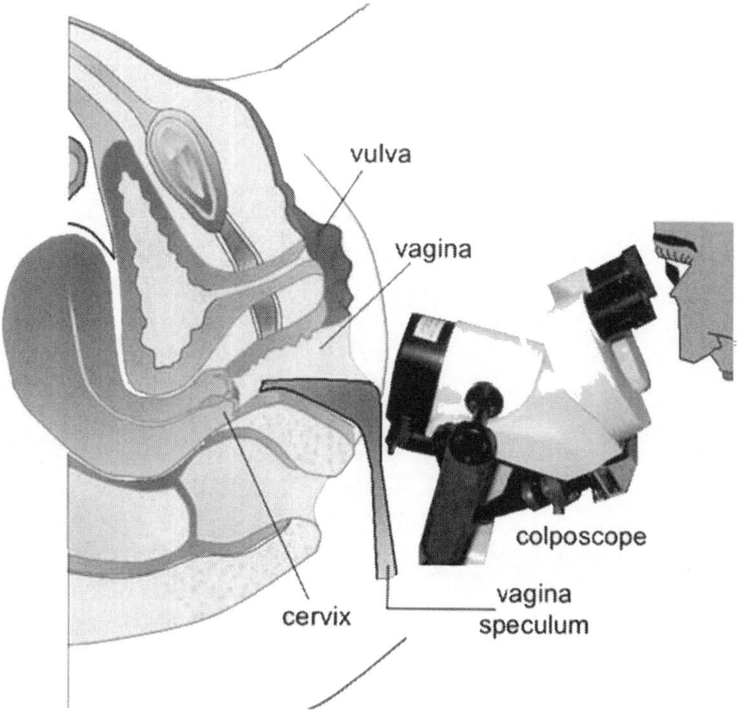

Figure 7.1 Colposcopy.

Table 7.2 Preparation, equipment and step-by-step colposcopy

(1) Colposcope machine, monitor, printer ± workstation (computer, printer, etc.)
(2) Colposcope couch
(3) Speculum, cotton swabs, sponge holding forceps, 20 cm dissecting forceps
(4) Vaginal side wall retractor
(5) Endocervical speculum
(6) Endocervical curette
(7) Biopsy forcep (e.g. Tischler-Morgan, Townsend, etc.)
(8) Single-toothed tenaculum
(9) Acetic acid 3–5%, Lugol's iodine solution

Step-by-step colposcopic procedures
▪ Counselling and explaining regarding the procedure ▪ Obtained an informed consent ▪ Modified lithotomy position ▪ Instrument tray with essential instruments for colposcopy is placed beside the couch ▪ Inspect the vulva ▪ Insertion of speculum ▪ If the vaginal wall is too lax, used vaginal wall retractor or applied a latex condom (from the glove) on the speculum blades with opening at the tip. ▪ While inserting the speculum, inspect the vaginal wall ▪ Identify the cervix and remove any excess mucous ▪ Repeat Pap smear may be necessary if it was not done earlier or the colposcopist interested to know the repeat test ▪ Swab for culture is taken if indicated ▪ Inspect the cervix quadrant by quadrant on a normal light source and then switch to green filter to look for abnormal vessels ▪ Return to normal light ▪ Identify squamo-columnar junction and transformation zone ▪ Spray or soaked the cervix with acetic acid 3–5% for 1–2 minutes ▪ Inspect the cervix for any abnormal epithelium characterized by white epithelium with well-demarcated margin, looks also for abnormal vessels such as punctation, mosaicism, etc.; please note that apart from the abnormal epithelium, light white epithelium can also be observed in the epithelium undergoing metaplasia ▪ Lugol's iodine application is an option, especially if colposcopist is decided to perform treatment at the same setting; normal squamous epithelium contains stores of glycogen will give a mahogany brown or nearly black stain; abnormal epithelium and columnar epithelium do not contain glycogen and therefore, does not take up the iodine ▪ Biopsy is taken from the abnormal epithelium ▪ Haemostasis is secured by applying Monsel's solution ▪ Endocervical biopsy or curettage is performed if necessary: (a) Normal colposcopy but abnormal cells were seen on cytology (b) If cytology reported the presence of abnormal glandular cells (c) If colposcopic examination is unsatisfactory ▪ Colposcopy is considered as unsatisfactory when the upper limit of transformation zone or squamo-columnar junction is not seen ▪ Endometrial biopsy/sampling is indicated if abnormal endometrial cells were detected on cytology or presence of endometrial cells in postmenopausal women

(*Continued*)

Table 7.2 (*Continued*)

- Withdrawn the speculum and perform a bimanual pelvic examination
- Explain the findings to the patient
- Document the findings
- Diagnostic accuracy of colposcopy is assessed based on the correlation between colposcopic findings and final histological reports; in a large retrospective analysis by (Benedet GL, 2004), involving more than 84,000 women, the accuracy of colposcopy was found to improve by the severity of the lesion (85% accuracy in high-grade lesion).

Indications for Colposcopy

Following are the indications for colposcopic examination:

- recurrent unexplained postcoital bleeding
- suspicious looking cervix
- invasive carcinoma on cytology
- persistent LSIL on cytology of more than 12 months
- persistent unsatisfactory smears (3 consecutively)
- three consecutive smears showing borderline nuclear changes
- high-grade lesion (HSIL/CIN 2, 3) on cytology
- CIN 1 or LSIL on cytology in a poorly compliant patients
- evidence of infection by oncogenic type of HPV
- VIA positive
- VILI positive
- Truscreen/Truscan/Polarprobe positive
- positive results in other screening tests

Objectives of Colposcopy

(1) to further assess abnormalities detected on cytology
(2) to confirm the diagnosis by directed biopsy
(3) to exclude invasive disease
(4) to aid in outpatient management of preinvasive disease
(5) follow-up after treatment

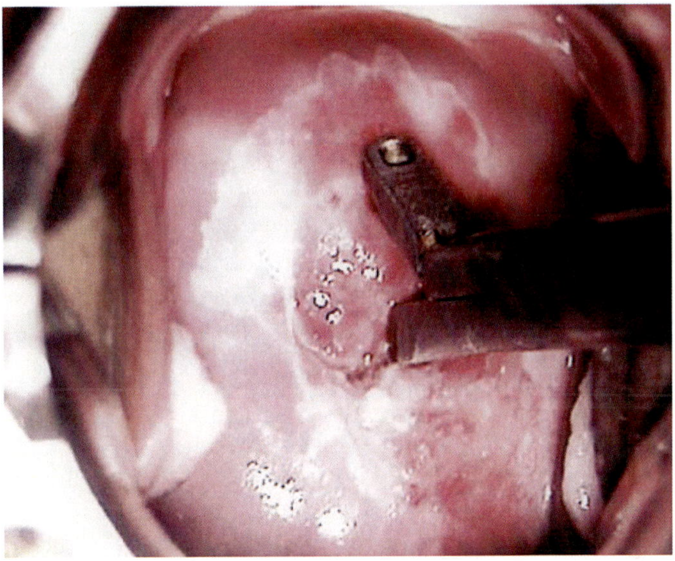

Figure 7.2 Cervical biopsy to confirm the CIN.

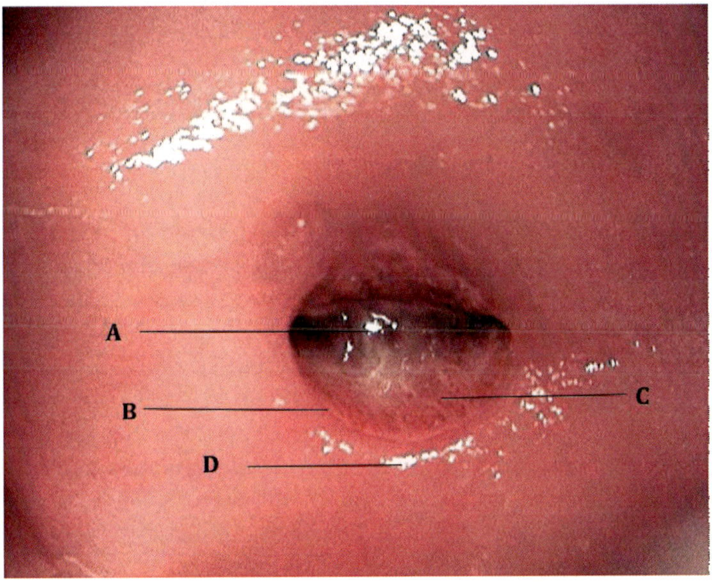

Figure 7.3 Normal cervix. A: cervical mucus from the endocervical canal, B: squamo-columnar junction, C: endocervical epithelium, D: ectocervical epithelium.

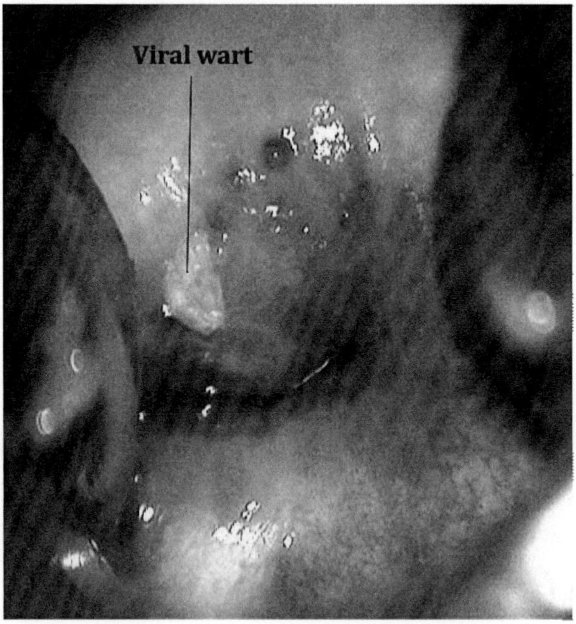

Figure 7.4 Viral wart or condylomata acuminata. Watch a raised lesion, white and well-defined margin without acetic acid application. The lesion is located just outside the transformation zone.

HPV Testing and Colposcopic Referral

It is widely accepted that women with high-grade abnormalities on cytology should be referred for colposcopy. Management of women with borderline or minor cytological abnormalities, e.g. ASCUS, AGUS and LSIL, is controversial although they constitute up to 10% of total cytological reports from screened population. Current evidence suggests that 5–47% of those borderline abnormalities, will, in fact reveal occult high-grade lesions in final histological reports. Studies have shown that women with borderline or minor cytological abnormalities on cytology and at the same time positive to high-risk HPV is at the higher possibility of having co-existing high-grade lesions on histology.

One of the most important trials that address the role of HPV testing in patients with borderline smear is ASCUS-LSIL Triage Study or ALTS. ASCUS-LSIL Triage Study (ALTS) initiated by National Cancer Institute is a randomized controlled trial to compare between immediate colposcopy versus HPV testing followed by colposcopy if positive to oncogenic HPV versus conservative management (N = 5060); the subjects were women with ASCUS and LSIL. The following are the results of ALTS study: (a) HPV triage is not suitable for LSIL because 83% of patients were positive (b) The most cost-effective approach to ASCUS is to perform reflex HPV testing (63% positive and require colposcopy), (c) HPV testing reduced the need for referral for colposcopy by 44% among women with ASCUS.

Meta-analysis by Arbyn et al. to compare an approach between repeat cytology versus HPV testing (Hybrid capture-2) as a triage method for women with ASCUS/AGUS on initial cytology have shown that HPV testing had a significantly higher sensitivity (95% versus 82%) in predicting high-grade lesions histologically. However, specificity of both approaches was comparable. In LSIL and above, HPV testing did not improve the sensitivity; in fact it had lower specificity.

The Trial of Management of Borderline and Other Low Grade Abnormal Smear (TOMBOLA) is a multicentre randomized controlled trial conducted in Scotland and England, compared the effectiveness and efficiency of cytological surveillance and immediate colposcopy in dealing of patients with low-grade abnormality of cervical smear. The results from this study have shown that (a) immediate colposcopy leads to overtreatment and more women experienced pain, bleeding, etc., (b) 30% of women with mild dyskaryosis were found to have CIN 2 and worse after colposcopy and biopsy, (c) approximately, 40% of patients with low-grade cervical abnormalities have evidence of high-risk HPV infection, (d) cytology surveillance might result in some cases of high-grade disease being missed because of non-attendance or limited sensitivity and (e) there is still uncertainty regarding the best form of follow-up either colposcopy or continued cytological surveillance.

Management of Cervical Intraepithelial Neoplasm

Cervical intraepithelial neoplasm must be diagnosed based on histological examination either from cervical punch biopsy or excisional biopsy. There are three types of CIN, i.e. CIN 1, CIN 2 and CIN

3. CIN (Fig. 7.5) 1 is considered low-grade lesion, while CIN 2 and CIN 3 are high-grade lesions and are true precancerous state of cervical cancer (Fig. 7.6). Majority of CIN 1 disappears spontaneously and needs no treatment; however, treatment is recommended if patients meet the following criteria: (a) poor compliance, (b) persistent CIN 1 for more than 12 months, (c) women older than 30 years and (c) positive to oncogenic HPV or high-risk of cervical cancer.

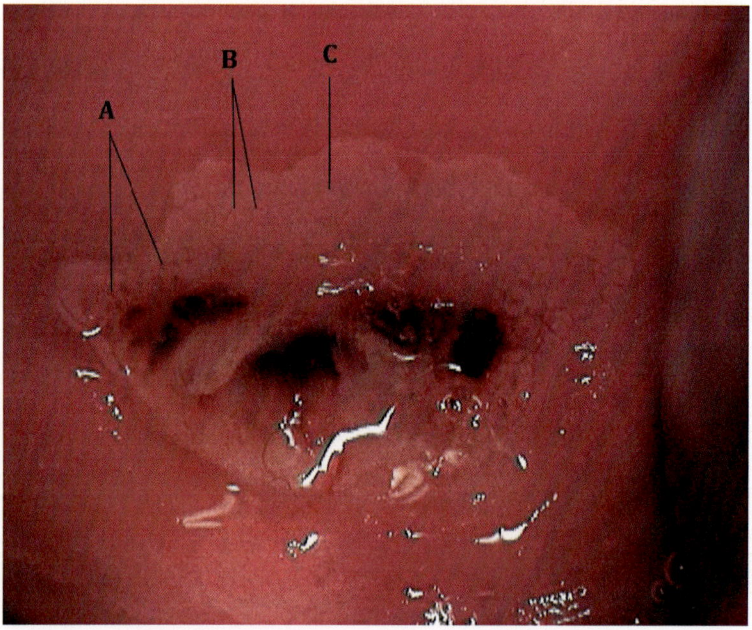

Figure 7.5 Abnormal cervix after application of acetic acid. A: punctation, B: acetowhite epithelium, C: fine mosaicism. Cervical biopsy-proven CIN 1.

All women with CIN 2 and CIN 3 must be treated. There are two main modality of treatment for preinvasive disease of cervix: (1) **local ablative treatment** and **(2) excisional treatment**.

Following are the types of local ablative treatment:

(a) cryotherapy (see below)
(b) electrodiathermy
(c) cold coagulation
(d) carbon dioxide laser

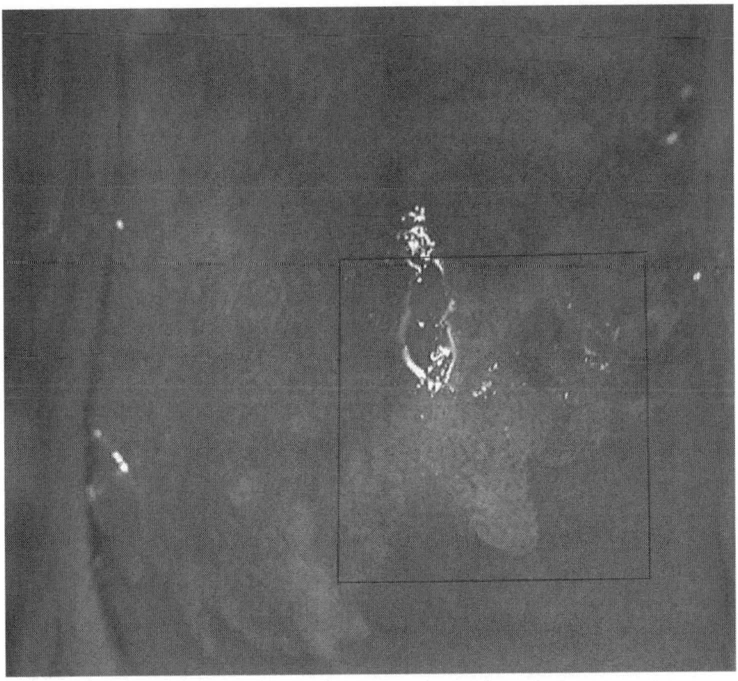

Figure 7.6 Abnormal cervix, high-grade lesion. Watch the significant acetowhite, punctuation and mosaicism seen in the box.

Local ablative treatment is indicated in persistent low-grade lesions (CIN 1). This treatment is not suitable if squamo-columnar junction and the limits of the lesions are not seen on colposcopy. Local ablative treatment is also not recommended if invasive disease cannot be ruled out. The disadvantage of local ablative treatment is there is no tissue specimen for histological examination.

In selected patients, local ablative treatment may be acceptable for high-grade lesions (CIN 2 and CIN 3) provide, they have fulfilled the following criteria:

(1) The treatment is performed by trained colposcopist.
(2) The entire lesions are seen.
(3) The lesions are small.
(4) There is no suspicion of microinvasive, invasive and glandular lesions.
(5) The patient is in good compliance.

Following are the types of excisional treatment:

(a) loop electrosurgical excision procedure (LEEP) or large loop excision of transformation zone (LLETZ)
(b) laser conization/laser excision of transformation zone
(c) cold-knife cone biopsy
(d) trachelectomy
(e) hysterectomy

Excisional treatment is the treatment of choice for high-grade lesions (CIN 2, 3) and also for cervical adenocarcinoma in situ. With excisional treatment, tissue samples are obtained for histological examination. LEEP/LLETZ is the most commonly performed excisional treatment for preinvasive lesions of the cervix. Laser conization has an advantage for being more precise, less lateral thermal injuries and better haemostasis. However, laser treatment requires special training, expensive equipment and stringent safety precautions. The other excisional method is cold-knife cone biopsy. Cold-knife cone biopsy is an excision of a cone-shaped area from the cervix, using scalpel. Cold-knife conization has to be done in the operating theatre under regional or general anaesthesia. It is indicated if the lesions are unable to be excised completely by LEEP/LLETZ. Some Gynaecologists prefer to do cold-knife conization in a patient with suspicious of endocervical lesions and endocervical adenocarcinoma in situ. Cold-knife conization carries slightly higher rate of complications as compared to LEEP/LLETZ and laser conization.

Risk of bleeding is small; Nuovo et al., had reported that the risk of bleeding is 4.6% in cold-knife conization, laser ablation (1.75%), LEEP (1.35%) and cryotherapy (0%). Systematic review and meta-analysis by (Kyrgiou M, Koliopoulus I, Vrekoussis T, et al. 2006) have shown that all three types of excisional treatment for preinvasive disease of cervix (LEEP, cold-knife conization and laser conization) was associated with a small but real increase risk of pregnancy-related morbidity such as preterm delivery, premature rupture of membranes, low birth weight and caesarean section. However, there was no significant risk to neonatal morbidity.

Study by Klaritsch on the obstetrics outcome after cold-knife conization of the cervix had found that, this surgery was associated with an increased risk of delivery before 37 weeks (22.4% versus 6.6%) and preterm premature of membranes (17.1% versus 2.6%). There was no difference in terms of mode of delivery, duration of labour and perinatal outcome (Klaritsch P, et al. 2006).

Trachelectomy is excision of the cervix. Partial or total trachelectomy has been successfully performed in selected patients with recurrent high-grade lesions following conization and fertility preserving procedure.

The patients who have completed their family and are presented with recurrent high-grade lesions following conservative surgery may be offered hysterectomy if repeat conization is not feasible or inappropriate. Hysterectomy is also recommended in patients with endocervical adenocarcinoma in situ when the fertility is not anymore an issue.

Loop Electrosurgical Excision Procedure

Loop electrosurgical excision procedure is also known as large loop excision of the transformation zone (LLETZ) in UK and Europe. It is the removal of abnormal areas from the cervix using a thin heated wire by constant low voltage current from the electrosurgical unit (Fig. 7.7). The wire is in the form of loops that is very fine stainless steel or tungsten wire and come with different shapes and sizes. The loop cuts and coagulates at the same time. For the purpose of haemostasis, ball diathermy is also available. LEEP can be done as an outpatient procedure under local anaesthesia. Please refer to Table 7.3 for step-by-step LEEP or LLETZ.

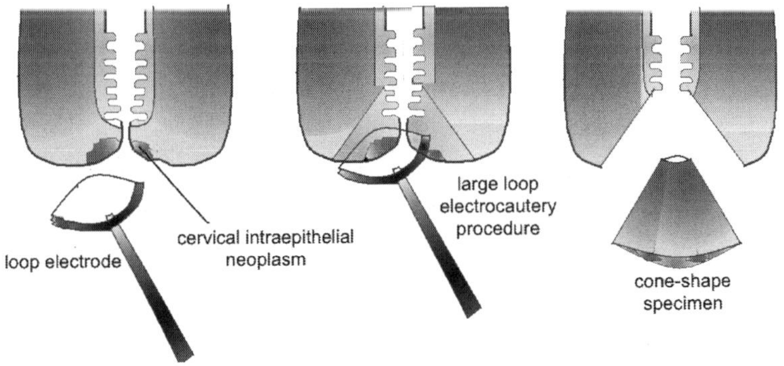

Figure 7.7 Basic principle of LEEP.

Table 7.3 Step-by-step LEEP/LLETZ

- Counselling and consent
- Provide oral analgesic, e.g. paracetamol/NSAIDs; to be taken 1 hour prior to the procedure
- Prophylactics antibiotic is optional and may be warranted in patients with higher risk of infection (e.g. immunosuppressive) or who had a history of vaginitis/cervicitis
- Ensure the equipment is available and is in good condition
- The patient is placed in the lithotomy position
- Insert the speculum and connected it with tubing to smoke evacuator
- Clean the vagina and cervix from mucous and discharge
- Re-examine the cervix and apply Lugol's iodine to determine the location and borders of the lesions
- Infiltrate local anaesthetic agents, i.e. xylocaine 1% with 1:80,000 dilution of adrenaline diluted in normal saline (using 5 mL syringe and 25–27G needle). Infiltrate 1 mL in each quadrant, total maximum of 5 mL. Wait for 1–2 minutes
- Choose appropriate loop based on the size of lesions and type of transformation zone. Loop must be wider than the lesions and the transformation zone to be removed
- Used cutting current 35–60 W
- The loop is introduced into the tissue 5 mm outside the margin of a lesion. The loop is directed gradually into the cervix until the horizontal bar nearly comes to the contact of the epithelial surface. Then swipe across from left to right preferably in a single pass
- Any bleeding from the raw area can be tackled by ball diathermy using spray mode 50–60 W. Monsel's solution can be applied to further secure the haemostasis
- If a lesion involves the endocervical canal and is not likely to have been removed with single pass, endocervical tissue can be excised via second pass using smaller loop either smaller oval loop or square loop (top-hat technique)
- The specimen must be orientated and marked at 12 o'clock position to guide the pathologist
- Observe the patient for 15–30 minutes after the procedure and allow home with oral analgesic
- Follow up the patient after 1–2 weeks

Counselling after LEEP/LLETZ

Following are most important informations that should be given to patient following the LEEP:

- mild cramping pain for a few hours

- dark brownish vaginal discharge for a week
- mild vaginal spotting for 1–2 weeks
- avoid vaginal douching and tampon
- to return back if having heavy bleeding, severe pain, foul smelling vaginal discharge and fever
- avoid sexual intercourse for 3–4 weeks

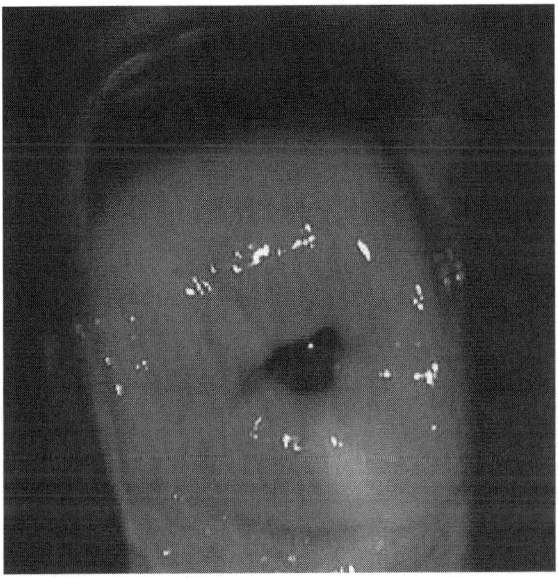

Figure 7.8 Complete healing after LEEP.

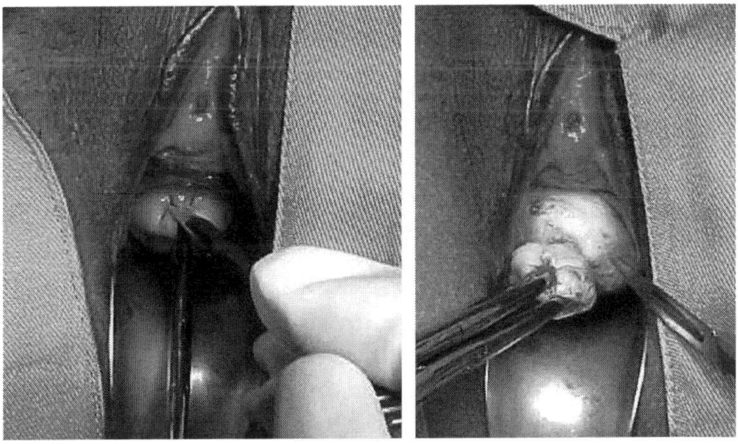

Figure 7.9 Cold cone knife conization.

Cryotherapy

Cervical cryotherapy is a procedure which involves freezing an area of abnormal tissue on the cervix. Cryotherapy is done by placing a small freeze-probe known as a cryoprobe against the cervix that cools the cervix to at least –20°C. The cells destroyed by freezing (cryonecrosis). The advantage of cryotherapy is cheap and can be done without anaesthesia. Cryotherapy relies on a steady supply of compressed refrigerant gases (N_2O or CO_2) in transportable cylinders. However, cryotherapy is not recommended to treat lesions in endocervix. The reported success rate is from 88–94%.

The preparation and step-by-step cryotherapy procedures are shown on Table 7.4.

Cryotherapy unit consists of three components: (1) cryoprobe and cryogun, (2) gas conveying tube and (3) gas cylinder.

Table 7.4 The preparation and step-by-step cryotherapy procedures

Material and equipment for cryotherapy
(1) Speculum (2) Glove (3) Cotton swab (4) Normal saline solution (5) Acetic acid solution (6) ± Colposcope (7) Cryotherapy Unit
Step-by-step cryotherapy procedures
• Counsel the patient • Inserting the speculum • Wipe the cervix with saline to wash the discharge and mucus • Apply acetic acid to outline the abnormalities • Explain to women that they may feel discomfort • Wipe the cryoprobe surface with saline • Apply the cryoprobe tip to the cervix with a tip in the internal os • Set timer and release the gas trigger to cool the probe • Observe the freezing, when a frozen area extends 4–5 mm beyond the edge of the cryoprobe, freezing is adequate • Allow two cycles of freezing and thawing: 3 minutes' freezing, followed by 5-minute thawing, followed by a further 3-minute freezing • Once the second freezing is complete, allow time for thawing before attempting to remove the probe from the cervix. Removing it early will pull tissue off the cervix

- Frozen area will appear white
- Observe for any bleeding
- Do not pack the cervix
- Remove the speculum
- Clean and sterilized the cryoprobe with alcohol 60–90%, followed by boiling with water and disinfect with 2% glutaraldehyde

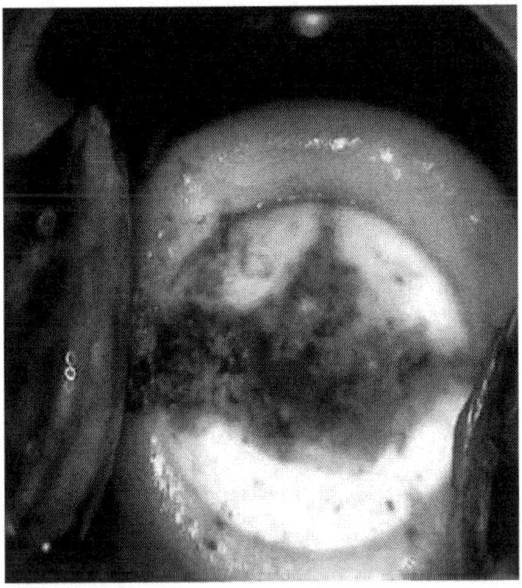

Figure 7.10 Ice-ball formation immediately after cryotherapy, the lesions and transformation zone undergoing cryonecrosis.

Post-Cryotherapy Care

Cryotherapy is a safe procedure; studies have shown that the complication's rate of this procedure is low. To ensure that any complications are kept at the minimal rate and detected at an early stage, post-cryotherapy care is important. Following are the counselling and recommendation of post-cryotherapy care:

- Explain to a patient regarding watery and blood stained discharge for up to 4 weeks
- No sexual intercourse for 4 weeks
- Advice not to use vaginal douches and tampons
- Cryotherapy may increase the transmissibility of HIV infection and using condoms is an effective means of after treatment
- To return if one has vaginal bleeding, severe pain, fever and foul smelling discharge
- Healing will take place 6 weeks after cryotherapy

- Follow-up in 6 weeks and then 3–6 months
- Repeat cytology or VIA during follow-up

Side Effects of Cryotherapy (Very Rare)

(1) profuse vaginal discharge
(2) cramping pain
(3) vaso-vagal attack during the procedure
(4) infection
(5) bleeding
(6) incomplete treatment (5–10%)
(7) cervical stenosis <1%
(8) reduced mucus discharge in 5–10% of women
(9) no adverse effect on subsequent pregnancy

Laser Treatment for Preinvasive Lesions of Cervix

Albert Einstein first discovered the key mechanism of action of laser in the 1990s. The word LASER is an acronym for Light Amplification of Stimulated of Radiation. Dr. Teodore Maiman first created laser with a synthetic ruby crystal in 1960. Laser radiation is an electromagnetic wave, which is not mutagenic, and it can be generated by many media but in gynaecology, CO_2 laser is most commonly used. The use of laser technology is limited in some areas because of the cost of laser treatment; it requires trained personnel and stringent safety precaution. When CO_2 laser is applied to the tissue, it will selectively absorb by extracellular and intracellular water leading to steam formation and vaporization of cellular and nuclear substances.

There are three different forms of laser therapy: (a) vaporization (b) excisional biopsy and (c) combination. Laser vaporization is indicated for patients with CIN lesions with no suspicion of invasive disease. The area of vaporization includes the entire transformation zone, including surrounding tissue up to 3 mm. The depth of tissue vaporization is set to 7 mm because more than 90% of CIN lesions do not extend into cervical glandular crypts for more than 4 mm. Laser excisional biopsy (laser conization) is performed under local anaesthesia. It involves the use of a high power density laser beam to excise a piece of cylindrical or conical tissue around the cervical os.

Laser has an advantage over electro-diathermy for being more precise in the depth of tissue destruction, better haemostasis and lesser collateral thermal injuries. Laser treatment is also a preferred method in treatment of extensive and multifocal preinvasive lesion of cervix, vulva and vagina. It can also be used for treatment of condylomata acuminata.

The desired power-density range for adequate ablation of excision with minimal thermal damage to an adjacent area is 750–2000 W/cm^2 (generally, 20–30 W at a continuous setting), with an effective beam diameter of 1.5–2 mm to maximize ablation and haemostasis while minimizing lateral thermal damage.

Complications of laser therapy are similar to LEEP and cold-knife conization, such as bleeding, pain, infection, cervical stenosis, anaesthetic and long-term obstetrics complications. The rate of bleeding after laser therapy had been reported to be similar to LEEP but less than cold-knife conization. A randomized trial to cryotherapy, carbon dioxide laser vaporization and LEEP for CIN reveals relatively equal rates of disease persistence and recurrence. Risk factors for recurrent CIN are large lesions, positive margin, presence of high-risk HPV infection and older women (age > 30 years old). A large retrospective cohort analysis done by Kalliala, involving 7466 women treated for CIN using cold-knife conization, LEEP/LLETZ, cryotherapy and Laser conization have shown that there was no difference between LEEP, cryotherapy and laser in reducing the risk of future CIN 3 and invasive cervical cancer.

Types of Transformation Zone

Treatment of CIN requires skill in assessing the extent of the lesion and ensures complete destruction or excision of the lesions together with transformation zone. The depth and width of excision/destruction must be adequate to prevent residual disease and recurrent CIN. Appropriate size of the loop is important to ensure complete excision with good surgical margin preferably with single pass.

In order to achieve above objectives and to standardize the description, the International Federation of Cervical Pathology and Colposcopy (IFCPC) has adopted a classification of the transformation zone (TZ) into three types:

(1) **Type 1**: TZ is completely ectocervical, fully visible, can be small or large.
(2) **Type 2**: TZ has an endocervical components, fully visible, may have ectocervical component which may be small or large.
(3) **Type 3**: TZ has an endocervical components, not fully visible, may have ectocervical component which may be small or large. Type of treatment and size of instrument can be based on the type of TZ. Low-grade lesion with type 1 TZ can be treated safely with local ablative therapy, whereas it is entirely inappropriate to choose this treatment for any type 3 TZ.

Management of Abnormal PAP Smear, CIN and Colposcopy during Pregnancy

Pap smear can be done during pregnancy, although the cervical cancer-screening program during pregnancy is still controversy. Pap smear taken during pregnancy is more likely to be unsatisfactory and can detect cytologically normal variants, which can cause unnecessary intervention and anxiety. Abnormal Pap smear detected during pregnancy should be managed similarly, colposcopic examination is indicated in high-grade lesion or if there is evidence of infection with oncogenic HPV. The indications for colposcopy in pregnancy are similar with non-pregnant women. Colposcopy during pregnancy is not easy and should be performed by experience colposcopist. Physiological changes during pregnancy can alter the colposcopic appearance of the cervix, i.e. increase vascularity, hypertrophy of the cervical stroma leading to eversion of the endocervical epithelium, transformation zone displaced more laterally, increased mucus production by endocervical glands and decidualization of the cervix (in 20% of cases) making the epithelium looks suspicious.

For pregnant women, the primary objective of the colposcopic examination is to rule out invasive cancer. A technique of colposcopy in pregnant women is also similar to non-pregnant women and biopsy is taken from the most suspicious area. If colposcopy is normal, repeat examination should be done at 8 weeks postpartum. If CIN is diagnosed, repeat colposcopy must be performed once in every trimester and 8 weeks postpartum.

Cervical conization is indicated if microinvasive or invasive cancer is suspected. The other indication for conization is in unsatisfactory colposcopy with high suspicious of high-grade lesions. Ablative treatment is not recommended during pregnancy. Treatment for pregnant women with all grades of CIN can be delayed until 6–8 weeks postpartum provided there is no suspicious of invasive cancer. If the patient is breast-feeding, local application of oestrogen may facilitate colposcopic re-evaluation. The management of labour is not influenced in any way by the presence of CIN, irrespective of severity.

Cervical Adenocarcinoma in situ

According to Bethesda 2001, endocervical glandular cell abnormalities (on cytology) are classified into four categories: (a) atypical glandular cells (AGC) not otherwise specified (NOS), (b) AGC favour neoplastic (FN), (c) adenocarcinoma in situ and (d) invasive adenocarcinoma. In patients with cytology AGC favour neoplastic, 29–68% of them were found to have high-grade lesions on histology. Women with AGC-FN must be referred for immediate colposcopy and endocervical evaluation.

Cervical adenocarcinoma in situ and invasive adenocarcinoma must be diagnosed by biopsy and histological examination. Cervical adenocarcinoma in situ (AIS) had been established as a precursor of invasive endocervical adenocarcinoma. However, the rate of progression to invasive adenocarcinoma is unknown. HPV16 and HPV 18 were found in an average of 89.8% cases of AIS. The diagnosis of AIS is based on the presence of cellular stratification, nuclear atypia, mitosis and apoptosis in two most active glands. Approximately, 50% of patients with AIS have co-existing squamous dysplasia/carcinoma. Patients with cervical AIS diagnosed by histology must be referred for cervical conization. Cervical conization preferably cold-knife cone biopsy is done to exclude invasive adenocarcinoma.

Margin involvement after conization is common in AIS averaging 25% of cases. Even with negative margin, the probability of residual AIS can be as high as 15–43% (hysterectomy and repeat cone specimens) and co-existing invasive adenocarcinoma in 1.6%. In a patient with positive resection margin on cone specimens, the risk of residual AIS is very high ranging from 12.5%–100% with the average of 55%. In same patient, the risk of co-existing invasive adenocarcinoma is 6%. Therefore, currently the gold standard for treatment of AIS is hysterectomy (following cervical conization regardless the status of resection margin). However, if the patient is keen to preserve her fertility, she must be counselled regarding the risk of recurrent disease, co-existing invasive adenocarcinoma and the important of close monitoring. Repeat colposcopy and endocervical evaluation (including endocervical curettage) must be done regularly. In this patient, repeat conization can be recommended if the surgical margin is positive.

HPV Testing and Other Markers in the Follow-Up after Treatment for CIN

Approximately, 10% of women may develop recurrent CIN within 4 years after excisional treatment. Early detection and treatment of recurrent CIN is important. Repeat cytology ± colposcopy was a common practice in following up the patient following treatment (e.g. UK NHS Clinical Guidelines recommended cervical cytology at 6 and 12 months followed by annual cytology for next 5 years, in some country (France), first follow-up after treatment is 3 months (colposcopy and cytology) then 3-monthly cytology for a year and annually thereafter).

Arbyn and colleagues found that HPV testing was more sensitive than cytology in detecting recurrent CIN although the specificity was comparable. Women with negative high-risk HPV was found to have higher chances of cure and lesser chances of recurrence as compared to women with positive high-risk HPV. The other potential markers to identify women at higher risk of recurrence are HPV viral load, L1 protein expression, E6/E7 RNA, human telomerase (hTERT), topoisomerase IIα, Cdc6 (DNA replication licensing protein), etc.

References

ALTS Group. Comparison of three management strategies for patients with atypical squamous cells of undetermined significance: baseline results from a randomized trial. *J Nat Cancer Inst* 2001; **93**(4): 293–299.

Arbyn M, Paraskevaidis E, Martin-Hirsch P, Prendiville W, Dillner J. Clinical utility of HPV-DNA detection: triage of minor cervical lesions, follow up of women treated for high grade lesions: an update of pooled evidence. *Gynecol Oncol* 2005; **99**(3 Suppl 1): S7–S11.

Arbyn M, Buntinx F, Van Ranst M, Paraskevaidis E, Martin-Hirsch J, Dillner J. Virologic versus cytologic triage of women with equivocal Pap smears: a meta-analysis of the accuracy to detect high-grade intraepithelial neoplasia. *J Natl Cancer Inst* 2004; **96**: 280–293.

Arbyn M, Sasieni P, Meijer CJ, et al. Clinical applications of HPV testing: a summary of meta-analyses. *Vaccine* 2006; **24**(Suppl 3): S78–S89.

ASCUS-LSIL Triage Study (ALTS) Group. Results of a randomized trial on the management of cytology interpretations of atypical squamous cells of undetermined significance. *Am J Obstet Gynecol* 2003; **188**(6): 1383–1392.

Bacon JL. Carbon dioxide laser surgery in cervical dysplasia. *E-Med Obstet Gynaecol* Dec 5, 2007.

Baggish MS. *Basic and Advanced Laser Surgery in Gynecology*. 2nd ed. Norwalk, Conn: Appleton & Lange; 1985: 207–216.

Benedet JL, Miller DM, Nickerson KG. The results of cryosurgical treatment of cervical intraepithelial neoplasia at one, five, and ten years. *Am J Obstet Gynecol* Aug 1987; **157**(2): 268–273.

Benedet JL, Matisic JP, Bertrand MA. An analysis of 84244 patients from the British Columbia cytology-colposcopy program. *Gynecol Oncol.* 2004; **92**: 127–134.

Bull-Phelps S, Garner EIO, Walsh CS, et al. Fertility-sparing surgery in 101 women with adenocarcinoma in situ of the cervix. *Gynecol Oncol* 2007; **107**: 316–319.

Colposcopy and programme management: guidelines for the NHS cervical screening programme. NHSCSP publication no. 20; 2004.

Flannelly G. The management of women with abnormal cervical cytology in pregnancy. *Best Pract Res Clin Obstet Gynaecol* 2010; **24**: 51–60.

Gordon HK, Duncan ID. Effective destruction of cervical intraepithelial neoplasia (CIN) 3 at 100 degrees Celcius using the Semm cold coagulator: 14 years experience. *Br J Obstet Gynaecol* Jan 1991; **98**(1): 14–20.

Hernadi Z, Szoke K, Sapy T, et al. Role of human papillomavirus testing in the follow-up of patients after treatment for cervical precancerous lesions. *Eur J Obstet Gynecol Reprod Biol* 2005; **118**(2): 229–234.

International Agency for Research on Cancer (WHO), IARC screening group website (http://screening.iarc.fr/index.php).

Jeng CJ, Shen J, Huang SH. Partial trachelectomy: a new treatment choice for persistent or recurrent high grade cervical intraepithelial neoplasia. *Gynecol Oncol* Feb 2006; **100**(2): 231–232.

Kalliala I, Nieminen P, Dyba T, Pukkala E, Anttila A. Cancer free survival after CIN treatment: comparisons of treatment methods and histology. *Gynecol Oncol* 2007; **105**: 228–233.

Klaritsch P, Reich O, Giuliani A, Tamussino K, Haas J, Winter R. Delivery outcome after cold-knife conisation of the uterine cervix. *Gynecol Oncol* 2006; **103**: 604–607.

Kyrgiou M, Tsoumpou I, Vrekoussis T, et al. The up-to-date evidence on colposcopy practice and treatment of cervical intraepithelial neoplasia: the Cochrane colposcopy and cervical cytopathology collaborative group (C5 group) approach. *Cancer Treat Rev* 2006; **32**: 516–523.

Kyrgiou M, Koliopoulos G, Hirsch PM, Arbyn M, Prendiville W, Paraskevaidis E. Obstetrics outcomes after conservative treatment for intraepithelial or early invasive cervical lesions: systematic review and meta-analysis. *Lancet* 2006; **367**: 489–498.

Keyserling HV, Kaufmann AM, Shneider A. Conference Report: HPV testing in the follow-up after treatment of women with CIN. *Gynecol Oncol* 2007; **107**: S5–S7.

Kim JH, Park JY, Kim DY, et al. The role of loop electrosurgical excisional procedure in the management of adenocarcinoma in situ of the uterine cervix. *Eur J O&G Reprod Biol* 2009; **145**: 100–103.

Loffe OB. Review: recent advances in the diagnosis and classification of endocervical glandular lesions. *Curr Diagn Pathol* 2004; **10**: 404–412.

Mathevet P, Dargent D, Roy M, Beau G. A randomized prospective study comparing three techniques of conization: cold knife, laser, and LEEP. *Gynecol Oncol* Aug 1994; **54**(2): 175–179.

Mitchell MF, Tortolero-Luna G, Cook E, et al. A randomized clinical trial of cryotherapy, laser vaporization, and loop electrosurgical excision for treatment of squamous intraepithelial lesions of the cervix. *Obstet Gynecol* Nov 1998; **92**(5): 737–744.

Moscicki AB, Shiboski S, Hills NK, Powell KJ, Jay N, Hanson EN. Regression of low-grade squamous intra-epithelial lesions in young women. *Lancet* Nov 6–12 2004; **364**(9446): 1678–1683.

Nobbenhuis MA, Helmerhorst TJ, van den Brule AJ, Rozendaal L, Voorhorst FJ, Bezemer PD. Cytological regression and clearance of high-risk human papillomavirus in women with an abnormal cervical smear. *Lancet* Nov 24 2001; **358**(9295): 1782–1783.

Nuovo J, et al. Treatment outcomes for squamous intraepithelial lesions. *Intl J Gynecol Obstet.* 2000; **68**(1): 25–33.

Prendiville W. Recent innovations in colposcopy practise. *Best Pract Res Clin Obstet Gynaecol* 2005; **19**(5): 779–792.

Ostor AG. Natural history of cervical intraepithelial neoplasia: a critical review. *Int J Gynecol Pathol* Apr 1993; **12**(2): 186–192.

Quint KD, de Koning NC, Geraets DT, Quint WGV, Pirog EC. Comprehensive analysis of Human Papillomavirus and Chlamydia trachomatis in in situ and invasive cervical adenocarcinoma. *Gynecol Oncol* 2009; **114**: 390–394.

Schlecht NF, Platt RW, Duarte-Franco E, Costa MC, Sobrinho JP, Prado JC. Human papillomavirus infection and time to progression and regression of cervical intraepithelial neoplasia. *J Natl Cancer Inst* Sep 3 2003; **95**(17): 1336–1343.

TOMBOLA group (Cruickshank M, Murray G, Parkin D, et al.). Cytological surveillance compared with immediate referral for colposcopy in management of women with low grade cervical abnormalities: multicentre randomised controlled trial. *BMJ* 2009; 339: b2546 doi: http://dx.doi.org/10.1136/bmj.b2546.

Westin MC, Derchain AF, Rabelo-Santos SH, et al. Atypical glandular cells and adenocarcinoma in situ according to the Bethesda 2001 classification: cytohistoligical correlation and clinical implication. European *J O&G Reprod Biol* 2008; **139**: 79–85.

WHO Integrated Health Care for Sexual and Reproductive Health and Chronic Diseases. Comprehensive Cervical Cancer Control. *Guide Essent Pract* 2006.

Chapter 8

Cancer of Cervix

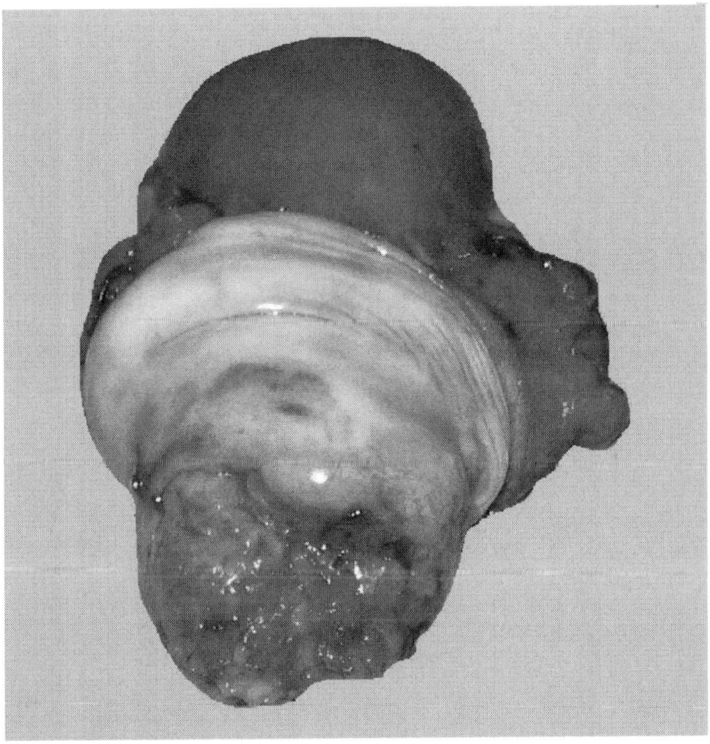

Gynaecologic Cancer: A Handbook for Students and Practitioners
Rushdan Noor, Eng Hseon Tay, and Jeffrey Low

ISBN 978-981-4463-06-5 (Hardcover), 978-981-4463-07-2 (eBook)
www.panstanford.com

Anatomy

The cervix is the lower constricted segment of the uterus. Cervix is divided into two portions, a supravaginal and vaginal portion (portio vaginalis). Portio vaginalis is the portion of the cervix that projecting into the vagina. The average size of portio vaginalis is 3 cm long and 2.5 cm wide. Supravaginal portio is separated in front from the bladder by fibrous tissue known as parametrium that extends from the sides between the broad ligaments. Posteriorly supravaginal cervix is covered by peritoneum. The portion of the cervix exterior to the external os is called ectocervix while the passage between external os and endometrial cavity is referred to the endocervical canal. Upper limit of the endocervical canal is internal os (Fig. 8.1).

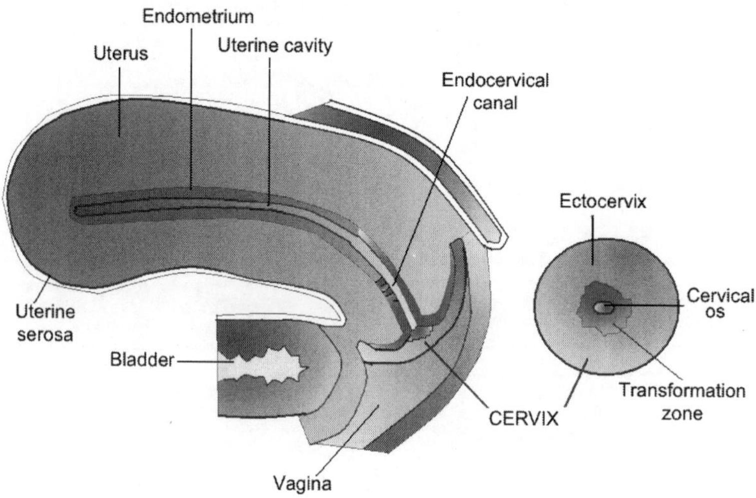

Figure 8.1 The cervix.

The main support structures of the cervix are the uterosacral and cardinal ligaments. Uterosacral ligaments are pair of support consisting of fibrous tissue with smooth muscle extending from the uterus to the sacrum and run along the recto-uterine-peritoneal fold. Cardinal ligament (transcervical/Mackenrodt's ligament) is a thickened connective tissue arising at upper lateral margins of the cervix and inserting into the fascia covering of the pelvic diaphragm.

Blood supply of the cervix is from the cervical and vaginal branches of uterine arteries. Uterine arteries are derived from the internal iliac arteries. Cervical branch of the uterine artery generally descends on the lateral aspects of the cervix at 3 and 9 o'clock positions. When the internal artery is ligated, many collateral blood supplies maintain the vascularization of the uterus. Following internal iliac ligations, blood supply to the uterus is maintained by collateral circulation via a **middle sacral** (lateral sacral), **inferior mesenteric** (middle haemorrhoidal) and **lumbar** (iliolumbar) **artery** (Bold arteries are from the aorta). The venous drainage of the cervix is parallel to arterial supply, eventually emptying into the hypogastric venous plexus.

Main nerve supply to the cervix is derived from the hypogastric plexus. Sensory, sympathetic and parasympathetic fibres are present in the cervix. The ectocervix has less sensory innervations as compared to endocervix and therefore, ectocervix can withstand a minor surgical procedure such as cryotherapy and biopsy without anaesthesia. Dilatation of the endocervical canal may result in vasovagal reaction with reflex bradycardia.

The lymphatic drainage of the cervix is complex and variable as shown in Fig. 8.2.

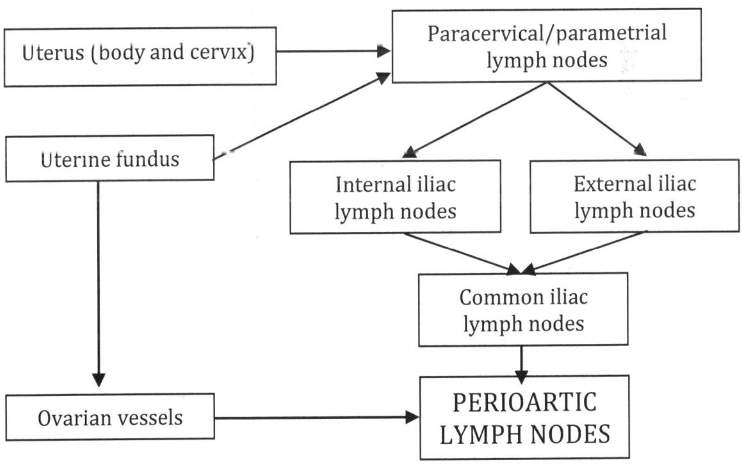

Figure 8.2 The lymphatic drainage of the cervix.

Cancer of Cervix

Epidemiology

More than 12 million new cases and 7.6 million cancer deaths estimated to have occurred in 2008. Approximately, 529,100 new cases of cervical cancer were reported leading to 275,000 deaths worldwide in 2008 (GLOBOCAN, 2008). Unfortunately, more than 80% of annual cervical cancer deaths occur in developing countries (50–60% occur in Asia and India alone, contributing 27% of the total number of cases). American Cancer Society most recently estimated that in 2009, there were approximately 11,000 new cases of cervical cancer and 4000 women will die in America. They also estimated that the death rate declines by nearly 4% each year mainly in developed countries due to their effective cervical cancer prevention program and better treatment of cervical cancer. Unfortunately, the death rate in under-developed and developing countries are still high. Globally, cervical cancer incidence and mortality rates have been declining since the 1960s in many developed countries due to their successful implementation of the organized screening program. However, the rate is still high in many parts of the Central and South America, Africa and Asia.

Regions with high-risk cervical cancer are Eastern Africa (ASR 34.5 per 100,000), Western Africa (ASR 33.7), Southern Africa (ASR 26.8), South Central Asia (ASR 24.6), Middle Africa (ASR 23.0) and South America (ASR 23.9), whereas the risk of cervical cancer is lowest in Western Asia (ASR 4.5), Northern America (ASR 5.7), Australia (ASR 5.0) and New Zealand (ASR 5.0). Age-standardized incidence of cervical cancer in South East Asia is 15.8 per 100,000 population. The peak age of developing cervical cancer is 45–60 years, declines in the incidence for older age groups but peaks again in the early 80 years of age.

Aetiology of Cervical Cancer

The scientific evidence obtained from virological, molecular, clinical and epidemiological data had demonstrated conclusively that cervical cancer is due to persistent infection of high-risk human papillomavirus (Bosch et al., 1995). Largest series by IARC (International Agency Research in Cancer) using standard protocol, recruiting approximately 1000 women with confirmed cancer of the cervix have detected HPV-DNA in 99.7% of the tumour (Bosch et al., 1995, 2002; Walboomers et al., 1999). The associations observed between the infection by HPV and cervical cancer is among the highest ever identified in research of human cancer.

The human papillomavirus (HPV) is a double-stranded DNA virus that belongs to the Papillomaviridae family. They are very small viruses with the diameter of 40–60 nm. The outer layer of this virus is covered by shell or capsid comprising 70 capsomers, and each capsomer consists of five molecules. The inner portion of this virus consists of 8000 base-pair long circular DNA molecules. There are three regions in the HPV DNA: **early protein regions** (E1–E7), **late protein regions** (L1, L2) and **long control regions**. Long control regions do not have coding potential. Early protein regions are genes responsible in virus replication and for the assembly of newly produced viruses within the infected cells. Late protein regions encode viral particle L1 proteins (VP L1) and viral particle L2 proteins (VP L2) which form the capsomer. Capsomer is the building block of the viral capsid. VP L1 is known as major capsid protein while VP L2 is known as minor capsid protein. VPL1 is the main epitope of HPV virus.

Within the early protein regions, there are E6 and E7 genes, which are the oncogenes. Both genes are controlled by E2 gene. Based on the differences of DNA sequence in E6, E7 and L1 coding regions, there are more than 100 different types of human papillomavirus identified. The HPV virus is divided into two groups: (a) Low-risk HPV (LRHPV) and (b) high-risk HPV (HRHPV).

Low-risk HPVs are associated with benign viral warts. Among LRHPVs are HPV 6, 11, 40, 42, 43, 44, 54, 61, 72 and 81. More than 90% of anogenital warts were due to HPV 6 and HPV 11. High-risk HPVs are oncogenic viruses closely linked to pre-cancerous and cancer of male and female genital organs. Some of these viruses were also linked with head and neck cancers. According to International Agency for Research on Cancer, there was sufficient evidence that HPV 16, 18, 31, 33, 35, 39, 45, 51, 52, 56, 58, 59 and 66 are carcinogenic (high risk) while HPV 26, 68, 73 and 82 are probably carcinogenic. More than 35 types of HPV have been isolated in neoplastic lesions of the anogenital tract and the WHO has recognized HPV 16 and HPV 18 as carcinogenic agents for human. Both HPV 16 and 18 are responsible for 70–80% of invasive cervical cancer.

Transmission of HPV is almost exclusively through a sexual contact. Low-risk HPV can also be transmitted through vertical transmission from mother to baby leading to respiratory papillomatosis. HPV infections are very common, especially in young women; however, 70% of new infections resolve within 1 year and almost 90% resolve within 2 years.

HPV and Cervical Carcinogenesis

Viruses reach the basal cells of the epithelium through microabrasion or small breaks in the epithelium. Virus enters the cell via an endocytic pathway and localized in the endosome, the virus uncoats within the endosome and the genome is released. Viral genome may remain in the basal cells for 2–5 years without any cellular or tissue reactions (Fig. 8.3). This period is called the latent period. Following the latent period, HPV viruses start to replicate and viral protein E1 and E2 are essential for this process. Infected basal cells are then push to the suprabasal compartment, and the viruses are then released into the environment. During these processes, infected epithelial cells become enlarged with perinuclear halo appearance. These cells are also known as koilocytes. Other features of koilocyte are nuclear enlargement and nuclear hyperchromasia.

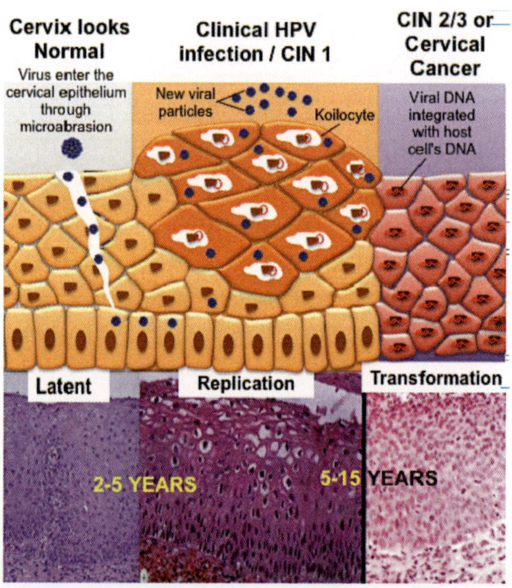

Figure 8.3 HPV infections and cervical pathology. Adapted from Goodman A, Wilbur DC. *N Engl J Med* 2003; **349**: 1555–1564.

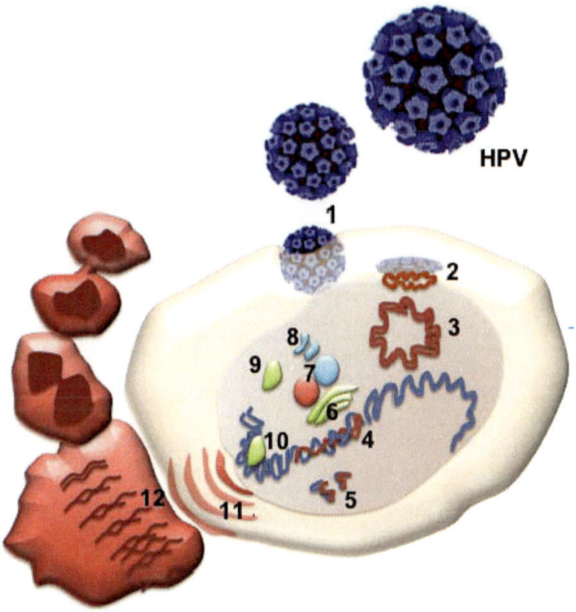

Figure 8.4 Pathogenesis of HPV infection and malignant transformation of the cervical epithelial cell. (1) Virus enter the host cell, (2) release of HPV DNA, (3) HPV DNA enters the nucleus towards the host DNA, (4) HPV DNA integrated with host DNA, (5) integration leads to partial deletion of E2 and E4 genes, (6) deletion of E2 and E4 leads to overexpression of E6 and E7 genes, (7) overexpressed E6 and E7 bind to tumour suppressor protein p53 and Rb (retinoblastoma), (8) degradation of P53 and Rb proteins, (9) disruption of normal cell cycle and release of transcription factors, (10) transcription factors bind to the host DNA, (11) stimulation of cell synthesis, (12) unregulated and uncontrolled cell proliferation (neoplasm).

In some cells, viral genome is integrated into host DNA, leading to partial deletion of E2 and E4 genes, which are essential in controlling the E6 and E7 oncogenes. Factors that trigger these phenomena are believed to be related to host immune system, smoking habit, persistent infection by high-risk HPV, etc. Partial deletion of E2 and E4 will lead to overexpression of E6 and E7 oncogenes. Subsequently, E7 oncoproteins bind to protein pRB (tumour suppressor protein) leading to activation of the E2F transcription factors which triggers the expression of proteins necessary for DNA replication. Normally, this unscheduled replication will not proceed. Instead the cells will undergo apoptosis by the action of tumour suppressor proteins known as p53. However, in this situation, p53 proteins have already undergone degradation following the binding with E6 oncoproteins. The binding of E7 to protein pRB and degradation of p53 by E6 oncoproteins lead to an increase in genomic instability, accumulation of oncogene mutations, loss of cell-growth control and ultimately malignant transformation (Fig. 8.4).

Types of HPV in Cervical Cancer

Based on the PCR test to identify HPV DNA, at least 70% of invasive cervical cancers are due to HPV 16 and HPV 18. HPV 16 is the most common HPV-related cervical cancer accounting for 54.6% of all cases (Smith et al., 2007). Combined HPV 16/18 prevalence among invasive cervical cancer cases was slightly higher in Europe, North America and Australia (74–77%) than Africa, Asia and South/Central America (65–70%) (Smith et al., 2007). The next six most important types of HPV related to invasive cervical cancer are HPV 31, 33, 35, 45, 52 and 58. In their meta-analysis involving more than 9000 cases of squamous cell carcinoma (SCC) of the cervix and almost 2000 cases of adenocarcinoma of the cervix, Smith et al. found that HPV 16 and HPV 18 were responsible in 68% of SCC (HPV 16: 55%, HPV 18: 13%) and 70% in Adenocarcinoma of the cervix (HPV 16: 33%, HPV 18: 37%). HPV 16 was more common in SCC cervix while HPV 18 was more common in adenocarcinoma of the cervix.

Risk Factors for Cervical Cancer

Invasive carcinoma of the cervix can be considered as sexually transmitted disease. Early age of sexual activity predisposed to invasive cervical cancer because the transformation zone in early reproductive age is believed to be more susceptible to a carcinogen. The relative risk of having cervical cancer is 2.5 if the age of first sexual exposure was <18 years old. Women with history of HPV infection are also at higher risk, the causal relationship between high-risk HPV infection and cervical cancer are the highest of all other cancers. Women with multiple sexual partners have a relative risk of 2.8 if the number of partners ≥5. Multiparous women are at higher risk of cervical cancer as compared to low parity or nulliparous women. Women in lower socioeconomic class are at higher risk of cervical cancer as compared to women from upper socioeconomic class. Women who married to a man with multiple sexual partners are also at higher risk of cervical cancer.

Cigarette smoking has been identified as a significant risk factor for cervical cancer by 2–5 folds. Oral contraceptive pills (OCPs) use increased the risk of cervical cancer (relative risk of 1.6) probably indirectly through increased sexual activity. Following are the compounding factors that create a bias regarding the relation between OCPs and cervical cancer risk:

(a) OCP usage has been linked with behaviour, low-risk women less practicing OCP.
(b) Patients can protect themselves from cancer by barrier contraception.
(c) Cancer can be detected earlier in OCP usage because women are under more frequent and regular follow-up.

Patients with immunodeficiency are at higher risk of developing cancer, including cervical cancer. This association is probably due to increase susceptibility to persistent HPV infection.

In utero exposure to DES increases the risk of clear cell adenocarcinoma of the cervix (Risk 0.14–1.4/1000 exposure).

Women with an uncircumcised sexual partner may be at higher risk of invasive cervical cancer. Based on seven case-control studies involving 3790 women, circumcised men had lower prevalence of HPV infection (5.5% vs. 19.6%) and female partners of circumcised men had a moderate but non-significant decrease in risk of cervical cancer (OR 0.72, 95% CI 0.49–1.04). However, when the circumcised sexual partner has low-risk sexual behaviour, circumcision does not have an impact on cervical cancer risk on their female partner (Castellsague et al., 2002). In other meta-analysis by Van Howe RS to determine the relationship of circumcision and risk of genital infection with HPV, he found that there is no strong evidence that circumcision reduces the risk for genital HPV infection. The relation of circumcision and risk of cervical cancer remain controversial.

Histopathological Subtypes of Cervical Cancer

The most common histologic variant of invasive cervical cancers is squamous cell carcinoma (Table 8.1). The second most common histological type is adenocarcinoma. The prevalence of adenocarcinoma of the cervix appears to increase (15–25%) probably a relative increase due to declined in the incidence of squamous cell carcinoma, especially in developed countries with a more effective cervical cancer prevention program. The increase may also be absolute, partly due to increase in detection rate. Most of our knowledge on the management of cervical cancer comes from the studies where the majority of the patients had squamous cell carcinoma. Pathological subtypes of cervical cancer are shown in the Table 8.1.

Table 8.1 Histopathological subtypes of cervical cancer

Squamous cell carcinomas
Squamous cell carcinoma
Verrucous
Papillary squamous
Lymphoepithelioma-like carcinoma
Adenocarcinomas (WHO classification)
Mucinous adenocarcinoma (most common)
Endocervical type
Intestinal type
Clear cell adenocarcinoma
Endometrioid adenocarcinoma
Serous adenocarcinoma
Mesonephric adenocarcinoma
Other carcinomas of cervix
Adenosquamous
Glassy-cell carcinoma
Adenoid cystic carcinoma
Adenoid basal carcinoma
Neuroendocrine tumour of cervix
Carcinoid tumour
Small cell carcinoma
Large cell neuroendocrine carcinoma
Undifferentiated carcinoma
Other malignant tumours of cervix
Leiomyosarcoma, rhabdomyosarcoma, stromal sarcoma, lymphoma

Natural History and Pattern of Spread

Cervical carcinoma originates in the transformation zone, frequently preceded by cervical intraepithelial neoplasm, 10–20 years before. Thirty percent of carcinoma in situ progresses to invasive cancer after 10 years, at 30 years, and 80% develop invasive carcinoma. Local spread is common in cervical cancer. The tumour may invade laterally into the parametrium, inferiorly into the vagina, anteriorly into the bladder and rectum, posteriorly. Invasion of tumour laterally may obstruct the ureter and leads to hydroureter and subsequently hydronephrosis (Fig. 8.5). Bilateral ureteric obstruction can lead to obstructive nephropathy. Renal failure secondary to obstructive nephropathy is one of the most important causes of morbidity and mortality in a patient with cervical cancer. Ten to thirty percent of invasive cervical carcinoma has spread to lower uterine segment or uterine cavity at presentation.

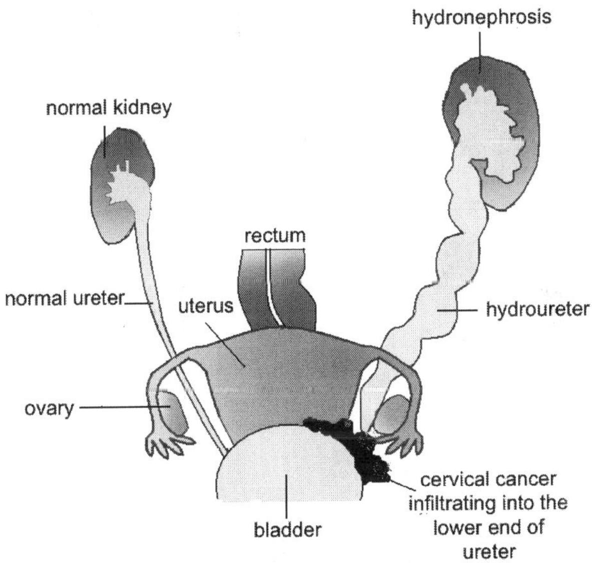

Figure 8.5 Direct invasion of the cervical cancer to the ureter leads to hydroureter and hydronephrosis. Obstructive nephropathy is one of the most common causes of morbidity and mortality in cervical cancer.

Lymphatic spread is important as the lymph node metastasis is one of the independent prognostic factors for survival. The risk of nodal metastasis is related to staging of the disease, depth of invasion, size of tumour, grade and presence of lymphovascular space invasion. The risk of pelvic lymph node metastasis is 0–0.6% in stage 1A1. However, in stage 1A2, the risk of nodal metastasis increases to be 4.8–11% (average 7% but higher if present of lymphovascular space invasion). Involvement of para-aortic lymph node without pelvic lymph nodes is unusual. Parametrial lymph nodes are the most commonly affected lymph nodes. Approximately, 80% of patients with positive parametrial lymph node also have positive pelvic lymph node. Generally, the risk of parametrial lymph node metastasis is approximately 10% in stage 1B and 20% in stage 2B. The risk of pelvic lymph node metastasis increases from 16% in stage 1B to 25–31% in stage 2 disease. The cancer can also spread through a blood stream to distant organs such as liver, spleen, kidney, lung, brain, bone, and others.

Presentations

In an early stage, many patients do not have any symptoms (asymptomatic). The most common presenting symptom is postcoital bleeding. Patients can also present with irregular vaginal bleeding, passing out blood stained mucus per vagina, pelvic pain and constitutional symptoms. Pelvic pain, urinary problems and constitutional symptoms are the strong indications of advanced stage disease. If the disease has obstructed the uterine outflow tract, menstrual blood will be accumulated in the uterine cavity (haematometra) and subsequently secondary bacterial infection leading to the formation of pus in the cavity (pyometra). Patients with pyometra often presented with pelvic pain, purulent vaginal discharge and fever. Invasion of the tumour posteriorly may cause tenesmus and per-rectal bleeding. In late-stage disease, patients may be presented with shortness of breath, bone pain, severe headache, neurological problems, loss of appetite and loss of weight. Lymphatic obstruction may result in lower limb lymphoedema. Venous outflow obstruction can lead to deep vein thrombosis, and patients will present with unilateral leg swelling. Both of these presentations are strong indications of advanced cervical cancer. In developed countries, 70–80% of patients presented at an early stage (stages 1 and 2); however, in underdeveloped regions only 30–40% of patients presented at an early stage.

Diagnosis

Patients who presented with symptoms suggestive of cervical cancer must undergo complete physical and pelvic examinations. If the lesion is not well-visualized, colposcopic examination must be performed to identify the abnormalities. Confirmation of the diagnosis is made via histological examination of the cervical biopsy. Cervical biopsy can be in the form of directed punch biopsy or cervical cone biopsy. The optimal site to take the biopsy is from the edge of the tumour, where the transition from invasive to non-invasive can be clearly seen. Avoid taking biopsy from the middle of the lesions because this will only reveal necrotic cells/tissues.

Staging Carcinoma of Cervix

Cervical cancer is staged clinically using radiographic examination and clinical examination under anaesthesia. Surgical staging may be more accurate. However, since 80% of cancers are diagnosed in developing countries, clinical staging is more affordable and remains practical until today. During an examination under anaesthesia, cystoscopy and thorough clinical assessment of the tumour are performed. According to the latest FIGO recommendation, cystoscopy and procto-sigmoidoscopy are not mandatory, especially in an early stage, these procedures are indicated if the patient is suspected to have bladder and rectal infiltration (Fig. 8.6). Suspected lesions in the bladder and rectum should be biopsied. Bullous oedema of the bladder and swelling of the rectal mucosa are not accepted as definitive criteria for staging. Chest radiography is a routine investigation in the staging processes.

Computed tomography scans (CT scan) with contrast may replace intravenous urogram to assess the urinary tract. CT scans is also useful in assessing the nature of primary tumour and extends of the disease. The other imaging techniques are MRI and PET scan. See Chapter 19 to learn more about imaging techniques in gynaecological malignancies.

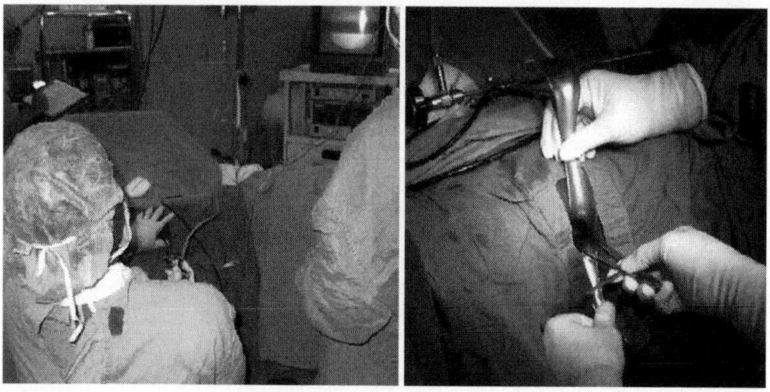

Figure 8.6 Clinical staging for cervical cancer. Examination under anaesthesia and cystoscopy.

Baseline investigations such as full blood count, renal function test, liver function test, tumour markers and urinalysis are important.

Abnormal or suspicious lymph nodes on CT scan or MRI should be confirmed with CT-guided FNAC (fine needle aspiration cytology), if feasible. In some centres, lymph node assessment is done through laparoscopic examination and biopsy. Retroperitoneal lymph node dissection is a preferred approach to avoid intra-abdominal adhesions and subsequent risk of radiation injuries to the bowels. Risk of major radiation injuries following intraperitoneal and retroperitoneal lymphadenecomy were 11% and 4%, respectively. Sentinel node biopsy is very promising but at present still investigational. Tables 8.2 and 8.3 show the old FIGO staging and new FIGO staging 2009 for comparisons.

Table 8.2 FIGO staging of cervical cancer 1994

Stage	Description
Stage 1	The carcinoma is strictly confined to the cervix (extension to the corpus should be disregarded)
Stage 1A	Invasive Ca diagnosed only by microscopy. All visible lesion is stage 1B. Stroma invasion with a maximum depth of 5 mm measured from the base of the epithelium and horizontal spread of 7 mm or less. Vascular space involvement, venous or lymphatic, does affect classification.

Stage 1A1	Stroma invasion ≤3 mm and ≤7 mm horizontal spread
Stage 1A2	Stroma invasion >3 mm and ≤5 mm and ≤7 mm horizontal spread
Stage 1B	Clearly visible lesion confined to cervix or microscopic lesion greater than in stage 1A2
Stage 1B1	Lesion ≤4 cm in greatest diameter
Stage 1B2	Lesion >4 cm in greatest diameter
Stage 2	Cervical carcinoma invades the uterus, but not to the pelvic wall or to the lower third of the vagina
Stage 2A	No parametrium invasion
Stage 2B	Parametrium invasion
Stage 3	Carcinoma extends to the pelvic wall and/or involves lower third of vagina or causes hydronephrosis/non-functioning kidney
Stage 3A	Tumour involves lower third of vagina, no extension to pelvic wall
Stage 3B	Tumour extends to pelvic wall or causes hydronephrosis or non-Functioning kidney
Stage 4A	Tumour invades bladder mucosa or rectum and/or extends beyond true pelvis
Stage 4B	Distant metastases

Note: The above old FIGO staging 1994 is purposely highlighted to guide the readers to compare with the latest FIGO staging 2009 in the next page.

Table 8.3 Latest FIGO staging 2009

Stage	Descriptions
Stage 1	The carcinoma is strictly confined to the cervix (extension to the corpus should be disregarded)
Stage 1A	Invasive cancer diagnosed only by microscopy. All visible lesion is stage 1B. Stroma invasion with a maximum depth of 5 mm measured from the base of the epithelium and horizontal spread of 7 mm or less.
Stage 1A1	Stroma invasion ≤3 mm and ≤7 mm horizontal spread
Stage 1A2	Stroma invasion >3 mm and ≤5 mm and ≤7 mm horizontal spread
Stage 1B	Clearly visible lesion confined to cervix or microscopic lesion (preclinical cancer) greater than in stage 1A[a]

(*Continued*)

Table 8.3 (*Continued*)

Stage	Descriptions
Stage 1B1	Clinically visible lesions ≤4 cm in greatest diameter
Stage 1B2	Clinically visible lesion >4 cm in greatest diameter
Stage 2	Cervical carcinoma involving the upper 2/3 of vagina or parametrium but not to the pelvic side wall
Stage 2A	Involvement of upper 2/3 of vagina with no obvious parametrial involvement
Stage 2A1	Clinically visible lesions ≤4 cm in greatest diameter
Stage 2A2	Clinically visible lesion >4 cm in greatest diameter
Stage 2B	Parametrium invasion bilateral or unilateral without extension to the pelvic sidewall
Stage 3	Carcinoma extends to the pelvic wall and/or involves lower third of vagina or causes hydronephrosis/non-functioning kidney[b]
Stage 3A	Tumour involves lower third of vagina, no extension to pelvic wall
Stage 3B	Tumour extends to pelvic wall or causes hydronephrosis or non-Functioning kidney
Stage 4A	Tumour invades bladder mucosa or rectum and/or extends beyond true pelvis.
Stage 4B	Distant metastases

[a]All macroscopically visible lesions—even with superficial invasion—are allotted to Stage IB. Invasion is limited to a measured stromal invasion with a maximal depth of invasion 5.0 mm and a horizontal extension of 7 mm. Depth of invasion should be taken from the base of the epithelium of the original tissue—superficial or glandular. The involvement of vascular spaces—venous or lymphatic—does not change the stage. These rules now apply to adenoma carcinomas.

[b]On rectal exam there is no cancer-free space between the tumour and the pelvic side wall. All cases with hydronephrosis or a non-functioning kidney should be included, unless they are known to be due to other causes.

Prognostic Factors

Clinical stage is the most important prognostic factor. Overall 5-year survival rates are 95–100% in stage 1A disease and from 75% to 90% in stage 1B. Patients with stage 4 cervical cancer have only 5% chances to survive after 5 years. See Tables 8.4 and 8.5 for reported survival rate by Fletcher et al. and Pettersson. Depth of tumour invasion, lymphovascular space invasion and tumour volume or diameter are three important independent prognostic factors for recurrence. Lymphovascular space invasion correlates with the risk of lymph node metastasis. In stage 1A2 cervical cancer, presence of lymphovascular space invasion increased the rate of nodal metastases from 3.2% to 16.1%. Largest tumour diameter is also an important prognostic factor. Lesion of 4 cm or less, with two nodes positive carry 10-year survival rate of 56–70% as compared to 13% in patients with a tumour diameter of more than 4 cm and two positive nodes. Endometrial extension associated with decreased survival, greater incidence of peritoneal carcinomatosis and distant metastases.

Lymph node involvement is known to correlate with survival. Patients with early-stage cervical cancer treated with surgical treatment have 5-year survival of 90% if their lymph nodes were negative. Survival decreased to 50–60% if the tumour has spread to pelvic lymph nodes. The 5-year survival rate is further decreased to 20–45% if the tumour has spread to para-aortic nodes. Five-year survival rates were also influenced by the number of lymph nodes involved (single lymph node positive, 62% survival, two lymph nodes positive, 36% survival rate). Survival rate of cervical cancer is shown in Table 8.4 and 8.5.

Table 8.4 Five-year survival rate in cervical cancer (Fletcher)

Five-year survival rate of 2000 patients after treated with radiotherapy (Fletcher)	
Stage 1	91.5%
Stage 2A	83.5%
Stage 2B	66.5%
Stage 3A	45%
Stage 3B	36%
Stage 4	14%

Patients with aggressive histology type such as adenosquamous, small cell neuroendocrine, sarcoma and poorly differentiated tumour are known to have poorer prognosis. Other prognostic factors are age, general conditions, including co-morbidity and nutritional status.

Table 8.5 Survival by stage in patients with cancer of cervix (From larger study* involving more than 32,000 patients, Pettersson, 1991)

Stage	Survival rate	
	Three-year (%)	Five-year (%)
1	86.9	81.6
2	69.5	61.3
3	44.6	36.7
4	16.6	12.1

*Pettersson F: Annual Report on the Results of Treatment in Gynecologic Cancer, vol. 21. Statements on the results obtained in patients 1982–1986, inclusive 3- and 5-year survival up to 1990. *Int J Gynecol Obstet* 1991; (supp): 27–127.

Management of Cervical Cancer

Patients with cervical cancer should ideally be managed in a centre with complete expertise and facilities for treatment of gynaecological cancer. Final decision on the best treatment for a patient is made based on the information regarding the pathology and extends of the disease, taking a consideration of the patient's factors such as age, fertility wishes, co-morbidity, performance status and patient's personal choices.

Following are the principal steps for the management of cervical cancer:

(1) Confirm the diagnosis and thorough evaluation of histopathological features of the tumour.
(2) Determine the extent of the disease through investigations and staging.
(3) Determine the intention of treatment either for curative or for palliative.
(4) Review all treatment modalities and decide the best for patients based on above findings taking into consideration patient-specific factors, fertility wishes, performance status, co-morbidity, surgical and medical history, patient's personal choices and psychosocial background.
(5) Counsel the patient and her partner.

(6) Offer the patient the most appropriate treatment.
(7) Monitor.

Following are the treatment options for a patient with cervical cancer:

(1) surgery
(2) radiotherapy or chemoradiation
(3) chemotherapy
(4) combination therapy

Treatment for Early-Stage Cervical Cancer

Early-stage disease refers to stages 1 to stage 2A. Both surgery and radiotherapy are equally effective in the treatment of a patient in early stage. Although both surgery and radiotherapy are equally effective in early disease, controversies exist about the optimal primary treatment for patients with bulky tumours (tumour diameter larger than 4 cm) and positive regional lymph nodes. Positive lymph node does not change the staging.

In other groups with early disease, surgery is obviously more advantageous because the majority of women with cervical cancer are relatively young and sexually active. Following are the advantages of surgical treatment in early disease: (a) Ability to conserve the ovarian function in premenopausal women; (b) fertility preservation in selected patients; (c) avoidance of radiation toxicities such as vaginal stenosis, bladder and rectal radiation injuries; vaginal stenosis may lead to sexual dysfunction or even apareunia and (d) availability of tumour and tissue samples for assessment and determination of the risk of recurrence and rate of survival.

Surgical Treatment for Stage 1A1

The prognosis for stage 1A1 is excellent with 5-year survival of more than 95% and the risk of lymph node metastasis is only 0.5%, if no lymphovascular space invasion. Local excision (cone biopsy) or simple hysterectomy is sufficient but hysterectomy is considered as the standard of care. Local excision is best performed by cone biopsy, knife cone biopsy has advantages over the LEEP or laser cone because it causes less thermal damage, and therefore, the specimen is intact for better for pathological evaluation.

Simple hysterectomy with or without bilateral salpingo-oophorectomy is the preferred treatment for the following patients:

(a) postmenopausal women
(b) patients with other gynaecological diseases requiring treatment such as symptomatic leiomyoma, endometriosis, etc.
(c) poor compliance
(d) patients in whom local excision is not feasible or there is high possibility of incomplete resection
(e) patients with evidence of co-existing adenocarcinoma in situ (ACIS) and who have completed their family

In a patient with evidence of lymphovascular space invasion, the risk of nodal metastasis increases to 4%; therefore, pelvic lymphadenectomy may be justifiable. Hysterectomy can be performed either by open surgery (abdominal and vaginal hysterectomy) or laparoscopically.

Surgical Treatment for Stage 1A2

The risk of nodal metastasis in stage 1A2 is approximately 7% and the risk increases to 10% in a small subset of patients with lymphovascular space invasion. Pelvic lymphadenectomy is indicated in all patients with stage 1A2 cervical cancer. Surgery for primary tumour is individualized ranging from radical trachelectomy, modified radical hysterectomy to radical hysterectomy. In a patient whom the diagnosis of stage 1A2 is made following simple hysterectomy, they do not require parametrectomy instead pelvic lymphadenectomy alone is sufficient. Glandular lesions and poor histology type such as adenosquamous and small cell neuroendocrine tumour should be dealt with a more radical approach. In patients who keen to preserve her fertility, radical trachelectomy and pelvic lymphadenectomy can be offered. Trachelectomy can be accomplished via laparotomy, vaginally or laparoscopically. Surgical techniques will be discussed in the last section of this chapter. The role of sentinel node biopsy in stage 1A2 is under investigation and appears promising.

Surgical Treatment for Stage 1B1 and Stage 2A1 Cervical Cancer

The risk of lymph node metastasis in stage 1B and 2A is 16–25%. Under new FIGO staging, stage 2A is further subdivided into stage 2A1 and 2A2. Stage 2A1 is when the tumour's largest diameter is 4 cm and less, while stage 2A2, if the diameter is more than 4 cm. Radical hysterectomy and pelvic lymphadenectomy are the standard of treatment in patients with stage 1B1 and stage 2A1, although they can also be treated with primary radiotherapy/chemoradiotherapy. In a prospective randomized study to compare surgery and radiotherapy in patients with stage 1B–2A, both treatments were equally effective and had a comparable outcome (Landoni et al., 1997). Five-year survival rates were 75–100% in patients with stage 1 to 2A treated by either surgery or radiotherapy.

The primary aim of radical hysterectomy is to remove the tumour with adequate margin, including parametrium and upper part of the vagina. Microscopic margin must be at least 5 mm and pelvic node dissection should include obturator, internal iliac, external iliac and common iliac nodes. Para-aortic lymphadenectomy is not mandatory. Landoni and colleagues have published a prospective randomized study to compare radical hysterectomy class II (modified radical hysterectomy) versus class III involving 243 patients with small volume stage 1B and 2A cervical cancer. They have concluded that class II and class III radical hysterectomy are equally effective as surgical treatment for early-stage cervical cancer (comparable 5-year survival rate). Patients who underwent class II radical hysterectomy had fewer late complications mainly urologic morbidity (13% vs. 28%) as compared to class III radical hysterectomy.

Kim and colleagues evaluated 140 cases of early cervical cancer with depth of invasion ≤5 mm in relation of lymph nodes metastases and parametrial involvement. They found that depth of invasion was a more important determinant of nodal metastasis and parametrial involvement than the width of invasion. None of the patients with depth of invasion ≤5 mm had parametrial involvement despite horizontal spread of more than 7 mm (stage 1B1). Patients with invasion of >5 mm were found to have 15.3% risk of parametrial involvement. The rate of nodal metastasis in patients with depth of invasion ≤5 mm was 3.5% as compared to 23% if the invasion was more than 5 mm. They suggested that patients with stage 1B1 cervical cancer with depth of invasion ≤5 mm may be subjected to less radical surgery. If further prospective clinical trials confirm that parametrectomy can be safely omitted in low-risk patients, less radical surgery, such as simple hysterectomy with pelvic lymphadenectomy, could be a reasonable therapeutic option for superficially invasive stage IB1 cervical cancer.

Treatment for Stage 1B2 and 2A2

Patients with bulky (diameter larger than 4 cm) stage 1B and 2A are categorized as stage 1B2 and stage 2A2 disease, respectively. The later is based on the new FIGO staging. Patients presenting with bulky stage 1B and 2A cervical cancers represent a greater therapeutic challenge. Several authors categorized bulky stage 1B (1B2) and 2A (2A2) under locally advanced stage cervical cancer (Allen and Narayan, 2005).

Measurement of tumour size is best performed by MRI and perhaps most important diameter is the craniocaudal diameter of the tumour. Hayashi and Kato, using a 4 cm cut-off value for craniocaudal diameter reported a 5-year disease-free survival of 70% in tumours with a diameter of less than 4 cm and 37% in tumours more than 4 cm in diameter. Interestingly, there was no difference in a survival rate if the transverse diameter was taken.

Numerous studies have demonstrated that volume and size of tumour are independent prognostic factors for tumour recurrence and survival. Patients with bulky tumour tend to have higher risk of nodal metastasis and surgical margin involvement. In view of higher rate of postoperative adjuvant radiotherapy, some Oncologist preferred to treat these patients with primary radiotherapy/chemoradiotherapy. Although many oncologists prefer to treat patients with bulky disease with primary radiotherapy/chemoradiation, there is so far no concrete evidence that this approach is superior to primary surgery in terms of overall survival. Landoni et al. randomized 343 patients with stage 1B–2A into two groups (1) treated with primary surgery and (2) primary radiotherapy. Overall survival was comparable in both groups. However, on further evaluation of stage 1B2 disease, they found that 84% of these patients required adjuvant radiotherapy (as compared to 54% in stage 1B1). Although there was no difference in overall survival, patients who underwent surgery and adjuvant radiotherapy had higher morbidity rate.

The five-year survival rates for stage 1B2 are 60% compared to 85% in stage 1B1. Rutledge TL and colleagues compared stage 1B1 and 1B2 cervical cancers treated with radical hysterectomy, there found that stage 1B2 was associated with significantly higher rate of nodal metastasis (28% vs. 12.8%), para-aortic node involvement (8.1% vs. 1.8%), parametrial involvement and adjuvant radiotherapy (52% vs. 37%).

The main concern about primary surgery in bulky disease is treatment-related morbidity. However, with the advancement and improvement in the surgical techniques, e.g. nerve-sparing surgery, minimally invasive surgery and less radical surgery, treatment morbidity related to this approach may be minimized in near future.

Surgical treatment for stages 1B and 2A is Type III radical hysterectomy and bilateral pelvic lymphadenectomy. In bulky stage 1B and 2A disease, the risk of para-aortic lymph node metastasis is expected to be higher (Stage 2A, risk 11%), perhaps in these subgroups of patients, surgical assessment of para-aortic lymph nodes is justifiable. Following surgical treatment, patients with high risk of recurrence are subjected to adjuvant radiotherapy.

Besides primary surgery and primary radiotherapy, patients with bulky disease have also been subjected to extensive studies to evaluate the other therapeutic options. Following are the other options of treatment for patients with stage 1B2 and 2A2 cervical cancer (please refer to the sections sections "Radiotherapy in Cervical Cancer" and "Neoadjuvant Chemotherapy in Cervical Cancer" of this chapter to learn more about each option and some of these options required further evaluation):

(a) concomitant radiotherapy and chemotherapy (chemoradiation)
(b) radiation therapy/chemoradiation followed by extrafascial hysterectomy (controversial, some believe that an addition of extrafascial hysterectomy did not improve the survival, although it reduces the recurrence rate) or radical hysterectomy
(c) neoadjuvant chemotherapy followed by radical hysterectomy.

Treatment for Stage 2B-4

Advanced stage cervical cancer can be further divided into (1) locally advanced cervical cancer and (2) metastatic disease. Stages 2B–4A are locally advanced stage disease, while stage 4B is a metastatic disease. Intention of treatment in metastatic disease is palliation. A patient with locally advanced disease is treated with primary chemoradiation. Pelvic exenteration can be considered in a selected patient with stage 4A cervical cancer. Pelvic failure rate after irradiation ranges from 18–39% in stage 2B, 40–50% in stage 3B. There is sufficient evidence to conclude that concurrent chemoradiation therapy is more superior to radiotherapy alone. An updated RTOG trial (RTOG 90-01) on locally advanced cervical cancer had concluded that the addition of chemotherapy (cisplatin, 5-FU) to irradiation improved 5-year survivals from 55% to 79% and disease-free survival from 46% to 74% for stage 1B/2A. These were achieved by reducing the rates of both local recurrence and distant metastases. For stage 3/4A disease, chemoradiation improved 5-year survivals from 45% to 59% and disease-free survival from 37% to 54% (Eifel et al., 2004).

Role of Adjuvant Radiotherapy or Chemoradiation after Surgery

Surgery is the treatment of choice for stage 1–2A1 cervical cancer. Many of the patients with stage 1 disease do not require further treatment if they do not have adverse prognostic factors. However, in significant proportion of these patients, adjuvant treatment is necessary, as their risk of recurrence is higher.

Following are the indications for postoperative adjuvant radiotherapy/chemoradiation:

(a) lymph nodes metastases
(b) narrow surgical margin (<5 mm)
(c) involvement of surgical margin
(d) involvement of lower uterine segment
(e) parametrium infiltration

(f) high GOG score (score > 120) in patients with negative lymph nodes and clear surgical margin (Refer appendix on how to calculate GOG score)

(g) poor histology type such as adenosquamous, small cell neuroendocrine, etc.

GOG score of higher than 120 was correlated with 41% recurrence rate, and Sedlis et al. used a modification of the GOG scoring system and reported a 44% reduction of the risk of recurrences after adjuvant radiotherapy when a combination of three risk factors was present compared to without postoperative irradiation. In another study using a modification from original GOG score, patients with at least two of the three risk factors (pathologic tumour size >4 cm, depth of invasion >15 mm and presence of LVSI) received total pelvic radiotherapy has a lower rate of recurrence (12% vs. 41%) compared to without adjuvant radiotherapy. Adjuvant radiotherapy also leads to significantly longer 5-year cancer specific survival (86% vs. 57%) and 5-year disease-free survival (85% vs. 43%) (Pieterse et al., 2006). The Cochrane Collaboration had reviewed the role of adjuvant radiotherapy and chemoradiation after surgery for cervical cancer, and it was published in 2009 (Rogers et al., 2009). The objective of review was to evaluate the effectiveness and safety of adjuvant therapies (radiotherapy, chemotherapy followed by radiotherapy, chemoradiation) after radical hysterectomy for early-stage cervical cancer (FIGO stage 1B1, 1B2 and 2A). In GOG 92, phase III trial, patients with negative lymph node but who have any of the combinations of deep stromal invasion, large volume and lymphovascular invasion were evaluated. The authors found that adjuvant radiotherapy significantly reduces the risk of death, especially in patients with deep stromal invasion and tumour size of more than 4 cm. Women who received radiotherapy had a significantly lower risk of disease progression within 5 years than women who received no further treatment (HR = 0.5, 95% CI 0.4–0.9). Interestingly, only 9% of patients with adenocarcinoma and adenosquamous tumours in the radiotherapy arm had disease recurrence as compared to 44% in the control arm. The impact of adjuvant radiotherapy on overall survival is unknown. One of the main concerns about adjuvant radiotherapy is the higher rate of toxicity.

Radical Hysterectomy for Cervical Cancer

Radical hysterectomy is indicated as primary surgical treatment in early-stage cervical cancer. Radical hysterectomy must be combined with pelvic lymphadenectomy; besides cervical carcinoma, it is also indicated in endometrial cancer with cervical involvement.

Clark published the first radical hysterectomy in 1895. Wertheim subsequently reported the outcome of abdominal radical hysterectomy in 1912, but during that time, the mortality rate was 19%. Mortality rate was reduced with vaginal radical hysterectomy introduced by Schauta. However, due to overall high operative morbidity and mortality, surgery was replaced by radiotherapy until it was re-introduced by Meigs in 1951. In original Wertheim's hysterectomy, lymphadenectomy was not a routine procedure; however, in Meigs radical hysterectomy, lymphadenectomy was performed routinely. Therefore, the current radical hysterectomy and pelvic lymphadenectomy are actually a combination of Wertheim's and Meigs' methods or Wertheim–Meigs radical hysterectomy.

The primary aim of radical hysterectomy is to remove the primary tumour with adequate surrounding tissues, including parametrium, paracolpus and vaginal cuff in order to reduce the recurrence rate (Fig. 8.7). Piver and Rutledge first published their five classifications of hysterectomy for cervical cancer in 1974, as shown in Table 8.6.

The type 1 Piver–Rutledge–Smith (extrafascial hysterectomy) is not a radical hysterectomy; it is almost similar to simple hysterectomy except in extrafascial hysterectomy, ureter has to be lateralized to enable clamping of the paracervical tissue avoiding cervical stroma and the cervix is removed in total. Extrafascial hysterectomy is recommended in stage 1A1 cervical cancer or in cancer of the endometrium. At present, there are no standard and universally accepted techniques and descriptions of radical hysterectomy. Various methods of radical hysterectomy have been described in the literature and demonstrated by gynaecological oncologists around the world such as Wertheim's radical hysterectomy, Meigs radical hysterectomy, Okabayashi radical hysterectomy, Nerve-sparing radical hysterectomy, total laparaoscopic radical hysterectomy, and others.

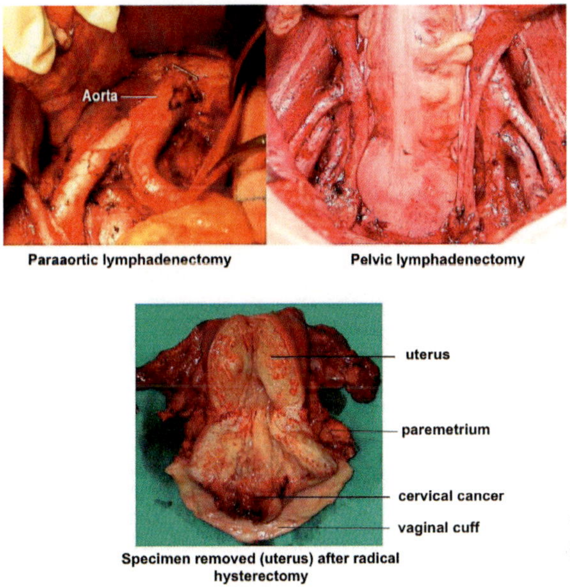

Figure 8.7 Radical hysterectomy and lymphadenectomy (pelvic and para-aortic) for cervical cancer.

Table 8.6 Classification of hysterectomy for cervical cancer (Piver–Rutledge–Smith classification)

Type	Description
1	Extrafascial hysterectomy; removal of all cervical tissue
2	Modified radical hysterectomy; removal of medial half of the cardinal and uterosacral ligaments; the uterine vessels are divided medially to the ureter
3	Equivalent to the classical Wertheim–Meigs operation; wide radical resection of the parametrium and paravaginal tissues with ligation of uterine vessels lateral to ureter; ureter dissected completely to bladder entry; uterosacral ligaments divided at origin; cardinals divided at pelvic side-wall
4	Ureter divided from pubovesical ligament; superior vesical artery ligated and upper two third of the vagina excised
5	Extended radical hysterectomy with possible bowel, bladder or ureteric dissection

The Piver–Rutledge–Smith classification of radical hysterectomy is the most commonly used classification until today. However, this classification has its own limitations:

(a) The classification does not refer to clear anatomical landmarks or international anatomical definitions.
(b) Vaginal resection is excessive from a third to two-thirds of the vagina.
(c) Type 1 is not radical hysterectomy.
(d) The rationale and anatomy to differentiate between types 3 and 4 are unclear.
(e) The classification does not take into account the idea of nerve preservation.
(f) It does not include other types of ultra-radical surgery and fertility sparing surgery.
(g) It applies only to open surgery and does not take into account the development of laparoscopic techniques and the revival of vaginal surgery.

New classification of radical hysterectomy was proposed during International Conference on Radical hysterectomy in Kyoto, Japan in 2007 ("Kyoto declaration"). This new classification is based on only the lateral extent of resection. Table 8.7 shows the proposal of new classification of radical hysterectomy.

Table 8.7 Newly proposed classification of radical hysterectomy

Type	Description
Type A	Minimum resection of paracervix • This is an extrafascial hysterectomy. The paracervix is transected medial to the ureter but lateral to the cervix. The uterosacral and vesicouterine ligaments are not transected at a distance from the uterus. Vaginal resection is generally at a minimum, routinely less than 10 mm, without removal of the vaginal part of the paracervix (paracolpos)
Type B	Transection of the paracervix at the ureter • Partial resection of the ureterosacral and vesicouterine ligaments, ureter is unroofed and rolled laterally, permitting transaction of the paracervix at the level of the ureteric tunnel. At least 10 mm of the vagina from the cervix or tumour is resected • Type B has two subtypes: Type B1: without removal of lateral paracervical lymph nodes and Type B2: additional removal of the lateral paracervical lymph nodes[c]

Type	Description
Type C	Transection of paracervix at junction with internal iliac vasculature system • Transection of the uterosacral ligament at the rectum and vesicouterine ligament at the bladder. The ureter is mobilized completely. 15–20 mm of vagina from the tumour or cervix and the corresponding paracolpos is resected routinely, depending on vaginal and paracervical extent • Type C has two subcategories: Type C1: with nerve preservation[b] and Type C2: without preservation of autonomic nerve
Type D	Laterally extended resection • Rare operations features additional ultraradical procedures. The most radical corresponds to the laterally extended endopelvic resection (LEER) procedure
Lymph node dissection	
Level 1	External and internal iliac up to bifurcation of common iliac
Level 2	Common iliac (including presacral) up to bifurcation of aorta
Level 3	Aortic infra-mesenteric (bifurcation of aorta up to inferior mesenteric artery
Level 4	Aortic infrarenal (inferior mesenteric artery to infrarenal vessels)

[a]This classification can be applied to fertility-sparing surgery and can be adapted to open, vaginal, laparoscopic and robotic surgery.

[b]Nerve preservation surgery involved transaction of uterosacral ligament after separation of hypogastric nerve. The nerve is identified systematically and preserved by transaction of only the uterine branches of the pelvic plexus. The bladder branches of the pelvic plexus are preserved in the lateral ligament of the bladder (i.e. lateral part of bladder pillar).

[c]Tissues that are medial and caudal to obturator nerve are classified as paracervix, tissues that are cranial and lateral to obturator nerves are classified as iliac.

The decision to remove both ovaries during radical hysterectomy is individualized similar to surgery for benign gynaecological conditions. Generally, bilateral salpingoophorectomy is recommended in perimenopausal and postmenopausal women. Bilateral salpingoophorectomy is not mandatory in young patients with early-stage adenocarcinoma of the cervix. A review of almost 1000 women with stage 1B cervical cancer found that the risk of ovarian metastasis was 0.5% in squamous cell carcinoma and 1.7% in adenocarcinoma (Sutton et al., 1992).

Radical hysterectomy carries the higher risk of bladder dysfunction, anorectal dysfunction and sexual dysfunction believed to be due to surgical trauma to sympathetic and parasympathetic innervations of the pelvic organs. Autonomic pelvic nerve injuries can be encountered at superior hypogastric plexus (para-aortic node dissection), hypogastric nerve (resection of uterosacral ligament), pelvic splanchnic nerve (during the transaction of cardinal ligament) and bladder branch of inferior hypogastric plexus (during resection of paracolpus and vesicovaginal ligament.

The pelvic nerve damage can be minimized by two main approaches: (a) less radical surgery and (b) nerve-preserving surgery.

Nerve-Preserving Radical Hysterectomy

Nerve sparing radical hysterectomy was pioneered by Japanese. Some believe that it was first inspired by Okabayashi since 1961 and subsequently popularized by Fujiwara in 1983, Yabuki et al. in the 1990s and later Fujii et al. Hockel et al. from Germany described the first non-Japanese method of nerve-sparing radical hysterectomy in 1998.

There are various methods of nerve-preserving surgery published either from Eastern or from Western countries.

The main steps of nerve sparing radical hysterectomy described by Prof Shingo Fujii from University of Kyota are as follows:

(1) isolation and separation of the deep uterine vein from the pelvic splanchnic nerve
(2) isolation and separation of the hypogastric nerve
(3) separation of the cut end of the deep uterine vein from the pelvic splanchnic nerve
(4) separation of blood vessels in the posterior leaf of the vesicouterine ligament
(5) isolation and division of the inferior vesical vein
(6) separation/division of the uterine branch from the inferior hypogastric plexus
(7) separation and division of the paracolpium

Pelvic lymphadenectomy was often performed first prior to nerve sparing radical hysterectomy. Raspagliesi et al. evaluated the role of nerve sparing radical hysterectomy by comparing type

2 RH, nerve-sparing type 3 RH and classical type 3 RH. They conclude that type 3 nerve-sparing RH seems to be comparable to type 2 RH and more superior than type 3 RH in terms of early bladder dysfunction.

Nerve sparing radical hysterectomy appears to be a feasible alternative to the classic technique of radical hysterectomy. However, at present the technique still needs further evaluation and revision before it can be accepted as a standard procedure. Furthermore, there are several concerns related to this relatively new surgical technique, such as the following:

(a) The procedure may lead to unintentionally incomplete or inadequate tumour resection.
(b) Only experienced and trained surgeon can perform this complex surgery.
(c) The complexity of this technique together with the requirement of special instruments and equipment may pose a hindrance for this technique to be performed in under-developed and developing countries due to cost factor.
(d) Lack of uniformity in the understanding of the anatomy and technique
(e) Prolonged operating time.

Complications of Radical Hysterectomy

Complications related to radical hysterectomy and pelvic lymphadenectomy can be divided into early complications and late complications. See Table 8.8 for the lists of early and late complications.

Table 8.8 Complications of radical hysterectomy and pelvic lymphadenectomy

Early complications	Late complications
1. Intraoperative complications such as anaestheticrelated complications, blood loss, injuries to the ureter (0.6–1.7%), bladder, rectum, pelvic vessels and nerve (genitor-femoral, obturator nerve). 2. Postoperative complications such as early deep vein thrombosis (0.3%), urinary tract infections (10–16%), voiding problem and wound infection (4–6%) and vesicovaginal or ureterovesical fistula. 3. Lymphocoele	1. Chronic bladder dysfunction 2. Rectal sphincter dysfunction 3. Ureteric stricture 4. Late fistula 5. Lymphoedema 6. Sexual dysfunction

Fertility-Preserving Surgery in Cervical Cancer

Approximately, 45% of patients with operable early-stage cervical cancer were diagnosed in women under the age of 40. Many of these women wish to preserve their fertility.

Following are the options for fertility-preserved surgery in cervical cancer:

(a) radical trachelectomy and pelvic lymphadenectomy
(b) cone biopsy or simple trachelectomy
(c) neoadjuvant chemotherapy followed by fertility-preserving surgery

Radical Trachelectomy

Radical trachelectomy is total excision of the cervix with surrounding tissues, including paracervical, paracolpus and vaginal cuff while retaining the uterine body and adnexae. Radical Vaginal trachelectomy was first described by Daniel Dargent in 1994. Radical Vaginal trachelectomy and laparoscopic lymphadenectomy is perhaps the most common fertility-preserved procedure for early cervical cancer reported in the literatures. Until 2008, there were more than 700 cases of RVT, and over 250 pregnancies had been reported.

Apart from the vaginal approach, trachelectomy can also be accomplished through different techniques such as

(a) radical abdominal trachelectomy
(b) total laparoscopic radical trachelectomy
(c) robotic radical trachelectomy

Not all patients with operable cervical cancer are suitable for radical trachelectomy. Patient selection is extremely important and the criteria for RVT are as follows (Ramirez et al., 2008):

(1) a desire for future fertility
(2) proven diagnosis of invasive cervical cancer
(3) squamous cell carcinoma and adenocarcinoma; unfavourable histology such as small cell neuroendocrine tumour and adenosquamous are excluded.
(4) stage 1A1 with lymphovascular space invasion, stage 1A2 or stage 1B1

(5) tumour size ≤2 cm and limited to the cervix (preferably by pre-operative MRI)
(6) no evidence of pelvic node metastasis
(7) no previous documentation of infertility

When the tumour size is difficult to assess, magnetic resonance imaging (MRI) is the best imaging technique to determine the size and volume of tumour. MRI is also useful to assess the degree of paracervical and parametrium involvement.

Laparoscopic lymphadenectomy is performed either prior to or after radical trachelectomy, preferably through retroperitoneal approach. If sentinel node mapping and biopsy are performed, frozen section of the sentinel node will determine the direction of subsequent management. If pelvic nodes are positive, trachelectomy should be abandoned.

Following radical trachelectomy, frozen section is done on the cervical specimen to assess the superior margin. The aim is to achieve at least 5 mm free margin. A cerclage is placed either with Mersilene, Prolene or Ethibond suture. The placement of cerclage at the time of radical trachelectomy is debatable, there has been increasing concern that cerclage at the same setting may lead to cervical stenosis, bladder irritation, erosion and chronic discharge.

Radical vaginal trachelectomy needs training and not many gynaecological oncologists are competent to perform this surgery. Perhaps many surgeons are more familiar with radical abdominal trachelectomy (RAT) because the surgery is almost similar to radical hysterectomy. Indications for RAT are similar to RVT, but RAT is a preferred approach in the following cases: (a) patients with distorted vaginal anatomy, (b) cervical cancer in paediatric, young and unmarried patients and (c) cancer of a cervical stump after subtotal hysterectomy.

The number of surgeons performing robotic radical trachelectomy is increasing; several case reports have demonstrated that robotic radical trachelectomy is a safe and feasible procedure if performed by the trained surgeon.

Results from several published papers (Ramirez et al., 2008; Olawaiye et al., 2009; Gien and Covens, 2010) reviewing the role of radical trachelectomy have concluded that radical trachelectomy is safe and feasible and pregnancy outcomes are favourable. Pregnancy rates of 41–79% were achieved, and 40% of them resulted in term delivery (Beiner and Covens, 2007; Plante, 2008).

Reported complications of radical trachelectomy are dysmenorrhea, irregular vaginal bleeding, problems related to cerclage suture, premature delivery in more than 40% of cases, excessive vaginal discharge, isthmic stenosis (10%), dyspareunia and amenorrhea.

Neoadjuvant Chemotherapy Followed by Fertility-Preserving Surgery

Neoadjuvant chemotherapy in cervical cancer is still controversial, and this topic will be discussed in the later section of this chapter. Neoadjuvant chemotherapy may reduce the tumour size and facilitates subsequent fertility-preserving surgery. Maneo and colleagues have reported 21 patients with stage 1B1 cervical cancer treated with neoadjuvant chemotherapy (platinum-based regimen) followed by cold-knife conization and pelvic lymphadenectomy. Twenty-one patients underwent conization and pelvic lymphadenectomy; after a median follow-up of 5 years 9 months, no relapses were observed.

Cone Biopsy or Simple Trachelectomy

The role of cone biopsy in stage 1A1 cervical cancer was discussed in earlier section. The use of cone biopsy and simple trachelectomy plus pelvic lymphadenectomy in selected patients with stage 1A2 and 1B1 is very controversial and warrant further investigation.

Radiotherapy in Cervical Cancer

There are two types of radiation therapy in cervical cancer: (a) External photon beam (delivered by linear accelerator) and (b) Brachytherapy.

External beam radiotherapy (EBRT) is irradiation delivered to the whole pelvis, parametrium, pelvic and para-aortic lymph nodes (extended beam). Brachytherapy is in the form of intracavitary radiotherapy targeting the cervix, vagina and medial parametrium. The most commonly used applicator is the Fletcher–Suit intrauterine tandem and vaginal ovoid. External pelvic irradiation is given prior to intracavitary insertion in: (a) bulky cervical lesions, (b) exophytic, easily bleeding tumour, (c) tumour with necrosis or infection and (d) parametrial involvement. The entire processes of radiotherapy are demonstrated in Figs. 8.8, 8.9 and 8.10.

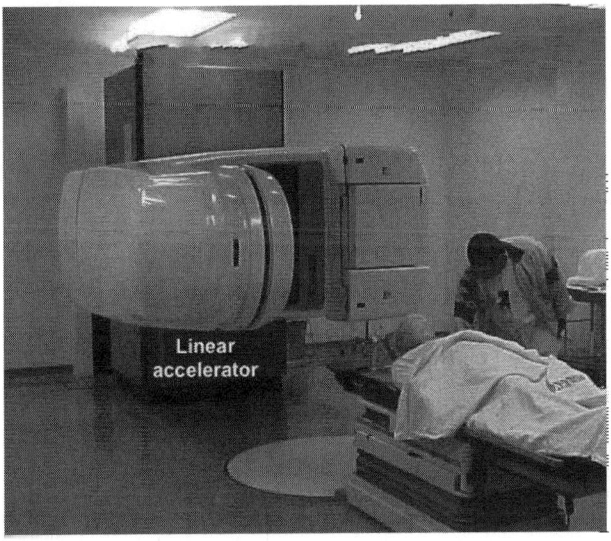

Figure 8.8 Linear accelerator delivers the high-voltage x-ray, as an external beam radiotherapy.

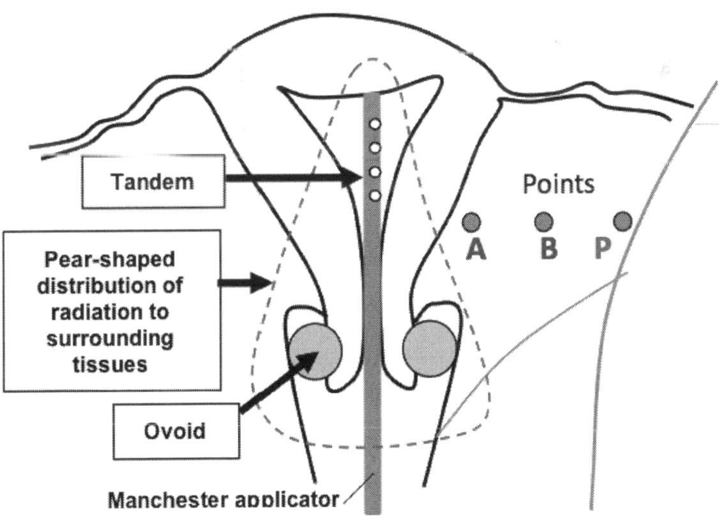

Figure 8.9 Brachytherapy technique using Manchester applicators.

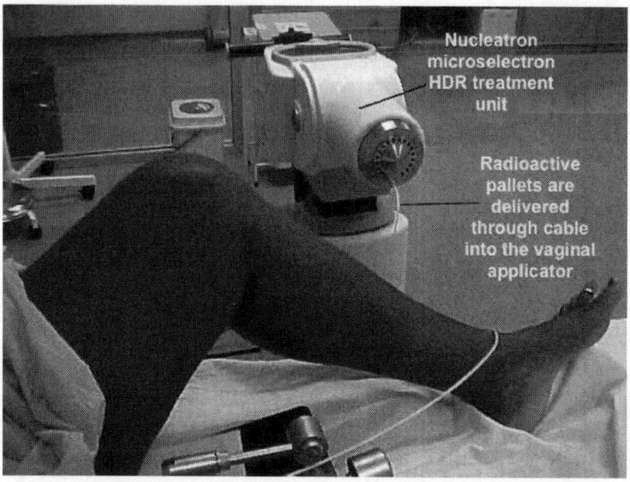

Figure 8.10 Brachytherapy delivered from the nucleatron microselectron (the radiation source is from iridium).

Stage 1A1 can be treated with intracavitary therapy alone with 60 Gy single insertions to point A. External pelvic irradiation is given to a patient with stage 1A2 and more (as an alternative to surgical treatment or as postoperative adjuvant therapy). Inoperable stage IB1 cervical cancer patients should be treated with both EBRT and brachytherapy. Concurrent chemotherapy may be considered at the Oncologist's discretion and based on the presence of high-risk features.

Clinical stage 1B2-4A cervical cancer should be treated with concurrent chemoradiation followed by brachytherapy.

Stage 4B cervical cancer may be palliatively treated with brachytherapy with or without EBRT to decrease the risk of haemorrhage or other life-threatening symptoms.

External pelvic irradiation is given in 20–25 fractions within 5 weeks and brachytherapy is inserted two to three insertion within one week at the end of EBRT treatment. The GOG has defined three standard pelvic points where dose designation can be planned and correlated with clinical effect (see Fig. 8.9):

(a) **Point A**: 2 cm from the midline of the cervical canal and 2 cm superior to lateral vaginal fornix/cervical os. The dose at the point A represents of the dose to paracervical triangle that correlates well with the incidence of sequelae and 5 years' control rate. This point is an also approximate point at which the ureter and uterine artery cross.

(b) **Point B**: 3 cm lateral to point A or 5 cm lateral to the centre of the pelvis at the same level as point A. This point is of significance in considering the dose to the node bearing tissue, especially obturator nodes or lateral parametrium.

(c) **Point P**: located along the bony pelvic sidewall at its most lateral point and represents the minimal dose to the external iliac lymph nodes.

Various techniques have been developed to improve the effectiveness of radiotherapy and minimized radiation toxicity to adjacent organs such as CT simulation, conformal blocking and intensity-modulated radiation therapy (IMRT). External pelvic irradiation is often given prior to brachytherapy. There are two types of brachytherapy, i.e. (1) low dose rate brachytherapy (LDR) and (2) high dose rate brachytherapy (HDR). In LDR brachytherapy, intracavitary insertion delivered 50–70 cGy/hour to point A in stage 1B and 70–75 cGy/hour in stage 2A, 2B and 3. Patients have to stay 2–3 days in the hospital. One or two treatment sessions are required. HDR brachytherapy has become more popular and increasingly used in many Oncology centres. Dose rate is typically 200 to 300 cGy/minute given within <30 minutes. HDR is administered as outpatient procedures. Studies have shown that HDR and LDR were equally effective in terms of a relapse-free survival and overall survival rates. Two to ten insertions are required.

If para-aortic nodes metastases are suspected, 45–50 Gys is given to para-aortic areas (extended external beam) plus 5 Gys boost to any enlarged nodes. The RTOG trial had found that para-aortic EBRT conferred a survival benefit in patients with bulky stage 1 disease (>4 cm) and stage 2 cervical cancer as compared to standard pelvic irradiation alone. There is no strong evidence regarding the role of hyperbaric oxygen, hypoxic sensitizer (Metronidazole, Misonidazole) and hyperthermia (microwave) in potentiating radiation therapy.

The radiotherapy is curative for cervical cancer up to stage 4A disease. However, in metastatic disease, radiotherapy provides symptomatic relief or palliative radiotherapy. Palliative radiotherapy may be indicated in (a) stage 4B and recurrent carcinoma presented with pelvic pain and bleeding and (b) single intracavitary insertion of tandem and colpostats delivering 55 Gy to point A may control the vaginal bleeding.

Concurrent Chemoradiation in Cervical Cancer

The combination of concomitant chemotherapy and radiation therapy is currently recognized as standard of care in many cancer treatments, including for locally advanced cervical cancer.

The rationales of chemoradiation are

(a) to sensitized the tumour cells to radiation (radiopotentiator)
(b) attack the different phases of the cell cycles and give synergistic effect.
(c) decrease tumour re-population
(d) increase tumour cell oxygenation
(e) shortened treatment time
(f) inhibition of repair of sublethal radiation damage
(g) to eradicate microscopic systemic disease and micrometastasis

The introduction of chemoradiotherapy into routine clinical practice for locally advanced cervical cancer is one of the significant medical discoveries in history of cancer treatment. In US, National Cancer Institute had first issued the support of using chemoradiation in cervical cancer in 1999.

The current recommendation of chemoradiation as the standard treatment for cervical cancer is based on the results of five landmark phase III randomized controlled trials listed below (see Table 8.9 for the summaries):

(1) Gynae Oncology Group (GOG) Protocol 85
(2) Gynae Oncology Group Protocol 120
(3) Gynae Oncology Group Protocol 123
(4) Southwest Oncology Group (SWOG): 1 study with GOG and RTOG (SWOG Protocol 8797)
(5) Radiation Therapy Oncology Group (RTOG): RTOG 90-01

An updated of RTOG Protocol 90-01 trial (refer to the original trial in Table 8.9) had reported that an addition of chemotherapy to radiation therapy improved disease-free survival from 46% to 74% and five-year survivals from 55% to 79% for stage 1B-2A.

Chemoradiation also improved disease-free survival from 37% to 54% and 5-year survival rates from 45% to 59% in stage 3/4A disease. After median follow time of 6.6 years, the overall survival rate for patients treated with chemoradiation was significantly greater than radiotherapy alone (67% vs. 41%, $p < 0.0001$). The overall reduction in the risk of recurrence was 51%. Disease-free survival (DFS) and overall survival (OS) in patients with stage 1B–2B treated with chemoradiation was significantly longer. In stages 3 and 4A, chemoradiation improves PFS but not OS ($p = 0.07$). The rate of serious late complications was similar (Eifel et al., 2004).

Table 8.9 Summary of five phase III randomized controlled trials on chemoradiation versus radiotherapy for cervical cancer

Trial	Summary
GOG 85 (Whitney CW, et al. GOG study. *J Clin Oncol* 1999; 17: 1339)	**Subjects**: Stage 2B-4A ($n = 368$), all para-aortic nodes negative **Study**: Irradiation + cisplatin (50 mg/m^2)/5-FU (1g/m^2/d vs. Hydoxyurea (80 mg/kg twice weekly) + irradiation. **Results**: Cisplatin/5FU more superior in progression free interval and survival ($p < 0.05$)
GOG 120 (Rose PG, Bundy BN, et al. *N Engl J Med* 1999; 340: 1144)	**Subjects**: Stage 2B, 3 and 4A ($n = 526$), all para-aortic nodes -ve. **Study**: Irradiation + weekly cisplatin (40 mg/m^2 weekly for 6 weeks (during ext radiation) vs. irradiation + hydroxyurea vs. irradiation + cisplatin/5FU/hydroxyurea vs. irradiation + hydroxyurea. **Results**: Cisplatinum based regimen more superior in survival and progression free survival with single agent cisplatin has almost similar result with combined regimes (45% vs. 43% reduction in risk of progression). Because of an improved therapeutic ratio, weekly cisplatin is the favoured regimen.
GOG 123 (Keys HM, Bundy BN, et al. *N Engl J Med* 1999; 340: 1154)	**Subjects**: Stage 1B to 2A ($n = 369$), all had surgical assessment of para-aortic nodes **Study**: Irradiation + extrafascial hysterectomy vs. cisplatin single agent weekly + irradiation + extrafascial hysterectomy. (GOG 71 study showed no benefit of added hysterectomy)

(Continued)

Table 8.9 *(Continued)*

Trial	Summary
	Results: Concurrent chemoradiation shows more superior in reduction of progression (49%) and survival (46% reduction of death, and 3-year survival 83% vs. 74%). Chemoradiation is treatment of choice in stage 1B and 2A.
RTOG Protocol 90-01 (Morris M, et al. *N Engl J Med* 1999; 340: 1137)	**Subjects**: Stage 1B to 4A (n = 389) **Study**: Irradiation + cisplatin/5-FU vs. RT alone. Not all had surgical staging for para-aortic nodes.
	Results: Chemoradiation is more superior in reduction of disease progression, survival, locoregional and distant relapses. (52% reduction in risk of progression, 41% reduction in risk of death and 5-year survival rate from 73% (stage 1B-2A), all statistically significant)
SWOG Protocol 8797 (SWOG + GOG + RTOG) (Peter WA, Liu PY, et al. *Gynecol Oncol* 1999; 72: 443)	**Subject**: Stage 1A2, 1B and 2A (n = 243), subjects had pelvic/para-aortic LN +, positive parametrial involvement, positive surgical margin after radical hysterectomy. Negative common iliac and/or para-aortic nodes were also included. **Study**: Irradiation + cisplatin (70 mg/m^2)/5-FU vs. irradiation alone. **Results**: Chemoradiation is more superior in progression free survival and survival (51% reduction in risk of death), 3-year survival rate was 87% vs. 77%.

The Royal College of Radiologists (RCR) in the United Kingdom had recently published retrospective audit of cervical cancer patients during chemoradiation era involving 1075 patients from 42 centres in the United Kingdom. The audit showed that chemoradiation increases overall 5-year survival rates by 11% (44% vs. 55%) as compared to radiation alone (Vale, 2008).

The Gynecologic Oncology Group 165 trial (randomized trial) by Lanciano et al. comparing single agent cisplatin versus single agent 5-FU infusion in combination with radiation for advanced cervical cancer had shown that single agent cisplatin was a better combination. Rose PG et al. also obtained a similar result in extended follow-up GOG 120 trial comparing single agent cisplatin, cisplatin-

5-hydroxyurea and radiotherapy in advanced cervical cancer. Nugent et al. did an analysis of the cisplatin dosing in a chemoradiation regimen and they found that patients who received less than six cycles of cisplatin had a worse progression free survival and overall survival.

The most popular and acceptable chemotherapy regimen in chemoradiation protocol is a cisplatin-based regimen. Single agent weekly cisplatin is the most commonly practiced followed by a combination of cisplatin with 5-FU. However, Kim and colleagues have found that combination cisplatin-5-FU was associated with higher rate of grades 3 and 4 haematologic toxicity (26% vs. 43%) with no survival advantage as compared to single agent cisplatin. The role of other agents in combination with cisplatin was also being evaluated such as topotecan (Long et al., 2005) and gemcitabine (Gonzalez et al., 2005); the results were encouraging. There are more than 20 randomized control trials on concurrent chemoradiation versus radiation alone for cervical cancer involving nearly 5000 patients, the trials have shown that chemoradiation improve progression-free survival, reduction in local recurrence and overall survival (Green et al., 2005; Vale, 2008).

Despite encouraging results from chemoradiation trials, there are at least three main concerns related to this treatment: (a) toxicity (60% risk of premature ovarian failure, higher haematological and gastrointestinal toxicity); (b) approximately, 20% of patients still develop pelvic failure and recurrence despite therapy; and (c) chemotherapy in chemoradiation protocol may not be sufficient to tackle distance diseases.

The long-term analysis of the clinical outcome of surgery following primary chemoradiation (cisplatin-5FU given every 4 weeks in three cycles during EBRT) was analyzed by Ferrandina et al. Out of 174 patients who underwent radical hysterectomy following chemoradiation for locally advanced cervical cancer, 71.3% showed a complete pathological response. After a median follow-up of 68 months, 5-year disease-free survival (DFS) was 75.5% and 5-year overall survival (OS) was 77.4%. Patients with no residual disease showed a significant longer DFS than a patient with microscopic and macroscopic residual tumour after treatment. Residual tumour and stage of disease were the most relevant prognostic factors for DFS and OS. The potential advantages of surgery after chemoradiation are removal of potential chemo and radioresistant clone and obtaining important prognostic information via histopathogical examination. However, the potential disadvantages of this approach are the side effects (13–20% risk of grade 3/4 complications), operative difficulties and impairment quality of life. Colombo PE et al. Compared total laparoscopic radical hysterectomy (TLRH) with abdominal radical hysterectomy (ARH) following chemoradiation for patients with bulky stage 1B, 2A and 2B; TLRH was associated with shorter hospital stay, less blood loss and lower morbidity rate (including urinary complications) without compromising the oncological outcome (PFS and OS were similar). The role of surgery following chemoradiation warrant further evaluation by phase III randomized control trial.

Chemotherapy in Cervical Cancer

Chemotherapy has becoming more important in the treatment of cervical cancer especially in the chemoradiation setting. Before 1983, cervical cancer was thought to be a chemoresistant tumour. There are five areas where chemotherapy play an important role in the management of cervical cancer: (a) management of recurrent and metastatic disease not amenable to be controlled with surgical or radiation therapy, (b) concurrent use of chemotherapy with radiation therapy (refer to an earlier section), (c) neoadjuvant chemotherapy for locally advanced cervical cancer (mainly in bulky stage 1B and 2A disease), (d) other forms of combination therapy with surgery, radiotherapy and targeted therapy (mainly in locally advanced disease) and (e) palliative chemotherapy.

Despite the above roles in cervical cancer, chemotherapy still has a considerable limitations because of the following reasons: (a) good response to surgical and radiation therapy, (b) the patient with recurrence disease had been irradiated and delivery of chemotherapeutic drug to the tumour will be impaired due to radiation-induced fibrosis and poor vascularization, (c) prior irradiation also causes a tumour resistant to chemo drug, (d) prior irradiation also causes limited bone marrow reserve and (e) recurrent or advanced tumour often causes obstructive nephropathy.

Chemotherapy for Metastatic and Recurrent Cervical Cancer

Chemotherapy is one of the options for patients with metastatic cervical cancer and perhaps most common treatment offered to this patient. The intention of treatment in metastatic cervical cancer is palliation. Patients with metastatic disease may not require any form of treatment if they are asymptomatic or if their general health is so poor to withstand any form of therapy. In the later group of patients, supportive treatment is the only option available for them. Generally, platinum-based chemotherapy is the standard regimen for patients with metastatic disease.

At least three GOG phase III randomized controlled trials (see Table 8.10) evaluated the most effective chemotherapy regimens in metastatic and recurrent cervical cancer. The control arm was single agent cisplatin 50 mg/m^2. As shown in Table 8.10, the study arms were cisplatin-based combined regimens (doublet). The second cytotoxic agent included in the doublet was ifosfamide, paclitaxel or topotecan.

Table 8.10 Phase III trials on chemotherapy in recurrent and metastatic cervical cancer

GOG trials	GOG 110[a]	GOG 169[b]	GOG 179[c]
Chemotherapy	Cisplatin vs. cisplatin + ifosfamide	Cisplatin vs. cisplatin + paclitaxel	Cisplatin vs. cisplatin + topotecan
Response Rate (%)	19% vs. 31%	19% vs. 36%	13% vs. 27%[d]
PFS (months)	3.2% vs. 4.6%	2.8% vs. 4.8%	2.9% vs. 4.6%[d]
OS (months)	8 vs. 8.3	8.8 vs. 9.7	6.5 vs. 9.4[d]

Note: Cisplatin regimen in all trials was 50 mg/m^2 every 3 weeks.
GOG, Gynaecology Oncology Group; PFS, progression-free survival, OS, overall survival.
[a]Omura GA, et al. *J Clin Oncol* 1997; **15**: 165–171.
[b]Moore DH, et al. *J Clin Oncol* 2004; **22**: 3113–3119.
[c]Long III HJ, Bundy N, Grendys Jr EC, et al. *J Clin Oncol* 2005; **23**: 4626–4633.
[d]Statistically significant difference.

All GOG trials listed in Table 8.10 showed that cisplatin doublet produced higher rates of response and progression-free survival than cisplatin monotherapy but all except topotecan did not reach statistical significant. Please note that in GOG 179, overall survival in cisplatin monotherapy was lower than in other GOG trials. The lower rate of OS in the control arm in the GOG 179 trial led to a statistically significant survival benefit in the study arm. Furthermore, in GOG 179, there were more patients received prior chemoradiation as their primary treatment as compared to other GOG trials (two-fold increase, nearly 60% received prior cisplatin-based chemoradiation). Although FDA has given an approval for the use of topotecan following the outcome of this study, the superiority of topotecan is still questionable and GOG had initiated the subsequent trial known as GOG 204, which had been completed and presented (see Table 8.11). Toxicity was more in a doublet regimen as compared to cisplatin monotherapy. However, despite increased toxicity, combination of cisplatin/paclitaxel and cisplatin/topotecan arms did not significantly reduce the patient-reported quality of life (Monk et al., 2005; McQuellon et al., 2006). Although a higher dose of cisplatin (75 mg/m^2 and 100 mg/m^2) was associated with slightly better objective response rate compared to lower dose of 50 mg/m^2, there was no associated improvement in the complete response rate, progression-free survival and overall survival. Higher dose cisplatin was associated with greater nephrotoxicity and myelosupresssion (Bonomi et al., 1985).

Table 8.11 GOG protocol 204 trial (GOG 204: A randomized phase III trial of four cisplatin containing doublet combination in stage 4B, recurrent, or persistent cervical carcinoma: A GOG study[a])

Arm 1	Paclitaxel (135 mg/m^2 over 24 hours on day 1 + cisplatin 50 mg/m^2 on day 2) every 3 weeks
Arm 2	Vinorelbine (30 mg/m^2 on days 1 and 8) + cisplatin 50 mg/m^2 on day 2) every 3 weeks
Arm 3	Gemcitabine (1000 mg/m^2 on days 1 and 8) + cisplatin 50 mg/m^2 on day 2) every 3 weeks
Arm 4	Topotecan (0.75 mg/m^2 on day 1, 2 and 3) + cisplatin 50 mg/m^2 on day 2) every 3 weeks

Note: Eligibility criteria included ECOG performance status of 0 or 1, acceptable end organ function and measurable disease.

GOG, Gynecologic Oncology Group.

[a]Wenzel LB, Huang H, Cella D, et al. *J Clin Oncol* 2008; **26** (May 20 suppl: abstr LBA5504).

At present, there is no strong evidence to show that carboplatin is equally effective as cisplatin. Cisplatin remains the drug of choice for advanced squamous cell carcinoma of the cervix.

The other interesting cytotoxic agents evaluated in advanced cervical cancer are vinorelbine and gemcitabine. Both of these drugs have been evaluated in phase II trial, and their response rate was encouraging ranging from 30–95%. As a follow-up of the above studies (Table 8.10), GOG has initiated a phase III randomized control trial (**GOG protocol 204**) since 2003 evaluating four cisplatin-based doublets, i.e. cisplatin/paclitaxel, cisplatin/topotecan, cisplatin/vinorelbine and cisplatin/gemcitabine in stage 4B, recurrent or persistent carcinoma of the cervix. Summary of the regimens is shown in Table 8.11.

The results of GOG 204 trial were presented in annual American Society of Clinical Oncology (ASCO) meeting 2008. There were 513 patients recruited and following are the results:

(a) No difference in tumour response rate across all four arms (response rate between 23.4–29.1%)

(b) No significant difference in progression-free survival and overall survival across the four arms, although non-statistically significant benefit to cisplatin/paclitaxel arm on median survival (12.9 months vs. 10–10.3 months in others) and hazard ratios for death.

(c) Quality of life (QOL) assessment shows no significant difference in QOL observed between all four arms, although QOL demonstrated a non-statistically significant trend towards improvement of the outcome with cisplatin/paclitaxel as compared to others.

(d) Toxicities did not vary significantly across the four arms.

(e) The authors concluded that cisplatin/paclitaxel should remain the doublet of choice in the treatment of advanced or recurrent cervical cancer.

Overall, treatment for advanced and recurrent cervical cancer remains unsatisfactory with median progression-free survival less than 6 months and median overall survival ranging from 10–12 months. Given these circumstances, all systemic chemotherapy options for treatment of advanced or recurrent cervical cancer should be viewed as palliative.

To role of targeted therapy or biologic agent such as bevacizumab in combination with chemotherapy has been evaluated. Among targeted therapies that have been evaluated are Gefitinib (phase II trial by Goncalves et al.), Cetuximab (ongoing study, combination of cisplatin-cetuximab in persistent and recurrent carcinoma of the cervix), erlotinib, trastuzumab, sunitinib and bevacizumab (combination of bevacizumab with 5-FU or capecitabine, response rate 34% (Wright et al., 2006).

Neoadjuvant Chemotherapy in Cervical Cancer

Neoadjuvant chemotherapy is chemotherapy given prior to primary surgical treatment with the intention to reduce the bulk of tumour, facilitate surgical resection and improving the oncological outcomes (disease-free survival and overall survival). With a smaller tumour, surgery can also be less radical and result in lower rate of treatment-related morbidity. The concept of neoadjuvant chemotherapy in cervical cancer was first published in *Journal of Gynecologic Oncology* in 1983 by Friedlander et al. In cervical cancer, neoadjuvant chemotherapy can also be administered prior to radiotherapy. Neoadjuvant chemotherapy given before radiotherapy may reduce the tumour size and controls micrometastases. This approach may also reduce radiation toxicity (compared to concurrent chemoradiation), improve the effectiveness of radiotherapy by reducing distortion and decreasing hypoxic cells fraction.

The rationales of giving chemotherapy prior to primary surgery are as follows:

(a) to reduce the bulk and downstaging the tumour
(b) to increase operability (surgery may also remove the radioresistant cell clone)
(c) smaller tumour and downstaging may also reduce surgical radicality
(d) less radical surgery may reduce operative morbidity
(e) less radical surgery is also referred to fertility-preserving surgery
(f) theoretically, chemotherapy given prior to surgery may decrease intra-operative dissemination of tumour cells

(g) eradication of subclinical metastases
(h) reduction in adjuvant radiotherapy rate

In evaluating the role of neoadjuvant chemotherapy in cervical cancer, there are at least four areas of interest:

(1) neoadjuvant chemotherapy followed by radiotherapy versus radical radiotherapy
(2) neoadjuvant chemotherapy followed by radical surgery versus radical radiotherapy
(3) neoadjuvant chemotherapy followed by radical surgery versus radical surgery
(4) neoadjuvant chemotherapy followed by radical surgery versus concurrent chemoradiation.

The role of neoadjuvant chemotherapy prior to radiotherapy was evaluated in systematic review and meta-analysis by Tierney et al. involving 21 trials mostly stage 2–3 disease. After correcting the significant heterogeneity in this analysis, the authors have discovered that 5-year survival rates were affected by the frequency and dose intensity of cisplatin. Patients with longer chemotherapy interval of more than 14 days and cisplatin dose intensity of less than 25 mg/m^2 had lower 5-year survival by 8% and 11%, respectively. There were some survival benefits if the chemotherapy interval was ≤14 days and cisplatin dose ≥25 mg/m^2.

The Italian multicentre randomized study compared neoadjuvant chemotherapy followed by radical surgery versus primary radiotherapy in patients with stage 1B2-3 cervical cancer. Fourteen centres were involved with almost 300 participants. Chemotherapy was cisplatin-based with second agent bleomycin (majority), vinristine or ifosfamide. Nine percent received cisplatin monotherapy. This study had shown that the operability rate following neoadjuvant chemotherapy was 85.5% for stage 1B2–2B and 55% for stage 3 disease. There was no difference in toxicity while the survival benefits were only observed in patients with stage 1B2–2B receiving neoadjuvant chemotherapy; not in more advanced stage (Benedetti-Panici et al., 2002).

Chen and colleagues had evaluated the role of neoadjuvant chemotherapy followed by radical surgery versus radical surgery in locally advanced cervical cancer stage 1B2–2B. In this randomized trial, they found that patients in the neoadjuvant chemotherapy group had lower lymph node metastases (14.4% vs. 45.5%) and parametrial infiltration rate than in the primary surgery group. A similar result was obtained in a study done by Cai et al. neoadjuvant chemotherapy was given to stage 1B cervical cancer; fewer lymph nodes metastases were noted in the neoadjuvant group. In addition, there was also an improvement in survival and disease-free survival in patients treated with neoadjuvant chemotherapy.

Sardi and colleagues did a long-term follow-up (7 years) of the first randomized trial on neoadjuvant chemotherapy in stage 1B squamous cell carcinoma of the cervix. They have found that neoadjuvant chemotherapy can reduce a pelvic failure rate and improve survival in bulky stage 1B (>4 cm) disease. Several other studies, however, did not show same survival advantages in the neoadjuvant chemotherapy arm (Napolitano et al., 2003; Eddy et al., 2007) instead neoadjuvant chemotherapy may be detrimental in some patients (Katsumata et al., 2006).

Several studies have shown that squamous cell carcinoma responds better to chemotherapy than adenocarcinoma. Namkoong et al. reported that response to neoadjuvant chemotherapy was more favourable in squamous cell carcinoma (87%) than in adenocarcinomas (38%). These findings were similar to study done by Chen et al. (76.7% vs. 33.3%, p value 0.005).

Patients with large volume of tumour (>5 cm diameter) have poorer response rate to neoadjuvant chemotherapy. Patients with large residual tumours after neoadjuvant chemotherapy often respond poorly to subsequent treatment and had poorer survival.

Studies comparing neoadjuvant chemotherapy followed by surgery versus primary chemoradiation by EORTC (European Organization for Research and Treatment of Cancer) and Tata Memorial Hospital are still under way. Both studies are comparing neoadjuvant chemotherapy versus chemoradiation in stage 1B2, 2A2 and 2B cervical cancer (EORTC 55994). In this study (EORTC 55994), the main eligibility criteria are (a) squamous cell carcinoma, adenosquamous or adenocarcinoma, (b) FIGO stage 1B2, 2A2 or 2B, (c) WHO performance status 0–2, (d) Age 18–75 and (e) No prior irradiation or chemotherapy. The neoadjuvant arm received cisplatin-based chemotherapy with minimum cumulative cisplatin dose of 225 mg/m^2 and 25 mg/m^2 per week. The chemoradiation arm receives cisplatin 40 mg/m^2, maximum 80 mg and six administrations concurrently with EBRT (45–50 Gy) in fractions of 1.8 Gy to 2 Gy plus external boost or brachytherapy. The primary endpoint is overall survival and secondary endpoints are progression free survival, toxicity and quality of life.

The problems and difficulties in incorporating neoadjuvant chemotherapy into the treatment protocol still exist and require further evaluation. Among the difficulties and dilemmas related to this practice are the following:

(1) choice of the best chemotherapeutic agents and regimen
(2) time factors, i.e. (a) duration and interval of treatment (b) potential delaying primary treatment
(3) toxicity
(4) problem with tissue plane and dissection during radical hysterectomy due to chemotherapy-induced fibrosis and calcification
(5) treatment dilemma in a patient with chemoresistance
(6) chemotherapy agents could have cross-resistance with radiotherapy, including the development of radio-resistant cellular clones
(7) alteration of pathologic parameters by chemotherapy (smaller node making the metastatic deposits hard to detect by pathologist, which is called "concealing effect")
(8) "concealing effect" may also lead to the underestimation of the risk of recurrence and undertreatment
(9) cost effectiveness and psycho-social problems

Neoadjuvant chemotherapy in cervical cancer is still considered as investigational because (a) the number of studies and samples are still inadequate, (b) heterogeneity in the study design, chemotherapy regimens, tumour stage, and others, (c) chemotherapy regimen used in many trials are considered outdated and (d) radiotherapy in many published studies was radiotherapy alone and not chemoradiation. Chemoradiation is currently the standard treatment for cervical cancer and should be considered in a control arm.

Treatment for Non-Squamous Cell Carcinoma of Cervix

Almost 80% of cervical carcinoma is squamous cell carcinoma (SCC). Approximately, 10–20% of patients with advanced and recurrent cervical cancer are a non-SCC type. There are limited phase III trials of chemotherapy in non-SCC cervical cancer.

In recurrent adenocarcinoma of the cervix, various chemotherapy regimens have been evaluated in phase II trial either as a single agent or combination therapy. Single agent paclitaxel administered over 24-hour infusion was associated with 31% overall response rate (Curtin et al., 2001). In platinum-naïve patients, combination of cisplatin and taxanes are probably the most reasonable option for patients with recurrent adenocarcinoma of the cervix.

Neuroendocrine tumours of the cervix are uncommon and account for only 1–2% of all cervical cancers. They can be classified as typical carcinoid, atypical carcinoid, small-cell carcinoma and large-cell neuroendocrine carcinoma. Most of the reported cases are small-cell carcinomas. Small cell carcinoma, which exhibits no squamous differentiation, should not be confused with small cell non-keratinizing squamous cell carcinomas. The later belong to squamous cell carcinoma histotypes.

The diagnosis of small cell neuroendocrine tumour is based on histology and immunostaining. Up to 80% of haematoxylin and eosin-positive small cell neuroendocrine carcinomas are also staining positive to neuroendocrine markers such as synaptophysin, chromogranin and CD56. Neuroendocrine markers can be negative in 20–70% of cases. Patients with small cell neuroendocrine carcinoma of the cervix often do badly and have a very poor prognosis. It is characterized by frequent and early nodal and distant metastases. About 50% of the patients died of the disease, typically within 2–3 years of diagnosis. In a case series by Viswanathan et al., overall survival rates were 43% and 29% at 2 and 5 years, respectively, and none of the women who had the disease more extensive than stage 1B1 survived more than 30 months. Five -year survival rates for patients with stage 1 disease are 33%. Factors that correlate with a poorer outcome are stage, size of tumour, presence of lymph node metastases and chromogranin positive. The primary treatment for stage 1 and 2A disease is radical hysterectomy, and most patients will require adjuvant treatment such as concurrent chemoradiation, radiation therapy or chemotherapy. There is no standard adjuvant treatment for small cell neuroendocrine tumour of the cervix. Chemotherapy regimen for these patients is cisplatin and etoposide with or without doxorubicin. The other chemotherapy regimen found to be effective against small cell neuroendocrine tumours is vincristine/doxorubicin/cyclophosphamide.

Patients with advanced or recurrent glassy-cell carcinoma of the cervix can be treated with a paclitaxel and carboplatin combination; however, data are very limited.

Recurrent Carcinoma of Cervix

The prognosis for early-stage cervical cancer is very good but in advanced stage disease, most of the patients will experience recurrence. Patients with recurrent cervical cancer often have poor survival rate and 80% of recurrence is detected within 2 years of primary treatment. The 5-year survival for patients with recurrent cervical cancer is less than 5%. Clinical diagnosis of pelvic recurrence can nearly always be made by triad: (a) sciatic pain, (b) leg oedema and (c) hydronephrosis. The patterns of failure in carcinoma of cervix according to stages are shown in Table 8.12.

Table 8.12 Pattern of failure in carcinoma of cervix according to stages

	Stage of cervical cancer at presentation (FIGO 1994)					
Type of recurrence	**1A**	**1B**	**2A**	**2B**	**3**	**4A**
Pelvic failure rate (%)		10	17	23	42	74
Incidence of distance metastases (%)	3	16	31	26	40	75

In order to detect recurrence at an early stage, close monitoring after treatment is extremely important. Different oncology centres have different follow-up routines. Following is one of the examples of follow-up schedules for patients who have completed their treatment:

3 monthly for first year
4 monthly for second year
6 monthly from third to fifth year
yearly from sixth year onward

Although routine follow-up is important in detection of recurrent cancer, many studies have shown that detection at follow-up did not provide any survival benefit, this may relate to the limited therapeutic options available (Duyn et al., 2002; Gerdin et al., 1994). However, in a subset of patients where the option is available, early detection, and treatment may improve their survival. Common sites of metastasis according to frequency are lungs, para-aortic lymph node, abdominal cavity, supraclavicular lymph node.

Following are the principal steps for the management of recurrent cervical cancer :

(1) Confirm the diagnosis: recurrence should be confirmed by histology.
(2) Assess the extent of the disease (imaging technique such as chest x-ray, CT scan, MRI or PET scan).
(3) Determine the intention of treatment either for a cure or for palliation.
(4) Assess a patient's main symptom/s.
(5) Review the previous treatment.
(6) List the treatment options and decide the best one for a patient.
(7) Start the treatment and monitor the patient.

Patients with recurrent cervical cancer can be divided into two groups: (1) recurrence after definitive irradiation and (2) recurrence after surgical treatment.

Recurrence after Definitive Irradiation

Approximately, 70% of patients with cervical cancer receive radiation therapy at some point in the past. Up to 40% of them will develop a recurrent or persistent disease. Generally, the patient exhibiting complete tumour regression within 30 days after completion of radiation had a significantly lower incidence of pelvic recurrences and fewer distant metastases. Local recurrence responds poorly to chemotherapy due to postradiation effects of the pelvic tissues. Re-irradiation may be possible in highly selected patients after a long interval of disease-free; however, radiation toxicity is higher. Generally, re-irradiation is not advisable in patients who had been irradiated before.

Surgery is the most reasonable option for patients with local recurrence developed following primary treatment with radiotherapy. Surgery may involve a highly specialized surgery or ultra-radical procedure known as pelvic exenteration. Five-year survival rates after successful pelvic exenteration are more than

30%. Operative morbidity and mortality are the main concerns in pelvic exenteration.

Pelvic exenteration can be classified into three main categories according to Magrina's classification system:

(a) supralevator (type I)
(b) infralevator (type II)
(c) infralevator with vulvectomy (type III)

With the improvement of selection criteria (with better detection method such as PET scan), surgical techniques, better teamwork, better equipment and postoperative care, operative mortality of pelvic exenteration has been reduced to 5%. In order to achieve high cure rate after pelvic exenteration, surgery must achieve complete microscopic resection. The eligibility criteria for pelvic exenteration are (a) local recurrence, (b) no extrapelvic metastases, (c) tumour not infiltrating the pelvic wall and (d) the patient is fit for surgery. Para-aortic lymph node metastasis is an absolute contraindication for pelvic exenteration.

Recently, in some institutions, lateral pelvic wall infiltration is no longer an absolute contraindication for pelvic exenteration. They have implemented the so-called **laterally extended endopelvic resection procedure** (LEER). LEER permitted an excision of the tumour infiltrating to the muscle of the pelvic wall and obtaining free margin. Hoeckel has recently reported the success rate of LEER, 5-year disease-specific survivals were 55% and 97% of patients who underwent LEER had a clear margin. Recent review by Jurago and colleagues on resectability rate in patients with pelvic side wall recurrence concluded that around one third of the patients with clinically defined pelvic wall involvement can still undergo a complete macroscopic resection with negative margins. They also have reasonable chance of a long-term disease-specific survival rate of 33.3% at 10 years.

In pelvic exenteration, the patient may have to undergo urinary diversion procedure (anterior or total exenteration) or colostomy (posterior or total exenteration). An alternative to anorectal resection and permanent colostomy, colorectal re-anastomosis and temporary ileostomy is acceptable in selected patients. To improve pelvic vascularization and reduce the risk of fistula formation, the omental flap can be used to fill the pelvic cavity. If omentum is inadequate, rectus abdominis muscle or even a prosthetic material is a good alternative. High dose intraoperative radiotherapy (brachytherapy/implants) has been attempted in some centre to eradicate a residual disease during pelvic exenteration. The roles of this technique remain inconclusive and morbidity rate is high.

Recurrence after Previous Surgery

Local recurrence after surgery is increasingly less common due to early presentation and more effective treatment, including the use of adjuvant chemoradiation therapy in high-risk patients. Patients with bulky disease (more than 4 cm), deep tumour invasion, poor histology type and most important with nodal metastases are at higher risk of recurrence.

Local pelvic recurrence is best managed by radiotherapy (External irradiation + Intracavitary insertion/interstitial implants depend on tumour volume). Reported complete response rate was 88% for loco-regional recurrence and overall survival rate was 33–39%.

Surgical treatment (exenteration) is indicated in a selected patient if the tumour is resectable and the patient is fit for surgery.

Appendix

GOG Score for Patients with Negative Lymph Node and Clear Surgical Margin Following Radical Hysterectomy and Pelvic Lymphadenectomy

Relative Risk of Recurrence after Radical Hysterectomy for Stage I Cervical Cancer	
Variable	**Relative Risk**
Depth of tumour penetration (mm)	
Superficial	
3[a]	1.0
4	3.0
5	7.2
6	14
7	21
8	26
10	21

Relative Risk of Recurrence after Radical Hysterectomy for Stage I Cervical Cancer	
Variable	**Relative Risk**
Middle	
5	20
6	22
7	23
8	25
10	28
12	32
14	36
Deep	
7	28
8	30
10	34
12	37
14	41
16	45
18	49
20	54
Clinical tumour size	
Occult tumour	1.0
1	1.6
2	1.9
3	2.4
4	2.9
6	4.4
8	6.6
Capillary/Lymphatic spaceinvolvement	
No	1.0
Yes	1.7

Source: Delgado et al., *Gynaecol Oncol*, 1992; 38: 352.
Note: "GOG Score" is calculated by multiplying the relative risk for the depth × tumour size × capillary space involvement.
Example: 8 mm superficial tumour, measuring 2 cm with VSI would be 26 × 1.9 × 1.7 = 84.
GOG Score < 40: Low risk (no need of adjuvant RT).
GOG Score 40–120: Intermediate Risk (Individualized treatment).
GOG Score >120: High risk (require standard field RT).
[a]Arbitrary reference for depth invasion.

References

Allen D, Narayan K. Managing advanced stage cervical cancer. *Best Pract Res Clin Obstet Gynaecol* 2005; **19**(4): 591–609.

American Cancer Society. (2007) Global Cancer Facts & Figures 2007. American Cancer Society, Atlanta, GA.

Behtash N, Nazari Z, Ayatollahi H, et al. Neoadjuvant chemotherapy and radical surgery compared to radical surgery alone in bulky stage 1B-2A cervical cancer. *EJSO* 2006; **32**: 1226–1230.

Beiner ME, Covens A. Surgery insight: radical vaginal trachelectomy as a method of fertility preservation for cervical cancer. *Nat Clin Pract Oncol* 2007; **4**: 353–361.

Benedetti-Panici P, Greggi S, Colombo A, et al. Neoadjuvant chemotherapy and radical surgery versus exclusive radiotherapy in locally advanced squamous cell cervical cancer: results from the Italian multicenter randomised study. *J Clin Oncol* 2002; **20**(1): 179–188.

Bonomi P, Blessing JA, Stehman F, et al. Randomized trial of three cisplatin dose schedules in squamous cell carcinoma of the cervix: a Gynecologic Oncology Group study. *J Clin Oncol* 1985; **3**: 1079–1085.

Bosch FZ, Lorinez A, Munoz N, Meijer CJLM, Shah KV. The causal relation between human papillomavirus and cervical cancer. *J Clin Pathol* 2002; **55**: 244–265.

Bosch FX, Manos MM, Munoz N, et al. The IBSCC study group. Prevalence of human papillomavirus in cervical cancer: a worldwide perspective. *J Natl Cancer Inst* 1995; **87**: 796–802.

Burnett AF, Roman LD, Garcia AA, et al. A phase II study of gemcitabine and cisplatin in patients with advanced, persistent, or recurrent squamous cell carcinoma of cervix. *Gynecol Oncol* 2000; **76**: 63–66.

Cadron I, Gorp TV, Amant F, et al. Chemotherapy for recurrent cervical cancer. *Gynecol Oncol* 2007; **107**: S113–S118.

Cai HB, Chen HZ, Yin HH. Randomized study of preoperative chemotherapy versus primary surgery for stage 1B cervical cancer. *J Obstet Gynaecol Res* 2006; **32**(3): 315–323.

Castellsague X. Natural history and epidemiology of HPV infection and cervical cancer. *Gynecol Oncol* 2008; **110**: S4–S7.

Castellsague X, Bosch X, Munoz N, et al. Male circumcision, penile human papillomavirus infection, and cervical cancer in female partners. *N Engl J Med* 2002; **346**: 1105–1112.

Chemotherapy for Cervical Cancer Meta-analysis Collaboration (CCCMAC). Reducing uncertainties about the effects of chemoradiotherapy for cervical cancer: individual patient data meta-analysis. *Cochrane Database Syst Rev* 2010(1): CD008285.

Chen H, Liang C, Zhang I, et al. Clinical efficacy of modified preoperative neoadjuvant chemotherapy in the treatment of locally advanced (stage 1B2 to 2B) cervical cancer: a randomized study. *Gynecol Oncol* 2008, submitted on March 2008.

Chiva LM, Lapuente F, Cortijo LG, et al. Surgical treatment of recurrent cervical cancer: State of the art and new achievements. *Gynecol Oncol* 2008; **110**: S60–S66.

Cibula D, Velechovska P, Slama J, et al. Late morbidity following nerve-sparing radical hysterectomy. *Gynecol Oncol* 2010; **116**: 506–511.

Clark JG. A more radical method of performing hysterectomy for cancer of the uterus. *Johns Hopkins Med Bull* 1895; **6**: 120–124.

Colombo PE, Bertrand MM, Gutowski M, et al. Total laparoscopic radical hysterectomy for locally advanced cervical carcinoma (stage IIB, IIA and bulky stages IB) after concurrent chemoradiation therapy: Surgical morbidity and oncological results. *Gynecol Oncol* 2009; **114**: 404–409.

Covens A, Rosen B, Murphy J, et al. Changes in the demographics and perioperative care of stage 1a2/1b1 cervical cancer over the past 16 years. *Gynecol Oncol* 2001; **81**: 133–137.

Curtin JP, Blessing JA, Webster KD, et al. Paclitaxel, an active agent in non squamous carcinoma of the uterine cervix: a Gynecol Oncology Group study. *J Clin Oncol* 2001; **19**: 1275–1278.

deSouza NM, Soutter WP, Rustin G, et al. Use of neoadjuvant chemotherapy prior to radical hysterectomy in cervical cancer: monitoring tumour shrinkage and molecular profile on magnetic resonance and assessment of 3 years outcome. *Br J Cancer* 2004; **90**: 2326–2331.

Dreyer G, Snyman LC, Mouton A, Lindeque BG. Management of recurrent cervical cancer. *Best Pract Res Clin Obstet Gynaecol* 2005; **19**(4): 631–644.

Duenas GA, Lopez GC, Gonzalez A, et al. A phase II study of gemcitabine and cisplatin combination as induction chemotherapy of untreated locally advanced cervical carcinoma. *Ann Oncol* 2001; **12**: 541–547.

Dursun P, Ayhan A, Kuscu E. Nerve-sparing radical hysterectomy for cervical carcinoma. *Critical Rev Oncol/Hematol* 2009; **70**: 195–205.

Duyn A, Van Eijkeren M, Kenter G, Zwinderman K, Ansink A. Recurrent cervical cancer: detection and prognosis. *Acta Obstet Gynecol Scan* 2002; **81**: 351–355.

Eddy GL, Bundy BN, Creasman, et al. Treatment of (bulky) stage 1B cervical cancer with or without neoadjuvant vincristine and cisplatin prior to radical hysterectomy and pelvic/paraaortic lymphedenectomy: a phase III trial of the Gynecologic Oncology Group. *Gynecol Oncol* 2007; **106**(2): 362–369.

Eifel PJ, Winter K, Morris M, et al. Pelvic irradiation with concurrent chemotherapy versus pelvic and para-aortic irradiation for high-risk cervical cancer: An update of Radiation Therapy Oncology Group Trial (RTOG) 90-01. *J Clin Oncol* 2004; **22**: 872–880.

Ferrandina G, Margariti PA, Smaniotto, et al. Long-term analysis of clinical outcome and complications in locally advanced cervical cancer patients administered concomitant chemoradiation followed by radical surgery. *Gynecol Oncol* 2010; doi: 10.1016/j.ygyno.2010.08.004.

Fujii S. Original film of the Okabayashi's radical hysterectomy by Okabayashi himself in 1932, and two films of the precise anatomy necessary for nerve-sparing Okabayashi's radical hysterectomy clarified by Shingo Fujii. *Int J Gynecol Cancer* 2008; **18**(2): 383–385.

Gerdin E, Cnattingus S, Jognson P, Pertterson B. Prognostic factors and relapse factors in early stage cervical cancer after brachytherapy and radical hysterectomy. *Gynecol Oncol* 1994; **53**: 314–319.

Gien LT, Covens A. Fertility sparing options for early stage cervical cancer. *Gynecol Oncol* 2010; **117**: 350–357.

Gien LT, Beauchemin MC, Thomas G. Adenocarcinoma: a unique cervical cancer. *Gynecol Oncol* 2010; **116**: 140–146.

Goncalves A, Fabbro M, Lhomme C, et al. A phase II trial to evaluate gefitinib as second or third line treatment in patients with recurring locoregionally advanced or metastatic cervical cancer. *Gynecol Oncol* 2008; **108**: 42–46.

Gonzalez AD, Perez LC, Graniel CL, et al. Pathologic response and toxicity assessment of chemoradiotherapy with cisplatin versus cisplatin plus gemcitabine in cervical cancer: A randomied Phase II study. *Intl J Radiat Oncol Biol Phys* 2005; **61**(3): 817–823.

Green J, Kirwan J, Tierney J, Vale C et al. Chemoradiation in cervical cancer. *Cochrane Database Syst Rev* 2005 July 20; **3**: CD002225.

Hayashi T, Kato T. Usefulness of tumour size on MR imaging in assessing the prognosis of uterine cervical cancer treated with radiation. *Nippon Igaku Hoshasen Gakkai Zasshi* 1999; **59**: 250–255.

Hicks ML, Piver MS, Mas E, et al. Intraoperative orthovoltage radiation therapy in the treatment of recurrent gynaecologic malignancies. *Am J Clin Oncol* 1993; **16**: 497–500.

Ho GY, Bierman R, Beardsley L, Chang CJ, Burk RD. Natural history of cervico-vaginal papillomavirus infection in young women. *N Engl J Med* 1998; **338**(7): 423–428.

Hockel M, Konerding MA, Heussel CP. Liposuction-assisted nerve sparing extended radical hysterectomy: oncologic rationale, surgical anatomy, and feasibility study. *Am J Obstet Gynecol* 1998; **178**: 971–976.

Hoeckel M. Laterally extended endopelvic resection. Novel surgical treatment of locally recurrent cervical carcinoma involving the pelvic side wall. *Gynecol Oncol* 2003; **91**: 369–377.

Holland CM, Shafi MI. Radical hysterectomy. *Best Pract Res Clin O&G* 2005; **19**(3): 387–401.

IARC Monograph on the evaluation of carcinogenic risks to humans. *Human Papillomaviruses*, Vol. 90. Lyon: International Agency for Research on Cancer. In press.

Ijaz T, Eifel PJ, Burke T, Oswald MJ. Radiation therapy of pelvic recurrence after radical hysterectomy for cervical carcinoma. *Gynecol Oncol* 1998; **70**: 241–246.

Jemal A, et al. Cancer Statistic 2006. *CA Cancer J Clin* 2006; **56**: 1006–1030.

Jurado M, Alcazar JL, Monge RM. Resectability rates of previously irradiated recurrent cervical cancer treated with pelvic exenteration: Is still the clinical involvement of the pelvic wall a real contraindication? A twenty years experience. *Gynecol Oncol* 2010; **116**: 38–43.

Katsumata N, Yoshikawa H, Hirakawa T, et al. Phase III randomized trial of neoadjuvant chemotherapy followed by radical hysterectomy versus radical hysterectomy for bulky stage 1–2 cervical cancer (JCOG 0102). *Proc Am Soc Clin Oncol* 2006; 24(abstract 5013).

Keys H, Bundy B, Stehman F, et al. A comparison of weekly cisplatin during radiation therapy versus irradiation alone each followed by adjuvant hysterectomy in bulky stage IB cervical cancer: a randomized trial of the Gynecologic Oncology Group. *N Engl J Med* 1999; **340**: 1154–1161.

Kim K, Kim MJ, Chung HH, et al. Inadvertent potential risk of neoadjuvant chemotherapy in cervical cancer. *Med Hypotheses* 2009; **73**: 1005–1007.

Kim MK, Kim JW, Kim MA, et al. Feasibility of less radical surgery for superficially invasive carcinoma of cervix. *Gynecol Oncol* 2010, doi: 10.1016/j.ygyno.2010.06.027.

Kim YS, Shin SS, Nam JH. Prospective randomized comparison of monthly fluorouracil and cisplatin versus weekly cisplatin concurrent with pelvic radiotherapy and high-dose rate brachytherapy for locally advanced cervical cancer. *Gynecol Oncol* 2008; **108**: 195–200.

Kyrgiou M, Shafi MI. Invasive cancer of the cervix. *Obstet, Gynaecol Rep Med* 2010; **20**(5): 147–154.

Landoni F, Maneo A, Cormio G, et al. Class II versus Class III Radical Hysterectomy in Stage 1B-IIA Cervical Cancer: A Prospective Randomized Study. *Gynecologic Oncol* 2001; **80**(1): 3–12.

Landoni F, Maneo A, Colombo A, et al. Randomized study of radical surgery versus radiotherapy for stage 1B–2A cervical cancer. *Lancet* 1997; **350**: 535–540.

Lanciano R, Calkins A, Bundy BN, et al. Randomized comparison of weekly cisplatin or protracted venous infusion of fluorouracil in combination with pelvic radiation in advanced cervix cancer: A Gynecologic Oncology Group Study. *J Clin Oncol* 2005; **23**: 8289–8294.

Long HJ, Bundy BN, Grendys EC, et al. Randomized phase III trial of cisplatin with or without topotecan in carcinoma of the uterine cervix: A Gynecologic Oncology Group Study. *J Clin Oncol* 2005; **23**: 4626–4633.

Magierlo JS, Narog M, Kruczek A, et al. Radical hysterectomy during the transition period from traditional to nerve-sparing technique. *Gynecol Oncol* 2010; **116**: 502–505.

Magrina JF. Types of pelvic exenterations: a reappraisal. *Gynecol Oncol* 1990; **37**: 363–366.

Maneo A, Chiara S, Bonazzi C, Mangioni C. Neoadjuvant chemotherapy and conservative surgery for stage 1b1 cervical cancer. *Gynecol Oncol* 2008; **111**: 438–443.

Martinez Monge R, Jurado M, Aristu JJ, et al. Intraoperative electron beam radiotherapy during radical surgery for locally advanced and recurrent cervical cancer. *Gynecol Oncol* 2001; **82**: 538–543.

Martinez Monge R, Jurado M, Cambeiro M, et al. Perioperative high dose rate brachytherapy in locally advanced and recurrent gynaecologic cancer: initial results of a phase II trial. *Brachytherapy* 2006; **5**: 203–210.

McGuire WP, Arseneau JC, Blessing JA, et al. A randomized comparative trial of carboplatin and iproplatin in advanced squamous carcinoma of the uterine cervix: a Gynecologic Oncology Group study. *J Clin Oncol* 1989; **7**: 1462–1468.

McQuellon RP, Thaler HT, Cella D, Moore DH. Quality of life (QOL) outcomes from a randomized trial of cisplatin versus cisplatin plus paclitaxel in advanced cervical cancer: A Gynecologic Oncology Group study. *Gynecol Oncol* 2006; 101: 296–304.

Moore DH. Chemotherapy for recurrent cervical cancer. *Curr Opin Oncol* 2006; **18**: 516–519.

Monk BJ, Huang HQ, Cella D, Long HJ. Quality of life outcomes from a randomized phase III trial of cisplatin with or without topotecan in advanced carcinoma of the cervix: a Gynecologic Oncology Group Study. *J Clin Oncol* 2005; **23**: 4617–4625.

Morris M, Blessing JA, Monk BJ, et al. Phase II study of cisplatin and vinorelbine in squamous cell carcinoma of the cervix: a Gynecologic Oncology Group study. *J Clin Oncol* 2004; **22**: 3340–3344.

Meigs JV. Radical hysterectomy with bilateral pelvic lymph node dissections; a report of 100 patients operated on five or more years ago. *Am J Obstet Gynecol* 1951; **62**: 854–870.

Moore DH. Treatment of stage 1B2 (bulky) cervical carcinoma. *Cancer Treat Rev* 2003; **29**: 401–406.

Moore DH, Blessing JA, McQuellon MP, et al. Phase III study of cisplatin with or without paclitaxel in stage IVB, recurrent, or persistent squamous cell carcinoma of the cervix: a gynecologic oncology group study. *J Clin Oncol* 2004; **22**: 3113–3119.

Morris M, Eifel PJ, Lu J, et al. Pelvic radiation with concurrent chemotherapy versus pelvic and para-aortic radiation for high-risk cervical cancer: a randomized Radiation Therapy Oncology Group Clinical Trial. *N Engl J Med* 1999; **340**: 1137–1143.

Munoz N, Castellsague X, De Gonzalez AB, Gissmann L. HPV in the etiology of human cancer. *Vaccine* 2006; 24S3: S3/1–S3/10.

Munoz N, Bosch FX, Castellsague X, et al. Against which human papillomavirus types shall we vaccinate and screen? The international perspective. *Int J Cancer* 2004; **111**(2): 278–285.

Mutch DG. Meeting Report. The new FIGO staging system for cancers of the vulva, cervix, endometrium and sarcomas. *Gynecol Oncol* 2009; **115**: 325–328.

National Cancer Institute. Chemotherapy plus radiation improves survival (press release). Bethesda, MD: National Cancer Institute; 1999.

Namkoong SE, Park JS, Kim JW, et al. Comparative study of patients with locally advanced stage 1b and 2 cervical cancer treatment by radical surgery with and withut preoperative adjuvant chemotherapy. *Gynecol Oncol* 1995; **59**: 136–142.

Napolitano U, Imperato F, Mossa B, et al. The role of neoadjuvant chemotherapy for squamous cell cervical cancer (1b–3b): a long term randomized trial. *Eur J Gynaecol Oncol* 2003; **24**(1): 51–59.

Nugent EK, Case AS, Hoff JT, et al. Chemoradiation in locally advanced cervical carcinoma: An analysis of cisplatin dosing and other clinical prognostic factors. *Gynecol Oncol* 2010; **116**(3): 438–441.

Okabayashi H. Radical abdominal hysterectomy for cancer of the cervix uteri. *Surg Gynecol Obstet* 1921; **33**: 335–341.

Olawaiye A, Carmen MD, Tambouret R, et al. Abdominal radical trachelectomy: success and pitfalls in a general gynaecologic oncology practice. *Gynecol Oncol* 2009; **112**: 506–510.

Omura GA, Blessing JA, Vacarello L, et al. Randomized trial of cisplatin versus cisplatin plus mitolactol versus cisplatin plus ifosfamide in advanced squamous carcinoma of the cervix: a Gynecologic Oncology Group study. *J Clin Oncol* 1997; **15**: 165–171.

Peters WA, Liu PY, Barrett RJ, et al. Concurrent chemotherapy and pelvic radiation therapy compared with pelvic radiation therapy alone as adjuvant therapy after radical surgery in high-risk early-stage cancer of the cervix. *J Clin Oncol* 2000; **18**: 1606–1613.

Pettersson F: Annual Report on the Results of Treatment in Gynecologic Cancer, Vol 21. Statements on the results obtained in patients 1982–1986, inclusive 3 and 5 year survival up to 1990. *Int J Gynecol Obstet* 1991; (Supp): 27–127.

Pieterse QD, Trimbos JBMZ, Dijkman A, et al. Postoperative radiation therapy improves prognosis in patients with adverse risk factors in localized, early stage cervical cancer: a retrospective comparative study. *Intl J Gynecol Cancer* 2006; **16**(3): 1112–1118.

Piver MS, Rutledge F, Smith JP. Five classes of extended hysterectomy for women with cervical cancer. *Obstet Gynecol* 1974; **44**: 265–272.

Plante M. Vagina radical trachelectomy: an update. *Gynecol Oncol* 2008; **111**: S105–S110.

Possover M, Queakernack J, Chiantera V. The LANN technique to reduce postoperative functional morbidity in laparoscopic radical pelvic surgery. *J Am Coll Surg* 2005; **201**: 913–917.

Querleu D, Narducci F, Poulard V, et al. Modified radical vaginal hysterectomy with or without laparoscopic nerve-sparing dissection: a comparative study. *Gynecol Oncol* 2002; **85**: 154–158.

Querleu D, Morrow CP. Classification of radical hysterectomy. *Lancet Oncol* 2008; **9**: 297–303.

Ramirez PT, Schmeler KM, Malpica A, Soliman PT. Safety and feasibility of robotic radical trachelectomy in patients with early stage cervical cancer. *Gynecol Oncol* 2010; **116**: 512–515.

Ramirez PT, Schmeler KM, Soliman PT, Frumovitz M. Fertility preservation in patients with early cervical cancer: Radical trachelectomy. *Gynecol Oncol* 2008; **110**: S25–S28.

Raspagliesi F, Ditto A, Fontanelli R, et al. Type II versus type III nerve-sparing radical hysterectomy: Comparison of lower urinary tract dysfunction. *Gycecol Oncol* 2006; **102**: 256–262.

Raspagliesi F, Ditto A, Hanozet F, et al. Nerve-sparing radical hysterectomy in cervical cancer: Evolution of concepts. *Gynecol Oncol* 2007; **107**: S119–S121.

Rogers L, Siu SSN, Luesley D, Bryant A, Dickinson HO. Adjuvant radiotherapy and chemoradiation after surgery for cervical cancer (Review). The Cochrane Collaboration and published in The Cochrane Library 2009; **7**(4): CD007583. doi: 10.1002/14651858.CD007583.pub2.

Rose PG, Bundy BN, Watkins EB, et al. Concurrent cisplatin-based chemoradiation improves progression free and overall survival in advanced cervical cancer: results of a randomized Gynecologic Oncology Group study. *N Engl J Med* 1999; **340**: 1144–1153.

Rose PG, Ali S, Watkins E, et al. Long-term follow up of a randomized trial comparing concurrent single agent cisplatin, cisplatin-based combination chemotherapy, or hydroxyurea during pelvic irradiation for locally advanced cervical cancer. A Gynecologic Oncology Group Study. *J Clin Oncol* 2007; **25**: 2804–2810.

Rotman M, Sedlis A, Piedmonte MR, et al. A phase III randomized trial of postoperative pelvic irradiation in stage 1B cervical carcinoma with poor prognostic features: follow up of a gynaecologic oncology group study. *Intl J Radiat Oncol Biol Phys* 2006; **65**(1): 169–176.

Roy M, Plante M. Pregnancies after radical vaginal trachelectomy for early stage cervical cancer. *Am J Obstet Gynecol* 1998; **179**: 1491–1496.

Sardi JE, Giaroli A, Sananes C, et al. Long-term follow-up of the first randomized trial using neoadjuvant chemotherapy in stage 1b squamous cell carcinoma of the cervix: the final results. *Gynecol Oncol* 1997; **67**(1): 61–69.

Schiller JT, Day PM, Kines RC. Current understanding of the mechanism of HPV infection. *Gynecol Oncol* 2010; **118**: S12–S17.

Sedlis A, Bundy BN, Rotman MZ, et al. Randomized trial of pelvic radiation therapy versus no further therapy in selected patients with stage 1B carcinoma of the cervix after radical hysterectomy and pelvic lymphadenectomy: a gynaecologic oncology group study. *Gynecol Oncol* 1999; **73**: 177–183.

Simcock B, Shafi M. Invasive cancer of the cervix. *Obstet, Gynaecol Reprod Med* 2007; **17**(6): 181–187.

Smith JS, Lindsay L, Hoots B, et al. Human papillomavirus type distribution in invasive cervical cancer and high-grade cervical lesions: a meta-analysis update. *Int J Cancer* 2007; **121**(3): 621–632.

Steben M, Franco ED. Human papillomavirus infection: Epidemiology and pathophysiology. *Gynecol Oncol* 2007; **107**: S2–S5.

Sutton GP, Bundy BN, Delgado G, et al. Ovarian metastases in stage 1B carcinoma of the cervix: a Gynecologic Oncology Group Study. *Am J Obstet Gynecol* 1992; **166**: 50–53.

Tao X, Hu W, Ramirez T, Kavanagh JJ. Chemotherapy for recurrent and metastatic cervical cancer. *Gynecol Oncol* 2008; **110**: S67–S71.

Tierney J. Meta-analysis Group (Neoadjuvant Chemotherapy for Cervical Cancer Meta-analysis (NACCCMA) Collaboration. Neoadjuvant chemotherapy for locally advanced cervical cancer: a systematic review and meta-analysis of individual patient data from 21 randomised trials. *Eur J Cancer* 2003; **39**: 2470–2486.

Tierney JF, Vale C, Symonds P. Concomitant and neoadjuvant chemotherapy for cervical cancer. *Clin Oncol* 2008; **20**: 401–416.

Vale CI, Tierney JF, Davidson SE, Drinkwater KJ, Symonds P. Substantial improvement in UK cervical cancer survival with chemoradiotherapy: results of a Royal College of Radiologists audit. *Clin Oncol* (R Coll Radiol) 2010: 22.

Vale C. Meta-analysis Group: Reducing uncertainties about the effects of chemoradiationtherapy for cervical cancer: A systematic review and meta-analysis of individual patient data from 18 randomized trials. *J Clin Oncol* 2008; **26**: 5802–5812.

Van Howe RS. Human papillomavirus and circumcision: A meta-analysis. *J Infect* 2007; **54**: 490–496.

Viswanathan AN, Deavers MT, Jhingran A, et al. Small cell neuroendocrine carcinoma of the cervix: outcome and patterns of recurrence. *Gynecol Oncol* 2004; **93**: 27–33.

Walboomers JM, Jacobs MV, Manos MM, et al. Human papillomavirus is a necessary cause of invasive cervical cancer worldwide. *J Pathol* 1999; **189**: 12–19.

Wertheim E. The extended abdominal operation for carcinoma uteri. *Am J Obstet* 1912; **66**: 169–232.

Whitney CW, Sause W, Bundy BN, et al. A randomized comparison of fluorouracil plus cisplatin versus hydroxyurea as an adjunct to radiation therapy in stages IIB-IVA carcinoma of the cervix with negative para-aortic lymph nodes. A Gynecologic Oncology Group and Southwest Oncology Group Study. *J Clin Oncol* 1999; **17**: 1339–1348.

Willet CG, Czito BG, Tyler DS. Intraoperative radiation therapy. *J Clin Oncol* 2007; **25**: 971–977.

Wright JD, Viviano D, Powell MA, et al. Bevacizumab combination therapy in heavily pretreated, recurrent cervical cancer. *Gynecol Oncol* 2006; **103**: 489–493.

Yabuki Y, Asamoto A, Hoshiba T, Nishimoto H, Satou N. A new proposal for radical hysterectomy. *Gynecol Oncol* 1996; **62**: 370–378.

Yabuki Y, Asamoto A, Hoshiba T, et al. Radical hysterectomy: an anatomic evaluation of parametrial dissection. *Gynecol Oncol* 2000; **77**: 155–163.

Chapter 9

Carcinoma of Endometrium

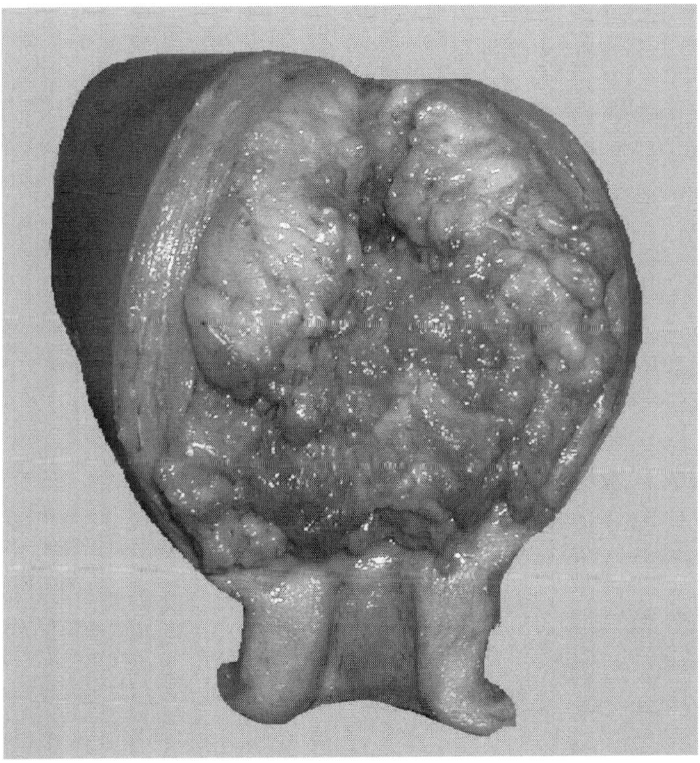

Gynaecologic Cancer: A Handbook for Students and Practitioners
Rushdan Noor, Eng Hseon Tay, and Jeffrey Low

ISBN 978-981-4463-06-5 (Hardcover), 978-981-4463-07-2 (eBook)
www.panstanford.com

Anatomy of the Uterus

The uterus is a hollow, thick-walled and muscular organ situated between the bladder anteriorly and rectum posteriorly. Uterus is the largest female reproductive organ in the pelvis weighing about 30–40 grams, 8 cm long, 5 cm wide and 2.5 cm thick. It serves as a site for the reception, retention and nutrition of the conceptus. The portion above the isthmus is termed as the body and that below, the cervix (Fig. 9.1). The cavity of the uterus is triangular in shape in a coronal section and mere slit, flattened antero-posteriorly. The total length of uterine cavity from external os to the fundus is approximately 6.25 cm.

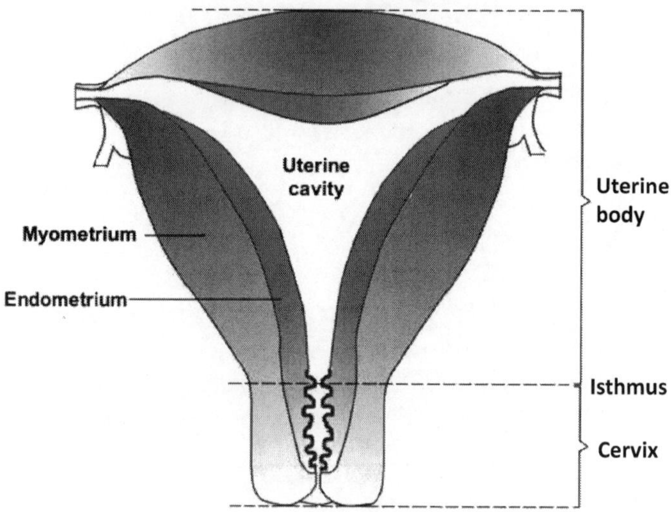

Figure 9.1 Uterine anatomy.

The uterus is composed of three layers: the endometrium, myometrium and perimetrium. The myometrium is composed of three layers of smooth muscle fibres. The most outer muscle layer placed beneath the peritoneum, it consists of fibres which pass transversely across the fundus, and converging at each lateral angle of the uterus, continued on to the uterine tube, round ligament and ovarian ligament. The middle layer of fibres presents no regularity in its arrangement, being disposed longitudinally, obliquely and transversely. The middle layer contains more blood vessels than other layers. The inner layer of myometrium consists of circular fibres arranged in the form of two hollow cones, the apices of which surround the orifices of the fallopian tubes, their bases intermingling with one another on the middle of the body of the uterus. Endometrium has two layers, the stratum basalis, a supporting layer, and the stratum functionalis, which proliferates then degenerates during the menstrual cycle, varying from 1–6 mm in thickness. Stratum functionalis is made up of stratum compactum and stratum spongiosum. Endometrium is the most active layer and responds to cyclic ovarian hormone changes and therefore is highly specialized and is essential to menstrual and reproductive function. Both the endometrium and myometrium exhibit substantial changes during pregnancy.

The uterus is usually bent anteriorly (anteflexed) between the cervix and body while the entire uterus is normally inclined anteriorly (anteverted). There are many structures that lie between the leaf of broad ligaments, i.e. fallopian tubes, round ligaments, ovaries, epoohoron and paroophoron, connective tissue, blood vessels and nerves.

The round ligament is fibromuscular bands represents the lower end of the gubernaculums extends from the superolateral angle of the uterus, through the inguinal canal to the labia majora. Round ligament helps to keep the uterus anteverted and anteflexed. There are three condensation of the pelvic fascia which formed three important ligaments supporting the uterus: (a) transcervical ligament (other name: cardinal, Mackenroth's ligament) extending from cervix and upper part of vagina to lateral pelvic wall, (b) uterosacral ligaments and (c) pubocervical ligaments.

The main blood supply to the uterus is from uterine artery a branch from internal iliac artery. The uterus is also supplied partly by ovarian artery, which forms an anastomotic trunk with the branches of uterine artery at the lateral wall of the uterus. The uterine artery gives off 6 to 10 arcuate arteries, which anastomose with one another in the myometrium. Branches from arcuate arteries or also known as radial arteries enter the basal layer of the endometrium, giving off straight arteries known as basal arteries, which supply this region, and continuing upward into the functional layer as the highly-coiled spiral arteries. Therefore, arcuate and radial arteries supply myometrium, while basal and spiral arteries supply the endometrium. The basal arteries are not responsive to hormones; they support the basal endometrial layer, which provides the proliferative cells for endometrial growth. Spiral arteries supply the functionalis layer and are hormonal sensitive blood vessels. In pregnancy, these spiral arteries lead to numerous arterioles, which anastomose to supply a rich capillary bed that includes thin-walled dilated spaces called lacunae. The lacunae or intervillous spaces provide the site for exchange of nutrients, wastes, hormones, and gases between the foetal and materal circulation. If the pregnancy does not occur, spiral arteries will constrict causing endometrial breakdown with desquamation of the glands and stroma. The venous supply of the uterus drains through uterine, ovarian and vaginal veins into the internal iliac vein.

Both sympathetic (T12, L1) and parasympathetic (S2, 3, 4) nerves supply the uterus. The lymphatic of the myometrium drains into the subserosal network. The lymphatic drainage of the uterus follows three main routes:

(a) **Fundus**: it mostly follows ovarian vessels to aortic lymph nodes, some to external iliac lymph nodes or runs along the round ligaments to superficial inguinal lymph nodes;
(b) **Body of a uterus**: mainly to external iliac lymph node;
(c) **Cervix**: internal iliac and sacral lymph nodes.

Epithelial Uterine Cancer

Epidemiology

The incidence of endometrial cancer is increasing and each year approximately 142,000 women have been diagnosed, and an estimated 42,000 woman die from this cancer every year. Endometrial cancer is fourth most common women cancer (after breast, bowel and lung) and the most common gynaecological cancer in America. More than 42,000 cases reported and 7780 deaths estimated in 2009. Endometrial cancer is more common in developed countries and mortality rate was higher in black than in white. The incidence is rising due to increase in life expectancy and rate of obesity as well as lack in physical activity. The highest incidence is in white North Americans have a rate seven times higher than Chinese. Asian women who migrate to the USA develop an incidence rate similar to the USA population. Most of the patients with endometrial cancer were aged 50–59 years old; 20–25% of cases were diagnosed before menopause. Approximately, 5% of women are diagnosed below 40 years of age. For all stages taken together, the overall 5-year survival rates is around 80% and 75% of patients presented at an early stage. Lifetime risk of developing Ca endometrium is a woman less than 75 year old is 1–3% (1% overall risk, GLOBOCAN 2008).

Type of Endometrial Cancer

Endometrial cancers are broadly classified into two main categories (first described by Bokhman in 1980s):

(a) **Type I endometrial cancer**: It is related to exposure to unopposed endogenous or exogenous oestrogen. The cancers frequently arise on a background of atypical hyperplasia and have an association with obesity, nulliparity, insulin resistance and hyperoestrogenism. Type I is usually well differentiated and has a better prognosis.

(b) **Type II endometrial cancer**: Type II has no association with predisposing factors as in Type I. Uterine papillary serous and clear cell carcinoma is the example of Type II endometrial cancer. Unlike type I, patients with type II endometrial cancer tend to be elderly and thin and have a poorer prognosis.

Approximately 80% of endometrial cancers are type I and the most common histologic subtype is endometrioid adenocarcinoma accounting for 75–80% of endometrial cancer. The differences between Type I and Type II endometrial cancer are shown in Table 9.1.

Uterine serous carcinoma of the endometrium is the most common type II endometrial cancer. Serous carcinoma accounts for less than 10% of endometrial malignancies with poor prognosis. Median age for patients with serous carcinoma is 5 years older than those with endometrioid endometrial carcinoma. They often spread intra-abdominally similar with ovarian cancer. Overall 5- year survival rates for patients with serous carcinoma of the endometrium were 52.6% as compared to 83.2% in endometrioid adenocarcinoma (Creasman et al., 2006). Clear cell carcinoma is the second most common type II endometrial cancer accounts for about 5% of all endometrial cancers. Clear cell carcinomas are aggressive and have a tendency to spread beyond the pelvis (40% of patients with clinically confined to the uterus) and has high relapse rate.

Table 9.1 Characteristic of type I and type II endometrial cancer

Characteristic	Type I	Type II
Unopposed oestrogen	Present	Absent
Menopausal status	Pre- and perimenopausal	Majority postmenopausal
Obesity	Yes	No
Parity	Low parity or nulliparous	Multiparous
Grade	Low	High
Myometrial invasion	Minimal	Deep
Histology of adjacent endometrium	Hyperplastic	Atrophic/cystic polyp
Histology	Endometrioid, adenoacanthoma	Papillary serous (UPSC), Clear cell
Precursor lesion	Atypical hyperplasia (WHO) or EIN (EIN nomenclature)	Endometrial intraepithelial carcinoma (EIC)
Progesterone receptor +/Oestrogen receptor +	Higher positivity in grade 1 (>90%)	Negative or mildly positive (0–30%)
PTEN (deletion or mutation)	50–80%	10–11%
P53 overexpression	5–10%	80–90%
EGFR expression	46%	34%
P16 inactivation	10%	40%
Ploidy	67% diploid	40% diploid
Behaviour	Less aggressive, better prognosis	Aggressive

Source: Adapted from (a) Kuman RJ, Zaimo R, Norris HJ. Endometrial carcinoma in Kuman RJ (ed.): *Blaustein's Pathology of the Genital Tract*, pp. 439–486. 1994, NY, Springer-Verlag; (b) Zagouri et al., 2010.

Approximately, 10% of endometrial carcinoma shows a mixed histology, i.e. presence of more than one component, each must be at least 10% of the tumour. Presence of serous component in even 10% of the tumour is enough to influence the overall prognosis. The other variants of mixed histology type of endometrial carcinoma are adenocarcinoma with squamous cell differentiation or adenoacanthoma (squamous cell components are benign) and adenosquamous carcinoma (squamous component resembles a squamous cell carcinoma). Adenoacanthoma has the same prognosis as endometrioid adenocarcinoma. Histological classification of endometrial cancer is shown in Table 9.2.

Table 9.2 Histological classification of endometrial carcinoma by WHO (Silverberg, et al.)

Histology type	Subtype
Endometriod adenocarcinoma	(a) With squamous differentiation (b) Villoglandular (c) Secretory (d) With ciliated cells
Other adenocarcinomas	(a) Mucinous carcinoma (b) Serous carcinoma (c) Clear cell carcinoma (d) Mixed adenocarcinoma (includes adenosquamous)
Other carcinomas	(a) Squamous cell carcinoma (b) Transitional cell carcinoma (c) Small cell carcinoma (d) Undifferentiated carcinoma

Synchronous endometrium and ovarian carcinoma is rare phenomena and occur in 15–20% of endometrioid adenocarcinoma of the ovary. Differential diagnosis of synchronous tumour is ovarian metastasis; however, metastasis to the ovary is unlikely from the endometrium if the following features exist: (a) Ovarian tumour is bilateral, (b) Myoinvasion is less than middle third of endometrium, (c) There is no vascular space invasion and (d) Endometrial carcinoma is of well-differentiated type (grade 1).

In endometrial cancer, differentiation of tumour is expressed in grade. FIGO, the WHO and International Society of Gynaecological

Pathologist are using two methods of grading. The grading of endometrial cancer can be done preoperatively by histologic examination of endometrial tissues taken from the endometrial sampling procedure.

Two methods of grading are:

1. By architectural growth pattern (adenocarcinoma component)
    - **Grade 1**: ≤ 5% of tumour is in solid sheets
    - **Grade 2**: 6–50% of tumour is in solid sheets
    - **Grade 3**: >50% of tumour are in solid masses

Notable nuclear atypia (grade 3, nuclear features) will raises 1 grade.

2. By nuclear features (for non serous carcinoma)
    - **Grade 1**: Round to oval nuclei with even distribution of chromatin and inconspicuous nucleoli.
    - **Grade 2**: Irregular, oval nuclei with chromatin clumping and moderate size nucleoli
    - **Grade 3**: Large pleomorphic nuclei with coarse chromatin and large, irregular nucleoli.

Higher grade of tumour is associated with increased risk of myometrial invasion and lymph node metastases.

Risk Factors for Endometrial Cancer

Generally, type I endometrial cancer is due to prolonged exposure to oestrogen either exogenous or endogenous in origin. High level of endogenous oestrogen is often seen in obese women. Patients with polycystic ovarian syndrome and oestrogen-producing tumour are also known to have a high level of unopposed oestrogen and therefore, at higher risk of endometrial cancer. The summary of risk factors for type I endometrial cancer is shown in Table 9.3.

About 50% of patients with endometrial cancer were found to have a body mass index of >25 kg/m^2. In premenopausal women, obesity causes insulin resistance, ovarian androgen excess, anovulation and chronic unopposed oestrogen. The rate of obesity is increasing especially in developed countries due to eating habits and sedentary lifestyle. Obesity in known to increase the endogenous oestrogen because peripheral fat is responsible in converting the androstenedione to oestrogen compounds. Postmenopausal women with high BMI have a higher oestrogen level (mainly oestrone) due to excessive peripheral conversion from androstenedione by adipose tissues. Obese women with normal circulating oestrogen remain at higher risk because of an alteration in insulin-like growth factor. Diabetes and hypertension have been recognized as risk factors independent of their association with obesity.

Table 9.3 Risk factors for type I endometrial cancer

Risk factors	Increased risk
Obesity	
>30 lb ideal BW	3×
>50 lb ideal BW	10×
Nulliparous	2–3×
Late menopause (age>52)	2.5×
Heavy perimenopausal bleeding	4×
Diabetes Mellitus	2.8×
Hypertension	1.5×
Unopposed exogenous oestrogen	9.5×
Untreated Complex atypical hyperplasia	29% will developed adenocarcinoma
Tamoxifen given for breast cancer increased the risk of endometrial cancer • Greatest risk after 5-year use and the risk remains even after stopping the tamoxifen • 36% occur within 2 years • Excess risk of more aggressive histotype was noted in patient taking tamoxifen, including type II endometrial cancer and carcinosarcoma • Risk of endometrial cancer has to weigh with the benefit of reducing recurrent breast cancer (from 227/1000 to 123/1000 breast cancer) and preventing cancer in contralateral breast (40 reduced to 23 per 1000). The benefit outweighs the risk.	Relative risk 6.4–7.5-fold (40 mg/d)
Endometrial hyperplasia	Progressing to Cancer
Simple hyperplasia (no atypia)	1%
Complex (adenomatous, no atypia)	3%
Atypical	
Simple (cystic with atypia)	8%
Complex (adenomatous + Atypia)	29%

The use of combination oral contraceptive pills for 1 year decreased the risk of endometrial cancers by more than 40%. Women on combined hormone replacement therapy have also been found to have lower risk of endometrial cancer as long as their progestogen content is more than 10–12 days per cycle.

Approximately, 5% of endometrial cancer is hereditary associated with a hereditary non-polyposis colon cancer syndrome (HNPCC). The lifetime risk of having endometrial cancer is 40–60% in patients with HNPCC. HNPCC is an autosomal dominant inherited disorder caused by germ-line mutation in DNA mismatch repair genes. Defective MMR genes are identified in 85% of HNPCC-associated endometrial carcinoma.

Smoking is said to reduce the risk of endometrial cancer due to its effect on oestrogen level. Pregnancy has a natural protective effect against endometrial cancer because of high production of progesterone by placenta.

Pre-Malignant Lesions of Endometrium and Pathogenesis of Endometrial Cancer

Majority of patients with Type I endometrial cancers have co-existing endometrial hyperplasia. Endometrial hyperplasia can be divided into simple endometrial hyperplasia without atypia, complex endometrial hyperplasia without atypia and hyperplasia with atypia (WHO classification). Hyperplasia is thought to result from excessive or unopposed oestrogen stimulation of the endometrial glands. In some individual, hyperplasia can also be due to an abnormal endometrial response to normal hormonal stimulation. Cytogenetic analysis has found that the most common genetic alterations in endometrial hyperplasia are: (a) Micro-satellite instability (MSI) and (b) Mutation of tumour suppressor gene PTEN (phosphatase and tensin homolog) seen in 20–30% of atypical hyperplasia and 40% of endometrioid adenocarcinoma. MSI and PTEN mutation can coexist in some cases.

Endometrial hyperplasia without atypia responds better to progestogen therapy because of higher level of progesterone receptors as compared to endometrial hyperplasia with atypia. In simple hyperplasia, endometrium is thick with dilated, outpouchings, invaginating and crowded glands. While in atypical hyperplasia, the abnormalities are more prominent with the present of cytologic atypia of the glandular cell such as nuclear hyperchromatism, nuclear enlargement and increased nuclear-cytoplasmic ratio. Presence of cytologic atypia is a single most important predictor of malignant potential and resistance to medical therapy. Co-existing endometrial carcinoma was found in 40% of hysterectomy specimens taken from patients with a preoperative diagnosis of atypical endometrial hyperplasia.

Patients on tamoxifen therapy are also at higher risk of endometrial pathology. Tamoxifen is an oestrogen receptor-modulating hormone and has antioestrogen properties to breast. Despite antioestrogen properties on breast tissue, it also has paradoxical mild oestrogenic effects on the endometrium especially in postmenopausal women. Therefore, women taken tamoxifen are at higher risk of endometrial hyperplasia, endometrial polyps, endometrial cancer and even uterine sarcoma (carcinosarcoma). The study showed that the use of tamoxifen for 2 years was associated with an approximately twofold increased risk of endometrial cancer, while the use for 5 or more years produces a 4–8-fold excess risk. The overall risk of endometrial cancer in a patient with simple hyperplasia, complex hyperplasia and atypical hyperplasia is 1%, 2.4% and 46.2%, respectively (Baak et al., 1992; Horn et al., 2004; Kurman et al., 1985). See Table 9.4 for details.

Table 9.4 Risk of endometrial cancer in different types of endometrial hyperplasia

	Simple hyperplasia	**Complex hyperplasia**	**Atypical hyperplasia**
Kurman et al. (1985)	1/93 (1.1%)	1/29 (3.4%)	10/35 (28.6%)
Baak et al. (1992)	0/8 (0%)	1/6 (16.7%)	5/11 (45.4%)
Horn et al. (2004)	—	8/390 (2.0%)	58/112 (51.8%)
Overall risk	1/101 (1%)	10/425 (2.4%)	73/158 (46.2%)

The diagnosis of atypical endometrial hyperplasia and grade 1 endometrial adenocarcinoma are known to have a poor reproducibility event among experienced Pathologists. As an alternative to former classification of endometrial hyperplasia, recently a new classification of pre-malignant lesions of the endometrium has been proposed and currently is widely used in United State. The new terminology for pre-malignant lesion of the endometrium is known as endometrial intraepithelial neoplasia (EIN) (Table 9.5).

Table 9.5 Classification of endometrial pathology and premalignant lesions of endometrium

EIN nomenclature	Functional category	Management
Benign proliferative endometrium (benign endometrial hyperplasia)	Oestrogen effect	Hormonal therapy
Endometrial intraepithelial neoplasia (EIN)	Pre-cancerous	Hormonal or surgery
Adenocarcinoma	Cancer	Based on stage

Based on a new concept of premalignant lesions of endometrium, endometrial pathology is now classified into three categories:

(a) Benign endometrial hyperplasia (Disordered Proliferative Endometrium)
(b) Endometrial intraepithelial neoplasia (EIN)
(c) Endometrial adenocarcinoma

The diagnosis of EIN is based on five diagnostic criteria (see Table 9.6). EIN classification was found to be more reproducible and has a better correlation with prognosis. EIN lesions are non-invasive genetically altered neoplasms, which arise focally, and may transform to malignant phenotype upon acquisition of additional genetic damage. Patients with EIN have 45-fold increased risk of endometrioid endometrial carcinoma and the median interval from diagnosis of EIN to carcinoma is 4 years. Approximately, 40% of patients with EIN were found to have concurrent endometrial carcinoma within 1 year. A study by Hecht et al. to evaluate the correlation between EIN classification and WHO classifications of pre-malignant lesions of endometrium found that 78% of patients with atypical endometrial hyperplasia

(WHO classification) have enough criteria to diagnose EIN. Full correlation is shown in the Fig. 9.2.

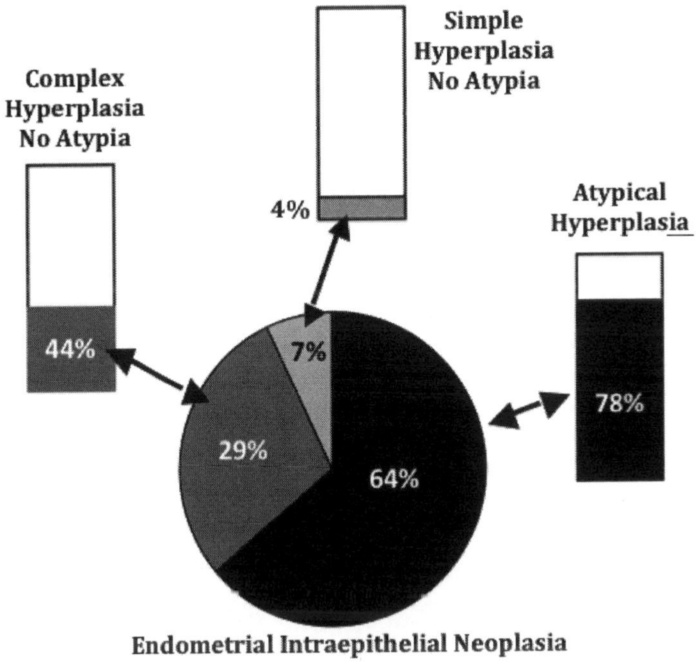

Figure 9.2 Correlation between WHO classification and EIN Nomenclature. Example: 78% of patients with atypical hyperplasia fulfilled the criteria for the diagnosis of EIN, while 64% of EIN was diagnosed as atypical hyperplasia (Hecht et al., 2005).

Table 9.6 EIN diagnostic criteria (Silverberg et al., 2003)

EIN Criteria	Comments
Architecture	Area of glands greater than stroma
Cytology	Cytology differs between architecturally crowded focus and background, or clearly abnormal.
Size > 1 mm	Maximum linear dimension exceeds 1 mm.
Exclude mimics	Benign conditions with overlapping criteria: basalis, secretory, polyps, repair, etc.
Exclude cancer	Carcinoma if mazelike glands, solid areas, polygonal "mosaic-like" glands, myoinvasion, or significant cribriforming

The EIN or endometrial intraepithelial neoplasia is the precursor for type I endometrial cancer. The precursor lesion for type II endometrial cancer is known as endometrial intraepithelial carcinoma (EIC). The EIC represents a non-invasive glandular lesion characterized by epithelial cells with marked nuclear abnormalities, resembling nuclei similar to those seen in serous carcinoma of the endometrium. In most cases, EIC is seen in the underlying atrophic endometrium of older postmenopausal women and not uncommon to detect this lesion within a polyp. The cells of EIC show negative reaction against oestrogen and progesterone receptor analysis but often positive to p53 and Ki-67. The Hypothetic model of the pathogenesis of type II endometrial cancer is shown in Fig. 9.4.

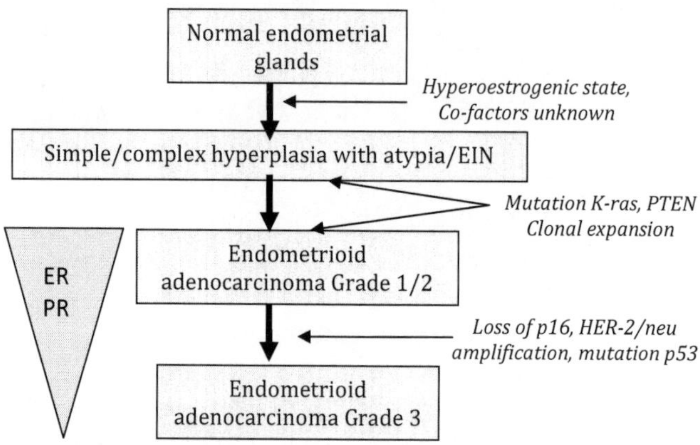

Figure 9.3 Hypothetic model of the pathogenesis of type I endometrial cancer (Horn et al., 2007).

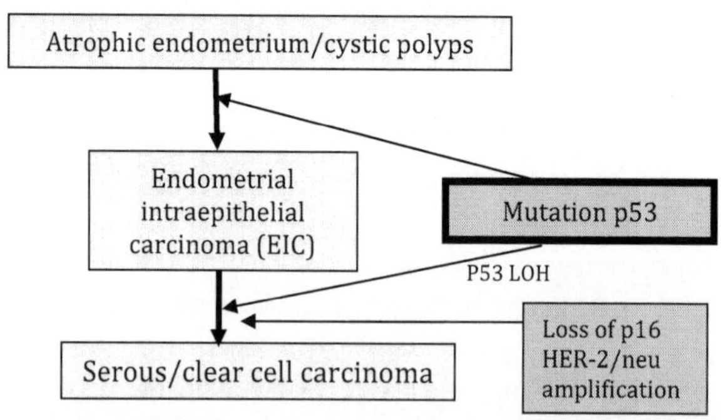

Figure 9.4 Hypothetic model of the pathogenesis of type II endometrial cancer (Horn et al., 2007).

Prevention of Endometrial Cancer

Treating the precursor lesions either by hormonal or surgical treatment can prevent endometrial cancer. Adding a progestogen for at least 10–12 days per cycle in hormone replacement therapy can reduce the risk of endometrial cancer, particularly if the hormone is taken continuously and in obese women. In contrast, if the oestrogen alone is given continuously for 2 years without progestogen, the risk of developing endometrial hyperplasia will be many folds higher according to dose. Women taking oestrogen 1.25 mg daily dose for 2 years has 32-fold increase risk of endometrial hyperplasia than 0.3 mg daily dose. Women with amenorrhea or oligomenorrhea (including women with PCOS) should be treated with cyclical progestogen to avoid prolonged exposure of the endometrium to a high level of oestrogen. Withdrawal bleeding of 3-monthly is sufficient to prevent endometrial pathology. There have been suggestions of a protective effect of high phyto-oestrogen consumption on risk of endometrial cancer among postmenopausal women (Goodman et al., 1997; Horn-Ross, 2003; Xu et al., 2004).

The use of intrauterine devices and tubal ligation has also been associated with a lower risk of endometrial cancer (Hubacher and Grimes 2002; Kjaer et al., 2004). Weight reduction and physical activities to achieve ideal body weight can reverse the effect of prolonged exposure to a high level of oestrogen. Pregnancy is a physiological protection against endometrial pathology due to a high level of hormone progesterone produced by placenta. The use of combination oral contraceptive pills for 1 year decreased the risk of endometrial cancers by more than 40%. Combined OCP is also known to reduce the incidence of ovarian cancer.

There is no effective screening method for endometrial cancer. Endometrial sampling, transvaginal ultrasound, endometrial brush sponge, endometrial aspiration, Pap smear and progestogen challenge test have been evaluated as a screening test but their accuracy in asymptomatic population is limited. For asymptomatic low-risk women, novel-screening approaches from epigenetics, proteomics and genomics are being explored. Small studies on the role of gene methylation patterns and telomerase assays have shown some promising results (Fiegl et al., 2004; Maida et al., 2002). Screening for high-risk women such as patients on tamoxifen therapy and long-term oestrogen replacement therapy using yearly transvaginal ultrasound have reported low sensitivity, specificity and positive predictive value in detecting endometrial cancer (Fung et al., 2003). American Cancer Society has suggested annual screening with endometrial biopsy for women above 35 years old with HNPCC and having lifetime risks of endometrial cancer between 40–60% (Smith et al., 2007). In women presented with postmenopausal bleeding, transvaginal ultrasound showing ET of ≤5 mm and negative endometrial sampling have nearly 100% negative predictive value.

Presentation and Diagnosis

Majority of patients with endometrial cancer are postmenopausal women. Most common presenting symptom is postmenopausal bleeding. Other presenting symptoms are (a) abnormal vaginal discharge, (b) abnormal vaginal bleeding in 80% (including postmenopausal bleeding and irregular menses in premenopausal women), (c) symptoms due to uterine enlargement including pressure symptoms and (d) symptoms indicative of extra-uterine spread.

Full evaluation of the endometrium (ultrasound and endometrial biopsy) must be performed in women presented with postmenopausal bleeding. Women with postmenopausal bleeding have 10–15% probability of endometrial cancer. The initial diagnosis of endometrial cancer is often made by transvaginal ultrasound and office endometrial sampling. In postmenopausal women, normal endometrial thickness is ≤5 mm (myometrium to myometrium). Transvaginal ultrasound is non-invasive with sensitivity and specificity of 91% and 96%, respectively (using cut-off point endometrial thickness of 5 mm). Endometrial carcinoma is seen in varieties of sonographic features, including a prominent thickened endometrium, polypoidal lesion and mixed echogenicity. Endometrial hyperplasia and grade 1 endometrial cancer usually showed hyperechoic features while grade 2–3 endometrial cancers tends to be hypoechoic on transvaginal ultrasound. Hysteroscopy and hysterosonography are not recommended in patients with highly suspicious of endometrial cancer because of potential risk of tumour spread from uterine cavity into the peritoneal cavity.

A meta-analysis on the value of pipelle endometrial sampling for the diagnosis of atypical hyperplasia or endometrial cancer has reported the sensitivity of 81–99% and specificity of 98%. There are many more endometrial samplers available in the market such as Kauman cannula, Tis-U-trap, Vabra aspirator and z-sampler. Pipelle endometrial sampler is perhaps the most commonly used method to assess the endometrium (Fig. 9.5). Office endometrial sampling using pipelle sampler was found to be valuable in terms of cost, high patient's acceptability and high percentage of diagnostic agreement (96%). However, result from office endometrial sampling technique has a poor correlation in tumour grading with final histological diagnosis (from a hysterectomy specimen). Study by Leitao Jr et al. (evaluating 490 patients with a preoperative diagnosis of grade 1 endometrial adenocarcinoma) have found that 15% of patients with preoperative grade 1 lesions were actually had a higher grade lesions (mostly grade 2 and some grade 3) on hysterectomy specimen. Combined analysis on same correlation was done by other authors, and they found that the rate of upgrading was even higher, up to 30% (Larson et al., 1995; Obermair et al., 1999; Frumovitz et al., 2004; Eltabbakh et al., 2005). Eltabbakh et al. also reported that 12.6% of patients diagnosed as grade 1 endometrial cancer preoperatively (total 182 patients) were found to have advanced stage disease. In most of the patients, pipelle endometrial sampling or other office endometrial sampling is as good as endometrial curettage (DD&C) in detecting endometrial cancer (Stovall, Dijkhuizen et al., 2000). However, in some patients, due to atrophic changes of the cervix and endometrium, endometrium is better evaluated by fractional DD&C (curetting the endocervix should be done prior to the endometrium). Diagnosis, dilatation and curettage was found to be more accurate in predicting grade of tumour as compared to office endometrial biopsy. The FIGO grade in the hysterectomy specimen was upgraded in only 15% of the cases after D&C as compared to 27% after office endometrial biopsy (Leito Jr et al., 2008; Larson et al., 1995; Frumovitz et al., 2004; Daniel and Peters, 1988). Hysteroscopy is indicated if a patient has persistent symptoms despite normal endometrial biopsy. Hysteroscopy can diagnose endometrial polyp or small focus of endometrial lesions in which hysteroscopic-directed biopsy can be performed (Fig. 9.6).

Hysteroscopy is also useful in patients taking tamoxifen when transvaginal ultrasound showed evidence of endometrial lesions suggestive of polyps and if the endometrial sample is insufficient.

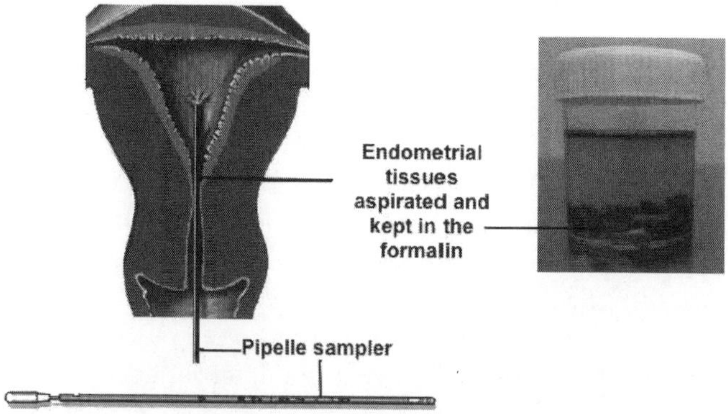

Figure 9.5 Office endometrial sampling.

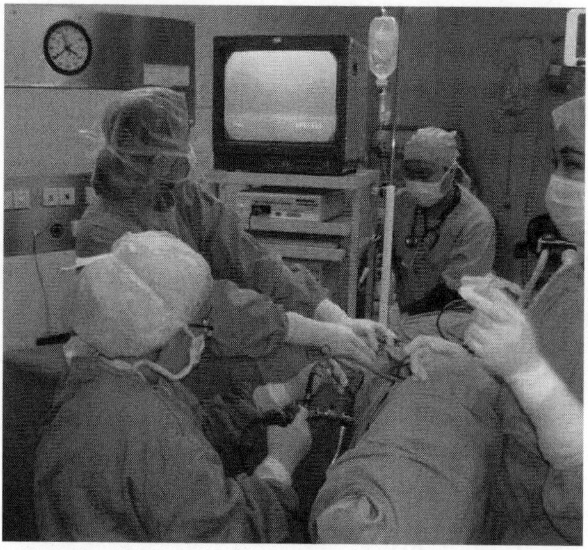

Figure 9.6 Hysteroscopy for the diagnosis of endometrial pathology.

Investigations and Staging

Once the diagnosis of endometrial cancer has been made, blood count, renal profiles and liver function tests are performed. There are no established tumour markers for endometrial cancer; CA125 level is elevated mainly in advanced stage disease (65–80%). In stage 1 and stage 2 endometrial cancers, CA125 is elevated only in 15% and 33%, respectively. CA125 is perhaps more useful in type II endometrial cancer. Raised Ca125 in an apparent early stage may indicate the presence of micrometastases. CA125 level is useful only in follow-up setting; almost 60% of patients with recurrent endometrial cancer showed elevated CA125.

Chest x-ray and CT scan are useful to evaluate the extent of the disease preoperatively. MRI is increasingly used in endometrial cancer, especially to evaluate the myometrial invasion, while CT scan is more superior in assessing retroperitoneal lymph nodes.

The final staging of endometrial cancer is determined after thorough histopathological assessment of the surgical specimens (surgico-pathological staging). Preoperative assessment of the tumour in terms of tumour grading and the degree of myoinvasion are important to determine the extent of surgical treatment. The surgical staging surgery for endometrial cancer includes exploratory laparotomy, peritoneal wash for cytology, extrafascial hysterectomy and bilateral salpingoophorectomy, excision of suspicious nodule or lymph nodes and omentectomy in advanced stage or in type II endometrial cancer. The role of routine systematic lymphadenectomy will be discussed later in this chapter.

Intraoperative assessment of myometrial invasion was found to be difficult and often inaccurate. Frumovitz and colleagues have evaluated 122 patients with endometrial cancer and reported that a frozen section diagnosis of no myometrial invasion is not accurate in 72% of cases. Furthermore, 26% of cases with a frozen section reported >50% myometrial invasion was actually had deeper invasion, cervical involvement, and/or extra-uterine disease. In another study by Mao and colleagues evaluating the accuracy of gross examination of the uterus intraoperatively, they found that intra-operative gross examination correctly identified the depth of microscopic myometrial invasion in 90.3% of patients. The sensitivity in detecting myometrial invasion was 80.6% and the specificity was 92.4%. With regard to cervical involvement, gross examination had an overall accuracy of 84.3%. The sensitivity in detecting cervical involvement was 32.6% and the specificity was 99.0%. However, in this study, specimen was examined by four members of experts comprising of two gynaecologic pathologists and two experienced gynaecologic oncologists.

FIGO Staging of Endometrial Cancer

FIGO has recently revised the new staging to replace FIGO staging 1988. FIGO with the collaboration of several other International bodies such as IGCS, Gynecologic intergroup, Society of Gynecologic Oncologists, the International Society of Gynecologic Oncologist, International Society of Gynecologic Pathologist and AJCC have come out with new FIGO staging for endometrial cancer (Mutch, 2009). For the purpose of comparison, both old and new FIGO staging are shown in the Tables 9.7 and 9.8, respectively.

Table 9.7 Corpus cancer staging, FIGO 1988 (old staging)

Staging	Descriptions
Stage 1	**Tumour confined to corpus uteri**
Stage 1A G123	Tumour limited to endometrium
Stage 1B G123	Invasion ≤ 50% of myometrium
Stage 1C G123	Invasion > 50% of myometrium
Stage 2	**Tumour invades cervix but not outside uterus**
Stage 2A G123	Endocervical gland involvement only
Stage 2B G123	Cervical stroma invasion
Stage 3	**Local and/regional spread**
Stage 3A G123	Tumour invades serosa and/or adnexae or positive peritoneal fluid cytology.
Stage 3B G123	Vaginal involvement (direct or metastases)
Stage 3C G123	Metastasis to pelvic and/or para-aortic nodes
Stage 4	**Tumour invades bladder and/or bowel mucosa, and/or distant metastases**
Stage 4A G123	Tumour invades bladder mucosa and/or bowel mucosa.
Stage 4B	Distant metastasis including intra-abdominal LNs (other than para-aortic) and/or inguinal lymph nodes.

Table 9.8 Corpus cancer staging, FIGO 2009

Staging	Descriptions
Stage 1	**Tumour confined to corpus uteri**
Stage 1A G123	No or less than half myometrial invasion
Stage 1B G123	Invasion ≥ 50% of myometrium

Stage 2	**Tumour invades cervical stroma but not outside uterus**[a]
Stage 3	**Local and/or regional spread of tumour**
Stage 3A G123	Tumour invades serosa and/or adnexae[b]
Stage 3B G123	Vaginal and/or parametrial involvement[b]
Stage 3C G123	Metastasis to pelvic and/or para-aortic nodes[b]
Stage 3C1 G123	Positive pelvic nodes
Stage 3C2 G123	Positive para-aortic lymph nodes with or without positive pelvic lymph nodes
Stage 4	**Tumour invades bladder and/or bowel mucosa, and/or distant metastases**
Stage 4A G123	Tumour invades bladder mucosa and/or bowel mucosa
Stage 4B	Distant metastasis including intra-abdominal metastases and/or inguinal lymph nodes

[a]Endocervical glandular involvement only should be considered as stage 1 and no longer as stage 2.
[b]Positive cytology has to be reported separately without changing the stage
G123: grade 1, grade 2 or grade 3.

The changes in new FIGO staging are based on the following issues:

(a) There was little survival difference between no myometrial invasion and less than 50% invasion; therefore these are combined.
(b) Parametrial involvement is now included.
(c) Peritoneal fluid for cytology was found to be highly variable based on sampling of washing hence it has been eliminated as a staging criteria.
(d) Pelvic and para-aortic lymph nodes metastases carry different survival and have to be separated in the staging.

Treatment for Pre-Malignant Lesions of Endometrium

Patients with premalignant lesions of the endometrium should be treated by either hormonal or surgical treatment. Spontaneous regression is possible in simple hyperplasia without atypia (72%

regression rate). Endometrial hyperplasia with atypia is less likely to regress spontaneously. The most important criteria to determine the choice of treatment is presence of nuclear atypia. The modality of treatment in premalignant condition of endometrium is depending on age, need for future fertility, co-morbidities and surgical risk.

Patients with simple or complex hyperplasia without atypia often respond well to hormonal treatment. In general, more than 90% of the endometrial hyperplasia without atypia showed complete regression following hormonal treatment. The risk of recurrence is approximately 10%.

Endometrial hyperplasia with atypia has lower response rate ranging from 50% to 80% and the lesions tend to persist in 50% of cases. There were also cases of progression to cancer despite the hormonal treatment. The choices of progestogens include megestrol acetate, medroxyprogesterone acetate, levenorgestrel-releasing devices and vaginal micronized progesterone. Patients with endometrial hyperplasia and atypia are often treated with high-dose progestogen for 3–6 months followed by maintenance low dose for another few months' once complete regression has been confirmed histologically. These patients should be followed up with transvaginal ultrasound scan and endometrial sampling.

Patients diagnosed as premalignant lesions of the endometrium using EIN classification should be treated similar to atypical endometrial hyperplasia (WHO classification). Concurrent endometrial carcinoma with atypical hyperplasia or EIN has been reported in many studies and in some patients, invasive cancer was discovered later during the follow-up. The study found that 40% of patients with EIN have concurrent carcinoma diagnosed within 1 year. The GOG study reported the rate of concurrent carcinoma with atypical endometrial hyperplasia to be 42.6% and Giede et al. reported an incidence of 35.7%. The high rate of concurrent carcinoma discovered in these studies was probably due to high incidence of endometrial cancer in the studied population (Western countries including America). Similar study done in Korea by Hahn et al., however, reported lower rate of concurrent carcinoma in patients with complex atypical endometrial hyperplasia, i.e. 12.7% (simple atypical hyperplasia was excluded). One of the explanations by the authors regarding this finding was probably related to the accuracy of preoperative diagnosis of endometrial hyperplasia in their study. In the majority of cases, the diagnosis was done via DD&C (78%) as compared to previous studies that mostly via office-based endometrial biopsy.

The effectiveness of oral progestogen therapy has been evaluated in few studies and generally the regression rate for non-atypical hyperplasia was more than 90% while in atypical hyperplasia in approximately 50%. Varma et al. evaluated the role of the levonorgestrel-releasing intrauterine system (LNG-IUS) in the treatment of endometrial hyperplasia and they found that treatment with LNG-IUS achieved endometrial regression in 90% of cases within 2 years. The regression rate was higher in patients with non-atypical hyperplasia as compared to atypical hyperplasia (92% versus 67%). In this study, follow-up pipelle endometrial biopsy was done 3-monthly for 6 months and subsequently 6-monthly.

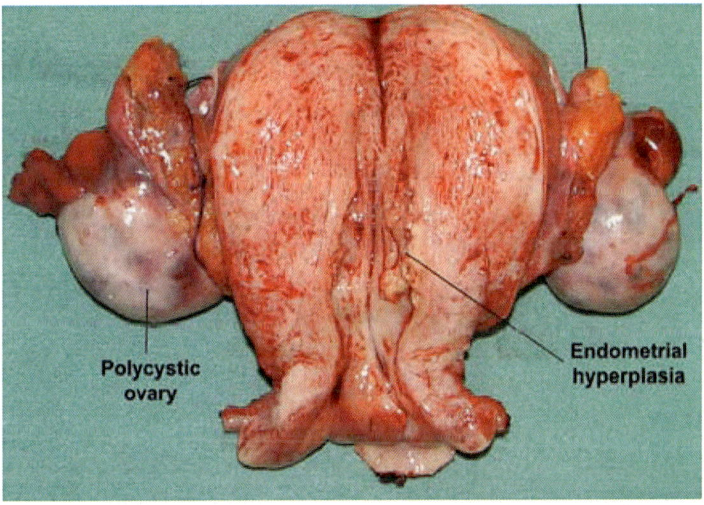

Figure 9.7 Endometrial hyperplasia associated with polycystic ovarian syndrome.

Patients with atypical endometrial hyperplasia presented after menopause, and those who had failed to respond to conservative treatment are best treated with simple hysterectomy. In premenopausal women, the treatment choice is individualized. In patients who are not medically fit for major surgical treatment, endometrial resection or endometrial ablation has been advocated.

They can also be treated with hormonal treatment either in oral form or with LNG-IUS. The German Working Group of Gynaecology Oncology has proposed a treatment guideline for patients with endometrial hyperplasia; please refer to Fig. 9.8.

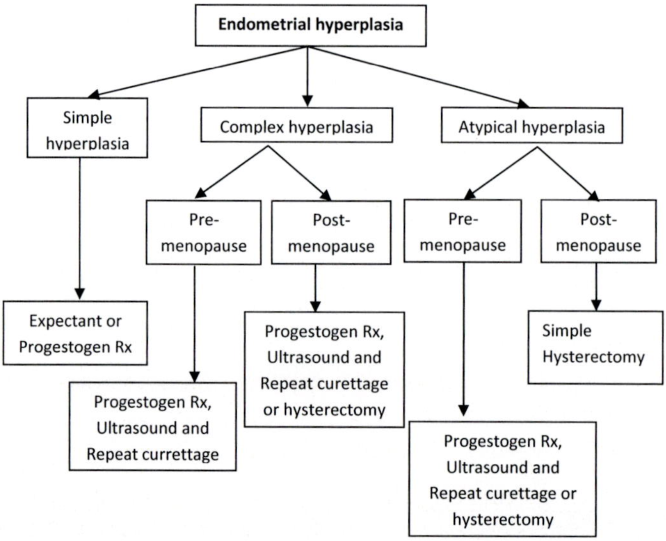

Figure 9.8 Treatment guideline for endometrial hyperplasia by German Working Group of Gynecologic Oncology (Horn et al., 2007).

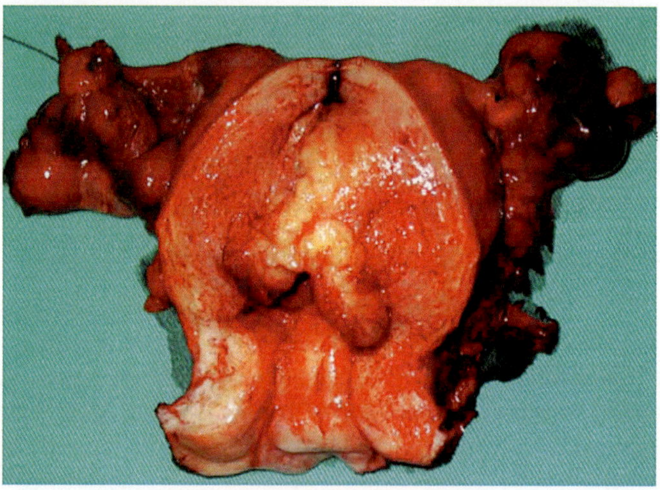

Figure 9.9 Endometrial carcinoma.

Treatment for Endometrial Carcinoma

Surgery

Surgery is the most important mode of treatment in endometrial cancer. Following are the principles of surgery for endometrial cancer:

(a) Maylard's incision (for early stage) and midline incision for advanced stage when upper abdominal surgery is likely to be performed.
(b) Thorough intraperitoneal exploration
(c) Peritoneal washing for cytology
(d) Extrafascial hysterectomy and bilateral salpingoophorectomy
(e) Pelvic ± Para-aortic lymphadenectomy
(f) Omentectomy in selected cases (in advanced type I endometrial cancer in which the omentum is involved or in type II endometrial cancer, i.e. serous carcinoma and clear cell carcinoma)

Comprehensive surgical staging for endometrial cancer as mentioned above will define disease biology and facilitate triage of tailored adjuvant therapy. The obturator lymph nodes (above the obturator nerve) and iliac lymph nodes are the most common sites for lymph node metastasis. Exploration and lymphadenectomy of the lymph nodes over this area will allow identification of 90% of node-positive patients. The role of routine lymphadenectomy will be discussed later in this chapter. Patients with positive pelvic nodes have a higher incidence of para-aortic lymph node metastasis and therefore require para-aortic lymphadenectomy. Para-aortic nodes were positive in 47% of patients who had disease documented in their pelvic nodes. Patients with deep myometrial invasion and grade 3 tumour have at least 5% (some reported up to 18%) risk of pelvic lymph node metastasis. Patients with pelvic node metastases are categorized as stage 3 disease and 5-year survival rate is 60% as compared to 97% in patients with stage 1 disease.

Patients with superficial myometrial invasion, grade 1 or 2 and tumour's greatest dimension of <2 cm have lower risk of pelvic lymph nodes metastases. Lymphadenectomy may be omitted in this group of patients if the diagnosis can be made accurately (via preoperative and intraoperative evaluation).

The routine systematic pelvic lymphadenecomy in apparent stage 1 endometrial cancer remains controversial. The purpose of this procedure is to establish the staging and to eradicate the metastatic lymph nodes, which may carry a therapeutic benefit. The first large randomized control trial evaluating the role of routine pelvic lymphadenectomy in apparent stage 1 endometrial cancer was performed by Panici et al. The study accrued 524 patients at 31 centres over 10 year's period. In study arm, systematic pelvic lymphadenectomy was performed while in control arm; lymphadenectomy was not performed; however, removal of bulky nodes (>1 cm) was allowed in the control arm. After almost 6 years, there was no difference in the adjusted hazard ratio for relapse and death between study and control arm. However, the results

From this trial were scrutinized with the following arguments:

(a) The trial did not meet the requirement to detect a difference due to insufficient samples.
(b) There was no standardization of postoperative adjuvant therapy and the Cox regression was not adjusted for postoperative therapy.
(c) More patients received adjuvant treatment in the control group (25.2% versus 16.7%, $p = 0.033$).
(d) Lymph node dissection was performed in some proportion of patients in control arm (16% had >6 lymph nodes removes and 11% had 10 lymph nodes removed).
(e) There was no standard definition of "adequate" lymphadenectomy.

The second randomized trial funded by Medical Research Council and National Cancer Research Network known as **MRC ASTEC trial** (efficacy of systematic pelvic lymphadenectomy in endometrial cancer) was published. The main objective of this trial was to determine if lymphadenectomy increase survival independent of adjuvant radiation. The trial accrued over 1400 women (from 85 centres in four different countries) with endometrial cancer suspected to be confined to the uterus. There were two arms in this trial: (1) Control arm underwent standard surgery (hysterectomy, bilateral salpingoophorectomy, para-aortic lymph node palpation, with suspicious node removal at the surgeon's discretion) and (2) Study arm underwent above procedures plus iliac and obturator nodes dissection. The primary outcome was overall survival. Patients who were unfit to undergo lymphadenectomy or whom the centre did not offer the procedure subsequently underwent standard surgery. If postoperatively they were found to be in an intermediate risk or high-risk early stage (stage 1A, 1B, grade 3, papillary serous or clear cell histology or stage 1C or 2A), they were randomized either receiving external beam radiotherapy ± brachytherapy or observation ± brachytherapy. MRC ASTEC trial also concludes that there was no evidence of benefit in terms of overall or recurrent-free survival of pelvic lymphadenectomy in women with early endometrial cancer. Similar to Panici trial, MRC ASTEC trial was also criticized because of the following limitations: (a) Lymphadenectomy arm had significantly more patients with disease spread beyond the uterus (21% versus 19%). (b) Lymphadenectomy arm had clearer cell or serous subtype and more stage 1C disease compared to control arm. (c) The median number of lymph nodes removed was 12 in the lymphadenectomy arm and 12% had <5 nodes removed. Only 65% of patients in this arm had an "adequate" lymph node dissection (more than 10 nodes). (d) The rate of complications was inconclusive because the results were not adjusted for adjuvant therapy (radiotherapy). (e) Most women were low risk (49% in control and 42% in lymphadenectomy arm) and would not have benefited from lymphadenectomy or radiation. (f) The rate of node positivity was low, i.e. 3.1% in a lymphadenectomy arm, low node positivity will lead to the difficulty to detect any survival difference.

Seamon and Fowler commented that both Pacini and MRC ASTEC trials were not powered to solve the most important clinical question, i.e. do intermediate/high-risk patients benefit from lymphadenectomy. They suggested that the trial should enrol patients with preoperative endometrioid histology to an intraoperative assessment for intermediate high-risk features, randomize only these patients to aortic and pelvic lymphadenectomy or no lymphadenectomy. Following surgery, adjuvant therapy would be standardized, regardless of lymph node status to allow assessment of true independent "therapeutic" effects of lymphadenectomy.

At present, the accuracy of preoperative and intraoperative prediction of staging, tumour grade and myoinvasion is still inaccurate to triage patient for lymphadenectomy. There is an also poor correlation between intraoperative frozen section and final histological diagnosis. Furthermore, complete surgical staging for grade 1 patients was found to alter management postoperatively in 30% of cases (Ben-Shachar et al., 2005). Based on these reasons, complete surgical staging including systematic lympha-denectomy is still being practice and become a standard surgical treatment for endometrial cancer in many Gynaecology Oncology Centers.

Patients with gross cervical involvement (stage 2) required radical hysterectomy, pelvic and para-aortic lymphadenectomy followed by adjuvant radiotherapy (brachytherapy or external beam radiotherapy based on pathologic results). While, a patient with advanced endometrial cancer is treated with exploratory laparotomy and debulking surgery followed with postoperative chemotherapy or combination of chemotherapy and radiation therapy.

Type II endometrial cancer such as serous carcinoma is an aggressive tumour and has a similar pattern of spread to ovarian carcinoma. Type II endometrial cancer also has a greater tendency for the lymphatic spread. Therefore, women with such a tumour need the same surgical management as those with ovarian cancer such as midline abdominal incision, peritoneal biopsies, total hysterectomy bilateral salpingoophorectomy, omentectomy and lymphadenectomy. The other alternative is to offer neoadjuvant chemotherapy followed by interval cytoreduction.

Pelvic and para-aortic lymph node metastasis is an important prognostic factor in a patient with endometrial cancer. New FIGO staging 2009 has classified endometrial carcinoma with metastasis to pelvic and para-aortic lymph nodes as stage 3C1 and 3C2, respectively. The National Comprehensive Cancer Network (NCCN) Practice Guideline recommended pelvic and para-aortic lymph node dissection instead of nodal sampling in patients with endometrial cancer. Studies have shown that lymph node size is not a reliable indicator for tumour infiltration in endometrial cancer. Approximately, 40% of enlarged nodes are positive while 37% of lymph nodes measuring ≤ 2 mm in diameter were found out to be positive (Girardi et al., 1993; Mariani et al., 2000). At present, there is no standard method for selecting patients who do not need para-aortic lymph node dissection. Overall frequency of para-aortic lymph node metastasis is 3.4–11.5%. The risk of para-aortic node metastasis in a patient with pelvic node metastasis is approximately 28–66% while in 0.7–2.0% has isolated para-aortic node metastasis without evidence of pelvic node involvement. The 5-year survival rate correlates with nodal involvement; patients with pelvic node metastasis have 5-year survival rates of 60–70% (83–95% without nodal involvement) while only 35% for those with para-aortic metastasis. Karube and colleagues evaluated the role of para-aortic lymphadenectomy in early-stage endometrial cancer and they have recommended this procedure in a patient with ≥ 50% myoinvasion, grade 3 tumour and pelvic node metastasis (mainly obturator and common iliac nodes). In their retrospective cohort analysis (SEPAL study) involving 670 patients with early endometrial cancer treated with complete surgical treatment and systematic lymphadenectomy, Todo et al. found that patients (intermediate and high-risk group) who had systematic pelvic and para-aortic lymphadenectomy have significantly longer overall survival as compared to pelvic lymphadenectomy alone.

The role of sentinel lymph node mapping need further evaluation and it may play an important role in helping the surgeon to decide the extent of surgery, including lymphadenectomy.

Laparoscopic surgery for women with endometrial carcinoma was first reported in 1992 and since then, laparoscopic surgery has gained widespread acceptance in the treatment of early stage of this cancer. Laparoscopy offers less intraoperative blood loss, fewer complications, shorter hospital stays and faster recovery. Furthermore, patients with endometrial cancer were majority postmenopausal, obese and had co-morbidities, hence were classified as high-risk for major surgery. However, concerns have been raised regarding seeding of laparoscopic port sites, tubal spillage or tumour, or vaginal cuff metastases due to uterine manipulation. The results from phase III randomized controlled trial known as GOG LAP2 trial by Walker et al., comparing laparoscopy versus laparotomy in the management of patients with endometrial cancer stage 1-2A was published in *Journal of Clinical Oncology* 2009. Almost 1700 patients were recruited under laparoscopy arm while 920 patients in a laparotomy arm. As compared to laparotomy, laparoscopic surgery was found to reduce the length of hospital stay, similar intraoperative complications, fewer postoperative complications and no difference in overall detection of advanced stage. Laparoscopic surgery was, however, associated with longer operating time, lymphadenectomy was not being able to be performed in higher percentage of women (8% versus 4%) and conversion rate of 25.8% (conversion to laparotomy). Long-term outcome of laparoscopic surgery in terms of late complications, recurrence rate, disease-free survival and overall survival are yet to be determined.

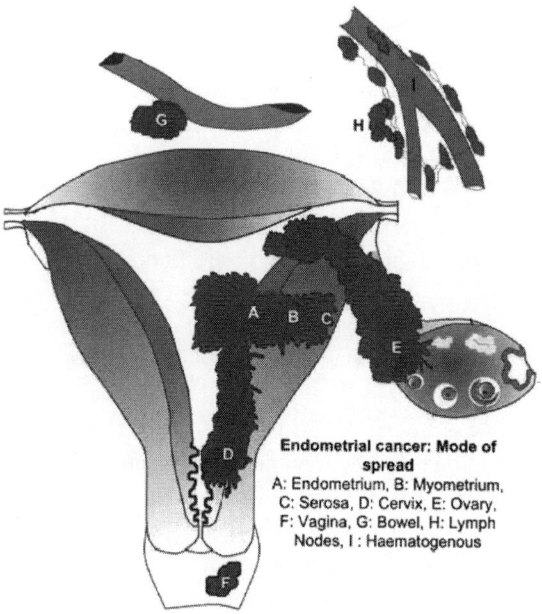

Figure 9.10 Mode of spread in endometrial cancer.

Radiotherapy

The main aim of radiotherapy in the majority of patients with endometrial cancer is as an adjuvant treatment. Primary radiotherapy is applied only in medically inoperable patients. The practice of neoadjuvant radiotherapy had been abandoned because of alteration in surgical staging and no survival benefits as compared to adjuvant radiotherapy.

The role of adjuvant radiotherapy in an early-stage endometrial cancer remains controversial. There are no standard guidelines in terms of indications of adjuvant treatment and type of radiotherapy (external beam or/and brachytherapy) for this group of patients. The aims of adjuvant radiotherapy are to treat the pelvic lymph nodes region and central pelvic region including the upper vagina. The precise benefit of adjuvant radiotherapy in early endometrial cancer is not clear unless prospective randomized control trial is conducted. Adjuvant radiotherapy may add to higher rate of treatment-related complications. The incidence of lymphaedema may approaches from 17–40% when lymphadenectomy and pelvic radiation are combined. External beam radiotherapy is more commonly used as adjuvant treatment in early endometrial cancer. The role of adjuvant radiotherapy in early endometrial cancer has been extensively evaluated in several phase III trials, as shown in Table 9.9. Staging was based on FIGO staging 1988.

Table 9.9 Randomized trials on clinical impact of the pelvic irradiation following surgery for early-stage endometrial cancer (Staging: FIGO 1988).

Authors and study profiles	Stage	Treatment arm	Outcome
Aalders et al., (1980) *N* = 540 No routine lymphadenectomy	Stage 1 Any grade and myoinvasion	Brachytherapy (60 Gy to vaginal mucosa) + Pelvic EBRT (40 Gy to pelvis) Versus Brachytherapy	5-year overall survival: 89% versus 91% Vaginal-pelvic recurrence: 1.9% vs. 6.9% ($p < 0.01$) Distance metastases: 9.9% vs. 5.4%
Creutzeberg et al., (2000) (**PORTEC-1**)[a] *N* = 715 No routine lymphadenectomy	Stage 1CG1, Stage 1BG3, Stage 1 G2 and any myoinvasion, Grade 3 Any histology	Pelvic EBRT (46 Gy to pelvis) versus observation	5 years overall survival: 81% versus 85% (non significant) 5 years risk of vaginal and pelvic recurrence rate: 5% vs. 19% ($p < 0.001$) Treatment-related complications rate more in radiotherapy arm (25% vs. 6%)

(*Continued*)

Table 9.9 *(Continued)*

Authors and study profiles	Stage	Treatment arm	Outcome
Nout RA, Putter H, Jurgenliemk-Schulz M, et al. (2008) (**PORTEC-2** trial) Multicentre phase III trial $N = 427$	Stage 1BG3, IC, any stage 2AG1, 2, 3 with < 50% myoinvasion, age > 60	EBRT (46 Gy in 23 fractions) versus BRT (21 Gy HDR in 3 fractions or 30 Gy LDR)	No significant difference in 5-year overall survival (79.6% in EBRT and 84.8% in BRT, $p = 0.57$) Disease-free survival (78.1% versus 82.7%, $p = 0.74$) 5 years vaginal relapse rate between EBRT and BRT (1.6% versus 1.8%), pelvic recurrence (0.5% vs. 1.5%), locoregional relapse (vaginal or pelvic recurrence, or both) were 2.1% for EBRT and 5.1% in BRT. No difference in rate of distant metastases. Patients with brachytherapy have better quality of life (lower grade 1–2 GIT toxicity 12.6% versus 53.8%).
Keys et al. (2004) **GOG 99** $N = 392$ Selective pelvic and para-aortic lymphadenectomy with the removal of any suspicious nodes	Endo-metrioid histology Stage 1B Stage 1C Stage 2A–2B (occult)	Pelvic EBRT (50.4 Gy to pelvis) versus observation	4 years overall survival: 92% versus 86% (non significant) Recurrence rate lower in radiation arm (3% vs. 12%, $p = 0.007$)

Authors and study profiles	Stage	Treatment arm	Outcome
ASTEC/EN.5[b] N = 905 Lymphadenectomy not required for randomization. Women with positive pelvic nodes were eligible for ASTEC but not for EN.5	Any histology Stage 1A–2A G3 endometrioid Stage 1C and any grade endometrioid Stage 1–2 serous or clear cell	EBRT (40–46 Gy to pelvis) ± Brachytherapy Versus Observation ± Brachytherapy	5 years overall survival: 83.5% versus 83.9% (non-significant)

Source: Adapted from Gadducci A, Greco C. *Critical Rev Oncol/Hematol* 2010, doi: 10.1016/j.critrevonc.2010.03.009.

Note: EBRT: External beam radiotherapy. Intermediate risk (old FIGO stage 1A, 1B G3, 1C G1, 2 and 2A G1, 2). High risk (old FIGO stage 1CG3, 2A G3 and all clear cell, papillary serous histology).

[a]PORTEC: Post-Operative Radiation Therapy in Endometrial Cancer.

[b]ASTEC/EN.5: Intergroup trial (combination of UK MRC ASTEC and National Cancer Institute of Canada (NCIC) Clincal Trial Group or EN.5).

In PORTEC-2 trial, 427 patients with endometrial cancer stage 1CG1-2, 1BG3 and age > 60, stage 2A G1-2 and stage 2AG3 (FIGO staging 1988) were randomized into two groups: (1) postoperative EBRT (46 Gy) and (2) postoperative vaginal brachytherapy (HDR: 21 Gy or LDR: 30 Gy). There was no significant difference in 5-year overall survival rates (79.6% vs. 84.8%,) in both arms. Five-year actuarial rates of pelvic recurrence for brachytherapy and EBRT were 1.8% and 1.6%, respectively (p = 0.3). Patients underwent brachytherapy were found to have a better quality of life (better social functioning, less likely to complaint of diarrhoea, faecal incontinence and bowel symptoms). Intravaginal brachytherapy may be a reasonable alternative to external beam radiotherapy for high-risk early-stage endometrial cancer if appropriate surgical staging (including lymph node assessment) is performed. Patients with nodal metastasis, presence of extensive lymphovascular space invasion and deep myometrial invasion are perhaps better being managed with external beam radiotherapy.

In PORTEC study (Nout et al., 2008), one of the important adverse prognostic factors for recurrent endometrial cancer was advancing age > 60 year old. Lymphovascular space invasion is also an important prognostic factor; Briet and colleagues evaluated the association between LVSI and recurrence rate in the total of 609 patients with stage 1 endometrial cancer. After a median follow-up of 58 months, 39% of patients with LVSI developed recurrence as compared to 19% without LVSI. The presence of LVSI was a significant predictor for both loco-regional and distant recurrence rate. Patients with LVSI were three times (43.8% versus 13.8%) as likely to have pelvic lymph node metastases (Briet et al., 2005).

The intergroup trial (combination of National Cancer Institute of Canada (NCIC) Clincal Trial Group or EN.5 and UK MRC ASTEC trial) evaluated the benefits of adjuvant external pelvic irradiation in patients with intermediate-high-risk endometrial cancer. A total of 905 women were involved and assigned into two groups: (1) surgery alone and (2) surgery + external pelvic irradiation; brachytherapy is allowed in either arm according to the policy of the respective centre. There was no difference in the incidence of distant failure, 5-year overall survivals, 5-year disease specific survivals and 5-year disease-specific recurrence-free survivals between both arms. The ASTEC/EN.5 writing committee concluded that external irradiation could not be recommended as routine adjuvant therapy for women in intermediate and high-risk early-stage endometrial cancer if the aim is to improve the survival. However, radiotherapy may have an effect on local control; and brachytherapy is perhaps a better option due to fewer side effects. Among the limitations of this study are that only 28–30% of patients in both arms underwent lymphadenectomy and 75–80% were an intermediate risk group (only 20–25% was high-risk group). Furthermore, 51% of patients in the control arm received brachytherapy.

The Cochrane database systematic review (Kong et al., 2007) analyzed all the trials related to adjuvant radiotherapy in early endometrial cancers (including most of the above trials) involving a total of 1770 patients. They have reported that external pelvic irradiation following surgery significantly reduced loco-regional recurrence rate, with a relative risk reduction of 72% (95% CI 56–83%, $p < 0.00001$) and absolute risk reduction of 6% (95% CI: 4–8%). However, there was no significant difference in the rate of distant metastases and endometrial cancer-related death. This meta-analysis concluded that external pelvic irradiation reduces the risk of loco-regional recurrence but does not significantly improve the overall survival, especially in stage 1C G1-2 or stage 1B grade 3 (formerly known as an intermediate risk group, in new FIGO staging, this group is now Staged 1B G1-2 and stage 1A G3). Pelvic irradiation appears to give a better clinical outcome in high-risk group (stage 1BG3 new FIGO staging).

Combination of Radiotherapy and Chemotherapy

In the analysis of pattern of recurrences following primary treatment for intermediate and high-risk early-stage endometrial cancer (without adjuvant), distant recurrences was accounted for half of the total recurrences while vaginal recurrences accounts for more than 50% of local recurrences. In order to overcome local and distance failure, the idea of incorporating chemotherapy with radiotherapy has been proposed. The role of this approach had been evaluated in a Radiation Therapy Oncology Group (RTOG) 9708 trial. In this trial, chemotherapy (single agent cisplatin 50 mg/m^2 given on day 1 and 28) was given concurrently with EBRT, and then followed by brachytherapy and four cycles of chemotherapy (paclitaxel/cisplatin). The participants were patients with intermediate-high risk early endometrial cancer who undergone primary surgical treatment. The results were encouraging with no recurrences after follow-up of 72 months. However, grade 3 and 4 toxicity was reported in 21% of cases (Grecen, et al). In a randomized phase III trial by Hogberg and colleagues (NSGO-EC-9501/EORTC 55991), patients who received adjuvant radiotherapy and chemotherapy showed better overall and progression-free survival than patients who underwent adjuvant radiation. In both studies, patients with stage 3 disease were also included and chemotherapy regimen in Hogberg trial was varying (Radiotherapy was given prior to chemotherapy). Further well design study is needed to evaluate the role of chemotherapy in patients with high-risk early disease as well as locally advanced endometrial cancer.

PORTEC-3 International collaboration is an ongoing large international intergroup phase III trial comparing concurrent chemoradiation (cisplatin 50 mg/m^2, two cycles) followed by adjuvant chemotherapy (paclitaxel/carboplatin) versus pelvic radiation (EBRT) alone (48.6 Gy) in high-risk early-stage and advanced-stage endometrial carcinoma (stage 1BG3 and LVSI, Stage

1C or 2AG3, 2B, 3A or 3C, stage 1B, 1C, 2 or 3 serous or clear cell carcinoma). Brachytherapy was given to a patient with cervical invasion. The aim of this trial is to see whether adding chemotherapy during and after radiotherapy has a survival advantage over the current standard treatment of radiotherapy alone.

The results from two randomized trials (NSGO-EC-951/EORTC 55991 and MaNGO ILIADE-III) on sequential combination of chemotherapy and radiotherapy versus RT alone following optimal cytoreductive surgery for stage 1–3 endometrial cancer were pooled and analysed. The authors found that overall survival approached statistical significance (HR 0.69, CI 0.46–1.03; *p* value: 0.07) and cancer specific survival was significantly better in study group (HR 0.55, CI 0.35–0.88; $p = 0.01$) (Hogberg et al., 2010). The sequential treatment in both studies was different (RT followed by chemotherapy in EORTC 55991 and chemotherapy followed by RT in MaNGO ILIADE III).

There are several other ongoing trials evaluating the role of chemotherapy and radiotherapy in early and advanced endometrial cancer. In GOG 249, whole pelvic radiation is compared to a combination of brachytherapy and chemotherapy (paclitaxel/carboplatin) in women with stage 1 to 2A endometrial cancer with intermediate or high risk factors (grade 2, 3, LVSI or outer third myoinvasion). Gynecology Oncology Group 258 trial evaluates carboplatin and paclitaxel given with or without cisplatin-sensitizing radiation therapy in women with stage 3 and 4A disease. Despite encouraging results from combined chemotherapy and radiotherapy approach, many important questions remain and need to be clarified by future studies. The results from GOG 249 and GOG 258 may provide some light on the optimal treatment modalities for endometrial carcinoma.

Pelvic intensify-modulated radiotherapy (IMRT) may one day play an important role in postoperative management of patients with high-risk endometrial cancer. IMRT to the pelvis and para-aortic nodes is feasible and can significantly reduce the incidence of radiation-related toxicities.

Systemic Treatment for Endometrial Cancer

The overall risk of treatment failure in endometrial cancer is 13%, and it is related to staging, histology type, myometrial invasion, tumour grade and lymph node status. Surgery and radiotherapy are used to control the local disease; however, approximately 60% of recurrence involves the distant sites. The most important independent predictor for distant failure is deep myometrial invasion and presence of lymphvascular space invasion.

Martin-Hirsch et al. in their analysis on more than 4000 patients with endometrial cancer treated with postoperative adjuvant progestogen therapy have reported that progestogen therapy did not significantly reduce the risk of recurrence, cancer-related death and did not improve survival. In advanced stage or metastatic disease, response rate to progestogen therapy was between 10% and 25%.

Chemotherapy is currently the first line treatment for advanced and metastatic endometrial cancer. The intention of chemotherapy in metastatic disease is for palliation. In a GOG 122 trial, 396 patients with stage 3–4 endometrioid adenocarcinoma of endometrium who underwent total abdominal hysterectomy were randomly assigned into two groups either whole abdominal radiotherapy (WAR) or chemotherapy (Doxorubicin and Cisplatin, 3-weekly for eight cycles). After a median follow-up of more than 6 years, chemotherapy significantly improved progression-free survival (HR: 0.71, 95% CI 0.55–0.91, $p = 0.007$) and adjusted death hazard ratio compared to radiotherapy (Randall et al., 2006).

The Japanese Gynecologic Oncology Group 2033 has compared whole pelvic irradiation to chemotherapy (cisplatin/doxorubicin/paclitaxel, 4-weekly) in patients with stage 1C –3 disease. Interestingly, 61% of patients were stage 1C. Overall, there was no difference in 5-year progression-free survival and overall survival. In a further analysis of patients with stage 1C, grade 3 and stage 2 with > 50% myoinvasion, both progression-free survival and overall survival were significantly better in the chemotherapy group (Susumu et al., 2008).

Gynecology Oncology Group 184 trial compared a doxorubicin/cisplatin regimen to cisplatin/doxorubicin/paclitaxel (CAP) in stage 3–4 endometrial carcinoma (88% stage 3 and 69% endometrioid histology) following debulking surgery. There was no difference in 3-year recurrence-free survival and overall hazard between both group and CAP regimen was associated with higher rate of toxicity (Homesley et al., 2009). Paclitaxel and carboplatin is less toxic combination and this regimen was evaluated in phase III randomized trial known as GOG 209 (stage 3 and 4 endometrial cancer), the standard regimen was CAP and results from this trial is pending.

Gynecology Oncology Group 163 trial, phase III randomized control trial compared cisplatin/doxorubicin versus doxorubicin/paclitaxel in advanced and recurrent endometrial cancers that were chemotherapy naïve (Fleming et al., 2004). There was no difference in overall response rate (43% versus 40%) and median overall survival. In GOG 177 phase III trial, paclitaxel/cisplatin/doxorubicin was compared to cisplatin/doxorubicin, a triplet was found to be associated with higher rate of toxicity mainly neurotoxicity and gastrointestinal toxicities (Fleming et al., 2004). The role of hormonal therapy in recurrent and metastatic endometrial cancer is discussed in the next section of this chapter.

Uterine Papillary Serous Carcinoma

Most of the studies in endometrial cancer were related to type I cancer and majority were endometrioid adenocarcinoma histotype. Although uterine papillary serous carcinoma (UPSC) represents approximately 10% of all endometrial cancer, its accounts for up to almost 40% of endometrial cancer related death (Fig. 9.11). Women with breast cancer who later develop endometrial cancer were 2.6 times more likely to develop UPSC as compared to endometrioid adenocarcinoma. The molecular genetics profiles of UPSC are different as compared to endometrioid type; UPSC is characterized by frequent p53 gene mutation and HER-2/neu gene amplification. Sherman et al. have proposed endometrial intraepithelial carcinoma (EIC) as the precursor lesions for UPSC. EIC was found in more than 90% of uterus with UPSC. The most common symptom in patients with UPSC is postmenopausal bleeding.

In most patients with UPSC, comprehensive surgical treatment including lymphadenectomy is believed to be beneficial. Because of its aggressive behaviour and pattern of recurrence, treatment of UPSC is often multimodal, incorporating surgery, chemotherapy and radiotherapy. The extent of surgical treatment cannot be based on uterine features such as myometrial invasion, lymphovascular invasion similar to type I cancer because in UPSC, high rate of extra-uterine disease (37–63%) were reported even in patients without myometrial invasion. Apart from pelvic and para-aortic lymphadenectomy, peritoneal biopsies and omentectomy are also advocated due to the tendency for UPSC to spread to peritoneal surfaces similar to ovarian serous carcinoma.

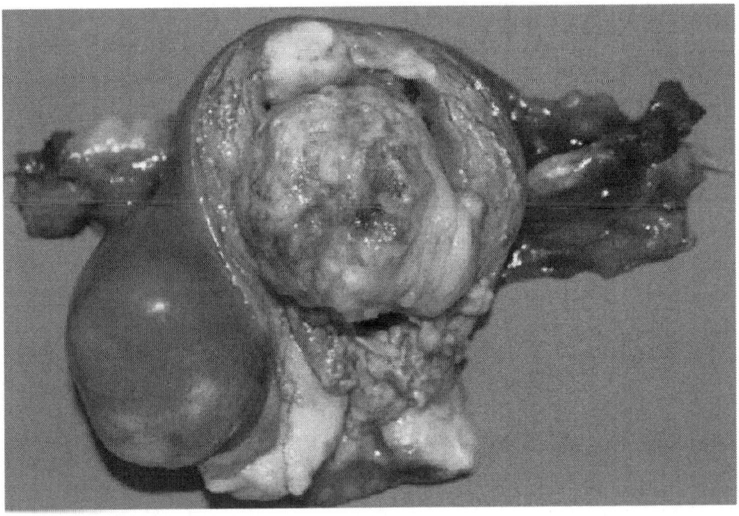

Figure 9.11 Uterine papillary serous carcinoma.

Majority of UPSC patients relapse outside of the pelvis, often in multiple sites. Due to high frequency of distant recurrence in stage 1 UPSC, along with treatment failures within the radiation fields, has led to increasing use of adjuvant chemotherapy. Chemotherapy regimen is a platinum-based regimen most often paclitaxel and carboplatin. Fader et al. demonstrated that while early-stage patients have a significant risk for extra-pelvic recurrence, recurrence and survival outcomes were significantly improved in patients who received platinum/taxane chemotherapy ± radiotherapy compared to women who received no adjuvant therapy or radiotherapy alone. Pelvic recurrence rate was 11.2% in chemotherapy arm as compared to 27% in patients who did not receive chemotherapy. The relative favourable prognosis of women with stage 1A UPSC with no residual uterine disease after comprehensive surgical staging may justify close observation but adjuvant chemotherapy and vaginal brachytherapy should be considered in other stage 1 patients. A society of Gynecologic Oncology (SGO) has published the UPSC management algorithm as shown in Fig. 9.12 (Boruta et al., 2009).

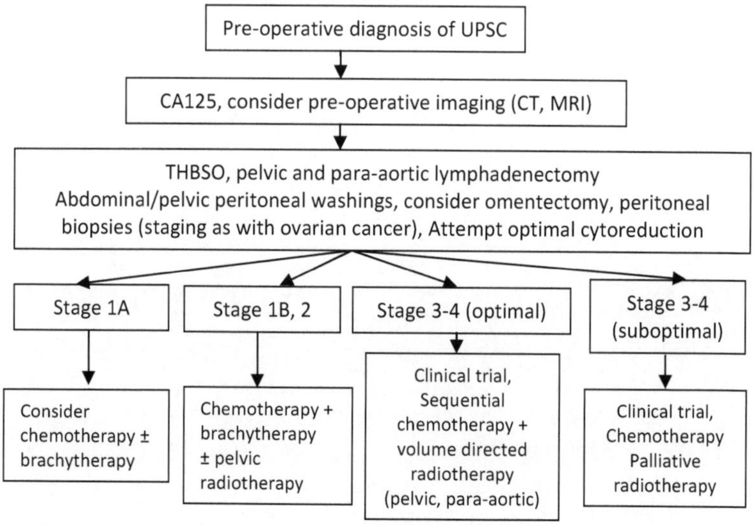

Figure 9.12 Management algorithm of UPSC (SGO).

Epithelial Endometrial Cancer: Prognosis and Recurrent Disease

Majority of patients with endometrial cancer are presented at an early stage. Overall 5-year survival rates in all histotype and grades are approximately 85–95%, 75%, 50% and 20% for surgical stage 1, 2, 3 and 4, respectively. In stage 1 endometrial cancer, 5-year survival depends on tumour grading, i.e. 92% for grade 1, 87% for grade 2 and 74% for grade 3. Serous carcinoma and clear cell carcinoma of the endometrium are an aggressive type and overall 5-year survival rates for both are 46% and 51%, respectively. Patients with more than 50% myoinvasion have 46% risk of recurrence as compared to 8–13% in patients with less than 50% invasion. The summary of 5-year survival rate in stage 1 endometrial cancer is shown in Table 9.10.

Overall, 25–30% of patients with endometrial cancer will develop recurrence and 80% occur during 3 years after treatment. In stage 1 endometrial cancer, patients with low risk factors (stage 1A, G1, G2) have 4% risk of recurrence while in a high-risk group (grade 3, deep myometrial invasion, presence of lymph vascular space invasion) have up to 23% risk of recurrence.

Table 9.10 Five-year survival rates in patients with stage 1 endometrial cancer

Depth of myometrial invasion	FIGO grade		
	1 (%)	2 (%)	3 (%)
No invasion (1A)	96	92	85
<50% invasion	95	90	69
>50% invasion	81	70	42

The risk of lymph node metastasis is 20–50% if the patient has lymphovascular invasion (Cohn et al., 2002); in a study done by Viani et al., lymphovascular invasion was associated with poor overall 5-year survival rates (81.1% versus 52.8%, $p = 0.043$).

Schink et al. evaluated 142 patients with stage 1 endometrial cancer treated with hysterectomy, BSO and lymph node biopsy. Only 4% of patients with tumour size ≤2 cm had lymph node metastasis but increased to 15% if the tumour size >2 cm. Furthermore, 5-year survivals for patients with tumour size ≤2 cm and >2 cm were 98% and 84%, respectively.

Localized pelvic recurrence is amenable to curative treatment either surgery or radiotherapy. Radiotherapy for vault recurrence can be considered for radiotherapy-naïve patients. Isolated small vaginal deposits can be removed surgically. Postradiation pelvic recurrence may be treated with more radical surgery such as pelvic exenteration. Most of the recurrences were associated with symptoms such as vaginal bleeding, pain and weight loss. The prognosis of local recurrences is better especially if it occurs more than 2 years after primary treatment. The most common extrapelvic sites for recurrences are lung, abdomen, para-aortic lymph nodes, brain, bone and liver. In many published data, the proportions of local and distant recurrence were similar. Patients who have surgical treatment alone tend to have a local recurrence while those who have adjuvant radiotherapy tend to have distanced disease.

In some patients with metastatic disease, progestogen therapy may be beneficial especially if the disease-free interval is more than 2 years, well-differentiated and receptor-positive tumour. There was no difference in terms of response rate among various types of progestogens (medroxyprogesterone acetate, megestrol acetate, hydroxy-progesterone caproate). Response rate was in the range of 10–30%. The problem with progestogen therapy is short duration of response; this could be due to down regulation effects of this drug on progesterone receptors. Oestrogenic compounds have been shown to increase progesterone receptors in endometrial cancers and could thus increase the effectiveness of progestational agents. Tamoxifen has oestrogenic properties and this provides the rationale for using this drug in combination with progestogen. GOG 119 trial evaluating medroxyprogesterone acetate (MPA) plus tamoxifen and GOG 153 studied alternating course of MPA and tamoxifen in patients with advanced or recurrent endometrial cancer. These studies have demonstrated the overall response rate of 33% and 27%, respectively. Median overall survival was 13 and 14 months, respectively (Fiorica et al., 2004; Whitney et al., 2004). Decruze and Green extensively evaluated the role of hormonal therapy in their meta-analysis involving 5 randomized trials and 29 phase II trials comprising a total of 2471 patients. The subjects were patients with advanced and recurrent endometrial cancer. They found that for the grade 1 or 2 tumour, the response rate for progestational agents was in the range of 11–56% with progression-free survival of 2.5–14 months. Higher response rate was observed in progesterone receptor-positive cases. They were also concluded that the most appropriate role for hormonal therapy in terms of combined modality with chemotherapy and/or radiotherapy remains unknown.

Targeted Therapy in Endometrial Cancer

Targeted therapy has been studied extensively in solid tumours and it has been approved for use in the treatment of colorectal, lung and breast cancer. Vascular endothelial growth factor (VEGF) is an important regulator of normal and abnormal angiogenesis. VEGF has been shown to be an important prognostic factor for some cancers, including endometrial cancer. There is a relationship between VEGF and steroid receptor in regulating angiogenesis. The presence and quantity of steroid receptors in endometrial cancer have been correlated with tumour grade, FIGO stage and survival. The GOG is currently evaluation the use of bevacizumab in patients with recurrent or persistent endometrial cancer (GOG

229E). Approximately, 10–52% of endometrial cancers are thought to overexpress HER2/neu. In this group of patients, targeting HER2/neu with anti-HER2/neu monoclonal antibody such as trastuzumab may be worthwhile exploring. GOG181B trial is looking into the use of trastuzumab in patients with advanced, recurrent or persistent endometrial cancer.

References

Aalders J, Abeler V, Kolstad P, Onsrud M. Postoperative external irradiation and prognostic parameters in stage I endometrial carcinoma: clinical and histopathologic study of 540 patients. *Obstet Gynecol* 1980; **56**: 419–27.

Amant F, Moerman P, Neven P, et al. Endometrial cancer. *Lancet* 2005; **366**: 491–505.

Anderson GL, Judd HI, Kaunitz AM, et al. Effects of estrogen plus progestin on gynecologic cancers and associated diagnostic procedures: the Women's Health Initiative randomized trial. *JAMA* 2003; **290**: 1739–1748.

Bailey J, Murdoch J. Endometrial cancer. *Curr Obstet Gynaecol* 2004; **14**: 337–342.

Benedetti Panici P, Maneschi F, Cutillo G, et al. Anatomical and pathological study of retroperitoneal nodes in endometrial cancer. *Int J Gynecol Cancer* 1998; **8**: 1837–1842.

Ben-Shachar B, Pavelka J, Cohn DE, et al. Surgical staging for patients presenting with grade 1 endometrial carcinoma. *Obstet Gynecol* 2005; **105**: 487–493.

Beral V on behalf on the Million Women Study Collaborators. Endometrial cancer and hormone-replacement therapy in the Million Women Study. *Lancet* 2005; **365**: 1543–1551.

Blake P, Swart AM, Orton J, et al. Adjuvant external beam radiotherapy in the treatment of endometrial cancer (MRC ASTEC and NCIC CTG EN.5 randomised trials): pooled trial results, systematic review, and meta-analysis. *Lancet* 2009; **373**: 137–146.

Bokhman JV. Two pathogenetic types of endometrial carcinoma. *Gynecol Oncol* 1983; **15**: 10–17.

Boruta II DM, Gehrig PA, Fader AN, et al. Review: management of women with uterine papillary serous cancer: A Society of Gynecologic Oncology (SGO) review. *Gynecol Oncol* 2009; **115**: 142–115.

Briet JM, Hollema H, Reesink N, et al. Lymphvascular space involvement: an independent prognostic factor in endometrial cancer. *Gynecol Oncol* 2005: **96**: 799–804.

Calle EE, Rodriguez C, Walker TK, Thun MJ. Overweight, obesity, and mortality from cancer in a prospectively studied cohort of US adults. *N Engl J Med* 2003; **348**: 1625–1638.

Cirisano Jr FD, Robboy SJ, Dodge RK, et al. Epidemiologic and surgicopathologic findings of papillary serous and clear cell endometrial cancers when compared to endometrioid carcinoma. *Gynecol Oncol* 1999; **74**: 385–394.

Clark TJ, Mann CH, Shah N, et al. Accuracy of outpatient endometrial biopsy in the diagnosis of patients with endometrial carcinoma: a systematic quantitative review. *BJOG* 2002; **109**: 313–321.

Clark TJ, Neelakantan D, Gupta JK. The management of endometrial hyperplasia: an evaluation of current practice. *Eur J Obstet Gynecol Reprod Biol* 2006; **125**(2): 259–264.

Cohn DE, Horowitz NS, Mutch DG, et al. Should the presence of lymphovascular space involvement be used to assign patients to adjuvant therapy following hysterectomy for unstage endometrial cancer? *Gynecol Oncol* 2002; **87**: 243–246.

Creasman WT, Odicino F, Maisonneuve P, et al. Carcinoma of the corpus uteri. *Int J Gynecol Obstet* 2006; **95**(Suppl. 1): S105–S143.

Creutzberg CL, van Putten WL, Koper PC, et al. Surgery and postoperative radiotherapy versus surgery alone for patients with stage-1 endometrial carcinoma: multicentre randomised trial. PORTEC Study Group. Post Operative Radiation Therapy in Endometrial Carcinoma. *Lancet* 2000; **355**: 1404–1411.

Creutzberg CL, van Putten WL, Koper PC, et al. Survival after relapse in patients with endometrial cancer: results from a randomized trial. *Gynecol Oncol* 2003; **89**: 201–209.

Curtis RE, Freedman DM, Sherman ME, Fraumeni JF Jr. Risk of malignantmixed Mullerian tumors after tamoxifen therapy for breast cancer. *J Natl Cancer Inst* 2004; **96**: 70–74.

Daniel AG, Peters III WA. Accuracy of office and operating room curettage in the grading of endometrial carcinoma. *Obstet Gynecol* 1988; **71**: 612–614.

Decruze SB, Green JA. Hormone therapy in advanced and recurrent endometrial cancer: a systematic review. *Int J Gynecol Cancer* 2007; **17**: 964–978.

Deligeoroglou E, Michailidis E, Creatsas G. Oral contraceptives and reproductive system cancer. *Ann N Y Acad Sci* 2003; **997**: 199–208.

Dijkhuizen FP, Mol BW, Brolmann HA, Heintz AP. The accuracy of endometrial sampling in the diagnosis of patients with endometrial carcinoma and hyperplasia: a metaanalysis. *Cancer* 2000; **89**: 1765–1772.

Dizon DS. Review: treatment options for advanced endometrial carcinoma. *Gynecol Oncol* 2010; **117**: 373–381.

Eltabbakh GH, Shamonki J, Mount SL. Surgical stage, final grade and survival of women with endometrial carcinoma whose preoperative endometrial biopsy shows well-differentiated tumors. *Gynecol Oncol* 2005; **99**: 309–312.

Fader AN, Drake RD, O'Malley DM, Gibbons HE, Huh WK, Havrilesky LJ, et al. Platinum/taxane-based chemotherapy with or without radiotherapy favourably impacts survival outcomes in stage I uterine papillary serous carcinoma. *Cancer* 2009; **115**(6): 2119–2127.

Fiegl H, et al., Methylated DNA collected by tampons—a new tool to detect endometrial cancer, *Cancer Epidemiol Biomark Prev* 2004; **13**(5): 882–888.

Fleming GF, Filiaci VL, Bentley RC, Herzog T, Sorosky J, Vaccarello L, et al. Phase III randomized trial of doxorubicin + cisplatin versus doxorubicin + 24-h paclitaxel + filgrastim in endometrial carcinoma: a Gynecologic Oncology Group study. *Ann Oncol* 2004; **15**: 1173–1178.

Fleming GF, Brunetto VL, Cella D, Look KY, Reid GC, Munkarah AR, et al. Phase III trial of doxorubicin plus cisplatin with *or witho*ut paclitaxel plus filgrastim in advanced endometrial carcinoma: a Gynecologic Oncology Group study. *J Clin Oncol* 2004; **22**: 2159–2166.

Fiorica JV, et al., Phase II trial of alternating courses of megestrol acetate and tamoxifen in advanced endometrial carcinoma: a Gynecologic Oncology Group study, *Gynecol Oncol* 2004, **92**(1): 10 14.

Frumovitz M, Singh DK, Meyer L, et al. Predictors of final histology in patients with endometrial cancer. *Gycecol Oncol* 2004; **95**: 463–468.

Fung MF, et al. Prospective longitudinal study of ultrasound screening for endometrial abnormalities in women with breast cancer receiving tamoxifen. *Gynecol Oncol* 2003; **91**(1): 154–159.

Gadducci A, Greco C. The evolving role of adjuvant therapy in endometrial cancer. *Crit Rev Oncol/Hematol* 2010, doi: 10.1016/j.critrevonc.2010.03.009.

Giede KC, Yen TW, Chibbar R, Pierson RA. Significance of concurrent endometrial cancer in women with preoperative diagnosis of atypical endometrial hyperplasia. *J Obstet Gynaecol Can* 2008; **30**: 896–901.

Girardi F, Petru E, Heydarfadai M, et al. Pelvic lymphadenectomy in the surgical treatment of endometrial cancer. *Gynecol Oncol* 1993; **49**: 177–180.

Goodman M, Wilkens LR, Hankin JH, et al. Association of soy and fiber consumption with the risk of endometrial cancer. *Am J Epedemiol* 1997; **146**: 294–306.

GOG 209: a randomized Phase III trial of doxorubicin/cisplatin/paclitaxel and G-CSF versus carboplatin/paclitaxel in patients with stage III & IV or recurrent endometrial cancer.

Gredmark T, Kvint S, Havel G, Mattson LA. Histopathological findings in women with postmenopausal bleeding. *BJOG* 1995; **102**: 133–136.

Greven KM, D'Agostino Jr RB, Lanciano RM, Corn BW. Is there a role for a brachytherapy vaginal cuff boost in the adjuvant management of patients with uterine-confined endometrial cancer? *Int J Radiat Oncol Biol Phys* 1998; **42**: 101–104.

Greven K, Winter K, Underhill K, et al. Final analysis of RTOG 9708: adjuvant postoperative irradiation combined with cisplatin/paclitaxel chemotherapy following surgery for patients with high risk endometrial cancer. *Gynecol Oncol* 2006; **103**(1): 155–159.

Hahn HS, Chun YK, Kwon Y, et al. Concurrent endometrial carcinoma following hysterectomy for atypical endometrial hyperplasia. *Eur J Obst Gynecol* 2010; **150**: 80–83.

Hannemann MH, Alexander HM, Cope NJ, Acheson N, Phillips A. Endometrial hyperplasia: a clinician's review. *Obstet, Gynaecol Reprod Med* 2010; **20**(4): 116–120.

Hecht JL, Ince TA, Baak JK, et al. Prediction of endometrial carcinoma by subjective endometrial intraepithelial neoplasia diagnosis. *Mod Pathol* 2005; **18**: 324–330.

Hogberg T, Rosenberg P, Kristensen G, et al. A randomized phase III study on adjuvant treatment with radiation (RT) ± chemotherapy in early stage high risk endometrial cancer (NSGO-EC-9501/EORTC 55991). *J Clin Oncol* 2007; **25**(18S): Abstract 5503.

Hogberg T, Signorelli M, de Oliveira CF, et al. Sequential adjuvant chemotherapy and radiotherapy in endometrial cancer: results from two randomised trials. *Eur J Cancer* 2010; **46**(13): 2422–2431

Holland C. Endometrial Cancer. *Obstet, Gynaecol Rep Med* 2007; **17**(11): 318–323.

Homesley HD, Filiaci V, Gibbons SK, Long HJ, Cella D, Spirtos NM, et al. A randomized phase III trial in advanced endometrial carcinoma of surgery and volume directed radiation followed by cisplatin and doxorubicin with or without cisplatin: a Gynecologic Oncology Group study. *Gynecol Oncol* 2009; **112**: 543–552.

Horn LC, Meinel A, Handel R, Einenkel J. Histopathology of endometrial hyperplasia and endometrial carcinoma: an update. *Ann Diagn Pathol* 2007; **11**: 297–311.

Horn LC, Schnurrbusch U, Bilek K, et al. Risk of progression in complex and atypical endometrial hyperplasia: clinicopathologic analysis in cases with or without progestogen treatment. *Int J Gynecol Cancer* 2004; **14**(2): 348–353.

Horn Ross PL, John EM, Canchola AJ. Phytoestrogen intake and endometrial cancer risk. *J Natl Cancer Inst* 2003; **95**: 1158–1164.

Hubacher D, Grimes DA. Noncontraceptive health benefits of intrauterine devices: a systematic review. *Obstet Gynecol Surv* 2002; **57**: 120–128.

Inoue Y, Obata K, Abe K, et al. The prognostic significance of vascular invasion by endometrial carcinoma. *Cancer* 1996; **78**: 1447–1451.

Jemal A, Siegel R, Ward E, et al. Cancer statistics 2009. *CA Cancer J Clin* 2009; **59**: 225–249.

Karube Y, Fujimoto T, Takahashi O, et al. Histopathological prognostic factors predicting para-aortic lymph node metastasis in patients with endometrioid uterine cancer. *Gynecol Oncol* 2010; **118**: 151–154.

Keys HM, Roberts JA, Brunetto VL, et al. A phase III trial of surgery with or without adjunctive external pelvic radiation therapy in intermediate risk endometrial adenocarcinoma: a Gynecologic Oncology Group study. *Gynecol Oncol* 2004; **92**: 744–751.

Kjaer SK, Mellemkjaer I, Brinton LA, et al. Tubal sterilization and risk of ovarian, endometrial and cervical cancer: a Danish population based follow up study of more than 65,000 sterilized women. *Int J Epidemiol* 2004; **33**: 596–602.

Kong A, Johnson N, Cornes P, et al. Adjuvant radiotherapy for stage I endometrial cancer. *Cochrane Database Syst Rev* 2007; (2): CD003916.

Larson DM, Johnson KK, Broste SK, et al. Comparison of D&C and office endometrial biopsy in predicting final histopathologic grade in endometrial cancer. *Obstet Gynecol* 1995; **86**: 38–42.

Leitao Jr MM, Kehoe S, Barakat RR, et al. Accuracy of preoperative endometrial sampling diagnosis of FIGO grade 1 endometrial adenocarcinoma. *Gynecol Oncol* 2008; **111**: 244–248.

Maida Y, et al. Is the telomerase assay useful for screening of endometrial lesions? *Int. J. Cancer* 2002; **100**(6): 714–718.

Mao Y, Wan X, Chen Y, Lv W, Xie X. Evaluation of the accuracy of intra-operative gross examination for the surgical management of endometrial cancer. *Eur J O&G Reprod Biol* 2008; **141**: 179–182.

Mariani A, Webb MJ, Galli L, et al. Potential therapeutic role of para-aortic lymphadenectomy in node positive endometrial cancer. *Gynecol Oncol* 2000; **76**: 348–356.

Martin-Hirsch PL, Jarvis G, Kitchener H, Lilford R. Progestagens for endometrial cancer. *Cochrane Database Syst Rev* 2000; (2): CD001040.

McMeekin DA, Lashbrook D, Gold M, et al. Nodal distribution and its significance in FIGO stage IIIc endometrial cancer. *Gynecol Oncol* 2001; **82**: 375–379.

Montejo M, Werner TL, Gaffney D. Current challenges in clinical management of endometrial cancer. *Adv Drug Deliv Rev* 2009; **61**: 883–889.

Mutch DG. Meeting Report: the new FIGO staging system for cancers of the vulva, cervix, endometrium and sarcomas. *Gynecol Oncol* 2009; **115**: 325–328.

Nout RA, Putter H, Jürgenliemk-Schulz IM, et al.Vaginal brachytherapy versus external beam pelvic radiotherapy for high-intermediate risk endometrial cancer: results of the randomized PORTEC-2 trial. *J Clin Oncol* 2008; 20(Suppl. 9): 26 [Absbstr LBA5503].

Nout RA, Putter H, Jürgenliemk-Schulz IM, et al. Quality of life after pelvic radiotherapy or vaginal brachytherapy for endometrial cancer: first results of the randomized PORTEC-2 trial. *J Clin Oncol* 2009; **27**: 3547–3556.

Nout RA, Smit BTHBM, Putter H, et al. Vaginal brachytherapy versus pelvic external beam radiotherapy for patients with endometrial cancer of high-intermediate risk (PORTEC-2): an open-label, non-inferiority, randomized trial. *Lancet* 2010; **375**(9717): 816–823.

Obermair A, Geramou M, Gucer F, et al. Endometrial cancer: accuracy of the finding of a well differentiated tumor at dilatation and curettage compared to the findings at subsequent hysterectomy. *Int J Gynecol Cancer* 1999; **9**: 383–386.

Panici PB, Stefano S, Maneschi F, et al. Systematic pelvic lymphadenectomy versus no lymphadenectomy in early-stage endometrial carcinoma: randomized clinical trial. *J Natl Cancer Inst* 2008; **100**: 1707–1716.

Parslov M, Lidegaard O, Klintorp S, et al. Risk factors among young women with endometrial cancer: a Danish case-control study. *Am J Obstet Gynecol* 2000; **182**: 23–29.

Potischman N, Hoover RN, Brinton LA, et al. Case-control study of endogenous steroid hormones and endometrial cancer. *J Natl Cancer Inst* 1996; **88**: 1127–1135.

Randall ME, Filiaci VL, Muss H, Spirtos NM, Mannel RS, Fowler J, et al. Randomized phase III trial of whole-abdominal irradiation versus doxorubicin and cisplatin chemotherapy in advanced endometrial carcinoma: a Gynecologic Oncology Group study. *J Clin Oncol* 2006; **24**: 36–44.

Rattanachaiyanont M, Angsuwathana S, Techatrisak K, et al. Clinical and pathological responses of progestin therapy for non-atypical endometrial hyperplasia: a prospective study. *J Obstet Gynaecol Res* 2005; **31**: 98–106.

Schink JC, Rademaker AW, Miller DS, Lurain JR. Tumor size in endometrial cancer. *Cancer* 1991; **67**(11): 2791–2794.

Scholten AN, van Putten WL, Beerman H, et al. Postoperative radiotherapy for Stage 1 endometrial carcinoma: long-term outcome of the randomized PORTEC trial with central pathology review. *Int J Radiat Oncol Biol Phys* 2005; **63**: 834–838.

Seamon LG, Fowler JM. Clinical Commentary. Lymphadenectomy for endometrial cancer: The controversy. *Gynecol Oncol* 2010; **117**: 6–8.

Silverberg SG, Mutter GL, Kurman RJ, et al. Tumors of the uterine corpus: epithelial tumors and related lesions. In: Tavassoli FA. Stratton MR, eds. WHO classification of Tumors: Pathology and Genetics of tumors of the breast and female genital organs. Lyon, France: IARC Press, 2003; 221–232.

Smith RA, Cokkinides V, Eyre HJ. Cancer screening in the United States, 2007: a review of current guidelines, practices, and prospects. *CA Cancer J Clin* 2007; **57**(2): 90–104.

Soderini A, Anchezar JP, Sardi JE. Role of adjuvant (RT) in intermediate risk (Ib-G2-3-1c) endometrioid carcinoma after extended staging surgery (ESS). Preliminary reports of a randomized trial. *Int J Gynecol Cancer* 2003; **13**(Suppl. 1) [78 Abstract P0147].

Stovall TG, Photopulos GJ, Poston WM, et al. Pipelle endometrial sampling in patients with known endometrial carcinoma. *Obstet Gynecol*, 1991; **77**(6): 954–6

Susumu N, Sagae S, Udagawa Y, Niwa K, Kuramoto H, Satoh S, et al. Randomized phase III trial of pelvic radiotherapy versus cisplatin-based combined chemotherapy in patients with intermediate- and high-risk endometrial cancer: a Japanese Gynecologic Oncology Group study. *Gynecol Oncol* 2008; **108**: 226–233.

Tabata T, Yamawaki T, Yabana T, et al. Natural history of endometrial hyperplasia. Study of 77 patients. *Arch Gynecol Obstet* 2001; **265**: 85–88.

Terakawa N, Kigawa J, Taketani Y, et al. The behaviour of endometrial hyperplasia: a prospective study. Endometrial Hyperplasia Study Group. *J Obstet Gynaecol Res* 1997; **23**: 223–230.

The Cancer and Steroid Hormone Study of the Centers for Disease Control and the National Institute of Child Health and Human Development. Combination oral contraceptive use and the risk of endometrial cancer. The cancer and Steroid Hormone Study of the Centers for Disease Control and the National Institute of Child Health and Human Developmen. *JAMA* 1987; **257**(6): 796–800.

The writing committee on behalf of the ASTEC study group. Efficacy of systematic pelvic lymphadenectomy in endometrial cancer (MRC ASTEC trial): a randomized study. *Lancet* 2009; **373**: 125–136.

Todo Y, Kato H, Kaneuchi M, et al. Survival effect of para-aortic lymphadenectomy in endometrial cancer (SEPAL study): a retrospective cohort analysis, *Lancet* 2010; **375:** 1165–1172

Trimble CL, Kauderer J, Zaino R, et al. Concurrent endometrial carcinoma in women with a biopsy diagnosis of atypical endometrial hyperplasia: a Gynecologic Oncology Group Study. *Cancer* 2006; **106**: 812–819.

Van Gorp T, Neven P. Endometrial safety of hormone replacement therapy: review of literature. *Maturitas* 2002; **42**: 93–104.

Van Leeuwen FE, Travis LB. Second cancers. In: DeVitaVT Jr, Hellman S, Rosenberg SA, eds. *Cancer Principles and Practice of Oncology*. Philadelphia: LippincottWilliams &Wilkins; 2005. pp. 2575–2602.

Varma R, Soneja H, Bhatia K, et al. The effectiveness of a levonorgestrel-releasing intrauterine system (LNG-IUS) in the treatment of endometrial hyperplasia: a long-term follow-up study. *Eur J Obstet Gynecol Reprod Biol* 2008; **139**: 169–175.

Viani GA, Patia BF, Pellizzon AC, et al. High risk surgical stage 1 endometrial cancer: analysis of treatment outcome. *Radiat Oncol* 2006; **1:** 24, doi: 10.1186/1748-717X-1-24.

Walker JL, Piedmonte MR, Spirtos NM, et al. Laparoscopy compared with laparotomy for comprehensive surgical staging of uterine cancer: Gynecologic Oncology Group Study LAP2. *J Clin Oncol* 2009; **27**(32): 5331–5336.

Whitney CW, et al. Phase II study of medroxyprogesterone acetate plus tamoxifen in advanced endometrial carcinoma: a Gynecologic Oncology Group study. *Gynecol Oncol* 2004; **92**(1): 4–9.

Wickerham DL, Fisher B, Wolmark N, et al. Association of tamoxifen and uterine sarcoma. *J Clin Oncol* 2002; 20: 2758–2760.

Xu WH, Zheng W, Xiang YB, et al. Soya food intake and risk of endometrial cancer among Chinese women in Shanghai: population based case-control study. *BMJ* 2004; 328: 1285 doi: http://dx.doi.org/10.1136/bmj.38093.646215.AE.

Zagouri F, Bozas G, Kafantari E, et al. Endometrial cancer:what is new in adjuvant and molecularly targeted therapy? *Obstet Gynecol Int* 2010; 749:579 doi: 10.1155/2010/749579.

Zeleniuch JA, Akhmedkhanow A, Kato I, et al. Postmenopausal endogenous oestrogens and risk of endometrial cancer: results of a prospective study. *Br J Cancer* 2001; 84: 975–981.

Chapter 10

Uterine Sarcoma

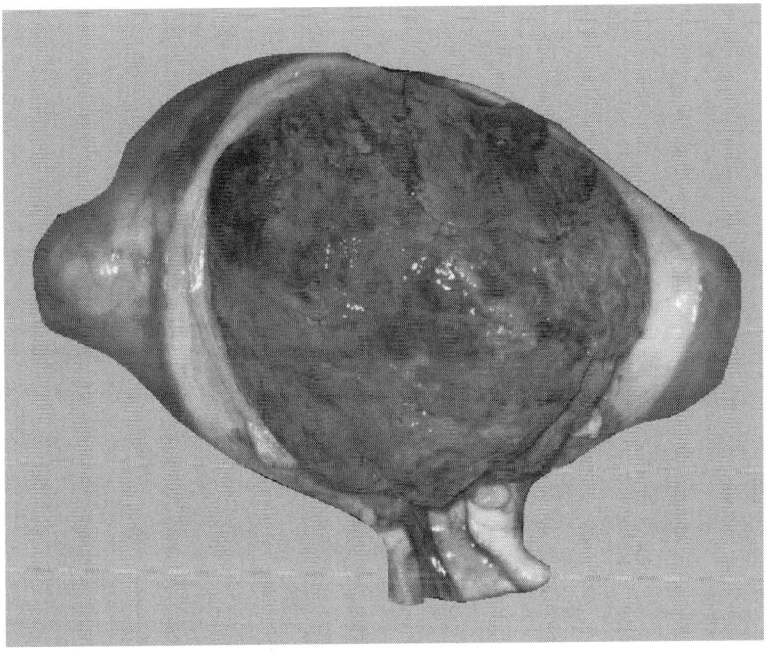

Gynaecologic Cancer: A Handbook for Students and Practitioners
Rushdan Noor, Eng Hseon Tay, and Jeffrey Low

ISBN 978-981-4463-06-5 (Hardcover), 978-981-4463-07-2 (eBook)
www.panstanford.com

Introduction

Uterine sarcomas are rare tumours that account for approximately 1% of female genital tract malignancies and 2–8% of uterine cancers. Despite representing a small proportion of uterine cancers, sarcomas account for a disproportionately high fraction of deaths. Data from a Norwegian cancer registry found that uterine sarcomas are responsible for 26% of mortalities from uterine cancers. The worldwide annual incidence of uterine sarcoma is between 0.5 and 3.3 cases per 100,000 women. According to SEER analysis of 2677 cases of uterine sarcoma in US, the overall age-adjusted incidence for black women was twice that of whites and more than twice that of women of other races. Overall, 45–54% of patients presented with stage 1 disease while overall 5-year survival was 40–50%.

The risk of uterine sarcomas had been linked with the used of oral contraceptive pill (leiomyosarcoma) and non-contraceptive oestrogen (carcinosarcoma). There is also an association of tamoxifen, previous exposure to pelvic irradiation and obesity with higher risk of uterine sarcoma.

Formerly, uterine sarcomas were classified into carcinosarcoma, leiomyosarcoma, endometrial stromal sarcomas (ESS), adenosarcoma and undifferentiated sarcomas. Based on this classification, carcinosarcoma is the most common type accounting for 40% of cases followed by leiomyosarcoma (30–40%), endometrial stromal sarcomas (10–15%) and undifferentiated sarcomas (5–10%). Carcinosarcoma was formerly known as malignant (MMMT). Recently there has been increasing evidence that carcinosarcoma is actually monoclonal as it is derived from a single stem cell. Therefore, this tumour may be better described as carcinomas with sarcomatous metaplasia as the carcinomatous element appears to be the central force while the sarcomatous element is a result of dedifferentiation. Carcinosarcoma should be classified under epithelial endometrial cancer rather than uterine sarcoma.

In the old classification system, endometrial stromal sarcomas were divided into low-grade and high-grade ESS. However, in the current classification, tumours previously termed high-grade ESS are now classified under poorly differentiated or undifferentiated uterine sarcoma. Endometrial stromal sarcomas are now classified as non-invasive (stromal nodules) and invasive (low-grade endometrial stromal sarcomas).

Presentation and Pre-Operative Diagnosis of Uterine Sarcoma

The most common presentations of uterine sarcoma are abnormal vaginal bleeding (80–90%), pelvic mass, mass pervagina and pelvic pain (30%). The triads of carcinosarcoma are painful postmenopausal bleeding, postmenopausal bleeding and prolapsing mass through endocervix.

Patients with uterine leiomyoma with sudden rapid increasing in size (double size within 3–6 months) may suggest sarcomatous transformation. Patients presented with abnormal bleeding need to be evaluated by pelvic examination and ultrasound pelvis. Endometrial sampling either by simple office procedures such as pipelle sampling or through dilation and curettage have high accuracy in the diagnosis of endometrial cancer. However, these diagnostic tests are less accurate in the uterine sarcoma due to the location of this tumour, which is predominantly within the myometrium. Bansal et al., evaluated the role of preoperative endometrial sampling (pipelle and D&C) for the detection of uterine sarcomas and they found that among women with uterine sarcomas, preoperative sampling suggested an invasive tumour in 86% and predicted the correct histologic diagnosis in 64%. The detection rate for sarcomas and endometrial cancer was similar but the prediction of histology was poorer for uterine sarcoma. Both pipelle sampling and curettage have similar accuracy (Bansal et al., 2008).

Imaging techniques such as ultrasound, CT scans and MRI are often performed preoperatively to evaluate the extent of the disease and also as the baseline investigation. The role of PET scans in uterine sarcoma is still being evaluated. In early-stage disease and low-grade sarcoma, sophisticated imaging technique may not be necessary as the risk of metastasis is low, less cost-effective and this preoperative imaging study may change management only in a minority (4–9%) of patients (Nugent et al., 2009; Bansal et al., 2008). CT scan is helpful in diagnosis and assessment of the extent of uterine sarcoma. CT scans with contrast enhancement showed relatively well-defined low-density myometrial mass that often difficult to differentiate with uterine leiomyoma or diffuse enlargement of uterus and several low-attenuation nodules. Among MRI findings suggestive of uterine sarcoma are markedly distended endometrial cavity with peripheral polypoidal masses on sagittal T2-weighted spin-echo image, irregular central non-enhancing necrotic portion, uterine enlargement with irregular central zones of low-intensity, well-marginated hyperintense mass in the left lateral wall of uterus or inhomogeneous contrast enhancement of uterine mass that extends through the myometrium. Imaging studies are also important to determine the extra-uterine spread of the tumour, such as to other pelvic organs, retroperitoneal lymph nodes, solid organs such as liver, bowels, kidney, spleen, lung, bone, and brain.

Staging for Uterine Sarcoma

Formally, staging of uterine sarcoma was according to the 1988 International Federation of Gynaecology and Obstetrics (FIGO) criteria for carcinoma of the corpus uteri. The FIGO Committee on Gynaecologic Oncology recognized that the old classification was no longer sufficient because more information on uterine sarcomas had become available and these malignancies justified independent staging.

According to new FIGO staging, three new classifications have been developed and approved:

(a) staging for leiomyosarcomas
(b) staging for endometrial stromal sarcomas and adenosarcomas
(c) staging for carcinosarcomas (formerly known as malignant mixed mullerian tumours, MMMT)

Carcinosarcoma is staged according to the new classification of endometrial carcinoma. The new FIGO staging 2009 is shown in Table 10.1.

Table 10.1 New FIGO staging 2009 for uterine sarcoma (leiomyosarcomas, endometrial stromal sarcomas, adenosarcomas and carcinosarcoma)

Stage	Definition
Leiomyosarcoma	
1	**Tumour limited to uterus**
1A	Less than or equal to 5 cm
1B	More than 5 cm
2	**Tumour extends to the pelvis**
2A	Adnexal involvement

2B	Tumour extends to extra-uterine pelvic tissue
3	**Tumour invades abdominal tissues (not just protruding into the abdomen)**
3A	One site
3B	>One site
3C	Metastasis to pelvic and/or para-aortic nodes
4A	Tumour invades bladder and/or rectum
4B	Distant metastasis
Endometrial Stromal Sarcomas and adenosarcoma[a]	
1	**Tumour limited to uterus**
1A	Tumour limited to endometrium/endocervix with no myometrial invasion
1B	Less than or equal to half myometrial invasion
1C	More than half myometrial invasion
2	**Tumour extends to the pelvis**
2A	Adnexal involvement
2B	Tumour extends to extra-uterine pelvic tissue
3	**Tumour invades abdominal tissues (not just protruding into the abdomen)**
3A	One site
3B	>One site
3C	Metastasis to pelvic and/or para-aortic lymph nodes
4A	Tumour invades bladder and/rectum
4B	Distant metastasis
Carcinosarcoma should be staged as carcinomas of the endometrium	

[a]Simultaneous tumours of the uterine corpus and ovary/pelvis in association with ovarian/pelvic endometriosis should be classified as independent primary tumours

Reference: FIGO Committee on Gynecologic Oncology: FIGO staging for uterine sarcoma. *Int J Gynecol Obstet* 2009; **104**: 179.

Leiomyosarcoma

Uterine leiomyosarcoma accounts for only 1–2% of uterine malignancies, most common in women older than 40 years old with median age of 54. Leiomyosarcoma represents about 30–40% of uterine sarcoma (if carcinosarcoma is included into the classification) and with exclusion of carcinosarcoma from the category of uterine sarcoma, leiomyosarcoma is the most common uterine sarcomas. The incidence of leiomyosarcoma in patients operated for presumed leiomyoma is approximately 0.1–0.3% and the incidence is higher in older women.

The most common presentation of leiomyosarcoma is abnormal vaginal bleeding (56%), palpable pelvic mass (54%) and pelvic pain (22%). Less often, the presenting signs and symptoms are related to tumour bleeding into the peritoneal cavity and extra-uterine metastasis. Almost 60% of patients with a leiomyosarcoma present with disease limited to the uterus.

The diagnosis of leiomyosarcoma can be difficult as there are many benign leiomyoma variants that mimic malignancy such as mitotically active leiomyoma, cellular leiomyoma, myxoid leiomyoma, leiomyoma with massive lymphoid infiltration, smooth muscle tumours of uncertain malignant potential (STUMP), etc. The typical gross appearance of leiomyosarcoma is a large tumour, poorly circumscribed mass with a soft, fleshy consistency and a variegated cut surface that is grey-yellow to pink, with foci of haemorrhage and necrosis.

Smooth muscle tumours of uncertain malignant potential is a benign tumour but frequently misdiagnosed as low-grade leiomyosarcoma. Recently, the WHO has suggested the following pathologic criteria for the diagnosis of STUMP:

(a) tumour cell necrosis in a typical leiomyoma
(b) necrosis of uncertain type with ≥10 mitotic features per 10 high power field
(c) marked diffuse or focal atypia with borderline mitotic counts
(d) necrosis which difficult to classify

The main histological criteria for the diagnosis of uterine leiomyosarcoma are

(a) presence of cytologic atypia
(b) high mitotic index (exceeding 10 mitotic figures per 10 high-power-field)
(c) coagulative tumour cell necrosis

O'Connor and Norris proposed diagnosis of leiomyosarcoma when a mitotic count >10/HPF plus any grade of atypia or if mitotic count 5–9/HPF plus grade 2 and 3 atypia. Hendrickson and Kempson add criteria of coagulative necrosis and/or atypia to diagnose sarcoma (mitotic count >10/HPF). Mitotic count of <10/HPF must have both diffuse atypia and coagulative necrosis to be categorized as leiomyosarcoma. In the GOG study on prognostic factors in an early-stage uterine sarcomas, mitotic count was found to be independent prognostic variable to progression-free survival and overall survival (Major et al., 1993; Gadducci et al., 2008).

Immunohistochemistry studies in leiomyosarcoma usually express smooth muscle markers such as desmin, h-caldesmon, smooth muscle actin and histone deacetylase 8 (HDCA8). Leiomyosarcomas are also often positive for CD10 and epithelial markers such as keratin and EMA. Oestrogen and progesterone receptors are positive in 26–87% and 17–80%, respectively. Recent studies have shown that uterine leiomyosarcoma has significantly higher levels of Ki67, overexpression and mutation of p16 and p53 (26–71%) as compared to benign leiomyoma including STUMP.

In comparison to other uterine cancers, leiomyosarcoma has some resemblance to type 2 endometrial cancers such as genetic instability, frequent p53 mutations, aggressive behaviour and resistance to chemotherapy.

Treatment for Uterine Leiomyosarcoma

Uterine leiomyosarcoma is a very aggressive tumour and even when diagnosed at an early stage, the recurrence rate has ranged from 53% to 71%. The overall survival rate ranged from 15% to 25%. Patients with leiomyosarcoma, limited to the uterus, had 5-year survivals of 51% in stage 1 and 25% in stage 2 disease.

Treatment of leiomyosarcomas includes total abdominal hysterectomy. Removal of ovaries is still controversial as metastases to these organs occur in less than 5% of cases. Some advocate bilateral salpingo-ophorectomy in low-grade leiomyosarcoma due to the higher percentage of hormonal receptor positive. Lymph node involvement is also rare (6–11%) in early disease and therefore, lymphadenectomy should not be routine procedures in uterine leiomyosarcoma. Lymph node metastases and ovarian involvement are often associated with more advanced stage. In advanced disease, tumour debulking is also performed to minimize residual disease.

There has been no consistency regarding a correlation between various prognostic factors (age, tumour grade, presence or absence of tumour necrosis, mitotic index and vascular invasion) with the outcome of leiomyosarcomas. In their retrospective review of 208 patients with leiomyosarcomas of the uterus, Giuntoli and colleagues reported that tumour size is one of the most important prognostic factors. None of the patients with tumour size >5 cm survive while the other two important prognostic factors are stage and tumour grade. Similar findings were also reported by Abeler et al.

In contrast to carcinosarcoma and endometrial stromal sarcoma, patients with leiomyosarcoma often have early recurrence of cancer and more frequently spread haematogenously especially to lung. Therefore, postoperative adjuvant radiotherapy alone may not be effective to control the disease without systemic therapy. In one of the largest retrospective analyses involving 3650 patients with uterine sarcoma, 5-year overall survival was 37% and among significant prognostic factors for local-regional failure free survival was stage, grade, histology and adjuvant radiotherapy. In this analysis, adjuvant RT was associated with 53% reduction in loco-regional failure; however, there was no improvement in overall survival (Sampath et al., 2010). Reed NS and colleagues had evaluated (phase III randomized trial) the role of adjuvant pelvic radiotherapy in patients with stage 1 and 2 uterine sarcomas in EORTC-GCG study (European Organisation for Research and Treatment of Cancer Gynaecological Cancer Group Study, protocol 55874). Patients in their study arm were given pelvic irradiation 51 Gy in 28 fractions. Initial analysis had shown that adjuvant radiotherapy reduces the rate of local recurrence but no effect on either overall survival or progression-free survival in patients with carcinosarcoma. However, adjuvant radiotherapy does not have beneficial effect on local control, progression-free survival and overall survival to patients with leiomyosarcoma (Reed et al., 2008).

The role of adjuvant chemotherapy in early stage remains unclear. Despite complete surgical resection, the recurrence rate is still high up to 61% and 80% of recurrence occurs outside the pelvis; the most frequent metastatic sites are lungs, liver and bone. Chemotherapy plays an important role in advanced and recurrent leiomyosarcomas. There are various combined chemotherapy regimens found to be effective in treating leiomyosarcomas such as doxorubicin/cyclophosphamide, doxorubicin/mitomycin/

cisplatin, hydroxyurea/dacarbazine/etoposide and ifosfamide/doxorubicin, while single agent chemotherapy regimens included topotecan, paclitaxel, cisplatin, etoposide and ifosfamide. Combined chemotherapy is better than a single agent in advanced leiomyosarcoma with response rate of 18–30% and 0–17%, respectively. Combination doxorubicin and ifosfamide show a response (partial plus complete) rate of 30%. Docetaxel and gemcitabine combination is increasingly used as the first line regimen for advanced or recurrent disease with response rates ranging from 27% to 36% (Hensley). There was so far no study to compare docetaxel/gemcitabine versus doxorubicin/ifosfamide; however, retrospective comparison shows an at least equivalent response with better toxicity profiles in docetaxel/gemcitabine combination. Similar to first line chemotherapy, second-line using combined regimen was associated with higher response rate than

Table 10.2 New drugs in advanced, persistent and recurrent uterine leiomyosarcoma

Author	Agent	Dose and schedule	Patients	Response rate
Sutton et al., 2005	Liposomal doxorubicin (Doxil)	50 mg/m^2 every 4 weeks	32[a]	5 (16%)
Look et al., 2004	Gemcitabine	1000 mg/m^2 days 1, 8,15 every 4 weeks	42[b]	9 (20%)
Hensley et al., 2009	Gemcitabine and docetaxel	900 mg/m^2 days 1 and 8, 100 mg/m^2 days 8 every 3 weeks	34[b]	18 (53%)
Anderson	Temozolomide	50–75 mg/m^2 daily 6 out of 8 weeks	12[c]	1 (8%)
Anderson	Temozolomide	150–300 mg/m^2 daily for 5 days every 4 weeks	7[c]	1 (14%)

[a]Chemonaive patients.
[b]Most patients had received prior chemotherapy.
[c]All patients had received prior chemotherapy.
References: Gadducci A, Cosio S, Romanini, Genazzani AR. The management of patients with uterine sarcoma: a debate clinical challenge. *Crit Rev Oncol/Hematol* 2008; **65**: 129–142.

a single agent. Combination of gemcitabine plus docetaxel given every 3 weeks was also shown to be effective in a patient with recurrent disease who had received chemotherapy with overall response rate of 53% (see Table 10.2). However, due to small samples and lacking in randomized controlled trials, there is still no universally accepted standard first line chemotherapy regimen for uterine leiomyosarcoma. New drugs tested in advanced and recurrent uterine leiomyosarcomas are shown in Table 10.2 (all phase II trials).

Table 10.3 Recommended postoperative chemotherapy in patients with stage 1–2 uterine sarcoma (Gadducci, et al.)

Histology type	Postoperative therapy
Leiomyosarcoma	Ifosfamide + doxorubicin/epidoxorubicin[a]
Undifferentiated endometrial sarcoma	Ifosfamide ± doxorubicin/epidoxorubicin
Carcinosarcoma	Cisplatin + ifosfamide ± doxorubicin/ epidoxorubicin
Low-grade endometrial stromal sarcoma	Progestin (medroxyprogesterone acetate, megestrol acetate)

Doses: Ifosfamide 3 g/m^2 days 1–3 every 3 weeks.
Doxorubicin 25 mg/m^2 days 1–3 every 3 weeks.
Cisplatin 25 mg/m^2 days 1–3 every 3 weeks.
Epidoxorubicin 25 mg/m^2 (alternative to doxorubicin).
[a]Alternative to ifosfamide/doxorubicin is gemcitabine/docetaxel regimen (gemcitabine: 900 mg/m^2 days 1 and 8, docetaxel 100 mg/m^2 day 8 every 3 weeks).

Endometrial Stromal Sarcoma

Endometrial stromal sarcoma is a rare uterine sarcoma accounting for 0.2–1% of all uterine malignancies. Excluding carcinosarcoma from the category of uterine sarcoma, ESS becomes the second most common uterine sarcoma after leiomyosarcoma. Formerly, ESS was divided into low-grade ESS and high-grade ESS. However, under current classification; ESS is referred to low-grade ESS while high-grade ESS is now classified under poorly differentiated or undifferentiated uterine sarcoma. This is important because the low-grade and high-grade variants have vastly different prognostic factors and therapeutic options. These high-grade tumours show similarity with uterine leiomyosarcoma in terms of clinical presentation, treatment modalities and prognosis.

According to the latest WHO classification, the term endometrial stromal sarcoma is applied to neoplasms typically composed of cells that resemble endometrial stromal cells of proliferative endometrium. In this chapter, ESS is referred to as the tumour that was formerly known as low-grade ESS.

Endometrial stromal sarcomas primarily arise from the endometrial stroma. They can also originate from adenomyosis or possibly from endometriosis. Endometrial stromal sarcomas usually have an indolent clinical course with good prognosis. The 5-year survival rate is 80–100% but recurrence can occur after many years of disease-free interval. In stage 1 disease, 5 years and 10 years actuarial survival rate is 98% and 89%, respectively. Most common sites of recurrence are pelvis and abdomen, and, less frequently, lungs. Approximately, 15–25% of patients will eventually die of the disease. Two important adverse prognostic factors are mitotic index and presence of tumour cell necrosis.

ESS was found to be a hormonally sensitive tumour and immunohistochemical study on paraffin-embedded material found oestrogen and progesterone receptors in 71% and 95%, respectively (Reich, et al.). However, the degree of receptor expression was variable and therefore some suggest that ER and PR status should routinely be quantified in patients with ESS. Hormonal therapy may play a role in the management of ESS but at the same time, oestrogen replacement therapy may also be detrimental to patients previously hysterectomized for ESS. Both oestrogen replacement therapy and tamoxifen are best avoided in a patient with ESS. Receptor status may have an important role in the management and prognosticating uterine sarcoma. Ioffe et al. have reported that 63% of their patients with uterine sarcoma were positive to ER and patients with ER positive demonstrated improved overall survival when compared with ER negative (median OS 36 months vs. 16 months, $p = 0.004$).

The diagnosis of ESS can be challenging especially in younger women, ultrasound features of ESS are hypoechogenic mass with irregular margins originating from the endometrium and Doppler study showed irregular central or circular vascularization. The other feature is a heterogenous pattern of the endometrium with high-intensity and hypoechoic areas scattered in the myometrium.

Typical MRI findings are invasive endometrial mass with extensive myometrial involvement and extension of the tumour along the vessels or ligaments. As compared to endometrial cancer, ESS is more frequently has irregular margin, nodular lesions at margin, intramyometrial nodular extension and multiple nodularity. Imunostaining of ESS showed positive staining for epidermal growth factor receptor (EGFR) in 70% but HER-2 is negative. Patients with ESS may be asymptomatic (25%) but the most common presentations are abnormal vaginal bleeding, pelvic pain and dysmenorrhea. Majority of patients presented at an early stage, while approximately 30% presented with extrapelvic extension most commonly involving the ovaries.

Treatment for Endometrial Stromal Sarcoma

Hysterectomy and salpingo-ophorectomy are the main treatment for a patient with endometrial stromal sarcoma. A thorough peritoneal exploration must be performed to search for any other lesions in the peritoneal cavity. The role of systematic lymphadenectomy is unclear but in a large population based analysis, involving more than 800 patients with all grades of ESS, nodal involvement was found in 6–8.9% of low-grade ESS, in the other recent small series, the rate of nodal involvement was 33–45%; however, lymphadenectomy had no effect on survival (Chan et al., 2008; Riopel et al., 2005; Reich et al., 2005). These findings were supported in a study done by Shah. The role of routine systematic lymphadenectomy is still unclear but lymphadenectomy should be done if the lymph node is enlarged as part of debulking surgery.

Adjuvant treatment in a high-risk patient must be strongly considered although the best adjuvant therapy is yet to be determined. Since this tumour is sensitive to hormones, adjuvant hormonal therapy either with progestogens or aromatase inhibitors is reasonable. The benefits of adjuvant medroxyprogesterone (250 mg daily) or megestrol (160 mg daily) over 2 years have been suggested in small studies. Among side effects of progestogens are weight gain and thrombosis while aromatase inhibitors are associated with osteoporosis, muscle and joint pain. Response rate has been reported to be 76% in 16 studies. Letrozole is the most frequently used aromatase inhibitors and the response rate was 88%, but the number of cases were limited (Amant et al., 2007).

A patient with recurrent ESS can be treated with repeat surgery if feasible. However, in a patient with resistance to hormonal treatment or if the surgery is not feasible, cytotoxic drugs such as ifosfamide and doxorubicin seem to be effective. Radiotherapy is effective in local control of ESS; however, in the majorities of studies conducted, it has no effect on overall survival.

Poorly Differentiated and Undifferentiated Uterine Sarcoma

Undifferentiated uterine sarcomas are very rare and represent less than 5% of all uterine sarcomas. They are characterized by an aggressive clinical behaviour, with a tendency to frequent and early recurrence. The stage and mitotic index are the most important prognostic variables. Treatment of undifferentiated uterine sarcoma is similar to other uterine sarcoma but adjuvant treatment should be given even in an early stage. There is no evidence from the literature that routine lymphadenectomy is necessary, and therefore this surgical procedure is optional. As this tumour is aggressive and has a high tendency of systemic spread, patients with undifferentiated uterine sarcoma often required multimodality treatment, which comprises surgery, chemotherapy and radiotherapy. Chemotherapy needs to be initiated early and hormonal therapy plays no role in undifferentiated uterine sarcoma. Undifferentiated uterine sarcomas have a very poor prognosis and most patients die of disease within 2 years of the diagnosis.

Adenosarcoma

In adenosarcoma, the essential feature is an epithelial lining that is well differentiated (benign) and a malignant mesenchymal component, thereby placing the tumour halfway along the spectrum of mixed mullerian tumours, with adenofibroma at one end and carcinosarcoma at the other. Majority of sarcomatous component in adenosarcoma is endometrial stromal sarcoma (56%). In 90% of sarcomatous component expressed oestrogen or progesterone receptors.

One of the most characteristic features of adenosarcoma is the manner in which the stromal cells concentrate about the glandular components, forming a cuff (periglandular cuffing) or so called "cambium" layer. Adenosarcoma is a slow-growing tumour and occurs mainly in the uterus of postmenopausal women. Adenosarcoma has also been reported in adolescents and young women. Adenosarcoma mostly originates from the endometrium and it can also arise from myometrium and endocervix. Adenosarcomas, in which more than 25% of the tumour is composed of pure sarcoma, are designated as adenosarcoma with sarcomatous overgrowth. This condition is always associated with more advanced disease and presence of deep myometrial invasion. The most common presenting symptom is abnormal vaginal bleeding, abdominal mass and vaginal discharge.

The treatment of choice is total hysterectomy and bilateral salpingo-ophorectomy. The role of adjuvant radiotherapy, chemotherapy or hormonal therapy has not been fully evaluated. Recurrent tumour can occur in up to 20–30% usually local recurrence. The presence of sarcomatous overgrowth and tumour cell necrosis are most important poor prognostic indicators. The majority of women with uterine adenosarcoma present with early stage and have favorable outcome. Five year survival is 79% for stage 1 adenosarcoma as compared to 51% in carcinosarcomas. Survival is only 63–69% for women with tumours invade into the wall of the uterus and less than 50% if the disease spread beyond the uterus. (Arend et al., 2010). There is no standard chemotherapy regimen for adenosarcoma, but some suggested cisplatin-ifosfamide-doxorubicin combination regimen to treat systemic disease. (Roman et al., 1993).

Uterine Carcinosarcoma

Uterine carcinosarcoma is a rare epithelial malignancy. In the United States, the incidence is approximately 7 per 100,000 women over age 35 and comprises only 1.2% of uterine cancers. Uterine carcinosarcoma is the disease of postmenopausal women with median age of 65 years old. However, it has also been reported in younger women less than 40 years old. Formerly, uterine carcinosarcoma was classified under uterine sarcoma, and it was also known as malignant mixed mullerian tumour or mixed mesodermal sarcoma.

Carcinosarcoma is an aggressive cancer and comprises both malignant epithelial and malignant sarcomatous components. The most common epithelial component is serous and endometrioid adenocarcinoma. Two third of epithelial component is serous carcinoma while one third is endometrioid carcinoma, in 80% of these carcinomas were high grade (poorly differentiated or grade 3). The stromal components may be homologous, similar to tissues normally present in the uterus or heterologous resembling tissue foreign to the uterus. Homologous stromal component may be represented by endometrial stromal sarcoma, or fibrosarcoma, whereas the heterologous stromal component may consist of rhabdomyosarcoma, chondrosarcoma, osteosarcoma or liposarcoma. The most common heterologous elements are rhabdomyosarcoma, and the majority are of high-grade tumour. The epithelial component has a dominant role for the biological behaviour of this malignancy. Therefore, uterine carcinosarcoma is now classified as high-grade endometrial carcinoma with metaplastic sarcomatous elements. This explains their clinical behaviour such as a relatively higher incidence of lymph node metastasis and higher sensitivity to cisplatin-based chemotherapy. Although they are more resembling endometrial carcinoma than sarcoma, carcinosarcomas have distinctive clinical and pathological features, which warrant their separation from endometrial carcinomas. Carcinosarcoma has a higher frequency of lymphovascular space invasion, higher vascular endothelial growth factor expression and worse prognosis when compared to high-grade endometrial carcinomas.

Patients with carcinosarcoma often presented with abnormal vaginal bleeding and bulky polypoidal mass protruding out from the endocervix into the vagina. The cut surface of this tumour is usually fleshy and often shows areas of haemorrhage, necrosis and cystic changes (Fig. 10.1). Carcinosarcoma can also arise from the cervix.

Immunohistochemistry study will show expression of cytokeratins, epithelial membrane antigen (EMA), vimentin and p53 for epithelial component. The tumour will also express rhabomyoblastic elements such as desmin and myogenin. They also have positive immunostaining for c-Kit, c-Kit expression was found to be associated with better prognosis. Overexpression of p53 has been reported in 28–68% of uterine carcinosarcoma.

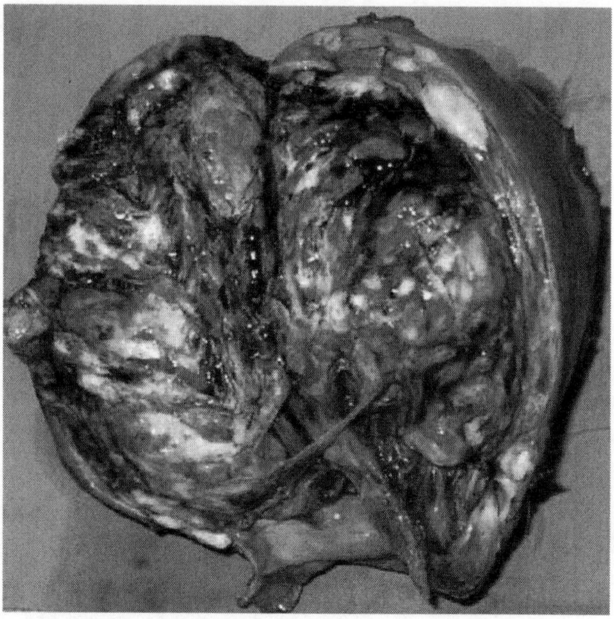

Figure 10.1 Carcinosarcoma.

The overall survival for patients with carcinosarcoma is about 30%. Overall 5-year survival for stage 1 disease is 50% and much lower than stage 1 endometrial cancer (>80%). Surgical stage and deep myometrial invasion are most important prognostic factors. Presence of heterologous elements is also found to be a statistically significant poor prognostic factor.

Treatment of Uterine Carcinosarcoma

Primary treatment for carcinosarcoma is surgery, which comprises exploratory laparotomy, extrafascial hysterectomy, bilateral salpingo-ophorectomy, peritoneal biopsies and pelvic ± para-aortic lymphadenectomy. Omentectomy is also indicated if the disease has spread beyond the uterus. In some institution, omentectomy is performed routinely even in an early stage. In advanced stage, tumour debulking should be done to attempt optimal cytoreduction. Pelvic and para-aortic lymphadenectomy is indicated in carcinosarcoma because the risk of lymph node metastasis is higher in this tumour as compared to other uterine sarcoma. A GOG study by Major reported that lymph node metastasis was observed in 15% of patients with early-stage homologous carcinosarcoma and in 21% of patients with heterologous carcinosarcomas.

Most of the patients with uterine carcinosarcomas required adjuvant therapy chemotherapy, radiotherapy or combination of both. Adjuvant therapy in an early-stage uterine carcinosarcoma is still controversial. Due to rarity of the disease, there was no large phase III randomized control trial to evaluate the role of adjuvant therapy for early-stage uterine carcinosarcoma. Wolfson AH and colleagues have evaluated the role of adjuvant therapy in patients with stage 1–4 uterine carcinosarcoma. Almost half of their patients were stage 1–2 and all patients must have no more than 1 cm residual disease. They compared whole abdominal irradiation (WAI) versus chemotherapy (3 cycles of cisplatin and ifosfamide/ mesna). Chemotherapy was associated with lower recurrence and death rate as compared to WAI although it was not statistically significant. Subsequently, EORTC-GCG (protocol 55874) reported their phase III randomized study evaluating the role of adjuvant pelvic radiotherapy in treatment of stage 1 and 2 uterine sarcomas. The total number of patients recruited were 224 and comprised all those with uterine sarcomas, including carcinosarcoma (91 patients). Adjuvant pelvic irradiation was 51 Gy in 28 fractions over 5 weeks was compared to no adjuvant treatment following total abdominal hysterectomy and bilateral salpingo-ophorectomy (lymphadenectomy was optional). In a subset of patients with carcinosarcoma, adjuvant radiotherapy was able to reduce the risk of local recurrence; however, there was no difference in overall survival and disease-free survival. Prognostic factor analysis shows that stage, age and histological subtype were important predictors of behaviour. In order to clarify the exact role of adjuvant treatment in carcinosarcoma especially in an early stage; further randomized trials are necessary and all patients should have complete surgical staging apart from incorporating systemic therapy (chemotherapy/hormonal/targeted therapy) into the adjuvant regimen. Table 10.4 showed the role of adjuvant pelvic irradiation in stage 1-2 uterine leiomyosarcoma and carcino-sarcoma.

Table 10.4 The role of adjuvant pelvic irradiation in stage 1–2 uterine sarcoma (EORTC-GCG protocol 55874)

Local Relapse Rate			
Local relapse in Carcinosarcoma		**Local relapse in Leiomyosarcoma**	
EBRT	Observation	EBRT	Observation
39%	53%	56%	47%
Median Progression-Free Survival and Overall Survival Following Adjuvant Pelvic Irradiation			
Progression free survival		**Overall survival**	
Carcinosarcoma	Leiomyosarcoma	Carcinosarcoma	Leiomyosarcoma
6.2 years	4.9 years	8.5 years	6.7 years

Reference: Reed NS, Mangioni C, Malmstrom H, et al. *Eur J Cancer* 2008; **44**: 808–818.

Table 10.5 Chemotherapy regimens in advanced, persistent or recurrent uterine carcinosarcoma

Author	Agent	Response rate
Leyvraz S et al., 2006	Doxorubicin/ifosfamide/G-CSF	77%
Sutton G et al., 2000	Cisplatin/ifosfamide	54%
Van Rijswijk REN et al., 2003	Cisplatin/doxorubicin/ifosfamide	54%
Curtin et al., 2001[a]	Paclitaxel	18%
Toyoshima et al., 2004[b]	Paclitaxel and carboplatin[c]	80%
Hoskin PJ et al., 2008	Paclitaxel and carboplatin	60%
Homesley et al., 2005[b]	Ifosfamide and paclitaxel	45%
Miller et al., 2005[a]	Topotecan	10%

[a]Most patients had received prior chemotherapy.
[b]Chemonaive patients.
[c]Small samples (5).
References: (1) Gadducci A, Cosio S, Romanini, Genazzani AR. The management of patients with uterine sarcoma: a debate clinical challenge. *Crit Rev Oncol/Hematol* 2008; **65**: 129–142. (2) Reed NS. The management of uterine sarcomas. *Clin Oncol* 2008; **20**: 470–478.

The most commonly used chemotherapy for uterine carcinosarcoma is cisplatin, doxorubicin and ifosfamide (Table

10.5); however, the role of adjuvant chemotherapy in early-stage carcinosarcoma is still unclear. Single agent cisplatin has response rate of approximately 20% while the combination of cisplatin-based and doxorubicin-based regimens yielded response rates ranging from 56%–75%. New drugs tested in uterine carcinosarcoma include paclitaxel, carboplatin and topotecan. Combination of paclitaxel and carboplatin obtained good response rate (80%); however, the samples were small (see Table 10.5 for details). The other promising combined regimen is paclitaxel and ifosfamide, which were evaluated in phase III GOG trial. In this trial, all patients were chemotherapy naïve and were suffering advanced, persistent or recurrent disease. Ifosfamide alone was compared to ifosfamide and paclitaxel; combined regimen was associated with higher response rate (45% versus 29%, p = 0.02), longer progression-free survival and overall survival (Homeslay HD, et al., 2005).

References

Abeler VM, Royne O, Thoresen S, et al. Uterine sarcomas in Norway. A histopathological and prognostic survey of a total population from 1970 to 2000 including 419 patients. *Histopathology* 2009; **54**: 355–364.

Akhan SE, Yavuz E, Tecer A, et al. The expression of Ki-67, p53, estrogen and progesterone receptors affecting survival in uterine leiomyosarcomas. A clinic-pathologic study. *Gynecol Oncol* 2005; **99**: 36–42.

Amant F, Coosemans A, Debiec-Rychter, Timmerman D, Vergote I. Clinical management of uterine sarcomas. *Lancet Oncol* 2009; **10**: 1188–1198.

Amant F, De Knijf A, Van Calster B, et al. Clinical study investigating the role of lymphadenectomy, surgical castration and adjuvant hormonal treatment in endometrial stromal sarcoma. *Br J Cancer* 2007; 97: 1194–1199.

Arend R, Bagaria M, Lewin SN, et al. Long-term outcome and natural history of uterine adenosarcomas. *Gynecol Oncol* 2010; **119**(2): 305–308.

Bansal N, Herzog TJ, Brunner-Brown A, et al. The utility and cost effectiveness of preoperative computed tomography for patients with uterine malignancies. *Gynecol Oncol* 2008; **111**: 208–212.

Benoit L, Arnould L, Cheynel N, et al. The role of surgery and treatment trends in uterine sarcoma. *EJSO* 2005; **31**: 434–442.

Brooks SE, Zhan M, Cote T, Baquet CR. Surveillance, Epidemiology, and End Results analysis of 2677 cases of uterine sarcoma 1989–1999. *Gynecol Oncol* 2004; **93**: 204–208.

Chen L, Yang B. Immunohistochemical analysis of p16, p53 and Ki-67 expression in uterine smooth muscle tumors. *Int J Gynecol Pathol* 2008; **27**: 326–332.

Chan J, Kawar N, Shin J, et al. Endometrial stromal sarcoma: a population-based study. *Br J Cancer* 2008; **99**: 1210–1215.

Chu MC, Mor G, Lim C, et al. Low-grade endometrial stromal sarcoma: hormonal aspects. *Gynecol Oncol* 2003; **90**: 170–176.

Curtin JP, Blessing JA, Soper JT, DeGeest K. Paclitaxel in the treatment of carcinosarcoma of the uterus: a gynecologic oncology group study. *Gynecol Oncol* 2001; **83**: 268–270.

D'Angelo U, Prat Jaime. Uterine sarcoma: a review. *Gynecol Oncol* 2010; **116**: 131–139.

Favette J, Coquard IR, Alberti L, et al. ET-743: a novel agent with activity in soft-tissue sarcomas. *Curr Opin Oncol* 2006; **18**: 347–353.

Gadducci A, Cosio S, Romanini A, Genazzani AR. The management of patients with uterine sarcoma: a debated clinical challenge. *Crit Rev Oncol Hematol* 2008; **65**: 129–142.

Gadducci A, Cosio S, Romanini A, Genazzani AR. The management of patients with uterine sarcoma: a debated clinical challenge. *Crit Rev Oncol/Hematol* 2008; **65**: 129–142.

Gadducci A, Landoni F, Sartori E, et al. Uterine leiomyosarcoma: analysis of treatment failures and survival. *Gynecol Oncol* 1996; **62**: 25–32.

Giuntoli II RL, Metzinger DS, DiMarco CS, et al. Retrospective review of 208 patients with leiomyosarcoma of the uterus: prognostic indicators, surgical management, and adjuvant therapy. *Gynecol Oncol* 2003; **89**: 460–469.

Hensley ML, Maki R, Venkatraman E, et al. Gemcitabine and docetaxel in patients with unresectable leiomyosarcoma: results of a phase II trial. *J Clin Oncol* 2002; **20**: 2824–2831.

Hensley ML, Blessing JA, Mannel R, et al. Fixed dose rate gemcitabine plus docetaxel as first-line therapy for metastatic uterine leiomyosarcoma: a gynecologic oncologic group phase II trial. *Gynecol Oncol* 2008; **109**: 329–334.

Hensley ML, Ishill N, Soslow R, et al. Adjuvant gemcitabine plus docetaxel for completely resected stage I-IV high grade uterine leiomyosarcoma: results of a prospective study. *Gynecol Oncol* 2009; **112**: 563–567.

Homesley HD, Filiaci V, Markman M, et al. Phase III trial of ifosfamide with or without paclitaxel in advanced uterine carcinosarcoma: a gynecologic oncology study. *Gynecol Oncol* 2005; **98**: 217–221.

Hoskins PJ, Le N, Hyde J, et al. Carboplatin plus paclitaxel for advanced or recurrent uterine malignant mixed mullerian tumors. The British Columbia Cancer Agency experience. *Gynecol Oncol* 2008; **108**(1): 58–62.

Ioffe YJ, Li AJ, Walsh CS, et al. Hormone receptor expression in uterine sarcomas: prognostic and therapeutic roles. *Gynecol Oncol* 2009; **115**: 466–471.

Jeffers MD, Farquharson MA, Richmond JA, McNicol AM. P53 immunoreactivity and mutation of the p53 gene in smooth muscle tumours of the uterine corpus. *J Pathol* 1995; **177**: 65–70.

Kanjeekal S, Chambers A, Kee Fung MF, et al. Review: Systemic therapy for advanced uterine sarcoma: a systematic review of the literature. *Gynecol Oncol* 2005; **97**: 624–637.

Leibsohn S, d'Ablaing G, Mishell DR Jr, Schlaerth JB. Leiomyosarcoma in a series of hysterectomies performed for presumed uterine leiomyomas. *Am J Obstet Gynecol* 1990; **162**: 968–974.

Leyvraz S, Zweifel M, Jundt G, et al. Long-term results of a multicenter SAKK trial on high-dose ifosfamide and doxorubicin in advanced or metastatic gynecologic sarcomas. *Ann Oncol* 2006; **17**: 646–651.

Look KY, Sandler A, Blessing JA, Lucci III JA, Rose PG. Gynecologic Oncology Group Study. Phase II trial of gemcitabine as second-line chemotherapy of uterine leiomyosarcoma. *Gynecol Oncol* 2004; **92**: 644–647.

Major FJ, Blessing JA, Silverberg SG, et al. Prognostic factors in early-stage uterine sarcoma: a gynecologic oncology group study. *Cancer* 1993; **71** (Suppl. 4): 1702–1709.

Miller DS, Blessing JA, Schilder J, et al. Phase II evaluation of topotecan in carcinosarcoma of the uterus: a gynecologic oncology study. *Gynecol Oncol* 2005; **98**: 217–221.

Mittal K, Demopoulos RI. MIB-1 (Ki-67), p53, estrogen receptor, and progesterone receptor expression in uterine smooth muscle tumors. *Hum Pathol* 2001; **31**: 984–987.

Nordal RR, Thoresen SO. Uterine sarcomas in Norway 1956–1992: incidence, survival and mortality. *Eur J Cancer* 1997; **33**(6): 907–911.

Nugent EK, Zighelboim I, Case AS, et al. The value of perioperative imaging in patients with uterine sarcomas. *Gynecol Oncol* 2009; **115**: 37–40.

O'Neill CJ, McBride HA, Connonlly LE, McCluggage WG. Uterine leiomyosarcomas are characterized by high p16, p53 and MIB1 expression in comparison with usual leiomyoma variants and smooth muscle tumours of uncertain malignant potential. *Histopathology* 2007; **50**: 851–858.

Pink D, Lindner T, Mrozek A, et al. Harm or benefit of hormonal treatment in metastatic low grade endometrial stromal sarcoma: single center experience with 10 cases and review of the literature. *Gynecol Oncol* 2006; **101**: 464–469.

Ramondetta L, Bodurka D, Deavers M, Jhingran A. Uterine sarcomas. In *MD Anderson Cancer Care Series, Gynecologic Cancer*, Eifel PJ, Gershenson DM, Kavanagh JJ, Silva EG, eds., Springer, New York; 2006: pp. 125–147.

Reed NS, Mangioni C, Malmstrom H, et al. Phase III randomized study to evaluate the role of adjuvant pelvic radiotherapy in the treatment of uterine sarcomas stages I and II: an European Organisation for Research and Treatment of Cancer Gynaecological Cancer group study (protocol 55874). *Eur J Cancer* 2008; **44**: 808–818.

Reed NS. The management of uterine sarcoma. *Clin Oncol* 2008; **20**: 470–478.

Reich O, Regauer S, Urdl W, et al. Expression of oestrogen and progesterone receptors in low-grade endometrial stromal sarcoma. *Br J Cancer* 2000; **82**: 1030–1034.

Reich O, Winter R, Regauer S. Should lymphadenectomy be performed in patients with endometrial stromal sarcoma? *Gynecol Oncol* 2005; **97**: 982–983.

Riopel J, Plante M, Renaud MC, et al. Lymph node metastases in low-grade endometrial stromal sarcoma. *Gynecol Oncol* 2005; **96**: 402–406.

Roman LD, Mitchell MF, Tornos C, et al. Dedifferentiated extrauterine adenosarcoma responsive to chemotherapy. *Gynecol Onco* 1993; **49**(3): 389–394.

Sampath A, Schultheiss TE, Ryu JK, Wong JYC. The role of adjuvant radiation in uterine sarcomas. *Int J Radiat Oncol Biol-Phys*, 2010; **76**(3): 728–734.

Schwartz SM, et al. Exogenous sex hormone use, correlates of endogenous hormone levels and the incidence of histologic types of sarcoma of the uterus. *Cancer* 1996; **77**: 717–724.

Shah JP, Bryant CS, Kumar S, et al. Lymphadenectomy and ovarian preservation in low grade endometrial stromal sarcoma. *Obstet Gynecol* 2008; **112**: 1102–1108.

Sutton G, Brunetto VL, Kilgore L, et al. A phase III trial of ifosfamide with or without cisplatin in carcinosarcoma of the uterus: a gynecologic oncology group study. *Gynecol Oncol* 2000; **79**: 147–153.

Sutton G, Blessing J, Hanjani P, Kramer P. Gynecologic Oncology Group. Phase II evaluation of liposomal doxorubicin (Doxil) in recurrent or advanced leiomyosarcoma of the uterus: a gynecologic oncology group study. *Gynecol Oncol* 2005; **96**: 749–752.

Toyoshima M, Akahira J, Matsunaga G, et al. Clinical experiences with combination paclitaxel and carboplatin therapy for advanced or recurrent carcinosarcoma of the uterus. *Gynecol Oncol* 2004; **94**: 774–778.

Van der Ven LT, Roholl PJ, Gloudemans T, et al. Expression of insulin-like growth factors (IGFs), their receptors and IGH binding protein-3 in normal, benign and malignant smooth muscle tissues. *Br J Cancer* 1997; **75**: 1631–1640.

Van Rijswijk REN, Vermorken JB, Reed N, et al. Cisplatin, doxorubicin and ifosfamide in carcinosarcoma of the female genital tract. A phase II study of the European Organization for Research and Treatment of Cancer Gynecological Cancer Group (EORTC 55923). *Eur J Cancer* 2003; **39**: 481–487.

Wolfson AH, Brady MF, Rocereto T, et al. A gynecologic oncology Group randomized phase III trial of whole abdominal irradiation (WAI) vs cisplatin-ifosfamide and mesna as post-surgical therapy in stage I-IV carcinosarcoma of the uterus. *Gycecol Oncol* 2007; **107**: 177–185.

Wickerham D, et al. Association of Tamoxifen and uterine sarcoma. *J Clin Oncol* 2002; **20**: 2758–2760.

World Healh Organization classification of tumours. In *Pathology and Genetics of Tumours of the Breast and Female Genital Organs*, Tavassoli FA, Devilee P, eds. IARC Press, Lyon; 2003.

Wysowski D, et al. Uterine sarcoma associated with Tamoxifen use. *N Engl J Med* 2002; **346**: 1832–1833.

Zagouri F, Dimopoulus AM, Fotiou S, Kouloulias V, Papadimitriou CA. Review: treatment of early uterine sarcomas: disentangling adjuvant modalities. *World J Surg Oncol* 2009; **7**: 38, doi: 10.1186/1477-7819-7-8.

Zelmanowicz A, Hildesheim A, Sherman ME. Evidence for a common etiology for endometrial carcinomas and malignant mixed mullerian tumours. *Gynecol Oncol* 1998; **69**: 253–257.

Chapter 11

Cancer of Fallopian Tube

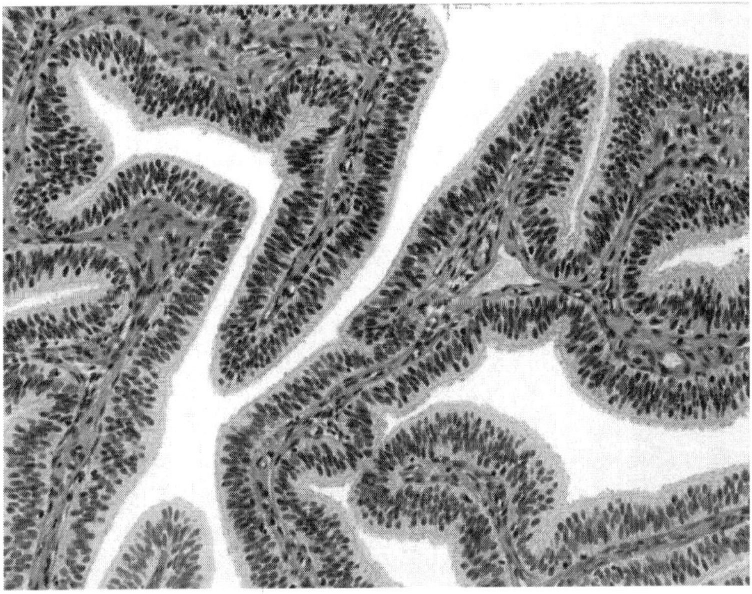

Gynaecologic Cancer: A Handbook for Students and Practitioners
Rushdan Noor, Eng Hseon Tay, and Jeffrey Low

ISBN 978-981-4463-06-5 (Hardcover), 978-981-4463-07-2 (eBook)
www.panstanford.com

Introduction

Fallopian tube is the least common site of malignant neoplasms of female genital tracts. Fallopian tube cancer can be classified into the following:

(a) primary fallopian tube cancer (either arising from tubal mucosa, pre-existing endometriosis or rarely from a mature teratoma)
(b) metastatic fallopian tube cancer from ovary, uterus or peritoneum
(c) synchronous tumour arising simultaneously from uterus, ovary or peritoneum

The most common type of fallopian tube carcinoma is metastatic, e.g. occurs in 50% of carcinoma of the ovary, 12% of uterine cancer and 4% of cervical carcinoma. Primary fallopian tube carcinoma is an uncommon tumour accounting for 0.14%–1.8% of female genital malignancies. Approximately, 1200 cases of primary fallopian tube carcinoma have been reported in the literature. Primary fallopian tube carcinoma is rare: one third presented at stage 1, one third at stage 2 while another one third presented at stage 3 and 4. The theoretical incidence of primary fallopian tube cancer is 3–3.6 per million women per year. Stroma and muscular walls of fallopian tube, uterine corpus and cervix are all formed from the mesenchyme that surrounds the paramesonephric duct. The US incidence rate for primary fallopian tube cancer was 0.41 per 100,000; similar to those reported in Denmark (0.3) and Finland (0.5).

Anatomy

Fallopian tube is a muscular tube average 12 cm length. The diameter of a fallopian tube is 2 mm proximally to 1.5 cm distally and the diameter of lumen is 1–2 mm proximally and 2–4 mm distally which opens into the peritoneal cavity. Ampulla is the widest and longest portion of the fallopian tube. The wall of the fallopian tube comprises the inner mucosa, intermediate muscular (outer longitudinal and inner circular) and serosa at the outer layer. The epithelium lining on the fallopian tube principally consists of 70% ciliated cells (motile) and 30% non-ciliated cells (secretory). Ciliogenesis or formation of the cilia occurs under oestrogen stimulation, most abundant during midcycle. Principal lymphatic drainage of the fallopian tube is via para-aortic lymph nodes. Histologic and physiologic features of fallopian tube cancer are similar to ovarian cancer.

Clinical Presentation

The peak age group is 60–69 years old. Fallopian tube cancer is more common in low parity and in white. Approximately, 47–65% presented at the localized stage (stage I and II).

The classical triad, pathognomonic of tubal carcinoma (but only in 11% of patients) is

- pelvic pain
- pelvic mass
- leukorrhea/vaginal bleeding/vaginal discharge

Syndrome of Hydrop tubae profluens (pain, sudden emptying of distended tube and reduction in size of pelvic mass associated with profuse watery serosanguineous vaginal discharge) is also pathognomonic.

Most common symptoms are abnormal vaginal bleeding (postmenopausal bleeding), pelvic mass and vaginal discharge. Approximately, 12–66% of patients presented with pelvic mass.

Diagnostic Work-Up

The diagnosis of fallopian tube cancer is seldom made preoperatively; most of the times the diagnosis is made on the operating table or in the pathological laboratory The method of staging for fallopian tube cancer is similar to ovarian cancer. FIGO staging for fallopian tube carcinoma is shown in Table 11.1. Pap smear and endometrial sampling have limited role: positive in only 0–18% of tubal carcinoma. Hysteroscopy and hysterosalpingography can be done but non-specific and theoretically can cause intraperitonel seeding if ampulla is patent. Transvaginal ultrasound with colour Dopplers is helpful but operator dependent. CT scan and MRI are superior to ultrasound scan in diagnosis of fallopian tube cancer. The most common radiological presentation is sausage-like cystic lesions with papillary projection or complex adnexal mass. Serum level CA-125 of >65 U/ml has specificity of 98% and sensitivity of 75%; it elevated significantly only in advanced stage. Various studies have linked mutations in the BRCA1 and BRCA2 genes to primary fallopian tube cancer while alteration in p53 may have an association with reduce in a survival rate.

Table 11.1 Staging of fallopian tube carcinoma (FIGO Staging, Singapore, 1991; no changes in new FIGO staging 2009*)

Stage 0	Carcinoma in situ
Stage 1	**Tumour confined to fallopian tube(s)**
1A	Tumour limited to one tube, without serosal invasion
1B	Tumour limited to both tube, without serosal invasion
1C	Tumour in one/two tubes, serosal invasion or/and peritoneal fluid/ascites cytology positive
Stage 2	**Tumour involves one or both tubes with pelvic extension**
2A	Extension and/or metastasis to uterus and/ovaries
2B	Extension to other pelvic structures
2C	Pelvic extension (2A or 2B) with malignant cell in ascites or peritoneal washout
Stage 3	**Tumour involves one or both tubes with peritoneal implants outside the pelvis and/or positive regional lymph nodes.**
3A	Microscopic peritoneal metastasis outside the pelvis
3B	Macroscopic peritoneal metastasis outside the pelvis 2 cm or less in greatest dimension
3C	Peritoneal metastasis more than 2 cm in greatest dimension and/ or positive regional lymph nodes
Stage 4	Distant metastasis (exclude peritoneal metastasis). Parenchymal liver metastases equals stage 4

*According to latest FIGO staging 2009, there are no changes in the staging of ovarian and fallopian tube cancer.

Pathology

Grossly, fallopian tube with cancer is enlarged, deformed with agglutination of the fimbriae end; it contains turbid fluid and friable mass in mucosal surface. Majority of primary fallopian tube cancer is adenocarcinoma (88.3%) and more than 90% of cases are papillary serous adenocarcinoma. The most common side is the ampulla followed by the infundibulum and 10% of fallopian tube cancer arises in fimbrial end. Extension to the ovary will result in tubo-ovarian complex. Fallopian tube cancer is presented more common as unilateral disease and diagnosed slightly more often at localized stage than advanced stage as compared to ovarian carcinoma. Bilaterality has been reported in 10–20% of cases but is more likely to be the metastatic tumour. Frequency of right side malignancy is equal to the left.

The mode of spread of fallopian tube cancer is similar with ovarian cancer, i.e. transperitoneal and lymphatic spread. Lymphatic spread depends on the tumour grade; grade 1 tumour rarely spread to the lymph nodes even in the advanced stage. About 10–30% has pelvic or para-aortic lymph node involvement at diagnosis. Capillary and lymphatic vascular permeation reduced the probability of 5-year survivals from 83% to 29%. Depth of invasion is another important prognostic factor, e.g. intramucosal invasion (91% 5-year survival), invasion of mucosal wall and serosal (25% 5-year survival).

Table 11.2 WHO classification of primary fallopian tube cancer

Serous carcinoma (Papillary serous is most common histotype of all primary carcinoma. Capillary and lymphatic vascular invasion is common)
Mucinous adenocarcinoma
Endometrioid adenocarcinoma (16% from all adenocarcinoma of fallopian tube and carry better prognosis than serous)
Clear cell adenocarcinoma (Rare)
Transitional cell carcinoma (Prognosis better or similar to serous)
Squamous cell carcinoma
Germ cell tumour
Gestational trophoblastic neoplasm
Mixed epithelial and mesenchymal (Poor prognosis, 5-year survival 15% with mean survival 17 months).

Ultrastructural appearance of fallopian tube carcinoma resembles that of ovarian serous papillary carcinoma. Gene's product of HER-2/neu and p53 were identified in 26% and 61%, respectively, similar to ovarian carcinoma. In contrast to ovarian carcinoma, overexpression of above oncogenes does not signify poor prognosis. Low malignant potential of fallopian tube tumour does exist. Table 11.2 shows a WHO classification of fallopian tube cancer.

Four Criteria for Pathologic Diagnosis of Primary Fallopian Tube Carcinoma (Sedlis A, 1961)

(1) The main tumour is in the tube and arises from the endosalpinx.
(2) The pattern histologically reproduces the epithelium of the mucosa and usually shows a papillary pattern.
(3) If the wall is involved, the transition between a benign and malignant tubal epithelium should be demonstrable.
(4) The ovaries and endometrium are either normal or contain lesser tumour than the tubes.

Pre-Invasive Carcinoma of Fallopian Tube

Preinvasive carcinoma of the fallopian tube has not been well described and has been reported rarely. Carcinoma in situ (CIS) is characterized with marked cytologic atypia, multi-layering, pleomorphic nuclei, prominent nucleoli and papillary configuration. Chronic salpingitis, including tuberculous salpingitis, can co-exist with carcinoma of the fallopian tube and granulomatous salpingitis can mimic CIS.

General Management

Surgery

The primary treatment is surgical resection/debulking surgery, similar to ovarian cancer. Surgical therapy should follow similar guidelines as used in ovarian carcinoma. Lymph node dissection (pelvic and para-aortic) is advocated, as the lymph node involvement is early in fallopian tube carcinoma. About 35–50% of a patient with apparent stage 1 disease has extrapelvic lymph node involvement. The amount of residual tumour left behind at primary resection (>1 cm) has major prognosis implications. Total unilateral salpingectomy may be indicated in selected young patients who wanted to preserve their fertility provided the tumour has not invaded beyond the mucosa. Radiation therapy has been used as adjuvant therapy for fallopian tube carcinoma. Second look laparotomy has more roles in fallopian tube carcinoma than in ovarian carcinoma because the negative predictive value of this procedure is higher in fallopian tube cancer. Only 19% of patients with a negative second look will develop recurrence in 4-year follow-up as compared to 50% in ovarian carcinoma.

Chemotherapy in Fallopian Tube Carcinoma

Chemotherapy is a preferred adjuvant therapy for fallopian tube carcinoma. Overall response rate is 81% using a cisplatin-based regimen. The indications for adjuvant therapy and chemotherapy regimen are similar to ovarian carcinoma. cisplatin/adriamycin/cyclophosphamide (PAC) regimen has similar response rate to ovarian carcinoma. Therefore, chemotherapy regimen is similar to ovarian cancer; paclitaxel and carboplatin combination is the first line regimen. Other antineoplastic drugs that show activity against fallopian tube cancer are

(a) doxorubicin
(b) cisplatin/carboplatin
(c) melphalan
(d) cyclophosphamide
(e) paclitaxel

There are no convincing clinical data to support the use progestational agents in the management of fallopian tube carcinoma. The five-year survival rate of primary fallopian tube carcinoma and ovarian carcinoma is shown in Table 11.3.

Table 11.3 Five-year survival for women with fallopian tube carcinoma and ovarian carcinoma

	Fallopian tube carcinoma			5-year survivals of ovarian carcinoma
FIGO stage	**Baekelandt et al. (N = 151)**	**Hentz et al. (N = 118)**	**Kosary and Trimble (N = 334)**	**(N = 9032)**
I	73%	69%	95%	88%
II	37%	58%	75%	65%
III	29%	20%	69%	31%
IV	12%	22%	45%	19%

Adjuvant Radiation Therapy

Radiotherapy has long been used on the ad hoc basis as adjunct therapy in fallopian tube cancer but less often than chemotherapy. Radiotherapy used as single or combination with chemotherapy has been reported. Irradiation technique is similar to ovarian carcinoma (refer to chapter Ovarian carcinoma). Among radiotherapy treatments given to patients with fallopian tube cancer are whole pelvic irradiation, whole abdomino-pelvic and intraperitoneal radioactive colloidal 32P. Irradiation was designed to deliver doses capable of eradiating microscopic residual foci to the original site of tumour and sites of possible occult metastases. The efficacy of whole abdominal irradiation and intraperitoneal 32P is unknown and controversial. The rational approach for occult microscopic disease in stage 1 to 3 with no residual disease is external irradiation to pelvis and para-aortic nodes followed by chemotherapy.

References

Aziz S, Kuperstein G, Rosen B, Cole D, Nedelcu R, McLaughlin J, et al. A genetic epidemiological study of carcinoma of the fallopian tube. *Gynecol Oncol* 2001; **80**: 341–345.

Baekelandt M, Nesbakken AJ, Kristensen GB, et al. Carcinoma of the fallopian tube. *Cancer* 2000; **89**: 2076–84.

Cormio G, Maneo A, Gabriele A, et al. Treatment of fallopian tube carcinoma with cyclophosphamide, adriamycin, and cisplatin. *Am J Clin Oncol* 1997; **20**: 143–145.

Gemignani ML, Hensley ML, Cohen R, et al. Paclitaxel-based chemotherapy in carcinoma of the fallopian tube. *Gynecol Oncol* 2001; **80**: 16–20.

Gungor T, Altundag OB, Ustunyurt E, Mollamahmutoglo L. Paclitaxel and carboplatin therapy in stage I fallopian tube carcinoma. *Int J Gynecol Obstet* 2006; **95**: 163–164.

Heintz APM, Odicino F, Maisonneuve P, et al. Carcinoma of the fallopian tube. *J Epidemiol Biostat* 2001; **6**: 87–103.

Hu CY, Taymor ML, Hertig AT. Primary carcinoma of the fallopian tube. *Am J Obstet Gynecol* 1950; **59**: 58–67.

Kosary K, Trimble EL. Treatment and survival for women with fallopian tube carcinoma: a population-based study. *Gynecol Oncol* 2002; **86:** 190–191.

Levine DA, Argenta PA, Yee CJ, Marshall DS, Olvera N, Bogomolniy F, et al. Fallopian tube and primary peritoneal carcinomas associated with BRCA mutations. *J Clin Oncol* 2003; **21**: 4222–4227.

Longacre TA, Oliva E, Soslow RA. Recommendations for the reporting of fallopian tube neoplasms. *Hum Pathol* 2007; **38**: 1160–1163.e3.

Rajabiani A, Vakili H. Case Report: Fallopian tube carcinoma: a case report and review of literature. *Iranian J Pathol* 2009; **4**(**4**): 190–193.

Rosen AC, Ausch C, Klein M, Graf AH, Metzenbauer M, Philipp K, et al. p53 expression in fallopian tube carcinomas. *Cancer Lett* 2000; **156**: 1–7.

Rosen AC, Klein M, Hafner E, et al. Management and prognosis of primary fallopian tube carcinoma. *Gynecol Obstet Invest* 1999; **47**: 45–51.

Sedlis A. Primary carcinoma of the fallopian tube. *Obstet Gynecol Surv* 1961; **16**: 209–226.

Stewart SL, Wike JM, Foster SL, Michaud F. The incidence of primary fallopian tube cancer in United State. *Gynecol Oncol* 2007; **107**: 392–397.

Zweemer RP, van Diest PJ, Verheijen RH, Ryan A, Gille JJ, Sijmons RH, et al. Molecular evidence linking primary cancer of the fallopian tube to BRCA1 germline mutations. *Gynecol Oncol* 2000; **76**: 45–50.

Chapter 12

Cancer of Ovary (Epithelial Ovarian Cancer)

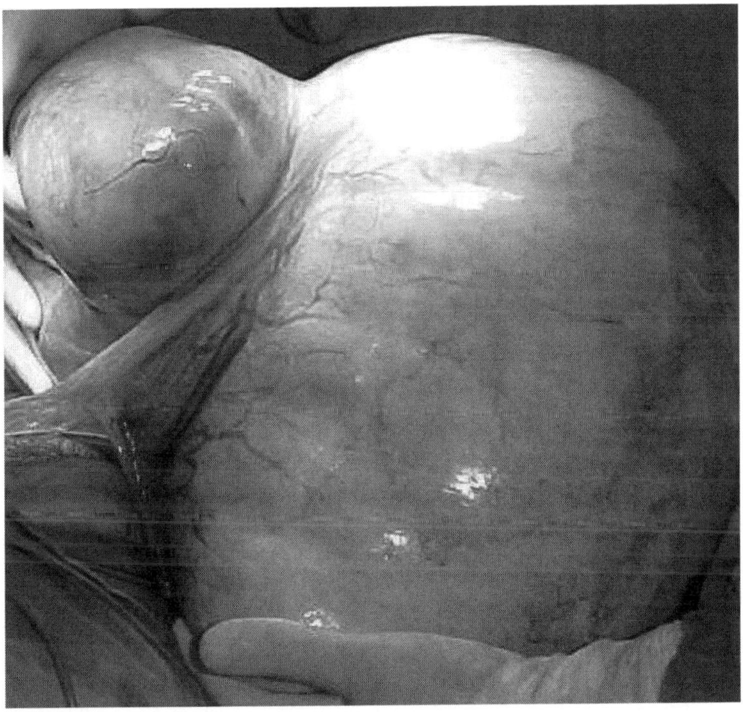

Gynaecologic Cancer: A Handbook for Students and Practitioners
Rushdan Noor, Eng Hseon Tay, and Jeffrey Low

ISBN 978-981-4463-06-5 (Hardcover), 978-981-4463-07-2 (eBook)
www.panstanford.com

Introduction

More than 220,000 women are estimated to develop ovarian cancer every year from around the world and about 140,000 died from this disease in 2008. Epithelial ovarian cancer results from malignant transformation of the ovarian surface epithelium that is in a continuum with peritoneum. Epithelial ovarian carcinoma is the leading cause of death from gynaecologic cancer in the United States. In the United States, cancer of ovary causes more mortality among women each year than all other gynaecologic malignancies combined. Estimated 21,650 new cases of ovarian cancer were diagnosed in the United States in 2008, and about 15,520 women will die to the disease and the lifetime risk of epithelial ovarian cancer is 1 in 70 women. Based on data from the American Cancer Society, the mortality rate of ovarian cancer has reduced significantly compared to the past few decades. Five-year survival rates have increased from 36% in the mid-1970s to 53% in the mid-1990s. Evidence suggests that the incidence of epithelial ovarian cancer in developed countries has been falling in all age groups since 1985. This may be attributed to widespread use of oral contraceptive pills (OCPs) and reduced fecundity.

Anatomy of Ovary

Ovary in females is homologous with testes in males. A normal ovary is pinkish grey or white in colour with smooth surface. The size of a normal ovary is 3–4 cm in length, 2 cm in width, 8–10 mm thick and weigh from 2 to 3.5 gm. Ovary lies in a shallow depression known as the ovarian fossa. Ovarian fossa is bounded above by the external iliac vessels, in front by the obliterated umbilical artery, and behind by the ureter. The surface of the ovary is covered by a layer of columnar cells, which constitutes the germinal epithelium of Waldeyer. The ovary consists of a number of vesicular ovarian follicles imbedded in the meshes of a stroma. The cross section of an ovary shows numerous round transparent vesicles of various sizes; they are the follicles containing the ova (Figure 12.1). Immediately, beneath the superficial covering is a layer of stroma, in which are a large number of minute vesicles, of uniform size, about 0.25 mm in diameter. These are the follicles in their earliest condition, and the layer where they are found has been termed the cortical layer. Medullary layer is the central portion of the ovary, which is highly vascular and continuous with the hilum through which the blood vessels enter and contain no follicles. Arterial supply of the ovary is from ovarian and uterine vessels; the right ovarian artery arises from the aorta while the left ovarian artery is from the left renal artery. The veins emerge from the hilum in the form of a plexus, the pampiniform plexus; the ovarian vein is formed from this plexus and leaves the pelvis in company with the artery. The nerve supply of ovaries is derived from the hypogastric or pelvic plexus, and from the ovarian plexus.

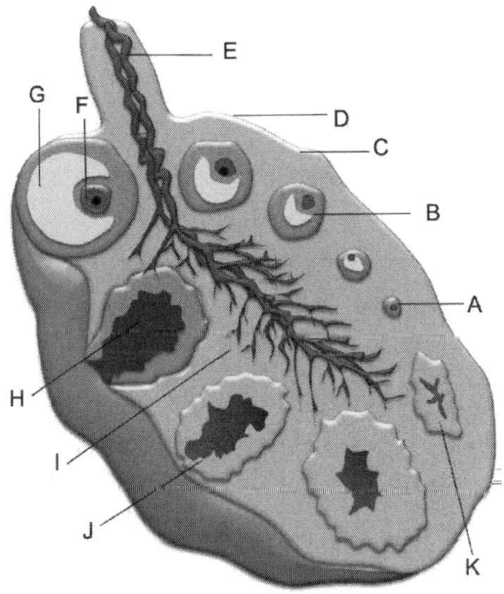

Figure 12.1 Anatomy of ovary. A: primary follicle, B: maturing follicle, C: tunica albugina, D: germinal epithelium, E: ovarian vein and artery, F: oocyte, G: mature Graafian follicle, H: empty follicle after ovulation, I: medulla of the ovary, J: corpus luteum, K: corpus albican.

Epidemiology

Incidence and Mortality

Epithelial ovarian cancer is infrequent in women younger than 40 years. The peak rate is at 70–74-year age group with the incidence of 57/100,000 population. Median age at diagnosis is 63 years old, and 48% of patients are >65 years old. Ovarian cancer among the older age group carries a poorer prognosis than in a younger age group. Incidence of epithelial ovarian cancer is highest in Europe, the United States and Israel and lowest in Japan (3/100,000) and developing countries. There was a total of 225,000 new cases of ovarian cancer reported worldwide in 2008, which is 3.7% of all women cancer and 140,000 deaths have been reported on the same year (4.2% of all cancer deaths in women). The cumulative risk of developing ovarian cancer is 0.7 (0.7 per 100 lifetime risk) (GLOBOCAN 2008). The incidence rates are higher in developed regions (overall ASR of 9.4 per 100,000 compared to 5.0 per 100,000 in less developed regions) and 100,254 new cases (45% from total cases worldwide) of ovarian cancer were reported in more developed regions in 2008. Highest risk of ovarian cancer among Jewish (17.2/100,000) probably related to high frequency of BRCA1 and BRCA2 mutation.

Aetiology

The risks factors for epithelial ovarian cancer can be classified into three broad categories: (a) reproductive factors, (b) genetic factors and (c) environmental factors.

Reproductive Factors

In general population, the birth of one live child reduces the risk of ovarian cancer, e.g., after their first pregnancy; women have a risk of 45% lower as compared to nulliparous women. Every further pregnancy reduces the risk by another 15%. Parous women have 30–60% less risk compared to nulliparous. Breastfeeding reduced the risk of epithelial ovarian cancer (OR 0.81, 95% CI 0.68–0.95) and tubal ligation is also associated with lower risk of ovarian cancer. In contrast, ovulation induction agent such as clomiphene increased the risk by two to three times if taken for >12 ovulatory cycles, although it is difficult to separate the increased risk related to the infertility itself from the risk carried by use of this agent. Oral contraceptive pills reduce the risk by 30–60% (RR 0.75). It is estimated that the routine use of oral contraceptives may prevent nearly 2000 cases of ovarian cancer yearly in United States. An analysis of 12 case-control studies done by Whittemore involving 2197 patients with ovarian cancer compared with 8893 control women, the protective effect of OCP was observed with an odd ratio of 0.66–0.7. The protective effect of oral contraceptives also applies to women carrying BRCA mutations. The factors that increase the risk of epithelial ovarian cancer are history of breast cancer increases the risk of ovarian cancer, early menarche and late menopause.

The association of hormone replacement therapy with the risk of epithelial ovarian cancer has been evaluated in many studies. Following are some of the results:

(a) Metanalysis by Garg et al. shows HRT used slightly increased risk of ovarian cancer (RR 1.15; CI 1.05–1.27).
(b) The Women's Health Initiative Trial, a randomized study of 16,608 postmenopausal women, also found an increased risk of ovarian cancer in women taking HRT with an OR of 1.58 (95% CI 0.77–3.24).
(c) Morch et al. conducted a prospective cohort study over 10 years (follow-up of almost 1 million women) and found that current users of hormone replacement therapy had incidence rate ratios for all ovarian cancers of 1.38 compared to women who never took hormone therapy. Incidence rate between current users and never-users of hormone was 0.52 and 0.4 per 1000 years, respectively.

Genetic Factors

The lifetime risk of ovarian cancer in the general population is 1.6%. The risk increases to 4% in women with a first-degree relative with ovarian cancer and 7% when two first-degree relatives are affected. About 5–10% of all epithelial ovarian cancer results from hereditary predisposition. Women under 40 years of age with a history of breast cancer have seven-fold increase in risk of future ovarian cancer if they have a first-degree relative with a history of breast, ovarian or both cancers.

The frequency of BRCA1 mutation in general population is estimated at approximately 1 in 800. Cancer associated with BRCA1 mutation has better prognosis and commonly serous cystadenocarcinoma. Oral contraceptive pills reduce the risk of ovarian cancer in patients with BRCA1 and 2 mutation (60% reduction).

Studies have shown that 62% of patients with epithelial ovarian cancer have a mutation of p53, and P53 expression was associated with decreased survival. Epithelial ovarian cancer has also been associated with an abnormality of oncogene c-myc (overexpression in 30% of cases), H-ras and Ki-ras. Ras protein is expressed in 40% of cases.

NIH consensus development panel suggested prophylactic oophorectomy in women older than 35 years with hereditary ovarian ovarian cancer syndrome or if they had completed their family.

Environmental Factors

The incidence of ovarian cancer is highest in industrialized countries (except Japan) and is lowest in underdeveloped and developing countries. High intake of meat and animal fat diet has been attributed to higher risk of ovarian cancer, while low-fat diet may reduce the risk of ovarian cancer in postmenopausal women. Hence, obesity has been attributed to higher risk of ovarian cancer. A population with high dietary intake of lactose but with lack of enzyme galactose-1-phosphate urinyltransferase was found to have an increased risk of ovarian cancer. Exposure to talc (hydrous magnesium trisilicate) used as dusting powder on diaphragms and sanitary napkins have been reported in some studies to increase the risk of ovarian cancer, although other studies have failed to find an association. There was no association between exposure to ionizing radiation and the risk of ovarian cancer.

Hereditary Ovarian Cancer Syndromes

There are three clinically distinctive type of hereditary ovarian cancer syndromes:

(a) Site-specific ovarian cancer
(b) Hereditary breast-ovarian cancer
(c) Hereditary non-polyposis colorectal syndrome
(d) Other hereditary syndromes

Site-Specific Ovarian Cancer

Site-specific ovarian cancer is recognized in families in which two or more first- and second-degree relatives are affected by epithelial ovarian cancer. The lifetime risk for ovarian cancer is about 4–5% (three-fold higher than general population). Some hypothesized that this disease could represent a variant of hereditary breast ovarian cancer syndrome. Site-specific ovarian syndrome is also known as familial ovarian cancer syndrome and there is no susceptibility gene has been identified.

Hereditary Breast-Ovarian Cancer

Hereditary breast-ovarian cancer (HBOC) syndrome constitutes 85–90% of all hereditary ovarian cancer syndromes. Women with HBOC have family history of both ovarian and breast cancer. Some individuals may even have family history of male breast cancer. The most common histologic type of ovarian cancer in patients with HBOC is serous adenocarcinoma. Hereditary breast-ovarian cancer is associated with mutation of tumour suppressor gene BRCA1 and BRCA2, and 75% of patients are associated with mutation of BRCA1. Both BRCA1 and BRCA2 genes are autosomal dominant with high penetrance. The lifetime risk for ovarian cancer is 40–50% in women with mutation of BRCA1 and 20–30% with mutation of BRCA2. They are also at increased risk (6–14%) of developing other types of cancer such as colon, prostate for man and pancreas. The remaining 10–15% of inherited ovarian cancer is related to Hereditary Non-polyposis Colorectal Syndrome (HNPCC).

Hereditary Non-Polyposis Colorectal Syndrome

Hereditary non-polyposis colorectal syndrome or HNPCC was formerly known as Lynch II syndrome. A patient with HNPCC has three-fold higher risk of ovarian carcinoma as compared to general population. Hereditary non-polyposis colorectal syndrome is an autosomal dominant condition and is cause by mismatch repair of MMR genes (hMLH1, hMSH2). A woman with MMR genes mutations has 9–12% risk of ovarian cancer (hMSH2 is more important). This gene is responsible for DNA repair. Ovarian cancer occurs in 5–10% of HNPCC with one of three germ line mutations (hMSH1, hMLH2 and pPMS2). Among HNPCC families, germ line mutations in hMSH2 and hMLH1 genes are found in more than 70% of the mutation carriers. The lifetime risk of ovarian cancer in HNPCC carrier is 12% and ovarian cancer in HNPCC is of epithelial type, often presented at a younger age, early stage and carry better prognosis as compared to sporadic type of ovarian cancer. BRCA mutation is associated mainly with serous histotype but MMR genes mutations in HNPCC have been found in various ovarian cancer histotypes. Synchronous endometrial cancer was reported in 21.5% of cases and patients with HNPCC are also at increased risk of cancer of endometrium, urogenital, pancreas and biliary tract.

Other Hereditary Syndromes Predisposing to Ovarian Cancer

An increase risk of ovarian cancer is also associated with several hereditary syndromes such as Gorlin's syndrome, Peutz–Jeghers syndrome, osteochondromatosis and Ollier's syndrome.

Somatic Mutation in Sporadic Ovarian Cancer

In approximately 10% of epithelial ovarian cancer, the mutation involved the DNA of somatic cells. Mutation of p53 tumour suppressor genes had been discovered in 40–60% of ovarian cancer and most commonly in serous histotype. About 50–80% of the tumour with high grade characteristic display mutation of p53. The other gene mutations identified were PTEN, CDKN2A, RAS/RAF, ERRB2, CMYC, HER2, HLA-G and MMR. Mutation of HLA-G and HER2 are also associated with high grade tumour. Whereas, mutation of RAS/RAF is associated with low grade or borderline tumour.

Mechanisms of Ovarian Carcinogenesis

The actual mechanism of ovarian carcinogenesis is unknown; however, several hypotheses have been proposed:

(a) **Incessant ovulation hypothesis**: Cancer developed from an aberrant repair process of the surface epithelium after frequent ovulation. Repeated ovulation also stimulates the formation of an invagination and inclusion cysts.

(b) **Gonadotropin theory:** Excessive LH/FSH secretion stimulates surface epithelium of the inclusion cyst in the ovary to undergo proliferation and malignant transformation.

(c) **Inflammation** and changes in redox potential in the setting of ovulation and surface epithelial repair may also involve in ovarian carcinogenesis. This may also be attributed to increased risk of ovarian cancer in talc and asbestos exposure, endometriosis and pelvic inflammatory disease.

(d) **Hormonal stimulation**: High concentration of androgens in the tumour microenvironment promote carcinogenesis; whereas progestins decrease risk. This is based on evidence that the risk of ovarian cancer in conditions of high circulating androgens (within inclusion cysts, PCOS etc). While, use of progestins decrease the risk and induces ovarian surface epithelium apoptosis.

Whatever the stimulus, repair of genomic damage is diminished in women with defective BRCA1 and BRCA2 function, leading to an increased risk of disease.

Prevention of Ovarian Cancer

Oral contraceptive pill (chemoprevention) has the highest protective effect against ovarian cancer. Evidence suggests that taking the OCP for at least 5 years, reduces the relative risk of developing epithelial ovarian cancer by 50%.

Following are two large trials evaluating the role of oral contraceptive practice as primary prevention of ovarian cancer, particularly hereditary ovarian cancer due to BRCA1 or BRCA2 mutations.

(a) **CASH (Cancer and Steroid Hormone) study** and **SEER data** (population based and case-control study to investigate the relationship between OCP and breast, endometrium and ovarian cancer among US women:

Results: (a) 5-year use of OCP in nulliparous women reduced the risk of ovarian cancer to similar with non user multi-para and (b) Ten years use of OCP reduced the risk in women with family history ovarian cancer to lower than those non users and has no family history.

(b) McLaughlin et al. published a case control study on 3223 women with BRCA mutation. OCP use lead to a highly significant reduction in ovarian cancer risk (BRCA1 odds ratio: 0.56, BRCA2 odds ratio: 0.39) in both univariate and multi-variate analyses. The maximum protective effect was seen with 3–5 years of OCP.

Although there is convincing evidence that use of the OCP reduces the risk of ovarian cancer, OCP may not be appropriate for chemoprevention in all age groups in the general population because the reduced mortality from ovarian and endometrial cancer is balanced by an increased mortality from cervical and ischaemic heart disease.

Carotenoids are natural pigments found in food, some of which have been studied in relation to ovarian cancer risk. The carotenoids are classified into: (a) alpha carotene, (b) beta carotene and (c) lycopene. They can be found in food such as yellow, orange and red vegetables, and xanthophyll, which is found in green vegetables. Carotenoids can also be synthetic such as fenretinide. The preliminary results from chemoprevention trial have shown that fenretinide protects breast cancer patients from developing new primary cancer, e.g., ovarian cancer. A reduced risk of ovarian cancer related to carotenoid intake (either in form of supplement or food intake) was demonstrated with an odds ratio of 0.33–0.64. However, data on carotenoids are complex and not fully consistent. Further study is needed to confirm this finding.

Tubal ligation (RR 0.33) and hysterectomy reduced the risk of ovarian cancer (RR 0.67) in general population probably by reducing the exposure of the ovary to ascending infection or chemicals. The odds ratio for ovarian cancer is 0.5–0.71 compared with women who have not had the procedure and there are also data that hysterectomy alone may reduces the risk of ovarian cancer (OR 0.7) due to altered ovarian blood flow or reduced exposure of the ovary to potential carcinogenic factors.

Prophylactic oophorectomy is often performed together with hysterectomy for benign conditions if the patient has higher risk of ovarian cancer. Prophylactic oophorectomy can be offered to women with BRCA1 and BRCA2 mutations after the age of 30–35 years old and preferably after completed their family. Finch et al.

evaluated the role of prophylactic oophorectomy in prospective study. They found that prophylactic oophorectomy reduces the risk of ovarian, fallopian tube and peritoneal cancer by 80% in patients with BRCA1 and BRCA2 mutations. Prophylactic oophorectomy, however, is not 100% protective as 5–10% of these patients will still develop intra-abdominal carcinomatosis (primary peritoneal carcinoma). For women with BRCA1 and BRCA2 mutations who opt not to undergo early oophorectomy, the task force of the Cancer Genetics Studies Consortium recommends transvaginal ultrasound (TVS) and CA125 levels performed every 6–12 months in these women aged 25–35 years.

Hereditary Ovarian Cancer and Genetic Testing

Germline mutation of BRCA1/2 (HBOC) and DNA mismatch-repair genes (HNPCC) are inherited in an autosomal dominant fashion. Each carrier has a 50:50 chances of passing the gene to a son or daughter, but it is uncertain whether anyone with the gene mutation will eventually develop an inherited cancer. Due to variable penetrance, Clinician has to take details family history and in selected individuals may be offered genetic testing. The geneticist and genetic counselor are able to calculate the risk of having ovarian cancer based on details family history and genetic risk assessment. The Society of Gynaecologic Oncologist recommended a genetic counseling and testing to women with personal risk exceeding 20–25% for HBOC (hereditary breast-ovarian cancer syndrome), however they also stated that it is reasonable to offer genetic risk assessment to individual with risk greater than 5–10% chance of having mutation. Patients with more than 20–25% chance of having HBOC and for whom genetic risk assessment is recommended are: (1) womwn with a personal history of both breast and ovarian cancer, (2) women with ovarian cancer and a close relative with breast cancer at 50 years and less or ovarian cancer at any age, (3) women with ovarian cancer at any age who are Ashkenazi Jewish ancestry, (4) women with breast cancer at 50 years and less, and a close relative with ovarian or male breast cancer at any age, (5) women of Ashkenazi Jewish ancestry and breast cancer at 40 years and less. Close relative is defined as a first, second, or third degree relative (i.e mother, sister, daughter, aunt, niece, grandmother, granddaughter, first cousin, great grandmother, great aunt (Lancaster et al., 2007).

Once the women (patient) is identified to undergo genetic counseling, they are offered to attend the genetic counseling clinic. This clinic is run by trained genetic counselor and geneticist. The counselor will take history and perform risk stratification. Genetic testing is only offered after appropriate counseling and consent has been obtained. It is most efficient to start by testing a cancer affected individual first; if she has an identified gene mutation, genetic testing of unaffected relatives are then recommended and done.

The genetic testing involved full testing of BRCA1 and BRCA2 mutation. The results of genetic testing are (a) positive, (b) negative or (c) uncertain significance. Uncertain significance is reported in approximately 5–12% of the result. The result is reported as uncertain significance when Geneticist discovered a pattern of mutation that is not fully understood. It may be pathogenic or just polymorphisms (normal variants that do not affect protein function). Subsequent management is most often based on the personal and family history. Women with tested negative will have the risk of ovarian cancer approaching that of the general population but false negative rate can be as high as 12% in very high risk families. Patient with any results but from extremely high risk families for HBOC, should be educated on risk-reduction strategies, including breast screening and chemoprevention options. For women with BRCA1 mutation, the risk of ovarian cancer begins to rise in the late 30s and early 40s, with an average age of 53 years at diagnosis. Risk-reducing salpingoophorectomy (RRSO) may be recommendedd. For BRCA2 mutation, the risk is only elevated 10 years later than BRCA1 mutation women. Women with BRCA2 mutation who delay RRSO until closer to the time of natural menopause may not entirely benefit from the breast cancer risk reduction of up to 70%.

Analysis of the BRCA1 and BRCA2 genes together consist of approximately 20,000 nucleotides. DNA is extracted from a patients blood sample and each exon of each gene is amplified by the PCR. Therefore, genetic testing is not a simple test and should not be offerred routinely. The failure to identify a pathogenic variant does not exclude the diagnosis of familial cancer. Majority of women with familial breast or ovarian cancer do not have an identifiable mutation in the BRCA1 or BRCA2 genes. On the other hand, once a mutation has been identified in the family, a normal test result means that the person has not inherited the family's predisposition to develop cancer and does not require special cancer surveillance. Genetic testing is very expensive test.

Screening for Ovarian Cancer

There is no effective screening method to detect early ovarian cancer in general population. The ideal tumour marker should have a 100% sensitivity, specificity and PPV; however, this is not achieved in practice. Approximately 90% of ovarian cancer is sporadic and mainly in women older than 50 years; therefore, the screening trials in the general population are focus in this group of women. Several screening methods have been evaluated in general population and following are some of those tests.

Pelvic Examination

Data are limited; there is no evidence that ovarian cancer detected in asymptomatic women on the basis of abnormal pelvic examination alters morbidity and mortality.

Ultrasound Scans

An autopsy study of 52 postmenopausal women who died from causes other than gynaecological or intraperitoneal cancer showed that as much as 56% of the women had an undetected small benign ovarian cyst measuring less than 5 cm in diameter. Transvaginal ultrasound has a sensitivity of 100% and specificity of 98.7%, and (PPV) 6.7% (15 laparotomy was needed to find 1 ovarian cancer). The risk of malignancy index (RMI) has been widely used in clinical practice for primary evaluation of individuals with an adnexal mass. The details on RMI are discussed later in this chapter. The newer approaches include three-dimensional ultrasound and three-dimensional power Doppler. Introduction of colour Doppler may reduce high false positive result.

Tumour Markers

CA125

The most limiting factor of a tumour marker is lack of specificity, as most markers are tumour-associated rather than tumour-specific, and are elevated in multiple cancers, benign and physiological conditions. The level of CA125 in body fluid or ovarian cysts does not correlate well with serum levels probably caused by the serum concentration is also contributed by the other factors that affect its release into the circulation. The widely adopted cut-off value of serum CA125 level is 35 kU/L based on the normal distribution of values in 99% of healthy individuals (in study involving 888 samples) (Bast, 1983). The level of CA125 is tend to be lower (<20 kU/L) in postmenopausal women. The level of CA125 can be elevated in physiological condition such as pregnancy, menstrual cycle, etc., and in many other benign gynaecological conditions such as endometriosis, uterine fibroid, inflammatory process that involved the peritoneum and others. It may also be elevated in non-gynaecological diseases such as inflammation of the pleura, pericardium, pancreatitis, hepatitis, cirrhosis, ascites, tuberculosis and other malignancies such as pancreas, breast, colon and lung cancers. The CA125 is not expressed or produced by 20% of ovarian cancers partly be caused by CA125 forming circulating immune antibodies containing complexes bound to the free antigen. Fifty percent of women with stage 1 and 2 ovarian cancer have CA125 more than 65 U/mL. Single reading is not strong; it needs at least annual measurement. For women age more than 50, CA125 of more than 35U/mL has a specificity of 97%. Specificity is increased to 99.8% if cut-off point level is set at 95 U/mL. However, the PPV was less than 10%.

Additional Markers

The performances of various other markers have been evaluated and among those markers are HE4, CA15-3, CA72-4, activin, inhibin, leptin, prolactin, transferrin, HER2 and others. At present, the most promising marker (other than CA125) is human epididymis protein (HE4). HE4 is a glycoprotein in the epithelial cells of the epididymis and increased serum levels and expression of the HE4 have been found in ovarian cancer. HE4 is also elevated in other cancers. The performance of 49 ovarian cancer biomarkers was assessed in pre-diagnostic specimens (within 6 months of cancer diagnosis) in asymptomatic women compared with clinical specimens obtained at diagnosis from a different set of individuals. Tumour markers that showed comparable performance with clinical samples were CA125, HE4, CA72-4 and CA15-3. CA125 remained the single best biomarker for ovarian cancer, with the second best marker being HE4 (sensitivity of 86% and 73%, respectively) Cramer DW et al., 2011. For all markers, the sensitivity declined in specimens more remote than 6 months from diagnosis. Although the combination of HE4 and CA125 has been found to increase sensitivity while maintaining high specificity, more recently it has been reported not to be of benefit in clinical settings. However, using algorithm of HE4 and CA125 can correctly classify 93.8% of women with epithelial ovarian cancer and triage women to Gynaecology Oncology Centre (Moore, 2009).

Multi-Modal Screening Tests

Specificity and positive predictive value (PPV) of screening has been improved by adding pelvic ultrasound as a second line test. Jacob et al. had evaluated the role of combined CA125 and TVS in detection of ovarian and fallopian tube cancer among more than 21,000 postmenopausal women. Women with CA125 ≥ 30U/mL were subjected to TVS and laparotomy was performed if abnormality was detected on TVS. Results: The PPV, specificity and sensitivity were 26.8%, 99.9% and 78.6%, respectively. However, there was no advantage in terms of overall survival (Jacob, 1993).

Interestingly, follow-up data from Jacob's trial have shown that elevated CA125 levels associated with malignancy tend to rise as compared to a flat or static profile or decreased with time in women without ovarian cancer. Using the computerized algorithm, the trend of CA125 levels was used to calculate the risk of ovarian cancer (ROC). The ROC of 2% indicates a risk of 1 in 50. Women are triaged into low, intermediate and high risk based on their ROC result (low risk, ROC less than 1 in 3500, intermediate risk, ROC between 1 in 3500 and 1 in 1000, high risk (or elevated risk, ROC more than 1 in 1000). Prospective evaluation of the ROC algorithm in a randomize-controlled trial of more than 13,000 postmenopausal women ages over 50 years, showed a high specificity (99.8%) and PPV of 19% for primary invasive epithelial ovarian cancer (Menon et al., 2009).

The United Kingdom Collaborative Trial of Ovarian Cancer Screening (UKCTOCS) has completed recruiting >200,000 postmenopausal women age 50–74 years old. Screening method was annual ultrasound or annual CA125 using ROC algorithm followed by ultrasound compared to control group (no intervention). The primary endpoint was ovarian cancer mortality. The ROC algorithm was used to triage the women into low, intermediate and elevated risk. Those with intermediate risk have to repeat CA125 in 12 weeks, whereas those in elevated risk group were referred for TVS and repeat CA125 in 6 weeks. Preliminary results showed that screening sensitivity was similar but specificity was slightly higher in multi-modality test, using CA125 followed by ultrasound scan (99.8% vs. 98.2%, p value <0.0001) and PPV of 35.1%, as compared to ultrasound alone (Menon et al., 2008; 2009). The effect of screening on mortality is still unavailable. The final results of this large trial (UKCTOCS) may be available by 2015.

An ongoing prospective randomized controlled trial sponsored by the National Cancer Institute USA known as National Institutes of Health PLCO (Prostate, Lung, Colorectal and Ovarian Cancer) Screening Trial has completed their recruitments of about 78,000 women in general population, age between 55 and 74 years. Screening was performed by annual CA125 for 6 years and TVS for 4 years. After the 13-year follow-up, ovarian cancer was diagnosed in 212 women in the intervention group and 175 in the control group. There were 118 deaths caused by ovarian cancer in the intervention group and 100 deaths in the control group. The study concluded that after 13-year follow-up, simultaneous screening with CA-125 and TVS compared with usual care did not reduce ovarian cancer mortality. Moreover, the excess morbidity of carrying out surgery in women with false-positive results was 5.1%. Since women will be followed up for at least 17 years, the final results (ovarian cancer mortality) are still unavailable (Buys et al., 2011).

Several other large ovarian screening trials were conducted for general population, such as the Kentucky Screening Study (KSS) and the Japanese Shizuoka Cohort Study of Ovarian Cancer

Screening (JSCSOCS). KSS is a single-arm annual ultrasound screening study involving more than 25,000 women had reported the sensitivity of 81% and specificity of 98.7% for epithelial ovarian cancer; 82% were stage 1 and 2 disease (Van Nagell et al, 2007). The Japanese Shizuoka Cohort Study of Ovarian Cancer Screening trial was randomized controlled trial of more than 82,000 low-risk postmenopausal women who were screened using an annual ultrasound and CA125. The screening strategy achieved a sensitivity and specificity of 77.1% and 99.9%, respectively (Kobayashi et al., 2008). The impact of these screening tests on ovarian cancer mortality rate is yet to be determined.

The problem with screening ovarian cancer is that the diagnosis has to be made via laparotomy. If the aim of PPV < 10% is to be achieved, the screening will result in a high number of instances of unnecessary laparotomy. Many of the trials mentioned above reported the benefits of ovarian cancer screening in terms of detection of cancer at an early stage and positive impact on the survival rate but none have confidently shown that it improved the incidence and mortality rate. Even in the high-risk group, there is no evidence that screening ovarian cancer reduced mortality. Both National Institutes of Health Consensus Conference and American College of Obstetricians & Gynaecologists have issued statements advising against routine screening for ovarian cancer due to its high false positive rate, leads to an unacceptable number of invasive interventions in women without significant disease. Study on proteomics as a screening ovarian cancer is ongoing and preliminary results were promising.

Histologic Classification of Ovarian Neoplasm (General)

Serous Tumour of the Ovary

Histologic classification of ovarian neoplasms is shown in Table 12.1 and 12.1. Serous tumour of the ovary is formed by cells that resemble those of the internal lining of the fallopian tube. It constitutes 46% of all epithelial tumours. In serous tumours, 33% are malignant (most commonly at sixth decade of life), 50% are benign (more common in fourth and fifth decade of life) and 17%, borderline tumour (on average diagnosed in the fifth decade of life). The mean age for malignant serous tumour is 56 years old. About 25% of serous adenoma is bilateral. Serous tumour of the ovary can be benign, borderline or malignant serous tumour (serous cystadenocarcinoma); 30% of serous borderline tumours are bilateral. The mean age at diagnosis for malignant serous tumour is 59.4 years old. In stage 1 serous cystadenocarcinoma, 1/3 is bilateral, while in advanced stage serous cystadenocarcinoma, 2/3 is bilateral. Serous tumour of borderline malignancy often secrete a fluid with higher mucin than benign lesion, it may be mistaken with mucinous tumour. Psammoma bodies are more abundant in malignant than benign tumour. In malignant serous tumour, higher psammoma bodies associated with low grade and better prognosis. Destructive invasion in a borderline tumour (invasion > 3 mm) indicates the presence of a serous carcinoma.

Table 12.1 General histologic classification of ovarian neoplasm

Classification	Sub-classification
A. Neoplasm derived from coelomic epithelium	1. Serous tumour 2. Mucinous tumour 3. Endometrioid tumour 4. Mesonephroid (Clear cell) 5. Brenner tumour 6. Carcinosarcoma and mixed mesodermal tumour
B. Neoplasm derived from Germ cell	1. Teratoma (a) Mature teratoma Solid adult teratoma Dermoid cyst Struma ovarii (b) Malignant neoplasms secondarily arising from mature cystic teratoma (c) Immature teratoma 2. Dysgerminoma 3. Embryonal carcinoma 4. Endodermal sinus tumour 5. Choriocarcinoma 6. Gonadoblastoma

C. Neoplasm derived from specialized gonadal stroma	1. Granulosa-theca cell tumours (a) Granulosa tumour (b) Thecoma 2. Sertoli–Leydig tumour (a) Arrhenoblastoma (b) Sertoli tumour 3. Gynandroblastoma 4. Lipid cell tumours
D. Neoplasms derived from non-specific mesenchyma	1. Fibroma, haemangioma, leiomyoma, lipoma 2. Lymphoma 3. Sarcoma
E. Metastatic tumour	From GIT, breast, endometrium, lymphoma, etc.

Table 12.2 Histopathological classification of common epithelial ovarian tumour (WHO classification)

Classification	Sub-classification
A. Serous tumours	1. Benign 2. Borderline malignancy 3. Malignant (Adenocarcinoma, surface papillary carcinoma, malignant adenofibroma and cystadenofibroma)
B. Mucinous tumours	1. Benign 2. Borderline malignancy 3. Malignant (Adenocarcinoma, Malignant adenofibroma and cystadenofibroma)
C. Endometrioid tumours	1. Benign 2. Borderline malignancy 3. Malignant (adenocarcinoma, adenocanthoma, adenosquamous carcinoma, malignant adenofibroma and cystadenofibroma, stroma sarcoma and carcinosarcoma)
D. Clear cell tumours	1. Benign 2. Borderline malignancy 3. Malignant
E. Transitional cell tumour	1. Brenner tumour 2. Brenner tumour of borderline malignancy 3. Malignant Brenner tumour 4. Transitional cell carcinoma

F. Squamous cell carcinoma
G. Mixed epithelial tumours
H. Undifferentiatied carcinoma

Both peritoneal lining and surface epithelium of the ovary is derived from mesothelial. Therefore, they can both undergo malignant or borderline transformation. Strong evidence suggests that many borderline tumours in the peritoneum were resulting from metastasis from primary serous borderline tumour of the ovary. Serous borderline tumour of the ovary can also metastasize to the peritoneum in the form of more invasive manners which carries a poorer prognosis.

Mucinous Tumour of the Ovary

Mucinous tumour is the second most common epithelial tumour of the ovary. In mucinous tumour, the tumour is formed by cells that resemble either those of the endocervical epithelium (endocervical or mullerian type) or those of the intestinal epithelium (intestinal type). Intestinal type is more common than endocervical type. Both endocervical and intestinal type may coexist.

Mucinous tumour constitutes about 36% of all epithelial ovarian tumours. Benign mucinous tumour account for up to 20% of all ovarian neoplasms, most frequently occur between third and fifth decades of life. About 75–85% of mucinous tumours are benign and majorities are unilateral, while, 14% of this tumour are borderline, while 5% are malignant. Borderline mucinous tumour of intestinal type may be associated with pseudomyxoma peritonei. Most case of pseudomyxoma peritonei may be originated from appendix.

The mean age of mucinous adenocarcinoma is 54.7 years old and it represents 5–10% of all malignant ovarian neoplasms. Six to 20% of mucinous cystadenocarcinomas are bilateral. Mucinous cystadenocarcinoma has a better prognosis than serous and endometrioid type.

Endometrioid Tumours

Endometrioid tumour of the ovary is characterized by the presence of epithelial elements, stromal elements or a combination of the two that resembles those of the endometrium. Eight percent of the epithelial tumours are an endometrioid type. Benign and borderline endometrioid tumours are rare. Majorities are malignant (80%) and histologically resemble the usual adenocarcinoma of the endometrium. Endometrioid adenocarcinoma of ovary constitutes 10–25% of all epithelial ovarian cancers and the mean age is 57 years old. Ten percent of cases (malignant) are associated with endometriosis. Ten to twenty percent of endometrioid tumour/cancer of the ovary is also associated with endometrial tumour/cancer. Many cases of endometriod adenocarcinoma of the ovary have co-existing endometriosis. Approximately 15% of borderline malignancy of endometrioid tumour associated with endometriosis. Compared to mucinous type, endometrioid tumour carries a better prognosis.

Clear Cell Tumours

Clear cell carcinoma of the ovary is uncommon and constitutes 3–5% of all ovarian cancer. It is characterized by presence of clear cells containing abundant cytoplasmic glycogen and hobnail (peg-shaped) cells. The hobnail cells are characterized by apical nuclei that protrude into the lumens of tubules and cysts beyond the cytoplasmic limits of the cells. About 50% of cases are associated with endometriosis. The malignant tissue has a white, yellow or light brown colour within the endometrotic cyst. The majority of clear cell tumour of ovary is malignant; few are benign or borderline tumours. Bilaterality is only found in 13% of cases and 60% of patients presented at an early stage. Clear cell adenocarcinoma of the ovary can resemble endodermal sinus tumour and dysgerminoma microscopically. The 5-year survival for stage 1 tumour is 60% and 12% for all other stages.

Transitional Cell Tumour (Brenner Tumour)

Transitional cell tumour, or Brenner tumour of the ovary, is the tumour of urothelial differentiation (cells resemble those of the internal lining of the urinary bladder). This tumour is very rare (2%) and is believed to derive from the ovarian surface epithelium that undergoes urothelium-liked transformation (urothelial metaplasia).

Majority is benign and small in size (more than 50% are smaller than 2 cm). Microscopically tumour cells are usually polygonal or ovoid and have clear cytoplasma with glycogen. The nuclei are oval and occasionally have grooves, giving them a **coffee-bean** appearance. In minority of cases, this tumour is either borderline or malignant in nature. Benign tumour is grossly small, mostly solid and well circumscribed, while malignant tumour is commonly more solid and often have a central lumen containing dense eosinophilic materials or mucin. There are two types of malignant tumour of transitional differentiation: (a) **malignant Brenner tumour** and (b) **transitional cell carcinoma non-Brenner type**. The tumour cells have pleomorphic, atypical nuclei and presence of stromal infiltration by malignant transitional cells. Malignant Brenner tumour is very rare, poorly differentiated and arising from benign Brenner tumour. The presence of benign or borderline Brenner tumour should be identified in or adjacent to these carcinomas to qualify the diagnosis of malignant Brenner tumour. Malignant Brenner tumours have an excellent prognosis when they are confined to the ovary. Majority of this tumour presented at an early stage (>80%). Transitional cells carcinoma non-Brenner type does not arise from existing benign lesion like malignant Brenner tumour. It resembles high-grade transitional cell carcinoma of bladder, more aggressive, majority presented at an advanced stage (>70%) but responsive to chemotherapy.

Undifferentiated Carcinoma of Ovary

Undifferentiated carcinoma of the ovary is very rare but the most aggressive form of epithelial ovarian cancer. The small cell carcinoma is a subgroup of undifferentiated carcinoma of the ovary. Small cell carcinoma is the most common type of undifferentiated carcinoma of ovary

There are at least two types of small cell carcinoma of ovary:

(a) Hypercalcaemic type
(b) Pulmonary type

Hypercalcaemic Type

The hypercalcaemic type occurs in the younger age group with mean age of 24 years old. Two-third of cases have hypercalcaemia, which may improve when the tumour is excised. Hypercalcaemia type is more common in young age (mean age: 24). In two-third of cases, the serum calcium is high and hypercalcaemia will reverse when the tumour is excised. Some patients presented with hypercalcaemic symptoms such as fatigue, lethargy, polydipsia and polyuria. The tumour is always unilateral and by the time of diagnosis, in 50% of patients, it has spread outside the ovary. Approximately 60% of patients with stage 1A disease will die of the disease.

Pulmonary Type

The pulmonary-type small cell carcinoma of ovary resembles small cell carcinoma of lung and it is more common in older women with the mean age of 59 years old. Fifty percent are bilateral and mean survival to death is 8 months.

The other type of undifferentiated carcinoma of the ovary is neuroendocrine tumour of the non-small cell type. This tumour also carries very poor prognosis.

Natural History and Patterns of Spread in Epithelial Ovarian Cancer

Epithelial ovarian cancer is a cancer arising from the ovarian surface epithelium. In an initial stage, it confines within the inclusion cyst in ovarian substances. The tumour then penetrates the capsule and enters peritoneum. Cancer cells follow the circulation of peritoneal fluid from the pelvis, right paracolic gutter, right hemidiaphragm and then whole abdomen. This transcoelomic implantation is one of two main spread of ovarian cancer.

The second most common mode of spread is via lymphatic channels: (a) retroperitoneal lymphatics: drain the ovary via ovarian vessel to para-aortic nodes up to the level of renal vessels, (b) parametrium and broad ligaments drain to pelvic lymph nodes and (c) round ligament to inguinal lymph nodes. Lymph node involvement indicates advanced stage of disease. Many cases of this spread are occult and subclinical. About 10% of apparent stage 1 disease has para-aortic lymph nodes metastasis; the incidence of subclinical metastases in apparent stage 1 disease is shown in Table 12.3.

Table 12.3 Incidence of subclinical metastases in apparent stage 1 ovarian cancer

Site of metastasis	Incidence of subclinical metastases detected after thorough surgical staging in apparent stage 1 ovarian cancer
Diaphragm	7.6%
Omentum	7.1%
Cytology	18.8%
Peritoneal	9.8%
Pelvic nodes	8.9%
Aortic nodes	12.3%

Diagnosis and Clinical Evaluation

Approximately 75–85% of a patient with ovarian cancer has peritoneal spread at the time of diagnosis. The Most common presentation is abdominal discomfort, pain and distension. Gastrointestinal symptoms are also common such as nausea, dyspepsis, constipation and others. The diagnosis of early-stage ovarian cancer is usually made by abdominal and pelvic palpation. In premenopausal women, functional cyst is rarely larger than 8 cm and will resolve after 2–3 months without treatment. Adnexal mass in a pre-menarchal and post-menopausal woman has a higher likelihood of being malignancy. Ultrasound scan can assist in the diagnosis of ovarian carcinoma; radiological features of malignancy are (a) irregular border, (b) solid component and papillary projection, (c) dense multiple irregular septae, (d) bilaterality, (e) ascites and (f) liver nodule, lymph nodes enlargement, which can be accurately assessed by CT scan or MRI.

Lymphangiography has 90% accuracy in detecting para-aortic lymph node involvement but suffers from poor patient acceptance and lack of experts. The brain scan, bone scan and barium study are only indicated if the patient has symptoms related to the respective organ. Mammography can exclude breast cancer secondary to the ovary. Pap smear may pick up ovarian cancer cells in advanced stage.

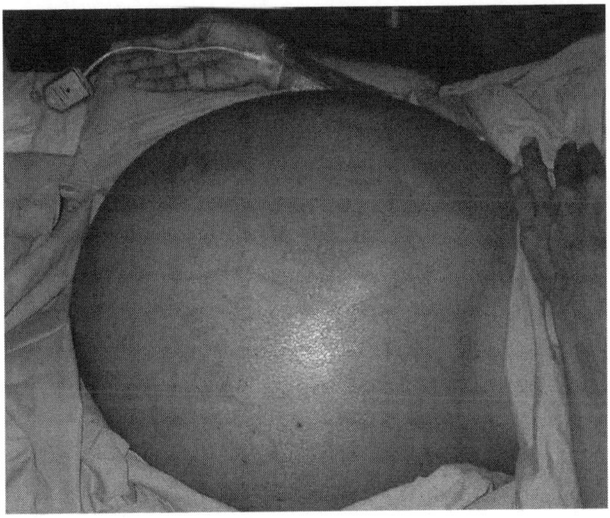

Figure 12.2 Abdominal distension is one of the most common presentations of patients with ovarian cancer.

Biomarkers and Risk Assessment

Ca125 is the most useful blood test for suspected epithelial ovarian cancer and 1% of normal non pregnant women have CA125 >35 U/mL. Overall, 80—85% of women with epithelial ovarian cancer has elevated CA125. Serum CA125 is elevated in 85% of women with serous tumour as compared to 69% in mucinous tumour. Pre-treatment of CA125 is an independent predictor of progression-free survival in advanced epithelial ovarian cancer treated with a standard chemotherapy regimen. In post-menopausal women with asymptomatic pelvic mass, elevation of CA125 >65 U/mL had a sensitivity of 97% and specificity of 78% for ovarian cancer.

Risk of Malignancy Index

Risk of malignancy index (RMI) is a scoring system based on the level of CA125, ultrasound findings and menopausal status. The score provides a prediction regarding the nature of ovarian cyst/tumour either benign or malignant (refer to Table 12.4). Risk of malignancy index score of 200 or greater gives a sensitivity of 85% and specificity of 97% for ovarian cancer. Using 200 as cut-off score, patients with score less than 200 can be reassured and managed by the general gynaecologist, while women with the RMI score >200 should be referred to a centre with experience in ovarian cancer surgery. This cut-off score can also be used to guide the surgeon, whether to perform intraoperative frozen section and staging surgery particularly in young patients who presented with suspicious ovarian cyst.

Table 12.4 Risk of malignancy index

Criteria	Score awarded	Score
Menopausal status		
Premenopausal	1	**A** (1 or 3)
Postmenopausal	3	
Ultrasound features	None of these features, score 0	
Multi-loculated	One feature, score 1	**B** (0,1 or 3)
Solid areas	More than one features, score 3	
Bilaterality		
Ascites		
Metastasis		
Serum CA125 concentration (IU/mL)	Absolute concentration of CA125	**C**
Risk of malignancy index (RMI) = A X B X C		

Source: *J Clin Pathol* 2004; **57**(11): 1232.

OVA1 Test

The other method to predict patients with ovarian cancer who presented with pelvic mass is OVA1 test, which was approved by the FDA in September 2009. OVA1 uses a blood sample to test for levels of five proteins that alter in ovarian cancer. The test combines five separate results into a single numerical score between 0 and 10 to indicate the likelihood of pelvic mass to be ovarian cancer. OVA1 is intended for women age more than 18 undergoing surgery for pelvic mass. The accuracy was 92% when combined with radiological test. OVA1 test, however, has high false positive test (64%). Five proteins involved in OVA1 test are apolipoprotein A1 (decrease in cancer), beta 2 microglobulin (increased in cancer), CA125 (increase), prealbumin (decrease) and transferrin (decrease in cancer).

Risk of Ovarian Malignancy Algorithm (ROMA)

Risk of ovarian malignancy algorithm (ROMA) is a qualitative serum test that combines the results of CA125, HE4 and menopausal status into a numerical score. Similar to OVA1 test, ROMA was also approved by FDA. The clinical usage of ROMA is similar to RMI and OVA1 test. Combination of CA125 and HE4 markers was found to be more accurate than either test alone in predicting the nature of adnexal mass. ROMA must be interpreted in conjunction with an independent clinical and radiological assessment. ROMA is indicated for women who meet the following criteria: (a) age more than 18, (b) ovarian mass present for which surgery is planned and (c) not yet referred to gynae oncologist. The test is not intended as a screening or stand-alone diagnostic assay. Patients classified as being at increased risk for ovarian cancer can be referred to a gynaecologic oncologist for optimal care. In a prospective multi-centre trial, the combination assay yielded a sensitivity of 94% with specificity of 75% (Moore et al., 2011). A new secondary analysis of trial data comparing patients with benign disease and all stages of epithelial ovarian cancer determined ROMA's sensitivity to be 94.3% vs. 83.7% for the (RMI), when specificity for both was set at 75%. ROMA also was more sensitive than RMI in a comparison of patients with benign disease, borderline tumours and epithelial ovarian cancer (89% vs. 80.7%).

New Tumour Markers in Ovarian Cancer

CA-19-9 is elevated in gastrointestinal, lung, ovarian, endometrial carcinoma, and most useful in pancreatic carcinoma. Mucinous ovarian cancer expresses the antigen more frequently than serous tumours (76% vs. 27%). The other potential tumour marker is ovarian carcinoma antigen (OCA): **NB/70K**, it has a sensitivity equal with CA125 but less specific. Macrophage colony-stimulating factor (**MCS**-F): MCS-F is secreted by ovarian carcinoma cell line and elevated in ascitic fluid and blood from women with ovarian cancer. MCS-F is also elevated in 40% of ovarian cancer patients with normal CA125. **OVX-1 or** murine monoclonal antibody is another new tumour marker in ovarian cancer. An elevated serum level (>7.2 U/mL) was reported in 5% of normal individuals and in 70% of patients with epithelial ovarian cancer. **Lysophosphatidic**

acid (LPA) stimulates proliferation of ovarian cancer cell in vitro. LPA has been shown to be a multi-functional signalling molecule in fibroblast and other cells. LPA has been found in the ascitic fluid of patients with ovarian cancer and is associated with the ovarian cancer cell proliferation. Further studies are needed to determine the role of these markers. **Topoisomerase II** expression was detected in a sample of ovarian cancer by immunohistochemistry and may be clinically relevant biomarker for survival in patients with advanced epithelial ovarian cancer. L1 (CAM) expression represents a noval diagnostic marker in serous ovarian neoplasms that shows characteristics of tumour progression. L1 expression is also associated with the chemotherapy response. Human epididymal protein 4 (HE4) test in combination with CA-125 can improve the sensitivity and specificity of CA125 alone in identification and monitoring of ovarian cancer.

Staging Carcinoma of Ovary

Carcinoma of the ovary is surgico-pathologically staged based on the understanding on the natural history and spread of ovarian cancer. See Table 12.5 for full new FIGO staging 2014. CT scan or MRI provides more information regarding the extent of the disease. Patients presented with abnormal vaginal bleeding should undergo endometrial sampling.

The staging surgery for ovarian cancer is exploratory laparotomy, adnexectomy or hysterectomy bilateral salpingoophorectomy, omentectomy, pelvic and para-aortic lymphadenectomy. Pre-operative counselling and bowel preparations are mandatory. Skin incision must always be midline and often extended midline incision above the umbilicus. Staging must include a complete evaluation of all visceral and parietal surfaces within the peritoneal cavity. Peritoneal fluid is taken (total: 100–150 mL), ideally should be sent in a separate container from the pelvis, right and left paracolic gutter and undersurface of right and left hemidiaphragms. Encapsulated cyst should be removed intact. Omentectomy and random peritoneal biopsy should be done. Pelvic and para-aortic lymph node dissections are recommended in an apparent early stage. Understaging of apparent early-stage disease occurs in 31% of cases, while 77% of understaged patients are actually in stage 3 disease.

Table 12.5 FIGO staging 2014 for cancer of ovary, fallopian tube and primary peritoneal carcinoma

Stage	Description
Stage 1	**Tumour confined to ovaries or fallopian tube(s)**
1A	Tumour limited to one ovary (capsule intact) or fallopian tube; no tumour on ovarian or fallopian tube surface; no malignant cells in the ascites or peritoneal washings
1B	Tumour limited to both ovaries (capsules intact) or fallopian tubes; no tumour on ovarian or fallopian tube surface; no malignant cells in the ascites or peritoneal washings.
1C	Tumour limited to one or both ovaries or fallopian tubes, with any of the following: 1C1: Surgical spill 1C2: Capsule ruptured before surgery or tumour on ovarian or fallopian tube surface. 1C2: Malignant cells in the ascites or peritoneal washings
Stage 2	**Tumour involves one or both ovaries or fallopian tubes with pelvic extension (below pelvic brim) or primary peritoneal cancer**
2A	Extension and/or implants on uterus and/or fallopian tubes and/or ovaries
2B	Extension to other pelvic intraperitoneal tissues
Stage 3	**Tumour involves one or both ovaries or fallopian tubes, or primary peritoneal cancer, with cytologically or histologically confirmed spread to the peritoneum outside the pelvis and/or metastasis to the retroperitoneal lymph nodes**
3A1	Positive retroperitoneal lymph nodes only (cytologically or histologically proven). 3A1 (i) : Metastasis up to 10 mm in greatest dimension 3A1 (ii): Metastasis more than 10 mm in greatest dimension
3A2	Microscopic extrapelvic (above the pelvic brim) peritoneal involvement with or without positive retroperitoneal lymph nodes
3B	Macroscopic peritoneal metastasis beyond the pelvis up to 2 cm in greatest dimension, with or without metastasis to the retroperitoneal lymph nodes
3C	Macroscopic peritoneal metastasis beyond the pelvis more than 2 cm in greatest dimension, with or without metastasis to the retro-peritoneal lymph nodes (includes extension of tumour to capsule of liver and spleen without parenchymal involvement of either organ)
Stage 4	**Distant metastasis excluding peritoneal metastases**
4A	Pleural effusion with positive cytology
4B	Parenchymal metastases and metastases to extra-abdominal organs (including inguinal lymph nodes and lymph nodes outside of the abdominal cavity)

Following is the summary of surgical staging of apparent early-stage ovarian cancer:

(1) vertical incision

(2) multiple cytologic washings (total 100–150 mL from pelvic, paracolic gutter, diaphragm)
(3) complete abdominal exploration and intact tumour removal
(4) removal of remaining ovaries, uterus, tubes
(5) omentectomy, lymph node dissection and random peritoneal biopsies
(6) scraping or sampling of undersurface of diaphragm

Prognostic Factors for Epithelial Ovarian Cancer

The prognosis of epithelial ovarian cancer is closely related to the following:

(a) **Tumour stage** (5-year survivals: stage 1 (90%), stage 2 (80%), stage 3 (15–20%), stage 4 (5%).

(b) **Volume of residual tumour**: Directly correlate with survival. Optimally a cytoreduced patient has 22-month improvements in median survival. Size and number of residual tumour are both important. Patients with small volume of disease are believed to have a less aggressive disease compared to large volume at presentation. Therefore, similar successful cytoreductive surgery (residual tumour <2 cm) does not mean similar response/survival after adjuvant therapy. Generally, optimally cytoreduced patient has mean survival of 39 months compared to 17 months after completion of adjuvant chemotherapy.

(c) **Histologic subtype and grade:** Histologic subtype has less prognostic significance than grade. Mucinous type has overall better survival than endometrioid and serous cancer. These findings may be due to the fact that a high-grade mucinous tumour is less common. Endometrioid cancer has overall survival rate better than serous histotype. Clear cell tumour has a poorer prognosis than others if compared stage by stage. In advanced stage, grade has no correlation with survival.

Tumour size, bilaterality and ascites without malignant cells are not significant prognostic factors for early stage. Tumour spillage, capsular penetration and positive peritoneal cytology are associated with worse prognosis.

CA125 as Prognostic Factor in Epithelial Ovarian Cancer

Pre-operative CA125 is not an independent prognostic factor. Debulking surgery or a paracentesis can, however, cause a temporary rise in CA125 levels. CA125 level reflects the volume of tumour and high CA125 may signify large volume and unresectable tumour. Post-operative CA125 may have stronger and independent prognostic significance. The rate of CA125 declining may correlate with the response to treatment and survival. Some study has demonstrated, CA125 of >100 U/mL after three cycles have median survival of 7 months as compared to 50% 5-year survival in patients with CA125 ≤10 units/mL. Studies have shown that a serial rise in CA125 of ≥25% over three samples is almost 100% specific for disease progression. Definition of CA125 response rate is as follows: (a) 50% response if level reduce 50% after two readings and (b) 75% response if >75% reduction after three samples. Sample has to be analysed at least 28 days after previous sample and the initial CA125 value must be ≥35 units/mL. In monitoring of the ovarian cancer treatment, clinical response is, however, more important.

Other Prognostic Factors for Ovarian Cancer

Ploidy Analysis

The use of ploidy analysis in prognosticating the epithelial ovarian cancer is controversial. The DNA content is more commonly aneuploid in advanced stage compared to early stage. Aneuploidy rate correlates with the grade of tumour. In early stage, diploid tumour has better prognosis than aneuploid tumour, negative second look laparotomy is more in diploid than aneuploid tumour.

Image Cytometry

One of the applications of image cytometry is to measure DNA content (ploidy analysis), to locate a specific areas in DNA for study and to analyse cell architectural organization and subcellular particles (e.g., mean nuclear area (MNA), mitotic index (MI), volume percentage of epithelium (VPE). In stage 1 disease, low MI and VPE is associated with better 5-year survival (91% vs. 38%) compared with high

MI and VPE, while MNA is higher in serous adenocarcinoma than borderline tumour (63 μm^2 vs. 30 μm^2).

Genetic and Biologic Factors

Following are the genetics and biologic factors that are currently evaluated in ovarian cancer:

(1) abnormalities in products of genes: (a) oncogene products, e.g. HER-2/neu, p20 and (b) suppressor gene products p53, p16, pRB.
(2) markers of proliferation: (a) DNA index, (b) S-phase fraction, (c) KI-67 index and (d) proliferating cell nuclear antigen
(3) markers of DNA repair: (a) leukocyte platinum, (b) DNA excision repair and (c) helicase complexes
(4) serum cytokine levels (CSF-1, IL-6)
(5) factors associated with tumour invasion and metastases (NM23)

Borderline Tumour (Tumour of Low Malignant Potential)

Borderline tumours comprise approximately 15% of all epithelial ovarian tumours. The aetiology of borderline tumour is still unclear. Some mucinous borderline tumours of ovary may actually represent metastasis from the appendix (based on molecular studies). Borderline tumour has good prognosis and majority (60%) presented at stage 1 disease. The mean age of occurrence is approximately 10 years younger than that of women with malignant ovarian cancer. Staging of borderline ovarian tumour is similar with malignant ovarian cancer. The 5-year survivals in stages 1 and 2A is 100%.

The histologic characteristics of borderline tumour described by Dietel and Hauptmann are as follows:

(a) epithelial multi-layering of more than four cell layers
(b) not more than 4 mitoses per 10 high-power fields
(c) nuclear atypia
(d) increased in nuclear: cytoplasmic ratio
(e) slight to complex branching of of epithelium resulting in papillary projection
(f) epithelial budding and cell detachment into the lumen

(g) no stromal invasion: a major component in differentiating malignant from borderline tumours

Micropapillary carcinoma is the variant of serous adenoma of borderline malignancy with more aggressive character than usual. Two histology types of borderline ovarian tumour are mucinous and serous type.

Currently, the newly proposed terms for borderline malignancy are (a) atypical proliferating tumour, (b) intraepithelial carcinoma or (c) epithelial atypia. Some have included the new subcategory of borderline tumour known as microinvasive tumour (invasion ≤3 mm), but the clinical features of microinvasive tumour is very much resemble borderline tumour. Approximately, 25% of borderline tumours have cell proliferations on the outer surface of the lesion with no evidence of growth from the inner surface. 90% of this will develop peritoneal implants. Peritoneal implants can be divided into two, i.e. (a) invasive and (b) non-invasive. Generally, invasive implants have similar characteristics with non-invasive type. Invasive implant is also has an additional characteristic, i.e. epithelial cell infiltration of the stroma.

The most common presenting symptoms are abdominal distension, abdominal pain and mass. Approximately, 23% of patients are asymptomatic.

Surgical staging is similar to ovarian cancer. More than 70% of patients with invasive implants were also found to have non-invasive implants. Exploration of peritoneum must be thoroughly done due to high possibility of co-existing invasive and non-invasive implants. Furthermore, there is also an association between surface proliferations and peritoneal implants.

Treatment is mainly surgical; fertility-preserved surgery is recommended in young patients. Borderline tumours are correctly diagnosed in 58–86% of the time by frozen section, depending on the experience of the pathologist. Only age at diagnosis and the presence of invasive implants are shown to influence prognosis. The DNA cytometry study found diploid DNA in 95% of cases. Diploid DNA carries excellent prognosis as compared to aneuploid DNA. The data on overexpression of certain oncogenes and tumour suppressor genes were conflicting. Chemotherapy (platinum-based) may be indicated in patients with evidence of invasive implants. CA125 is not helpful in the management and follow-up of a patient with borderline ovarian tumour.

Management of Tumours with Low Malignant Potential

Early-Stage Disease

Five-year survival rates for early stage is 90–100%. Surgery is the mainstay of treatment for a patient with early stage of tumour with low malignant potential or borderline tumour. Generally, borderline ovarian tumour will not respond to chemotherapy. Surgical staging is similar to invasive carcinoma. Unilateral salpingoophorectomy (SO) has a similar survival rate with TAHBSO, although recurrence rate is slightly higher in SO group (15% vs. 5%) in stage 1 borderline malignancy. In all stage 2 disease, TAHBSO with appropriate surgical staging is recommended. There is no evidence that postoperative adjuvant therapy decreases recurrence rate and prolongs survival in stage 2 borderline malignancy.

Stage 3 and 4 Borderline Tumour

Twenty percent of patients with borderline malignancy presented in stages 3 and 4. Primary surgery is identical to invasive ovarian cancer. The benefit of postsurgical therapy in this group has not been well established. Five-year survivals in this stage are 64–96% even without adjuvant therapy. This tumour tends to be less responsive to chemotherapy because of a low growth fraction in borderline malignancy. Some small subset of borderline malignancy has aggressive behaviour. Aneuploid borderline tumour tends to be more aggressive than diploid. Adjuvant chemotherapy in aneuploid borderline malignancy may be justifiable. Majority of borderline tumours is diploid (95%) associated with excellent prognosis.

Treatment for Invasive Epithelial Ovarian Cancer

Treatment for Early Stage of Epithelial Ovarian Cancer

Early-stage ovarian cancer can be divided into two categories:

(a) **favourable early stage**
stage 1A or 1B disease
well or moderately differentiated tumour

(b) **unfavourable early stage**
- stage 1A or 1B with poorly differentiated tumour (including clear cell carcinoma)
- tumour on external surface
- ruptured capsule
- ascites or positive peritoneal washing
- all stage 2

Therapeutic options

(a) cytoreductive surgery
(b) chemotherapy
(c) radiation therapy
(d) combination

Stage 1 and 2 diseases only represent 10–15% of ovarian cancer diagnosed but 1/3 of all cured patients are from this group. Detailed understanding of the most appropriate treatment for early-stage disease has been hampered by following facts:

(a) Early-stage disease has a better prognosis.
(b) Early stage is uncommon; therefore, the sample is insufficient.
(c) Current FIGO staging for early-stage disease is descriptive rather than prognostic. The prognostic significance of each category has not been established. Two large studies failed to show bilaterality, rupture or capsular penetration had any influence on the outcome.
(d) Different in staging methods and accuracy. Current methods of staging provides better and more accurate staging and therefore, retrospective comparison in unreliable.

Chemotherapy in Early Stage (Stages 1 and 2)

Surgery is the mainstay of treatment on all stages of ovarian carcinoma and in apparent stage 1 disease, thorough surgical staging must be performed. Patients with stage 1A, 1B and well-differentiated tumour do not require adjuvant chemotherapy. An earlier study by Italian Interregional Cooperative Group of Gynaecologic Oncology (1995) found that adjuvant chemotherapy (cisplatinum 50 mg/m^2) reduces recurrence rate (65%) but no improvement in overall 5-year survival (88% vs. 82%) in patients with early-stage disease (1A and 1B with grades 2 and 3) with poor prognostic factors when compared to no treatment. Gynaecologic Oncology Group Protocol 95 had completed a study comparing intraperitoneal irradiation (32P) versus intravenous cisplatin/cyclophosphamide in early stage with unfavourable prognostic factor. Chemotherapy was found to be more superior in reducing recurrence rate (31% lower) but 5-year disease-free interval was 66% versus 77%.

Combined results from trials of EORTC-ACTION and ICON reported that adjuvant chemotherapy improved recurrence-free survival but not overall survival. In subgroup patients who had complete surgical staging, both recurrence-free survival and overall survival were better. After a median follow-up of 10.1 years, analysis of the more mature data from the ACTION trial has concluded that completeness of surgical staging in patients with early ovarian cancer was found to be statistically significantly associated with better outcomes, and the benefit from adjuvant chemotherapy appeared to be restricted to patients with non-optimal surgical staging (Trimbos et al., 2009).

GOG 157 evaluated three versus six cycles of paclitaxel (175 mg/m^2) and carboplatin (AUC 7) in patients with early high-risk epithelial ovarian cancer. There was no difference in terms of survival between both arms; however, further analysis of this study found that in patients with serous carcinoma, six cycles, were better than three cycles (5-year recurrence-free survival 83% vs. 60%).

Analysis from GOG 157 showed patients who developed recurrence had a poor survival rate comparable with recurrent advanced ovarian cancer with median survival of 24 months.

Management of Patients with Advanced Epithelial Ovarian Cancer

Cytoreductive Surgery

Generally, in any solid tumour, aggressive surgical resection is justified only if all tumours can be removed. However, ovarian cancer is an exception as removal of bulky ovarian tumour masses even with residual disease in advanced stage has several benefits:

(a) improved patient's comfort
(b) reduced adverse metabolic consequences of tumour
(c) enhanced patient's ability to maintain nutritional status
(d) increased ability to tolerate intensive chemotherapy
(e) enhanced response of the remaining tumour to chemotherapy due to relatively poor blood supply in large tumour as a large tumour tends to have low growth fraction
(f) decrease in the development of chemoresistant secondary to mutation as a large tumour tends to have more dividing cells and higher possibility of mutation (Goldie and Coldman).
(g) enhanced immune function due to removal of tumour bulk (Morton).

NIH Consensus Development Conference on Ovarian Cancer in April 1994 concluded: "*Aggressive attempts at cytoreductive surgery as the primary management of ovarian cancer will improve the patient's opportunity for long-term survival.*"

To achieve optimal cytoreduction, surgery should be performed by a trained gynaecological oncologist. An analysis of more than 3000 ovarian cancer patients treated between 1992 and 1999 and monitored by SEER program showed the better outcome for patients treated by gynaecological oncologist (Earle, et al.).

Systematic review by Vernooij evaluating a surgical outcomes as well as systemic therapy has shown that patient outcomes are better when treatments are offered by gynaecological oncologist or in a specialized hospital.

The most important prognostic factor that influences the likelihood of achieving surgically confirmed complete remission is the volume of residual disease at the time of chemotherapy. Studies have long established that survival for advanced ovarian cancer improves by removing as much tumour volume as possible at surgery. Bristow et al. demonstrated that for each 10% decrease in residual volume, there is a 5.5% increase in median survival. About 30–50% of all patients who do not achieve a surgically confirmed complete remission will experience recurrence.

GOG definition of optimal cytoreduction is when the diameter of the residual tumour is ≤1 cm. Approximately, 30–45% (mean) of patients with stage 4 diseases can achieve optimal cytoreductive/debulking surgery. The target for optimal cytoreduction rate in a good centre as defined by Bristow is ≥75%. Currently, there is a trend to establish optimal cytoreduction to no visible residual diseases (microscopic diseases). GOG trial (Winter et al.) examining primary cytoreduction and adjuvant chemotherapy had found that patients with no visible residual disease had the best prognosis for survival. Winter et al. reported in their published GOG trial that progression-free survival (PFS) and overall survival (OS) for stage III disease with microscopic residual disease were 33 months and 71.9 months, respectively. The PFS and OS for patients with residual disease ≤1 cm were 16.8 and 42.4 months, respectively, while for patients with residual disease of >1 cm, PFS was 14.1 months and OS 35 months. The benefits were also observed in patients with stage IV disease.

Occasionally splenectomy has to be performed. Indications of splenectomy are (a) bulky tumour involving the splenic surface, hilum and/or contiguous with omental metastases, (b) isolated or confluent hilar and/or capsular metastases that could not be resected, ablated or aspirated and (c) parenchymal metastases.

Isolated diaphragmatic tumours can be ablated. Extensive diaphragmatic disease can be removed either by stripping the peritoneum away from the muscle or if the disease infiltrating deeper, full thickness resection and repair may be required.

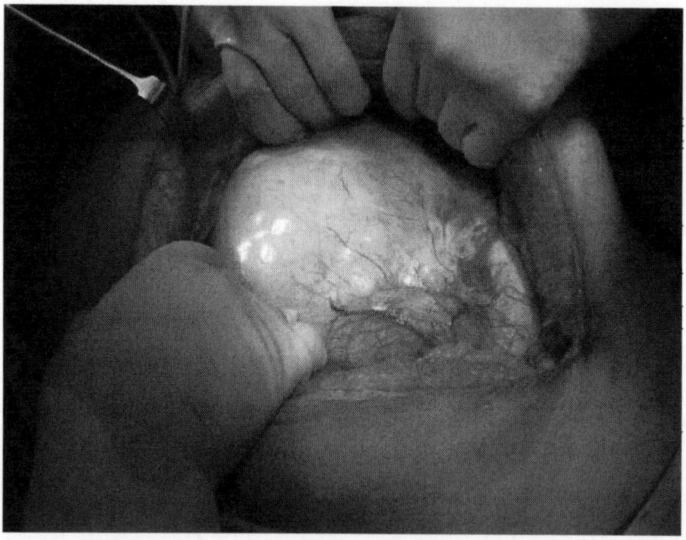

Figure 12.3 Midline laparotomy is the best approach for patient with ovarian cancer.

To increase the possibility of successful optimal cytoreduction, induction chemotherapy two to three cycles prior to surgery may be offered. Interval debulking can improve survival (median survival and progression-free interval) in advanced ovarian cancer. Interval debulking appears beneficial in patients who are not able to be optimally cytoreduced at their primary procedures. The concept of neoadjuvant chemotherapy and delayed surgery is currently being addressed by two international trials (EORTC-55971) and MRC-CHORUS. This topic will be further discussed later in this chapter.

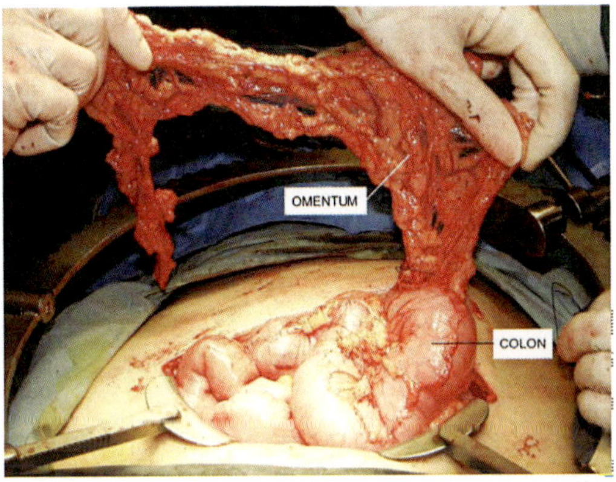

Figure 12.4 In advanced stage, omentum is one of the most common sites for malignant spread and omentectomy is the standard procedure for ovarian cancer.

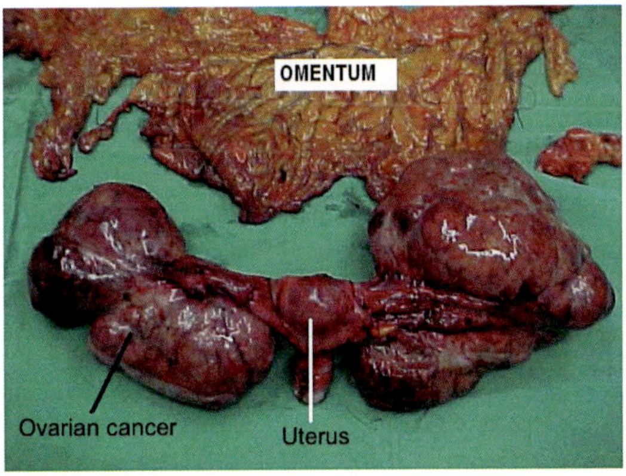

Figure 12.5 Total abdominal hysterectomy, bilateral salpingoophorectomy and omentectomy specimens.

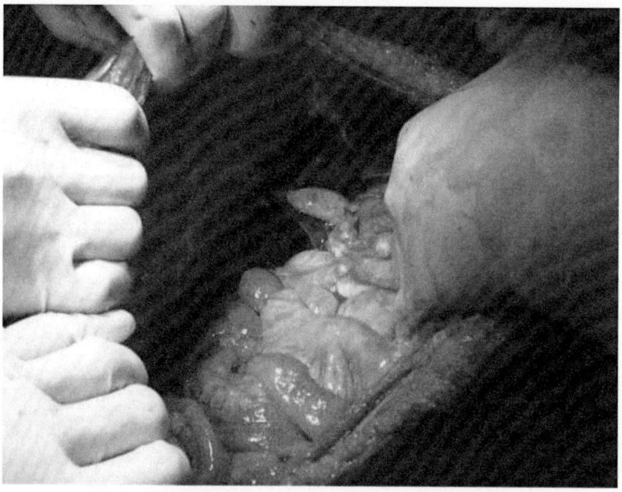

Figure 12.6 Tumour deposits over the liver surface and right hemidiaphragm.

Post-Operative Chemotherapy (First Line) in Ovarian Cancer

Ovarian cancer is highly chemosensitive cancer. Platinum compounds remain the most active agents. Currently standard of care for most patients with ovarian cancer consists of combination paclitaxel and carboplatin. Approximately, 50% of patients with advanced ovarian cancer will achieve a clinical complete response with this regimen.

Chemotherapeutic Drugs as First Line Regimen in Ovarian Cancer (Post-Operative Adjuvant Treatment)

Platinum Compounds

Gynaecologic Oncology Group 47 trial compared PAC (cisplatin/doxorubicin/cyclophosphamide) versus AC (doxorubicin/cyclophosphamide). PAC regime had better complete response rate (51% vs. 26%), better response duration, longer progression-free interval and overall survival (15.7 months vs. 9.7 months)

(Omura, 1986). In phase 1 trial, carboplatin was found to be less nephrotoxic, less neurotoxic and less emetogenic than cisplatin. However, carboplatin has dose-limiting myelotoxicity particularly thrombocytopenia. The haematologic toxicity of carboplatin correlates with AUC (area under the curve). Study had found that the tumour response to carboplatin plateauing at AUC 6–7. Ten out of 12 trials, including two meta-analyses, showed that single agent carboplatin had equivalent efficacy with cisplatin alone or combination therapy. A meta-analysis of 11 trials, involving more than 2000 patients, showed no difference in overall survival between carboplatin and cisplatin. In optimally cytoreduced cases, cisplatin combination shows the trend of better improvement in survival as compared to carboplatin combination regimens. However, there was difference in suboptimal diseases. An addition of platinum compound significantly improves survival with 12% reduction in risk of death (HR: 0.88) and 5% improvement in 2- and 5-year survival.

Doxorubicin and Platinum Combination

The GOG 52 trial compared PAC versus PC and this trial demonstrated that there is no difference in complete remission rate, progression-free interval and overall survival between both arms (Omura et al., 1989). A metanalysis of data from 10 trials in 1702 patients showed a modest but significant improvement in survival for PAC regimens as compared to the regimen without doxorubicin (overall HR: 0.85, p = 0.003). The difference was only 2 months and due to potential cardiotoxicity with doxorubicin; most investigators in the United States abandoned doxorubicin in favour of the cyclophosphamide-platinum regimen, while European researchers continued to retain the doxorubicin in their triplet regimen. Meta-analyses known as International Collaborative Ovarian Neoplasm Study (ICON 2) compared single agent carboplatin AUC 5 versus PAC (cisplatin 50 mg/m^2, doxorubicin 50 mg/m^2, cyclophosphamide 500 mg/m^2) and the study showed there was no difference in a survival rate, while ICON 3 trial had made comparison between single agent carboplatin versus PAC versus paclitaxel/carboplatin; single agent carboplating was found to be equally effective with better toxicity profile.

Taxanes

Taxane was reported to have significant activity in ovarian cancer in 1989. Gynaecologic Oncology Group 111 trial compared paclitaxel (135 mg/m^2)/cisplatin (75 mg/m^2) versus cyclophosphamide/cisplatin in stage 3 and 4 suboptimal disease. Study arm had better response rate (overall response rate, 73% vs. 60%; complete response rate: 51% vs. 31%) and overall survival (38 vs. 24 months); all with *p* value of less than 0.05 (McGuire, et al.). Piccart et al. confirmed the findings from GOG 111 study after follow-up review of 6.5 years. As the second line chemotherapy (previously treated), response rate of taxane is approximately 30–40%. Paclitaxel (Taxol, Anzatax) also shows an active action (overall response 37% and clinical complete remission rate 18%) as single agents in platinum-resistant ovarian cancer. Docetaxel (Taxotere) has a similar activity but slightly different spectrum of toxicity (primarily myelosuppression). Response rate in platinum resistance was 23–40%.

Paclitaxel 24 hour infusion (GOG 111 trial) was less neurotoxic than 3 hour infusions (European and Canadian trial (OV-10). Paclitaxel plus platinum based should be considered as the standard regime for subsequent clinical trial. The GOG 158, phase 3 trial in stage 3 optimal disease. The trial compared paclitaxel/carbo versus paclitaxel/cisplatin. An interim results shows a similar result (survival). Toxicity was less in **paclitaxel/carbo**, this combination therefore can be considered as standard of care. Two randomized trials by Ozol et al. and Du Bois et al. compared paclitaxel/carboplatin versus paclitaxel/cisplatin showed similar efficacy but paclitaxel/carboplatin arm was associated with lower toxicity.

Phase 3 trial (GOG 182/ICON 5) comparing doublets (paclitaxel/carboplatin) versus triplets (paclitaxel/carboplatin/gemcitabine or liposomal doxorubicin) versus two sequential doublets (topotecan/carboplatin + paclitaxel/carboplatin or gemcitabine/carboplatin + paclitaxel/carboplatin) showed no difference overall survival in all arms. Therefore, paclitaxel/carboplatin remains the first choice of adjuvant chemotherapy and has been adopted as a control arm in the next generation studies.

In the SCOTROC 1 trial (Scottish Gynaecological Cancer Trials Group, subject stage 1C, 2, 3 and 4), docetaxel/carboplatin regimens was found to be as efficacious as a paclitaxel/carboplatin regimen but with less neurotoxicity and greater improvement in some quality of life parameters (Vasey et al., 2004). In subsequent SCOTROC 2A and 2B trials, docetaxel-carboplatin based regimens were used as first line chemotherapy in ovarian cancer. In SCOTROC 2A, carboplatin was given 3 weekly for first four cycles followed by sequential treatment with docetaxel with or without gemcitabine (Vasey et al., 2006), while in SCOTROC 2B trial, study design was similar to SCOTROC 2A but instead of gemcitabine, iv irinotecan 200 mg/m^2 was used. Both studies showed an addition of third drug in sequential approaches was generally well tolerated but further exploratory studies are still needed (Clamp et al., 2006).

At present, paclitaxel and carboplatin are still the first line choice of adjuvant chemotherapy in epithelial ovarian cancer.

Dose of Platinum and Paclitaxel

Administering cisplatin with the dose of more than 100 mg/m^2 was often associated with unacceptable toxicity, mainly neurotoxicity. The GOG trial compared cisplatinum 50 mg/m^2 and cyclophosphamide 500 mg/m^2 versus double dose showed no significant difference in overall response rate and survival. There was, however, more toxicity associated with a double dose regimen (McGuire et al., 1995). Therefore, the recommended dose for cisplatinum is 75 mg/m^2. While, for carboplatin, the response rate plateuing at AUC 4–6 and in some study, 6–7. Many centres are using AUC 6 as the optimal starting dose for carboplatin.

In paclitaxel, higher dose gives better response and survival in recurrent disease. Some study used 250 mg/m^2 dose. Comparison study between 175 and 135 mg/m^2 either 24 hour or 3 hour infusions have shown the superiority of 175 mg/m^2 dosage (Eisenhauer, 1994). The Gynaecologic Oncologic Group evaluated the paclitaxel dose in recurrent ovarian cancer; they compared 250 mg/m^2 + GCSF versus 175 mg/m^2 24 hour infusions. Progression-free survival and overall survival were similar but higher dose were associated with higher toxicity. Recommended dose of paclitaxel is 175 mg/m^2, 3 hour infusions in recurrent disease.

SCOTROC 4 trial is a multi-centre randomized trial evaluating carboplatin flat dosing versus dose escalation in first line chemotherapy of ovarian, fallopian tube and primary peritoneal cancers (stage 1C, 2, 3 and 4 disease). Baanerjee et al. (2013) had published the report from SCOTROC 4 and ANZGOG trials comparing flat dosing versus dose escalation of single-agent carboplatin as first line chemotherapy for advanced ovarian cancer. In this multicenter phase III trial, 964 patients were recruited from 71 centers. Both arms were given an initial dose of carboplatin AUC 6, 3 weekly interval but for study group, dose escalation was given from cycle 2–6 based on nadir neutrophil and platelet counts. The median AUC received by study group was 7.2 compared to 6.0 for control group. There was no significant different in progression free survival and median overall survival for both group but grade 3/4 non-haematological toxicity was higher in study group (dose escalation).

Addition of Targeted Agents and Novel Agents to Platinum/Taxanes Regimen (Triplets)

One of the strategies to improve the effectiveness on first line therapy is to incorporate novel agents into the paclitaxel–carboplatin regimen. The addition of epirubicin as a third drug in a paclitaxel–carboplatin regimen failed to show any improvement as compared to paclitaxel–carboplatin alone (du Bois et al.). In GOG 182-ICON 5 Trial, other cytotoxic agents such as gemcitabine, topotecan and liposomal doxorubicin were added to the carboplatin–paclitaxel regimen in the five-arm randomized trial. As compared to carboplatin–paclitaxel, none of the experimental regimens tested showed any improvement in either progression-free or overall survival (Bookman et al.).

Anti vascular endothelial growth factor (anti-angiogenesis) is most promising targeted agent for ovarian cancer. An example of anti VEGF is bevacizumab. GOG 218 trial is the placebo controlled study of three arms involving 2000 participants (patients with stage III or IV ovarian cancer), i.e. paclitaxel–carboplatin for six cycles versus paclitaxel–carboplatin–bevacizumab versus paclitaxel–carboplatin–bevacizumab (maintenance with bevacizumab 15 mg/kg every 3 weeks for 48 weeks). GOG 218 completed accrual in June 2009. The results were presented in ASCO 2010; adding bevacizumab improved PFS in previously untreated women with advanced ovarian cancer (14.1 months versus 10.3 months, HR: 0.72; $p < 0.0001$). ICON 7 is another phase III trial (stage 1 and grade 3, stage 2, 3 or 4 epithelial ovarian cancer, primary peritoneal carcinoma, fallopian tube cancer) comparing paclitaxel–carboplatin versus paclitaxel–carboplatin–bevacizumab followed by 12 cycles of maintenance bevacizumab (7.5 mg/kg every 3 weeks). ICON 7 trial was closed to recruitment in Feb 2009 with a total number of 1528 patients involved. An addition of maintenance bevacizumab was found to improve PFS similar to GOG 218 trial. The progression-free survival (PFS) at 42 months was 22.4 months with standard therapy, as compared with 24.1 months with standard therapy plus bevacizumab (P = 0.04). In subgroup of patients with high risk for progression, the benefit was greater with bevacizumab; PFS of 14.4 months versus 18.1 months at 42 months. Bevacizumab was associated with more toxic effect (most often hypertension of grade 2 or higher); 18% versus 2%. In conclusion, bevacizumab improved progression-free survival in women with ovarian cancer (Perren et al., 2011).

ICON 6 is phase III trial evaluating the role of new antiangiogenesis (anti vascular endothelial growth factor receptor) known as Cediranib (Recentine) or AZD2171. Cediranib is an oral VEGF tyrosine kinase inhibitor. The subjects are patients with recurrent ovarian cancer (disease-free for more than 6 months). Study arm is the standard treatment (mostly paclitaxel/carboplatin or carboplatin) plus ceduranib with and without maintenance therapy (1 tablet daily for 18 months) and the control arm is standard therapy plus placebo. Maintenance therapy is given to all arms either in the form of ceduranib or placebo. The recruitment was started in 2007 and expected to be completed in December 2012. The median progression-free survival (PFS) was 8.7 months in the chemotherapy arm and 11.1 months in the Cediranib maintenance arm (HR, 0.57; p = 0.00001). When a restricted means analysis was done, the final result shows 3.1 month difference favoring Cediranib (9.4 months versus 12.5 months). Median overall survival was longer in Cediranib group, 20.3 months versus 17.6 months (p = 0.0042). However, Cediranib was associated with more treatment discontinuation, diarrhea and fatigue. Compared to bevacizumab, there was less hypertension in Cediranib.

EORTC 55041 or Tarceva Trial is phase III trial evaluating the role of an epidermal growth factor receptor inhibitors known as erlotinib in the management of high-risk stage 1, stage 2, 3 and 4 ovarian cancer. Erlotinib or Tarceva is EGFR inhibitor, given as once-daily, orally currently licensed for the treatment of advanced or metastatic Non small cell lung cancer and locally advanced, unresectable or metastatic pancreatic cancer. Patients in the control arm were given standard first line adjuvant chemotherapy, while in study group, apart from a standard chemotherapy regimen, oral Erlotinib 150 mg daily was given for up to 2 years. EORTC trial 55041 results show that maintenance erlotinib after first-line treatment in ovarian cancer did not improve progression-free survival (12.7 months in erlotinib versus 12.4 months in control) and overall survival. Due to the side-effects mainly rash, 26% of the patients in the erlotinib arm stopped maintenance treatment.

Trials on Alternative Regimen as First Line Chemotherapy in Ovarian Cancer

SCOTROC 1, 2A and 2B trials were evaluating the role of docetaxel as an alternative to paclitaxel in the treatment of patients with stage 1C, 2, 3 and 4 epithelial ovarian cancer, fallopian tube cancer and primary peritoneal carcinoma. SCOTROC 2A and 2B (phase II feasibility trial) were also evaluating the role of adding third drugs, i.e. gemcitabine (SCOTROC 2A) and irinotecan (SCOTROC 2B) to carboplatin–docetaxel regimens given in a sequential manner. Both trials were feasibility trial and further analysis, and studies need to be done in order to evaluate and identify the optimal sequence and drug combination (SCOTROC: Scottish Randomized Trial in Ovarian Cancer).

MITO2 Trial or Multi-Centric Italian Trials in Ovarian Cancer is the ongoing trial comparing carboplatin–paclitaxel (CP) versus carboplatin–liposomal doxorubicin (CD). Interim analysis showed carboplatin–liposomal doxorubicin regimen has similar activity with different toxicity profile compared to paclitaxel/carboplatin; haematological and neurological toxicities were more common in CP, while hair loss, skin toxicity and stomatitis were more common in CD (Pignata et al.).

Phase III trial by Japanese Oncologic Group compared carboplatin–weekly paclitaxel versus carboplatin–3-weekly paclitaxel showed significant improvement in PFS in a weekly-paclitaxel group. Dose for paclitaxel was 180 mg/m^2 (3 weekly regimen) and 80 mg/m^2 on Day 1, 8 and 15 for weekly regimen. Neutropenia and anaemia were more common in a weekly regimen (Isonishi et al.).

Triplets and sequential doublets are the other alternative that had been evaluated in the clinical trials. Combination of two cytotoxic drugs given once in a cycle is called a doublet. Triplet is when the third cytotoxic drug being added into the doublet. An addition of epirubicin to the carboplatin–paclitaxel regimen in at least three trials showed no improvement in overall survival (AGO-GINECO trial, NSGO-EORTC-NCIC trial). An addition of PLD every other course of carboplatin–paclitaxel in the GOG182 (ICON 5) trial also did not show any improvement in progression-free survival and overall survival. There was also no difference in PFS and OS in patients treated with topotecan and gemcitabine sequentially with a standard regimen. Study on the role of the triplet regimen was evaluated in AGO-OVAR-9-GINECO-NSGO study by du Bois et al. Paclitaxel 175 mg/m^2 and Carboplatin AUC 5 was given on day 1 versus Paclitaxel/Carboplatin plus Gemcitabine 800 mg/m^2, given on day 1 and day 8. The results of this study have shown that an addition of Gemcitabine into the standard Paclitaxel/Carboplatin regimen did not improve the progression-free survival and overall survival.

Bolis and colleagues have evaluated in multi-centre and randomized trial, the role of triplet in the postoperative management of patients with FIGO suboptimally (residual tumour ≥1 cm) resected stage III-IV epithelial ovarian cancer. The control arm was treated with a standard paclitaxel/carboplatin (every 3 weeks) regimen, while patients in the study arm were treated with topotecan/paclitaxel/carboplatin (topotecan 1.0 mg/m^2 daily for 3 days and paclitaxel/carboplatin on day 3, every 3 weeks). The authors concluded that based on the Cox regression model, there were no statistically significant differences in survival in both arms. Drug-related serious adverse events were higher in the triplets' arm. The findings were similar to analysis done by Gynaecologic Cancer InterGroup study (topotecan was given 1.25 mg/m^2) (Bookman et al., 2009). An addition of topotecan for four cycles following standard six cycles of the standard paclitaxel/carboplatin regimen was also found to have no impact on median survival

(Pfisterer et al., 2006). However, higher dose (1.25 mg–1.5 mg/m^2 given for 5 days) showed a tendency (although non-significant) of longer survival in patients with <1 cm residual disease.

Intraperitoneal Chemotherapy

Ovarian cancer is a disease that spread throughout the peritoneum and recurrent disease is generally confined to the peritoneum. Intraperitoneal chemotherapy is a rational strategy for a patient with no gross residual disease. Intraperitoneal chemotherapy was known since the 1950s and started to be implemented in 1978.

There are three methods of obtaining access to peritoneal cavity:

(a) single-use percutaneous catheter
(b) semipermanent percutaneous catheter
(c) implanted subcutaneous port and catheter

The catheter is inserted either at the time of primary debulking surgery or at delayed surgery by minilaparotomy or laparoscopy. The catheter is implanted in the left or right upper quadrant of the abdomen and tunnelled into the peritoneal cavity with the tip in the pelvis, cytotoxic drug (platinum or taxane is most commonly used) will be diluted with 2 L of saline (if using cisplatin) and infused into the peritoneal cavity followed by rolling the patients into four different positions every 15 minutes to disperse the drug (Walker et al., 2006; Gray et al., 2010). The drug reaches the tumours via direct exposure or through capillary flow after systemic absorption. The outer rim of peritoneal tumour will be exposed to a high level of drug by direct diffusion from the peritoneal surface while the inner core of tumour will be targeted by cytotoxic drugs in microcirculation.

The advantages of intraperitoneal chemotherapy are direct contact of the peritoneum with cytotoxic drug, expose to higher concentration, longer exposure and fewer systemic side-effects. The problem is to ensure even distribution of drug in the peritoneal cavity. This is always hindered (20–30% of cases) by adhesions. Examples of cytotoxic drugs that can be administered intraperitoneally are cisplatin and paclitaxel.

SWOG/GOG-104 trial (the **Abert study**, $N = 546$) compared IV cisplatin plus IV cyclophosphamide versus IV cyclophosphamide plus intraperitoneal cisplatin demonstrated survival advantage but higher complication rate in the intraperitoneal arm (Albert et al., 1996). The GOG-114/SWOG trial (the **Markman study**, $N = 462$) compared IV cisplatin-IV paclitaxel versus IV carboplatin followed by intraperitoneal cisplatin plus IV paclitaxel. There was a significant difference in progression-free survival but no significant improvement of overall survival. Due to different platinum dose higher toxicity, the authors concluded that this schedule should not be recommended (Markman 2001). GOG 172 trial (the **Armstrong study**, $N = 415$) studied the role of intraperitoneal chemotherapy (IV paclitaxel 135 mg/m^2 over 24 hours infusion followed by day 2 intraperitoneal cisplatin 100 mg/m^2 and day 8 intraperitoneal paclitaxel 80 mg/m^2 versus standard IV cisplatin 75 mg/m^2 plus IV paclitaxel 135 mg/m^2 in 24 hour infusions). This study had shown that intraperitoneal chemotherapy improved the overall median survival as compared to the standard regimen (16 months longer than the intravenous control arm) (Amstrong et al., 2006). A systematic review by Cochrane Collaboration showed that intraperitoneal chemotherapy when incorporate into the first line chemotherapy regimen was associated with a significant reduction in the risk of progression (HR: 0.79) and death (HR: 0.80) (Jaaback and Johnson).

Intraperitoneal chemotherapy, however, is associated with higher treatment-related complications, including catheter complications (obstruction, infection, bowel perforation, fistula), nausea, abdominal discomfort, systemic toxicity due to higher absorption into the blood stream, etc. There was significantly more grade 3 and 4 toxicity for leucopenia, neuropathy, gastrointestinal infection, fatigue and pain in an intraperitoneal therapy group. Patients receiving the intraperitoneal therapy regimen also had a worse quality of life during the first year of treatment as compared to the intravenous group. Studies on fewer toxic regimen (e.g., using paclitaxel in 3 hours instead of 24 hour infusions, using carboplatin instead of cisplatin, etc.) are still ongoing, including an addition of bevacizumab into the study arm. At present, women with ovarian cancer should not be subjected to intraperitoneal chemotherapy outside the context of a properly designed clinical trial.

Hyperthermia Intraperitoneal Chemotherapy (HIPEC)

The concept of hyperthermia intraperitoneal chemotherapy was first described by Dr. John Spratt from the University of Louisville in 1979. HIPEC was originally used for the treatment of pseudomyxoma peritonei. HIPEC is only suitable in patients who had complete cytoreductive surgery and the procedure is performed in the operating theatre after completion of cytoreductive surgery. Large volume of chemotherapy solution is instilled into the peritoneal cavity and the tumour beds in the peritoneal surfaces will be exposed to direct cytotoxic agents for 60–90 minutes. Heat is applied to the solution under temperature between 42–43°C. The advantage of hyperthermia is that it can increase the penetration of chemotherapy into the tissues. It also has a direct effect to cancer cells and the heat can increase the cytotoxicity of the selected chemotherapy agents.

There are two techniques in HIPEC: (a) Open abdominal technique and (b) Close abdominal technique.

Open Abdominal Technique

The open abdominal technique is also known as "Coliseum technique". The abdomen is left open and the chemotherapy solution will be perfused under high temperature maintained at 42–43°C. The duration of exposure is about 90 minutes and all the anatomic structure within the peritoneal cavity will be uniformly exposed to heat and chemotherapy. Before closure of the incision, the solution will be drained out from the peritoneal cavity and vaginal cuff must be closed to avoid leakage of the remaining chemotherapy solution. The advantages of open technique are better distribution of chemotherapy solution and tissue penetration. However, the open technique had higher systemic absorption of chemotherapy agent (Deballon et al., 2010).

Close Abdominal Technique

In the close abdominal technique, the inflow (with temperature probe) and outflow tubing will be placed into the peritoneal cavity and skin closure is done. Both tubings will be passed through the incision. With the wound closed, the inflow and outflow tubing is connected, and the preheated peritoneal dialysis solution is allowed to fill the cavity. When the temperature is maintained at approximately 42°C, the chemotherapy is added into the solution and allowed to circulate for 90 minutes. Subsequently, abdomen will be reopened and the chemotherapy solutions is drained out and irrigation of the peritoneal cavity is performed using saline solution. Abdomen is closed in layers. The advantages of closed technique are less exposure of the staff to chemotherapy solution, less potential contamination of environment to chemotherapy and better temperature control.

Maintenance Therapy

Maintenance therapy is an extension of chemotherapy to as long as 12 months in order to improve progression-free survival and overall survival. Maintenance therapy is also called consolidation therapy and the role of maintenance therapy is still controversial. SWOG-GOG phase III trial, randomized patients with advanced ovarian cancer who had achieved a complete response after five to six cycles of chemotherapy into two groups: The first group received additional three cycles and the second group received another 12 cycles. Significant improvement in PFS was observed in the second group. However, there were no differences in overall survival (Markman et al.). Paclitaxel is the most common cytotoxic drug used in maintenance therapy. Maintenance therapy was associated with higher rate of toxicity mainly neurotoxicity. A number of other treatments have been tested as maintenance therapies in ovarian cancer such as the INF-alpha, gefinitib, erlotinib, interleukin-2 and 13-cis-retinoic acid combination, goserelin, bevacizumab, liposomal doxorubicin and altretamine. The results from these studies were variable. More research is needed to determine the most efficacious and cost-effective approach. Ongoing trial such as GOG 212 will be the key in establishing overall survival benefits of paclitaxel maintenance therapy.

Neoadjuvant Chemotherapy

Nearly all retrospective and prospective studies have confirmed that the extent of cytoreductive surgery and the amount of residual disease are among the most important factors to determine the survival of women with advanced ovarian cancer. An optimal surgery which is defined as leaving residual tumour of less than 1 cm is not always possible, especially in old patients, patients with poor co-morbidity and extensive tumour bulks. Neoadjuvant chemotherapy is an approach to medically cytoreduced the tumour in order to increase the proportion of patients with advanced ovarian cancer to achieve optimal cytoreduction after subsequent surgical treatment. Cytoreduction performed after neoadjuvant chemotherapy is also called interval cytoreduction (IDS). Interval debulking surgery is usually performed after two to four cycles of chemotherapy. After IDS, chemotherapy will be continued.

The potential benefits of neoadjuvant chemotherapy are (a) reduced the risk of perioperative morbidity (e.g., lesser blood lost, a lower requirement of intensive care unit admission, shorter duration of hospital stay, etc.), (b) higher rate of optimal cytoreduction (ranging from 77–94%), (c) facilitation of the response of any residual tumour to subsequent chemotherapy and (d) better quality of life (Chan).

Despite above benefits, there is still no solid evidence that neoadjuvant chemotherapy and interval cytoreduction improved survival. Many systematic reviews and meta-analysis have shown conflicting results of neoadjuvant chemotherapy. This is probably due to lack of good prospective randomized control trials. Many of the trials were non-randomized and phase 1–2 trials. Apart from that, there was also an absence of widely accepted chemotherapy schedule and selection criteria.

The selection criteria for neoadjuvant chemotherapy reported in many studies are

(a) "unresectable" disease on CT scans, e.g., massive ascites, pleural effusion
(b) dense adhesion between bowel, mesentery and omentum
(c) omental disease extending to spleen
(d) large diaphragm disease
(e) multiple bowel involvement
(f) PERITONEAL carcinomatosis
(g) porta hepatis disease
(h) extensive disease in liver surface

Study had shown that CT scan is not reliable in predicting suboptimal cytoreduction. Laparoscopy is probably reliable and more accurate in assessing operability than CT scan, but it's required anaesthesia and invasive procedure. Furthermore, magnification of the tumour through laparoscopy can mislead the surgeon that the tumour is unresectable.

Diagnosis of ovarian cancer prior to neoadjuvant chemotherapy is important. The accuracy of cytologic diagnosis (from peritoneal fluid, pleural fluid or FNAC) was found to be as good as histologic diagnosis in the diagnosis of epithelial ovarian cancer prior to neoadjuvant chemotherapy (92–98% accuracy). Clinical prediction using imaging and tumour markers were less accurate (Freedman et al.). In gynaecologic oncology centres, when the selection is done by the gynaecologic oncologist, 10–20% of patients with advanced ovarian cancer fulfil the above criteria. Phase III randomized controlled trial by Rose et al. (GOG trial) involving 550 patients with stage 3 and 4 epithelial ovarian cancer that had a residual disease >1 cm after an initial attempt of surgical cytoreduction. All patients will be subjected to three cycles of chemotherapy. Those with no disease progression will be further assigned either secondary cytoreduction or continue with same chemotherapy. The study had shown that there was no difference in terms of PFS and risk of death in both groups. Few meta-analyses reported inferior survival rate among patients treated with neoadjuvant chemotherapy as compared to primary surgery. In their meta-analysis, Bristow et al. found that survival outcome was inversely proportional to an increasing number of preoperative chemotherapy cycles, with each additional cycle associated with a 4.1-month reduction in median survival. This could be due to increasing number of cycles will promote the development of chemo-resistant cell clones.

A Cochrane Systematic Review by Tangjitgamol et al. assessing the effectiveness of interval debulking surgery reported that they could not conclude whether interval debulking surgery following adjuvant chemotherapy would improve the survival of women with advanced epithelial ovarian cancer. IDS appeared to yield a benefit only in the patients whose primary surgery was not performed by expert surgeons. The results of EORTC 55971 trial was released in September 2010. In this trial, 670 patients with biopsy-proven stage 3C or 4 ovarian carcinoma, primary peritoneal carcinoma or fallopian tube carcinoma were randomly assigned to receive either primary debulking surgery followed by platinum-based chemotherapy or to receive neoadjuvant platinum-based chemotherapy followed by interval debulking surgery and then platinum-based chemotherapy. There was no difference in a survival rate between both study arms. However, neoadjuvant chemotherapy followed by interval debulking surgery was associated with a lower postoperative mortality, shorter operation time, less grade 3 haemorrhage, venous complications and infections. The authors note that whenever debulking surgery is performed either as primary treatment or following NACT, complete resection of all macroscopic tumours was the strongest independent variable predicting overall survival (Vergote et al.). At least two major studies (Randomized phase III trials) are conducted to evaluate the efficacy of neoadjuvant chemotherapy, i.e. CHORUS (Chemotherapy or Upfront Surgery) and Japan Clinical Oncology Group study (JCOG 0602). CHORUS is the second phase III randomized controlled trial to investigate timing of initial surgery in ovarian cancer presented at stage III-IV. The study arm was treated with 3 cycles of neo-adjuvant chemotherapy followed by surgery and continue another 3 cycles chemotherapy after surgery. The authors concluded that neoadjuvant chemotherapy was associated with increased optimal debulking, less early mortality and similar survival (progression-free survival and 3 years overall survival). This results are consistent with EORTC55971. In JCOG 0602, a total of 8 cycles of chemotherapy were given, in neoadjuvant chemotherapy arm, 4 cycles were given prior to interval surgery. This trial completed accrual in 2011. There are still remaining questions unanswered with regards to neoadjuvant chemotherapy (NACT) in ovarian cancer: (1) criteria for best candidate for NACT, (2) duration and number of cycles of chemotherapy prior to surgery, (3) duration and number of cycles of chemotherapy after surgery and (4) whether the failure to achieve optimal cytoreductive surgery is to due to the result of the surgeon's skill or cancer biology.

Recurrent Ovarian Cancer

At least 75% of patients with advanced disease will respond to first line therapy (clinical complete response in 50% of cases, i.e.

clinically, radiologically and biochemically (CA125). Only one third will have surgically confirmed complete response on second look laparotomy following platinum based chemotherapy. Even with surgically confirmed complete remission, 30–50% will ultimately experience recurrence. Almost 80% of recurrent ovarian cancer occurs during the first 2 years of diagnosis.

Among the patients with recurrent disease, only 30–40% will respond to second line chemotherapy but only 10% will achieve clinical complete remission and median survival <1 year. Approximately, 60% of patients with recurrent ovarian cancer will die within 5 years of diagnosis. The prognosis is poorer in platinum-resistant ovarian cancer.

Patients with recurrent ovarian cancer can be categorized into two groups:

(a) Platinum-sensitive group, when the disease-free interval is more than 6 months.

(b) Platinum-resistant group, when the disease-free interval is less than 6 months.

Refractory ovarian cancer is when the cancer is progressing despite treatment. Patients do not have a disease-free period. Both platinum-resistant and refractory ovarian cancers are managed in the same manner; however, the survival outcome is poor. A rising of CA125 level can predict tumour progression many months prior to clinical evidence of recurrence. This rising can accurately predict recurrence in 95% of patients. Treatment for patients with rising CA125 without clinical evidence of recurrence is unknown. Chemotherapy and hormonal therapy (antioestrogen, e.g., Tamoxifen) did not improve the survival in this group of patients.

Treatment of Platinum-Sensitive Patients

Patients are categorized as platinum-sensitive when their disease-free interval is ≥6 months. Some researchers use 12 months as cut-off point between platinum-sensitive and platinum-resistant ovarian cancer. Majority of patients with advanced ovarian cancer will develop recurrence within 2 years of treatment.

There are three options for patients with platinum-sensitive disease:

(a) secondary cytoreduction/debulking
(b) chemotherapy (re-challenging with a similar chemotherapy regimen)
(c) combination

Secondary Cytoreduction for Platinum-Sensitive Patients

Secondary cytoreduction is defined as an operative procedure performed at some time remote from the completion of primary therapy with the intended purpose of tumour reduction. The clinical utility of secondary cytoreduction is still controversial. Meta-analysis by Bristow et al. on the role of cytoreductive surgery for recurrent ovarian cancer had found that among patients undergoing operative intervention for recurrent ovarian cancer, the proportion of patients undergoing complete cytoreductive surgery is independently associated with overall post-recurrence survival time. Each 10% increase in the proportion of patients of undergoing complete cytoreductive surgery was associated with 3 months increase in median overall survival.

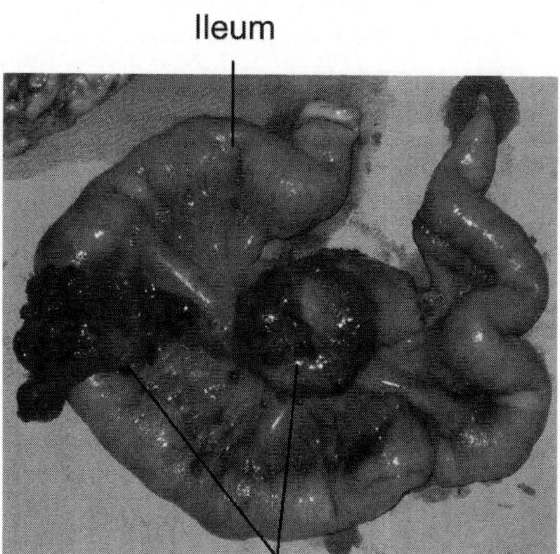

Figure 12.7 Resection of the small bowel to achieve completed surgical resection.

Based on available data, secondary cytoreduction is best considered in patients with following characteristics:

(a) disease-free interval at least 6–12 months
(b) response to frontline chemotherapy
(c) younger age group
(d) good performance status
(e) the tumour is potentially resectable with minimal residual diseases.

Chemotherapy for Platinum-Sensitive Patients

Patients with platinum-sensitive ovarian cancer can be re-challenged with the same chemotherapy regimen. Combination treatment with platinum–paclitaxel doublets shows better survival benefit compared to single-agent platinum. Response rate was 66% in doublet as compared to 54% in single agent platinum group. The hazard ratio for overall survival was 0.82, which was statistically significant. There was no difference in quality of life between study and control arm (ICON 4/AGO-OVA 2.2). The probability of response to re-challenging of chemotherapy is closely related to the duration of platinum-free interval, generally ranging from 20–30% if the disease-free was 6–12 months and >60% if disease-free was >12 months.

Options of chemotherapy for platinum-sensitive tumour

Combination of paclitaxel/carboplatin is the first choice regimen for patients who were treated with a paclitaxel and carboplatin during their first presentation. The overall response rate was ranging from 75% to 90% and median times to progression of approximately 9 months.

Docetaxel as a substitute to paclitaxel was proposed in the SCOTROC trial. Scottish Randomized Trial in Ovarian Cancer (SCOTROC) by Vasey et al., which recruited more than 1000 patients and compared carboplatin–paclitaxel versus carboplatin–docetaxel, showed no difference in PFS and overall survival. Paclitaxel was found to be more neurotoxic but docetaxel was more haematotoxic with higher rate of neutropenic sepsis (11%).

In Gynecologic Cancer InterGroup trial known as AGO-OVAR trial, carboplatin AUC 4 plus Gemcitabine 1000 mg/m^2 on days 1 and

8 was compared with single agent carboplatin AUC 5. The results showed combination carboplatin–gemcitabine had significantly higher response rate (47.2% versus 30.9%) and significantly longer progression-free survival (8.6 versus 5.8 months). Impact on overall survival was unknown (Pfisterer et al.).

Combination carboplatin plus PLD (doxorubicin encapsulated in liposomes and coated with methoxypolyethylene glycol) was evaluated in GINECO trial. In GINECO trial, platinum-sensitive patients were treated with combination of carboplatin AUC 5 and pegylated liposomal doxorubicin (PLD) 30 mg/m^2 every 4 weeks. Overall response rate was 63% with 38% of patients demonstrating a complete response (Ferrero et al.). The trial known as **CALYPSO/ AGO-OVAR 2.9 trial** was launched by Gynecologic Cancer InterGroup (GCIG) had completed recruiting 976 patients (carboplatin AUC 5 and liposomal doxorubicin 30 mg/m^2 versus carboplatin AUC 5 and paclitaxel 175 mg/m^2). Final analysis of CALYPSO study had found that median PFS was significantly more superior in PLD–carboplatin arm compared to paclitaxel–carboplatin arm (11.3 vs. 9.4 months, $p = 0.005$). Safety and toxicity profile in PLD–carboplatin arm was found to be better than paclitaxel–carboplatin arm (well tolerated and lower rates of severe and long-term (neuropathy) toxicities in PLD arm). Single agent PLD was found to be better than single agent topotecan as a second line chemotherapy in platinum-sensitive epithelial ovarian cancer in phase III trial by Gordon A.

The other combination chemotherapy is carboplatin plus topotecan that was evaluated in phase III trial (OV16). The study compared combination carboplatin–topotecan versus carboplatin–paclitaxel in platinum-sensitive patients; the results showed no difference in terms of progression-free survival but carboplatin-topotecan arm was associated with more toxicity, especially haematological toxicity (Bookman et al.). Reported rate of severe myelosupression in topotecan arm was grade 3–4 neutropenia (50–59%), grade 3 thrombocytopenia (12%) and grade 3 anaemia (24%).

GOG182/ICON 5 Phase III randomized controlled trial comparing standard carboplatin–paclitaxel versus carboplatin (sequence or combination) with either gemcitabine, topotecan or liposomal doxorubicin had found no improvements in progression-free survival or overall survival in all study arms as compared to standard combination carboplatin–paclitaxel (Bookman et al.).

The other systemic therapy that may have potential role in ovarian cancer is targeted therapy. ICON 6 is a phase III randomized control trial evaluating the role of new antiangiogenesis (anti-vascular endothelial growth factor receptor) known as Cediranib (Recentine) or AZD2171. The subjects are patients with platinum-sensitive recurrent ovarian cancer. Study arm is standard treatment (mostly paclitaxel/carboplatin or carboplatin) plus Cediranib with and without maintenance therapy (1 tablet daily for 18 months) and the control arm is a standard therapy plus placebo. Maintenance therapy is given to all arms either in the form of Cediranib or placebo. The results of this study have shown that patients in Cediranib group had slightly longer progression-free survival (3 months different) compared to standard chemotherapy group.

Treatment for Platinum-Resistant and Refractory Epithelial Ovarian Cancer

Ovarian cancer is recognized to be a chemosensitive malignant tumour as majority of patients will be experiencing both objective and subjective benefit following therapy with first line chemotherapy. However, recurrence rate is common and approximately 50% of these patients will develop resistance to first line chemotherapy.

Platinum-resistant epithelial ovarian cancer is when the disease-free is less than 6 months, while patients with refractory epithelial ovarian cancer have no disease-free, i.e. the disease persists or progress despite treatment. Patients with platinum-resistant ovarian cancer has poorer prognosis and median overall survival for 2 years is only 23%; only 5% will survive after 2 years (Markman et al., 2004). Patients who develop resistance and not responding to platinum and paclitaxel during initial chemotherapy have a lower response to second line therapy. For most patients, the appropriate choice of second-line treatment consists of single agents, while combined regimens reserved to patients who have prolonged disease-free interval.

The standard of care for platinum-resistant epithelial ovarian cancer is either one or combination of following options:

(a) second line chemotherapy
(b) biologic therapy/novel therapeutic approach
(c) palliative care

Chemotherapy for Platinum-Resistant and Refractory Ovarian Cancer

Topotecan

Topotecan is topoisomerase I inhibitor and has been approved by the FDA for the treatment of relapsed epithelial ovarian cancer. The dosage is 1.5 mg/m^2/day for 5 days as a single agent. Response rate was between 6–23%. In a phase III trial by Gordon et al., comparing topotecan and PLD in the treatment of platinum-resistant/refractory ovarian cancer, there was no difference in progression-free survival and overall survival but haematological toxicity were significantly higher with topotecan. Weekly topotecan has been evaluated to reduce the risk of neutropenia (4 mg/m^2 weekly). Sehouli et al. presented the results of TOWER trial (multi-centre trial of the North-Eastern German Society of Gynaecological Oncology) comparing weekly topotecan (4 mg/m^2, D1, 8, 15 every 28 days) versus topotecan 1.25 mg/m^2 day 1–5 every 21 days). Patients were with platinum-resistant tumour. Weekly administration was found to have lower likelihood of severe haematological toxicity without compromising the efficacy.

Gemcitibine

Gemcitabine was approved by the FDA for treatment of pancreatic cancer. Gemcitabine is administered in a weekly interval using a dose of 800–1000 mg/m^2. Response rate for platinum-resistant epithelial ovarian cancer is between 15–20%. Generally, gemcitabine is well tolerated but a major side effect is grade 3–4 neutropenia.

Pegylated Lyposomal Doxorubicin

Pegylated liposomal doxorubicin was approved by the FDA in 2005 for treatment of relapse epithelial ovarian cancer. Pegylated liposomal doxorubicin is a formulation of doxorubicin encapsulated in liposomes and coated with methoxypolyethylene glycol. This formulation will improve the drug delivery and reduce the toxicity profile of doxorubicin, mainly cardiotoxicity. The incidence of myelosuppression, vomiting and alopecia are also less than with PLD as compared to doxorubicin. However, PLD is associated with higher risk of mucositis and palmar-plantar erythrodysesthesia (PPE). The dose of PLD is 40–50 mg/m^2 every 4 weeks. A response rate is between 18–25% in the platinum-resistant group.

Oral Etoposide

Oral etoposide is given 50 mg/m^2/day for 21 days as a second line chemotherapy. GOG study by Rose PG reported response rate of 26.8% with oral etoposide as a second line chemotherapy for platinum-resistant epithelial ovarian cancer. However, the major toxicity or oral etoposide is bone marrow suppression with 45% of patients developed grade 3–4 neutropenia.

Paclitaxel and Docetaxel

The mechanism of drug resistance is different between paclitaxel and platinum. Patients with platinum-resistant tumour may still respond to non-platinum drug in the regimen. Single agent paclitaxel can be acceptable second line chemotherapy in patients with platinum-resistant/refractory ovarian cancer even if the first line chemotherapy was platinum–paclitaxel combination. Several studies using weekly paclitaxel 80 mg/m^2 in 1 hour infusion have achieved objective response rate 10–20% in a patient with platinum-resistant ovarian cancer. With this regimen, neurotoxicity was reported to be less common as compared to single higher dose regimen. Docetaxel is an alternative to paclitaxel. In phase 2 trial using Docetaxel (30–40 mg/m^2 weekly) in platinum-refractory ovarian cancer, the reported response rate was between 6.9% and 18.9% (Berkenblit et al., 2004; Markman et al., 2003; Tinker et al., 2007). Weekly administration with lower dose paclitaxel and docetaxel were found to be less neurotoxic and haematotoxic, respectively, as compared to a higher dose regimen at 3-weekly interval.

Second Look Laparotomy/Laparoscopy

Surgical treatment is a reasonable option for certain patients with recurrent ovarian cancer. However, there is no evidence that any type of surgical procedure after initial chemotherapy prolongs overall survival. In many patients, the signs of recurrent cancer manifested late and in some, increasing level of the biomarker is the earliest clue. Biomarkers in ovarian cancer are non-specific and further evaluation is needed to confirm the recurrent cancer.

Second look laparotomy is defined as "*systemic surgical exploration in asymptomatic patients who have completed a planned course of chemotherapy for ovarian cancer.*"

Second look surgery was formerly indicated in patients who have no monitoring parameter clinically, radiologically or biochemically. Formerly, laparotomy was the method of choice for second look surgery. Laparoscopy could be an alternative but 55% of patients with negative laparoscopic evaluation were found to have the residual disease on subsequent laparotomy. In contrast, about 62% of patients with normal CA125 on follow-up were found to have a residual/persistent tumour on laparotomy.

Techniques of Second Look Laparotomy

Following is the step-by-step technique of second look laparotomy:

(1) Just prior to surgery, perform examination under anaesthesia
(2) Cystoscopy and proctoscopy in selected patients with relevant symptoms and previously had bladder/rectal involvement
(3) Extended midline abdominal incision
(4) Peritoneal wash for cytology
(5) Frozen section done for suspected tumour recurrence
(6) Removed tumour as much as possible
(7) If no tumour, undertake a systematic and meticulous search
(8) Adhesion should be released and excised for HPE
(9) Random biopsies should be taken from
    Stumps of infundibular pelvic ligaments
    Other suspicious pelvic pedicles
    Hysterectomy
    Remaining omentum

Peritoneum

Pelvic and para-aortic lymphadenectomy

(10) A laparoscope can be used to inspect undersurface of the diaphragm

About 55% of patients with no clinical evidence of recurrence were found to have cancer presence at second look laparotomy. The main determinants to the positive second look are stage, initial tumour volume and residual tumour during primary surgery. Findings on second look laparotomy can forecast the patient's survival. Patients with microscopic disease have 2-year and 5-year survival rates of 96% and 71%, respectively. Of the patients with bulky tumour on the second look, 80% died within 3 years. Second look laparotomy, however, has very limited role because (a) invasive technique with potential complications, (b) false negative result, (c) treatment (second line therapy) in a patient with a positive second look does not prolong survival and (d) lack of prospective control trial. Retrospective trial had shown similar survival in patients with and without second look laparotomy. The benefit of secondary cytoreductive operation (in 40% of patients) at second look laparotomy has not been clearly demonstrated in terms of survival benefits. Secondary cytoreductive during second look laparotomy may be indicated in patients whose tumours remain sensitive to first line chemotherapy (platinum-sensitive ovarian cancer).

Novel Anticancer Agents for Platinum-Resistant/Refractory Epithelial Ovarian Cancer

In general, patients with recurrent ovarian cancer in particularly platinum-resistant group have poor prognosis and their response to second line chemotherapy is less than 30% despite dose modification, different combinations and schedules of existing anticancer drugs. Surgical treatment in ovarian cancer has improved and this has contributed to marginal improvement in progression-free survival and overall survival; however, major improvement will likely require new therapies using new cytotoxic drugs, biological agents or targeted therapy.

There are at least two new therapies undergoing evaluation for ovarian carcinoma:

(a) Novel cytotoxic agents
(b) Targeted agents

Novel Cytotoxic Agents

Epothilones

Epothilones are natural (bacterial) microtubule stabilization agents obtained from mycobacterium *S. cellulosum*. Epothilones have similar mode of action with taxanes. At least five epothilones are currently in clinical trial, i.e. patupilone, ixabepilone, BMS-310705, KOS-862 and ZK-EPO. In vitro study showed epothilone is more active than taxane. This new cytotoxic agent was investigated in patients with recurrent ovarian cancer resistant to taxane. Patupilone was evaluated in phase III trial compared with PLD in refractory/relapsed ovarian carcinoma (Study NCT00262990). A total of 829 patients were randomly assigned to received patupilone (10 mg/m^2 intravenously every 3 weeks) or pegylated liposomal doxorubicin (PLD) 50 mg/m^2 intravenously every 4 weeks. There was no significant improvement in overall survival between two groups. Frequently observed adverse events of any grade included diarrhea (85.3%) and peripheral neuropathy (39.3%) in the patupilone arm and mucositis/stomatitis (43%) and hand-foot syndrome (41.8%) in the PLD arm (Colombo et al., 2012).

Canfosfamide (Telcyta TLK286)

Overexpression of glutathione S-transferase P1-1 (GST P1-1) after an initiation of chemotherapy is associated with chemo-resistance to alkylating and platinum agent. Canfosfamide is a glutathione prodrug activated by GST capable of inducing apoptosis. ASSIST-3 phase III trial by Rose et al. evaluating canfosfamide plus carboplatin versus PLD as second line therapy for platinum-resistant ovarian cancer. Overall PFS was comparable. ASSIST-5 trial (ASSIST: Assessment of Survival In Solid Tumour) compared PLD versus PLD plus canfosfamide versus carboplatin–canfosfamide, results are pending. The results was presented at the 45th Annual Meeting of the

American Society of Clinical Oncology (ASCO). Patients with platinum refractory or resistant ovarian cancer with measurabl disease were eligible for enrollment in the trial. In study arm, intravenous Canfosfamide HCl (TELCYTA), 1000 mg/m^2, was combined with PLD (50 mg/m^2). This regime was compared with PLD alone. The median survival in the platinum refractory and primary platinum resistant population showed a positive trend in survival for the TELCYTA plus PLD arm (11.8 months versus 7.8 months). The TELCYTA plus PLD arm also achieved shorter median time to respose and longer duration of stable disease (7.4 versus 4.1 months, HR = 0.49, p = 0.0439). There was higher incidence of haematologic adverse events in patients on the TELCYTA plus PLD arm (66% vs 44%).

Yondelis (ET-743)

Yondelis is also known as trabectedin. Yondelis is a marine-derived compound from Ecteinascidia turinate. It can be now being produced synthetically. Yondelis binds to DNA and distorting its structure inducing apoptosis and cell cycle arrest. Yondelis has demonstrated clinical activity in soft tissue sarcoma, ovarian, prostate and breast cancer. Pooled phase II trials have shown that overall response rate of Yondelis for platinum-resistant and platinum-sensitive patients were 8% and 34%, respectively (McMeekin et al.; Del Campo et al.; Sessa et al.). Main toxicity was grade 3–4 neutropenia in more than 40% of patients. Phase III study NCT00113607 is ongoing and is evaluating single agent (PLD) versus PLD-Yondelis. Recent results from OVA-301 phase III randomized trial evaluating trabectedin plus PLD showed the longest medial overall survival ever reported in partially platinum-sensitive patients (23 months). Partially platinum-sensitive patients are patients with disease free interval between 6–12 months following first line chemotherapy (Sehouli et al., 2012).

Phenoxodiol

Phenoxodiol is an isoflavone analog, under new class of anticancer drugs known as multiple signal transduction regulators. It induces cancer cell death through inhibition of antiapoptotic protein, including XIAP (X-linked inhibitor of apoptosis protein). XIAP was shown to be overexpressed in chemo-resistant cells. Phenoxodiol can interfere with XIAP activity. OVATURE trial (Ovarian Tumour Response trial) is ongoing multi-centre, randomized phase III trial comparing phenoxodiol-carboplatin versus carboplati-placebo in patients with refractory/resistant ovarian cancer.

Targeted Agents

Targeted cancer therapies are drugs or other substances that block the growth and spread of cancer by interfering with specific molecules involved in tumour growth and progression. FDA has approved many targeted cancer therapies. Antioestrogen is perhaps one of the earliest targeted therapies approved by FDA. Tamoxifen was approved for the treatment of breast cancer by binding to the oestrogen receptor and promote destruction of cancer cells. Various targeted agents, have been explored in the management of ovarian cancer.

Angiogenesis is one of the most important processes in tumour invasion and metastasis. Angiogenesis is triggered by vascular endothelial growth factors (VEGF) released by cancer cells. Increased level of VEGF in ovarian cancer has been associated with poor prognosis. Agents targeting angiogenesis is called anti-angiogenesis.

There are at least three categories of anti-angiogenesis agents:

(a) monoclonal antibodies to VEGF ligand
(b) tyrosine kinase inhibitor
(c) soluble decoy VEGF receptors

The other group of targeted therapies is anti-epithelial growth factor Receptors (EGFR). Most of the targeted therapies have more than one mode of action.

In general, all targeted therapies can be classified into two main groups:

(1) Monoclonal Antibodies, which are large molecule inhibitors
(2) Small-molecule inhibitors

Monoclonal Antibody (Large Molecule Inhibitors)

Monoclonal antibody with larger molecules (Large molecule inhibitors) and targets extracellular component such as ligand and receptor. The route of administration of this group is intravenous.

Bevacizumab (Avastin)

Bevacizumab is a recombinant humanized monoclonal antibody against VEGF. At least 5 phase II prospective trials of bevacizumab (dosage: 10–15 mg/kg every 2–3 weeks) in recurrent ovarian cancer (both platinum-sensitive and platinum-resistant) have been conducted either as single agent or combination with cytotoxic chemotherapy. Overall response rate was between 15% and 24%. Two phase III randomized controlled trials comparing a standard first line regimen versus a first line regimen plus bevacizumab have completed their recruitment in 2009 (GOG 218 and ICON-7) GOG 218 and ICON 7 have demonstrated a modest improvement in progression-free survival when bevacizumab was added to initial chemotherapy and continued every 3 weeks for 16 and 12 additional cycles, respectively, as a maintenance phase. Another two phase III randomized trials evaluating the role of Bevaizumab in patients with platinum-sensitive recurrent diseases are GOG 213 and OCEANS trial. OCEANS trial (Ovarian Cancer Study Comparing Efficacy and Safety of Chemotherapy and Anti-Agiogenic Therapy) is double blind, placebo-controlled, phase III trial of chemotherapy (Gemcitabine plus carboplatin) with or without Bevacizumab. Patients were platinum-sensitive recurrent ovarian cancer, fallopian tube cancer and primary peritoneal carcinoma. Median PFS for patients receiving bevacizumab was 12.4 months versus 8.4 months for those receiving a placebo. Objective responses to chemotherapy were increased when combined with bevacizumab (78.5% vs. 57.4%, $p < 0.0001$) (Aghajanian et al., 2012). Bowel perforation is one of the most important life-threatening side-effect of bevacizumab and this complication is more common in ovarian cancer (5.4%). Bevacizumab is yet to be approved by the FDA for this indication.

Cetuximab (Erbitux)

Cetuximab is a monoclonal antibody that binds to EGFR, preventing the receptor from being activated by growth signals, which may inhibit signal transduction and lead to antiproliferative effects. Cetuximab is approved for head and neck cancer as well as some colorectal cancer. Few studies on the role of cetuximab in recurrent ovarian cancer and also as third agent in first line chemotherapy regimen were conducted and the results were promising.

Trastuzumab (Herceptin)

Trastuzumab is a monoclonal antibody that binds to the human epidermal growth factor receptor 2 (HER-2). HER-2 is expressed in high level in some breast cancer. Trastuzumab binds to HER-2 on the surface of cancer cell and prevents HER-2 from sending growth-promoting signals.

Small-Molecule Inhibitors

Small-molecule inhibitors enter cells, thereby blocking receptor signalling (mainly tyrosine kinase) and interfering with downstream intracellular molecules. Tyrosine kinase signalling initiates a molecular cascade that leads to cell growth, proliferation, migration and angiogenesis in normal and malignant tissues. As compared to large molecule Inhibitors, small-molecule inhibitors are commonly administered in oral form and cheaper than large molecule inhibitors.

Imatinib Mesylate (Gleevec)

Imatinib mesylate targets several members of a class of proteins called tyrosine kinase enzymes that participate in signal transduction. So far, Imatinib mesylate has been evaluated in several phase II trials on recurrent ovarian cancer but the activities were minimal. Combination with anticytotoxic or anti-angiogenic agents may produce better results. Imatinib is approved for treatment of gastrointestinal stromal tumour and certain leukaemia.

Gefitinib (Iressa)

Gefitinib is a small-molecule drug inhibits the tyrosine kinase activity of the epidermal growth factor receptor (EGFR). A pilot study by Hariprasad et al. showed that an overall response rate of the combination of gefitinib and paclitaxel/carboplatin regimen in patients with platinum-refractory and platinum-sensitive ovarian cancer was 19.2% and 61.9%, respectively.

Erlotinib (Tarceva, OS1774)

Erlotinib is the also small-molecule drug inhibits the tyrosine kinase activity of EGFR. Phase III multi-centric randomized trial evaluating the role of maintenance therapy with erlotinib after first line platinum-based chemotherapy for ovarian cancer had completed recruiting in 2008. In the study arm, Erlotinib is taken orally (150 mg daily) for up to 2 years. This phase III trial is known as EORTC trial 55041. Results from EORTC trial 55041 have shown that maintenance erlotinib after first-line treatment in ovarian cancer did not improve progression-free survival (12.7 months in erlotinib versus 12.4 months in control) and overall survival. Due to the side-effects mainly rash, 26% of the patients in the erlotinib arm stopped maintenance treatment. Side-effects of erlotinib are diarrhoea, skin rashes and neutropenic sepsis.

Sorafenib (Nexavar, BAY 43-0006)

Sorafenib is an oral small-molecule multi-kinase inhibitor that inhibits VEGF receptor 1/2/3. Sorafenib also blocks an enzyme that is involved in cell growth and division. Sorafenib is currently approved for the treatment of advanced renal cell carcinoma. Sorafenib was evaluated in a study by Welch et al. in phase II study in combination with gemcitabine in recurrent epithelium ovarian cancer. Overall response rate was 33%.

Sunitinib (Sutent)

Sunitinib is also small-molecule tyrosine kinase inhibitor approved for the treatment of metastatic renal cell carcinoma or gastrointestinal stromal tumour that is not responding to imatinib.

Pazopanib (Votrient)

Pazopanib is a small-molecule inhibitor of several tyrosine kinases, including VEGF receptors, c-kit and platelet-derived growth factor receptor.

Cediranib

Cediranib is a small-molecule tyrosine kinase inhibitors that target the VEGF. It is an oral formulation and was evaluated in ICON-6 phase III placebo controlled trial in recurrent ovarian cancer (platinum-sensitive). Cediranib was added in a carboplatin–paclitaxel regimen as maintenance therapy for 18 months. The median progression-free survival (PFS) was 8.7 months in the chemotherapy arm and 11.1 months in the Cediranib maintenance arm (HR, 0.57; p = 0.00001). When a restricted means analysis was done, the final result shows 3.1 month difference favoring Cediranib (9.4 months versus 12.5 months). Median overall survival was longer in Cediranib group, 20.3 months versus 17.6 months (p = 0.0042). However, Cediranib was associated with more treatment discontinuation, diarrhea and fatigue. Compared to bevacizumab, there was less hypertension in Cediranib.

Other Targeted Therapies

(1) Agents that modify the function of protein, which regulate gene expression and other cellular functions are:
   (a) Vorinostat
   (b) Romidepsin
   (c) Bexarotene
   (d) Alitretinoin
   (e) Tretinoin
(2) Agents that induce cancer cells to undergo apoptosis
   (a) Bortezomib interferes with the action of large cellular structure called proteasome, which degrades proteins.
   (b) Pralatrexate is an antifolate, interferes with DNA synthesis
(3) Agents that act by helping immune system to destroy cancer cells[1]
   (a) Rituximab is a monoclonal antibody that recognized molecule known as CD20 on the surface of B cells, it binds to these cells and triggers an immune response that destroys the cells.

[1]Agents 3 and 4 are mainly approved for haematological malignancies. Agents category 4b and 4b were linked to radioisotopes, which will deliver the radiation to cancer cells.

(b) Alemtuzumab is also monoclonal antibody bind to protein found on the surface of malignant B and T cells called CD52. It induces an immune response similar to rituximab.
(c) Ofatumumab

(4) Agents that deliver toxic molecules to cancer cells[1]
(a) Gemtuzumab ozogamicin is monoclonal antibodies against the protein CD33, antitumour substance called calicheamicin will be released and prevent DNA synthesis.
(b) Tositumomab
(c) Ibritumomab tiuxetan
(d) Denileukin diftitox consists of interleukin-2 protein fused to a diphtheria toxin. Cytotoxic action of diphtheria toxin will kill the cancer cells.

Special Consideration in Ovarian Cancer Management

Radiation Therapy in Ovarian Cancer

The role of radiotherapy in treatment of ovarian cancer is controversial. Radiation therapy has been used during the past 15 years in all stages and extents of ovarian cancer. For radiation to be of curative benefit, whole abdomino-pelvic radiation should be employed. Radiation therapy is primarily effective in patients who have no macroscopic residual disease after primary surgery. For patients with suboptimal cytoreductive leaving more than 2 cm tumour, the probability of cure is only 0–14%. There is little or no curative potential for abdominal irradiation in patients with bulky disease in the upper abdomen.

Choices of radiation techniques (both give similar survival rate) are

(a) **Moving strip technique**: small part of the abdomen is irradiated daily sequentially.
(b) **Open field technique**: whole volume is treated daily (standard in most oncology centres because of shorter duration of therapy, technical simplicity and reduced long-term toxicity).

The toxicities associated with abdomino-pelvic radiation therapy are: (a) Fatigue is the most common toxicity, (b) GIT toxicity, nausea, diarrhoea, abdominal cramps, etc., (c) Late effect: Basal pneumonitis and fibrosis in 15–20% and (d) Risk of late complications to bowel (malabsorption, abdominal pain, obstruction, fistula, etc.) is increased if the lymph node sampling was performed during initial operation.

The role of abdomino-pelvic radiation therapy is currently limited and the curative benefit of this treatment has not been established in stage 1 disease, however, in some institution, this treatment modality may be offered to the following patients: (a) in stage 1 disease with adverse prognostic factors including dense adhesion, (b) in stage 2 and 3 disease with no macroscopic disease in the upper abdomen and with small residual tumour (<2 cm) in the pelvis and (c) the most appropriate group, those with stage 1, grades 2 and 3, all stage 2 with residual tumour less than 2 cm and grade 1 and 2 and stage 3 with small residual tumour and grade 1.

Engelen and colleagues have evaluated the role of whole abdominal radiotherapy (WART) for high-risk early-stage ovarian cancer; WART was given to stage 1 and 2 ovarian cancer without residual disease. WART comprised 23.75 Gy of whole abdominal radiotherapy, in 19 fractions of 1.25 Gy daily for 5 days a week, followed by a pelvic boost of 20 Gy in 10 daily fractions of 2 Gy (similar protocol to Dutch University Clinics). WART was compared to adjuvant chemotherapy and without adjuvant treatment. There was no difference in 10 years overall survival in the study and control arm (62–65%). Patients who received adjuvant WART had higher risk of long-term gastrointestinal toxicities (28%) and 15% required surgery for radiation enteritis. The risk of secondary malignancies such as leukaemia and solid tumours (pancreas, bladder, rectum, etc.) were higher in WART group, especially if the patients survived more than 15 years.

Technical principles of curative radiotherapy are as follows (Dembo):

(a) Entire peritoneal cavity must be encompassed.
(b) Open-field technique is preferred.
(c) No liver shielding is used. This limit the upper abdominal dose to 2500–2800 cGy in 100–120 cGy daily fractions.
(d) Partial kidney shielding is used to keep the renal dose at 1800–2000 cGy.

(e) True pelvis is given a boost dose in 180–220 cGy.
(f) Use parallel-opposing portals, with beam energy sufficient to ensure a dosage variation no >5%.

Radiation Therapy after Chemotherapy in Advanced Disease

Thomas analysed the option of incorporating chemotherapy, surgery and radiotherapy for advanced ovarian cancer. They had evaluated the role of sequential cisplatin-based chemotherapy followed by secondary cytoreductive surgery and then whole abdomino-pelvic radiation. In their analysis, patients with no residual tumour had 76% survival, 49% in microscopic or <5 mm and 17% in macroscopic disease (Thomas, 1993).

A multi-centric study by Swedish Norwegian Ovarian Cancer Study had evaluated the approach of administering four cycles of cisplatin/doxorubicin followed by second look surgery then ± consolidation therapy (whole abdominal radiation versus chemotherapy (another six cycles) versus none). Improvement of survival was seen in radiation group but complications rate were higher. A better result was observed in those patients with microscopic or no residual disease.

Radiation is appropriate only as a sole postoperative therapy for patients with no macroscopic disease in the upper abdomen and small or no macroscopic residual disease in the pelvis. Radiation therapy is unsuitable in a patient who has a larger volume of tumour, had undergone secondary cytoreductive therapy and chemotherapy as most of this patient may already have a resistant tumour. Hyperfractionation (delivery of 2–3 small radiation fraction per day) is one of the proposed methods of radiation to minimize a complication in abdominalpelvic radiation technique. Cross resistance between radiation and cisplatinum therapy may occur and this sequential type of therapy is only indicated in small selected patients.

Radiation as Palliative Treatment for Ovarian Cancer

Recurrent or persistent ovarian cancer after first line chemotherapy is incurable. Second, third or fourth line chemotherapy is to prolonged life and for palliation.

Radiation therapy may play a role as palliation in the symptomatic patients with localized tumour at site and volume that may be safely targeted by radiation. Following are the examples:

(a) local fixed pelvic mass causing vaginal bleeding, bowel or urinary symptoms is an example where radiation can be used
(b) retroperitoneal lymph nodes
(c) supraclavicular or inguinal lymph nodes
(d) bony metastases
(e) brain metastases
(f) painful hepatomegaly (due to capsular distension)

Palliative irradiation is in the form of large single-fraction 1–3 fractions of 10Gy, overall response rates (pain and bleeding) are 55–71% (Anderson Cancer Center).

Palliative Surgery for Ovarian Cancer

Involvement of the intestine leading to obstruction can be very stressful for the patient and the caregiver. Surgical resection in selected patients may be indicated if conservative treatment fails (after weighing the risks and benefits). Advanced stage, ascites, poor nutritional status, big palpable tumour and previous radiation therapy were associated with poor outcomes postoperatively. Small intestine is the most common site for obstruction (44%) and those who successfully undergo laparotomy and released of obstruction, their mean postsurgical survival was 6.8 months. For those who are not a suitable candidate for surgery or found to be inoperable, percutaneous gastrostomy offer more comfortable alternative to prolong nasogastric drainage.

Hormonal Therapy and Receptors in Ovarian Carcinoma

Steroid receptor status in normal ovary and ovarian tumour is not completely known but epidemiologic studies indicate that steroid hormones play roles in ovarian organogenesis. Gonadotropins, oestrogen and androgen may be causative factors, while gonadotropin-releasing hormone and progesterone may be protective factors. Study on ER and PR in carcinoma of ovary and relation with tumour grade, histology grade and prognosis are conflicting. Trial has been done to evaluate the activity of tamoxifen in patients refractory to cytotoxic chemotherapy. In GOG trial, tamoxifen 20 mg twice daily was given to a patient with stage 3 and 4 ovarian epithelial carcinoma with persistent or recurrence after first line therapy; complete response rate of 10–15% was observed. Approximately, 89% of these patients had elevated oestrogen receptor. Highest response to tamoxifen was observed in endometroid histology. Review of 18 trials on hormonal therapy in advanced ovarian cancer showed 13% overall response rate (majority uses tamoxifen). Recent meta-analysis specifically on tamoxifen involving 14 studies showed overall response rate of 9.6% and stable disease in 31.9%.

Progestogen (50 mg tds) had also been use but complete response rate was less than 5%. Overall response rate only 8% in The Northern California Oncology Group study using high dose megestrol. Other potential hormonal treatments in recurrent ovarian cancer are aromatase inhibitors (letrozole and anastrozole) and GnRH analogue (response rate between 9% and 12%).

Biologic Therapy for Ovarian Cancer

Administration of non-specific immunostimulants is the most extensively studied immunotherapy in ovarian cancer. Majority of these trials is phase I or II and at the moment the role of biologic therapy in ovarian cancer is still unclear. Among immunostimulants (combination with chemotherapy or alone in small volume disease) that had been evaluated includes Corynebacterium parvum, BCG, interferon alpha and Interleukin II given intravenously, subcutaneously or intraperitoneal. There was no improvement in survival. Interferon alpha and IL-II had been given through intraperitoneal route. Response rate to immunotherapy alone and combination immunochemotherapy was 31% and 40%, respectively.

The role of monoclonal antibody against the surface marker (e.g., CA125, OC125) of epithelial ovarian cancer cell or transferrin receptor had been assessed. This antibody had been tag with radioisotopes (**radioisotope conjugates**), e.g., Iodine 125, or to the toxin (**immunotoxin**), e.g., endotoxin from pseudomonas. The main problem with this approach is toxicity.

Recombinant humanized anti-HER-2/neu had been administered to patients with recurrent ovarian cancer (HER-2/neu oncogene overexpression/amplification is associated with poor prognosis and exists in 30% of cases). The other group of biological therapy is known as immunopotentiator, which had been studied in ovarian cancer. The example of immunopotentiator is cytotoxic T-lymphocyte specific for HER-2/neu, CD4-positive and CD8 tumour infiltrating lymphocytes.

Reversal of Drug Resistance

Acquired drug resistance is a major problem limiting the drug effectiveness and 20–25% of patients have intrinsically drug-resistant tumour at the time of diagnosis. Resistance to first line chemotherapy always associated with a poor response to second line due to cross-resistance.

Mechanisms of resistance in the alkylating agents and platinum compound are multi-factorial:

(a) Alteration in drug accumulation
(b) Increased inactivation by detoxification enzymes such as glutathione-S-transferases (GST)
(c) Direct binding to non-protein thiols such as glutathione (GSH) or to protein thiol, e.g., metallothionein.
(d) Increased removal of lethal DNA adducts by activated DNA repair enzymes.

Drug-resistant ovarian cancer cell line was found to have higher level of GSH; inhibition of GSH synthesis is possible by inhibiting enzyme gamma glutamyl cysteine synthetase using buthionine sulfoximine (BSO). Therefore, BSO can be used to reduce drug resistance and increased effectiveness.

Ethacrynic acid can inhibit GST to restore the effectiveness alkylating agents, and aphidicolin inhibits DNA polymerase alpha (DNA repair enzymes) in cisplatin-resistant cancer cell line.

Decreased net accumulation due to increased expression/ amplification of MDRI gene is a major mechanism of multi-drug resistance frequently with natural products, e.g. doxorubicin, vincristine and VP16. MDRI gene code for a protein that acts as an efflux pump. This efflux pump can be inhibited by verapamil and therefore, increase drug accumulation.

Biricodar is another drug that can reverse multi-drug resistance conferred by overexpression of MDR1 and MRP. All drugs under this category are still experimental.

Gene Therapy

One of the approaches in gene therapy is the transduction of Herpes Simplex virus thymidine kinase (HSVTK) gene into tumour cells. Following the transduction, an antiviral drug (nucleoside gancyclovir) is administered to the patient in order to destroy the cancer cells.

Mutation compensation approaches is targeting the gene responsible in the development of cancer, e.g., targeted ablation of dominant oncogene (e.g., p53), replacement of an altered tumour suppressor gene and interference with the function of a growth factor or its receptors. Example of mutation compensation approaches is delivery of wild type p53 gene (using viral gene) to ovarian cancer cell to replace their p53 gene, which can reverse the malignant phenotype. Phase 1 trial combination paclitaxel/carboplatin with p53 gene replacement using adenoviral vector. BRCA1 gene replacement was also evaluated in a phase 1 and 2 trial in one of the phase 2 trial, intraperitoneal infusion of vector was used as a gene therapy.

The other approach of gene therapy is to modify the gene in bone marrow cells using genetic engineering, so they are more tolerance to chemotherapy and facilitates administration of higher dose of chemotherapeutic agents. The progenitor cells in bone marrow are transduced with retrovirus containing MDR gene then transplanted back into patients after high dose chemotherapy.

A number of investigators have used virus gene therapy as one possible route to supplement ovarian cancer conventional chemotherapy. Adenoviral vectors have been widely used for gene therapy because they can transfect many cell types. Adenovirus-mediated anti-angiogenesis gene therapy based of PEG-PE liposome can be used to inhibit the growth of ovarian cancer and liposome can synergize with endostatin. Endostatin is a potent endogenous vascular inhibitor.

Abbreviations Used in This Chapter

ACTION: Adjuvant Treatment in Ovarian Neoplasms
EORTC: European Organization for Research and Treatment of Cancer
GOG: Gynecologic Oncology Group

ICON:	International Collaborative on Ovarian Neoplasms
IICG:	Italian Interregional Cooperative Group
PLCO:	Prostate, Lung, Colorectal and Ovarian Trial
SCOTROC:	Scottish Randomized Trial in Ovarian Cancer
SNG:	Swedish-Norwegian Group
GINECO:	Groupe des Investivateurs Nationaux pour I'Etude des Cancers de I'Ovaire
GCIG:	Gynecolgic Cancer InterGroup

References

Aghajanian C, Blank SV, Goff BA, et al. OCEANS: a randomized, double-blind, placebo-controlled phase III trial of chemotherapy with or without bevacizumab in patients with platinum-sensitive recurrent epithelial ovarian, primary peritoneal, or fallpian tube cancer. *J Clin Oncol* 2012; **30**(17): 2039–2045.

Albert DS, Liu PY, Hannigan EV, et al. Intraperitoneal cisplatin plus intravenous cyclophosphamide versus intravenous cisplatin plus intravenous cyclophosphamide for stage III ovarian cancer. *N Engl J Med* 1996; **335**: 1950–1955.

Amstrong DK, Bundy B, Wenzel l, et al. Intraperitoneal cisplatin and paclitaxel in ovarian cancer. *N Engl J Med* 2006; **354**: 34–43.

Anderson GL, Judd HL, Kaunitz AM, et al. Effects of estrogen plus progestin on gynecologic cancers and associated diagnostic procedures: the Women's Health Initiative randomized trial. *JAMA* 2003; **290**: 1739–1748.

Ardekani AM, Liotta LA, Petricoin EF III. Clinical potential of proteomics in the diagnosis of ovarian cancer. *Expert Rev Mol Diagn* 2002; **2**: 312–320.

Banerjee S, Rustin G, Paul J, et al. A multicenter, randomized trial of flat dosing versus intrapatient dose escalation of single-agent carboplatin as first-line chemotherapy for advanced ovarian cancer: an SGCTG (SCOTROC 4) and ANZGOG study on behalf of GCIG. *Ann Oncol* 2013; **24**(3): 679–687.

Bast Jr RC, Klug TL, St John, et al. A radioimmunoassay using a monoclonal antibody to monitor the course of epithelial ovarian cancer. *N Engl J Med* 1983; **309**: 883–887.

Bergfeldt K, Rydh B, Granath F, et al. Risk of ovarian cancer in breast-cancer patients with a family history of breast or ovarian cancer: a population-based cohort study. *Lancet* 2002; **360**: 891–894.

Berkenblit A, Seiden MV, Matulonis UA, et al. A phase II trial of weekly docetaxel in patients with platinum-resistant epithelial ovarian, primary peritoneal serous cancer, or fallopian tube cancer. *Gynecol Oncol* 2004; **95**: 624–631.

Bolis G, Scarfone G, Raspagliesi F, et al. Paclitaxel/carboplatin versus topotecan/paclitaxel/carboplatin in patients with FIGO suboptimally resected stage III-IV epithelial ovarian cancer a multicenter, randomized study. *Eur J Cancer* 2010; doi: 10.1016/j.ejca.2010.06.124.

Bookman MA, Brady MF, McGuire WP, et al. Evaluation of new platinum-based treatment regimens in advanced stage ovarian cancer: phase III trial of the gynecologic cancer intergroup. *J Clin Oncol* 2009; **27**(9): 1419–1425.

Brewster WR. Temporal trends in ovarian cancer incidence and mortality across Europe. *Nat Clin Pract Oncol* 2005; **2:** 286–287.

Bristow RE, Tomacruz RS, Armstrong DK, et al. Survival effect of maximal cytoreductive surgery for advanced ovarian carcinoma during the platinum era: a meta-analysis. *J Clin Oncol* 2002; **20**: 1248–1259.

Bristow RE, Chi DS. Platinum-based neoadjuvant chemotherapy and interval surgical cytoreduction for advanced ovarian cancer: a metaanalysis. *Gynecol Oncol* 2006 [Jul 26 electronic publication ahead of print; PMID: 16875720].

Bristow RE, Eisenhauer EL, Santillan A, Chi DS. Delaying the primary surgical effort for advanced ovarian cancer: a systematic review of neoadjuvant chemotherapy and interval cytoreduction. *Gynecol Oncol* 2007; **104**: 480–490.

Bristow RE, Puri I, Chi DS. Review. Cytoreductive surgery for recurrent ovarian cancer: a meta-analysis. *Gynecol Oncol* 2009; **112**: 265–274.

Buys SS, Partridge E, Greene MH, et al. Ovarian cancer screening in the Prostate, Lung, Colorectal and Ovarian (PLCO) cancer screening trial: findings from the initial screen of a randomized trial. *Am J Obstet Gynecol* 2005; **193**: 1630–1639.

Buys SS, Partridge E, Black A, et al. Effect of screening on ovarian cancer mortality: the Prostate, Lung, Colorectal and Ovarian (PLO) Cancer Screening Randomized Controlled Trial. *JAMA* June 8 2011; **305**(22): 2295–2303.

Campos SM, Ghosh S. Review article: A current review of targeted therapeutics for ovarian cancer. *Hindawi Publishing Corporation Journal of Oncology* 2010; Article ID 149362, page 1–11. Doi: 10.1155/2010/149362.

Cannistra SA. Cancer of the ovary. *N Engl J Med* 2004; **351:** 2519–2529.

Chan JK, Tian C, Teoh D, et al. Survival after recurrence early stage epithelial ovarian cancer. A Gynecologic Oncologic Group Study. *Gynecol Oncol* 2010; **116**(3): 307–311.

Chan YM, Ng TY, Ngan HY, Wong LC. Quality of life in women treated with neoadjuvant chemotherapy for advanced ovarian cancer: a prospective longitudinal study. *Gynecol Oncol* 2003; **88**: 9–16.

Chen VW, Ruiz B, Killeen JL, Cote TR, Wu XC, Correa CN. Pathology and classification of ovarian tumours. *Cancer Suppl.* (Published by ACS) 2003; **97**(10): 2631–2642.

Clamp AR, Maenpaa J, Cruickshank D, et al. SCOTROC 2B: feasibility of carboplatin followed by docetaxel or docetaxel-irinotecan as first line therapy for ovarian cancer. *Br J Cancer* 2006; **94**: 55–61.

Collaborative Group on Epidemiological Studies of Ovarian Cancer. Ovarian cancer and oral contraceptives: collaborative reanalysis of data from 45 epidemiological studies including 23 257 women with ovarian cancer and 87 303 controls. *Lancet* 2008; **371:** 303–314.

Colombo N, Kutarska E, Dimopoulos M, et al. Randomized, open-label, Phase III study comparing Patupilone (EPO906) with Pegylated Liposomal Doxorubicin in Platinum-Refractory or Resistant Patients with Recurrent Epithelial Ovarian, Primary Fallopian tube or Primary Peritoneal Cancer. *J Clin Oncol* 2012, DOI: 10.1200/JCO.2011.38.8082.

Cramer DW, Welch WR. Determinants of ovarian cancer risk. II. Inferences regarding pathogenesis. *J Natl Cancer Inst* 1983; **71:** 717–721.

Cramer DW, Bast JR RC, Berg CD, et al. Ovarian cancer biomarker performance in prostate, lung, colorectal, and ovarian cancer screening trial specimens. *Cancer Prev Res* 2011; **4**(3): 365–374.

Daponte A, Kostopoulou E, Kollia P, et al. L1(CAM) (CD171) in ovarian serous neoplasms. *Eur J Gynaecol Oncol* 2008; **29**(1): 26–30.

Deballon PO, Facy O, Jambet S, et al. Which method to deliver hyperthermic intraperitoneal chemotherapy with oxaliplatin? An experimental comparison of open and closed techniques. *Ann Surg Oncol* 2010; **17**: 1957–1963.

Dembo AJ. Epithelial ovarian cancer: the role of radiotherapy. *Int J Radiat Oncol Biol Phys* 1992; **22**: 838.

Dietel M, Hauptmann S. Serous tumors of low malignant potential of the ovary. 1. Diagnostic pathology. *Virchows Arch* May 2000; **436**(5): 403–412.

Dinh P, Harnett P, Piccart-Gebhart M, Awada A. New therapies for ovarian cancer: Cytotoxics and molecularly targeted agents. *Crit Rev Oncol/Hematol* 2008; **67**: 103–112.

Du Bois A, Luck HJ, Meier W, et al. A randomized clinical trial of cisplatin/paclitaxel versus carboplatin/paclitaxel as first line treatment of ovarian cancer. *J Natl Cancer Inst* 2003; **95**: 1320–1330.

Du Bois A, Weber B, Rochon J, et al. Addition of epirubicin as a third drug to carboplatin–paclitaxel in first line treatment of advanced ovarian cancer: a prospectively randomized gynecologic cancer intergroup trial by the Arbeitsgemeinschaft Gynaekologische Onkologie Ovarian Cancer Study Group and the Groupe d'Investigateurs Nationaux pour l'Etude des Cancers Ovariens. *J Clin Oncol* 2006; **24**: 1127–1135.

Du Bois A, Sehouli J, Lund, et al. Paclitaxel–carboplatin–gemcitabine (TCG) as first line treatment of ovarian cancer: a prospective multicenter phase II study (AGO-OVAR 8) followed by a prospectively randomized phase III GCIG Intergroup study (AGO-OVAR 9, GINECO-TCG, NSGO-OC-0102) comparing TCG with standard TC. *Int J Gynecol Cancer* 2005; **15** (suppl 3): 224–225.

Earle CC, Schrag D, Neville BA, et al. Effect of surgeon specialty on processes of care and outcomes for ovarian cancer patients. *J Natl Cancer Inst* 2006; **98**: 172–180.

Eisenhauer EL, Abu Rustum NR, Sonoda Y, et al. The effect of maximum surgical cytoreduction on sensitivity to platinum-taxane chemotherapy and subsequent survival in patients with advanced ovarian cancer. *Gynecol Oncol* 2008; **108**: 276–281.

Engelen MJA, Snel BJ, Schaapveld M, et al. Long-term morbidity of adjuvant whole abdominal radiotherapy (WART) or chemotherapy for early stage ovarian cancer. *Eur J Cancer* 2009; **45**: 1193–1200.

Fathalla MF. Incessant ovulation—a factor in ovarian neoplasia? *Lancet* 1971; **298:** 163.

Finch A, Beiner M, Lubinski J, et al. Salpingo-oophorectomy and the risk of ovarian, fallopian tube and peritoneal cancers in women with a BRCA1 and BRCA2 mutation. *JAMA* 2006; **296**: 185–192.

Ferrero JM, Weber, Geay JF, et al. Second-line chemotherapy with pegylated liposomal doxorubicin and carboplatin is highly effective in patients with advanced ovarian cancer in late relapse: a GINECO phase II trial. *Ann Oncol* 2007; **18**: 263–268.

Foster T, Brown MT, Chang J, Menssen HD, Blieden MB, Herzog TJ. Review: A review of the current evidence for maintenance therapy in ovarian cancer. *Gynecol Oncol* 2009; **115**: 290–301.

Freedman OC, Dodge J, Shaw P, et al. Diagnosis of epithelial ovarian carcinoma prior to neoadjuvant chemotherapy. *Gynecol Oncol* 2010; **119**(1): 22–25.

Garg PP, Kerlikowske K, Subak L, Grady D. Hormone replacement therapy and the risk of epithelial ovarian carcinoma: a meta-analysis. *Obstet Gynecol* 1998; **92**: 472–479.

Garcia M, Jemal A, Ward EM, et al. Global cancer facts and figures 2007. Atlanta: *American Cancer Society*, 2007.

Gordon A, Tonda M, Sun S, Rackoff W. Long-term survival advantage for women treated with pegylated liposomal doxorubicin compared with topotecan in a phase 3 randomized study of recurrent and refractory epithelial ovarian cancer. *Gynecol Oncol* 2004; **95**: 1–8.

Gray HJ, Shah CA, Swensen RE, et al. Alternative intraperitoneal chemotherapy regimen in optimally debulked ovarian cancer. *Gynecol Oncol* 2010; **116**: 340–344.

Hankinson SE, Hunter DJ, Colditz GA, et al. Tubal ligation, hysterectomy, and risk of ovarian cancer. A prospective study. *JAMA* 1993; **270:** 2813–2818.

Hariprassad R, Kumar L, Patnaik R, et al. Maintenance therapy in epithelial ovarian cancer: could EGFR inhibitor–gefitinib be a candidate drug? A pilot study. *Proc Am Soc Clin Oncol* 2006; **24**(18s): 15046a.

Hayat MJ, Howlader N. Reichman ME, Edwards BK. Cancer statistics, trends, and multiple primary cancer analyses from the Surveillance, Epidemiology, and End Results (SEER) Program. *Oncologist* 2007; **12:** 20–37.

Houck K, Nikrui N, Duska L, et al. Borderline tumors of the ovary: correlation of frozen and permanent histopathologic diagnosis. *Obstet Gynecol* Jun 2000; **95**(6 Pt 1): 839–843.

Huncharek M, Geschwind JF, Kupelnick B. Perineal application of cosmetic talc and risk of invasive epithelial ovarian cancer: a metaanalysis of 11,933 subjects from sixteen observational studies. *Anticancer Res* 2003; **23**: 1955–1960.

ICON and EORTC-ACTION Investigators. International Collaborative on Ovarian Neoplasm Trial 1 and Adjuvant Treatment in Ovarian Neoplasm Trial: two parallel randomized phase 3 trials of adjuvant chemotherapy in patients with early stage ovarian cancer. *J Natl Cancer Inst* 2003; **95**: 105–112.

ICON. International Collaborative Ovarian Neoplasm Study. Paclitaxel plus carboplatin versus standard chemotherapy with either single agent carboplatin or cyclophosphamide, doxorubicin, and cisplatin in women with ovarian cancer: the ICON 3 randomized trial. *Lancet* 2002; **360**: 505–515.

Isonishi S, Yasuda M, Takahashi F, et al. Randomized phase III trial of conventional paclitaxel and carboplatin (c-TC) versus dose dense weekly paclitaxel and carboplatin (dd-TC) in women with advanced epithelial, fallopian tube or primary peritoneal cancer: Japanese Gynecologic Oncology. *J Clin Oncol* 2008; **26**(15 Suppl) 294s (abstract 5506).

Jaaback K, Johnson N. Intraperitoneal chemotherapy for the initial management of primary epithelial ovarian cancer. *Cochrane Database Syst Rev* 2006 (1): CD005340.

Jacobs I, Davies AP, Bridges J, et al. Prevalence screening for ovarian cancer in postmenopausal women by CA 125 measurement and ultrasonography. *BMJ* 1993; **306**: 1030–1034.

Jacobs I, Oram D, Fairbanks J, et al. The risk of malignancy index incorporating CA125, ultrasound and menopausal status for the accurate preoperative diagnosis of ovarian cancer. *BJOG* 1990; **97**: 922–929.

Kaku T, Ogawa S, Kawano Y, et al. Histological Classification of Ovarian Cancer. *Med Electron Microsc* 2003; **36**: 9–17.

Kehoe S, Wheeler S. CHORUS (Chemotherapy or Upfront Surgery). A randomized feasibility trial to determine the impact of timing of surgery and chemotherapy in newly diagnosed patients with advanced epithelial ovarian, primary peritoneal or fallopian tube carcinoma. Available at http://www.ctu.mrc.ac.uk/studies/CHORUS asp (accessed July, 2008).

Kobayashi H, Yamada Y, Sado T, et al. A randomized study of screening for ovarian cancer: a multicenter study in Japan. *Int J Gynecol Cancer* 2008; **18**: 414–420.

Lancaster JM, et al. Society of Gynecologic Oncologists Education Committee Statement on risk assessment for inherited gynecologic cancer predispositions. *Gynecol Oncol* 2007; **107**: 159–162.

Lin H, Changchien CC. Management of relapsed/refractory Epithelial ovarian cancer: current standards and novel approaches. *Taiwan J Obstet Gynecol* 2007; **46**(4): 379–388.

Marman M, Bundy BN, Alberts DS, et al. Phase III trial of standard-dose intravenous cisplatin plus paclitaxel versus moderately high-dose carboplatin followed by intravenous paclitaxel and intraperitoneal cisplatin in small-volume stage III ovarian carcinoma: an intergroup study of the gynecologic oncology group, South-Western Oncology Group, and Eastern Cooperative Oncology Group. *J Clin Oncol* 2001; **19**: 1001–1007.

Markman M, Liu PY, Moon J, et al. Impact on survival of 12 versus 3 monthly cycles of paclitaxel (175 mg/m^2) administered to patients with advanced ovarian cancer who attained a complete response to primary platinum–paclitaxel: follow-up of a Southwest oncology group and gynecologic oncology group phase 3 trial. *Gynecol Oncol* 2009; **114**: 195–198.

Markman M, Zanotti K, Webster K, Peterson G, Kulp B, Belinson J. Phase 2 trial of single agent docetaxel in platinum and paclitaxel-refractory ovarian cancer, fallopian tube cancer and primary carcinoma of the peritoneum. *Gynecol Oncol* 2003; **91**: 573–576.

Markman M, Webster K, Zanotti K, et al. Survival following the documentation of platinum and taxane resistance in ovarian cancer: a single institution experience involving multiple phase 2 clinical trials. *Gynecol Oncol* 2004; **93**: 699–701.

McGuire WP, Hoskin WJ, Brady MF, et al. Cyclophosphamide and cisplatin compared with paclitaxel and cisplatin in patients with stage III and stage IV ovarian cancer. *N Engl J Med* 1996; **334**: 1–6.

McLaughlin JR, Risch HA, Lubinski J, et al. Reproductive risk factors for ovarian cancer in carriers of BRCA1 or BRCA2 mutations: a case-control study. *Lancet Oncol* 2007; **8**: 26–34.

Morch LS, Lokkegaard E, Andreasen AH, Kruger-Kjaer S, Lidegaard O. Hormone therapy and ovarian cancer. *JAMA* Jul 15 2009; **302**(3): 298–293.

Moore RG, McMeekin DS, Brown AK, et al. A novel multiple marker bioassay utilizing HE4 and CA125 for the prediction of ovarian cancer in patient with a pelvic mass. *Gynecol Oncol* 2009; **112**: 40–46.

Moore RG, et al. Evaluation of the diagnostic accuracy of the risk of ovarian malignancy algorithm in women with a pelvic mass. *Obstet Gynecol* 2011; **118**(2 Pt 1): 280–288.

Morris CR, Rodriguez AO, Epstein J, Cress RD. Declining trends of epithelial ovarian cancer in California. *Gynecol Oncol* 2008; **108:** 207–213.

Omura G, Blassing JA, Ehrlich CE, et al. Randomized trial of cyclophosphamide and doxorubicin with or without cisplatin in advanced ovarian carcinoma. A Gynecologic Oncology Group Study. *Cancer* 1986; **57**: 1725–1730.

Omura GA, Bundy BN, Berek JS, et al. Randomized trial of cyclophosphamide plus cisplatin with or without doxorubicin in ovarian carcinoma: a gynecologic oncology group study. *J Clin Oncol* 1989; **7**: 457–465.

Onda T, Matsumoto H, Shibata K, et al. Phase III trial of upfront debulking surgery versus neoadjuvant chemotherapy for stage III/IV ovarian, tubal and peritoneal cancers: Japan clinical oncology group study JCOG0602. *Jpn J Clin Oncol* 2008; **38**: 74–77.

OVATURE (Ovarian Tumour Response) Study: a phase III study of weekly carboplatin with and without phenoxodiol in patients with platinum-resistant, recurrent epithelial ovarian cancer. Available at: http://clinicaltrials.gov/ct/show/NCT00382811.

Ovarian Cancer Metanalysis Project. Cyclophosphamide plus cisplatin versus cyclophosphamide, doxorubicin and cisplatin chemotherapy of ovarian carcinoma: a metanalysis. The Ovarian Cancer Meta-Analysis Project. *J Clin Oncol* 1991; **9**(9): 1668–1674.

Ozol RF, Bundy BN, Greer BE, et al. Phase III trial of carboplatin and paclitaxel compared with cisplatin and paclitaxel in patients with optimally resected stage III ovarian cancer: a gynecologic oncology group study. *J Clin Oncol* 2003; **21**: 3194–3200.

Palmar MK, Ledermann JA, Colombo N, et al. Paclitaxel plus platinum-based chemotherapy versus conventional platinum-based chemotherapy in women with relapsed ovarian cancer: the ICON 4/AGGO-OVAR-2.2 trial. *Lancet* 2003; **361**: 2099–2106.

Palo GD, Mariani L, Camerini T, et al. Effect of fenretinide on ovarian carcinoma occurrence. *Gynecol Oncol* 2002; **86**(1): 24–27.

Patupilone versus doxorubicin in patients with ovarian, primary fallopian, or peritoneal cancer. Available at: http://www.clinicaltrials.gov/ct/show/NCT00262990?order=7.

Perren TJ, Swart AM, Pfisterer J, et al. A Phase 3 trial of Bevacizumab in Ovarian Cancer (ICON 7). *N Engl J Med* 2011; **365**: 2484–2496.

Pfisterer J, Plante M, Vergote I, et al. Gemcitabine plus carboplatin compared with carboplatin in patients with platinum-sensitive recurrent ovarian cancer. *J Clin Oncol* 2006; **24**: 4699–4707.

Pfisterer J, Weber B, Reuss A, et al. Randomized phase III trial of topotecan following carboplatin and paclitaxel in first line treatment of advanced ovarian cancer: a gynecologic cancer intergroup trial of the AGO-OVAR and GINECO. *J Natl Cancer Inst* 2006; **98**: 1036–1045.

Piccart MJ, Bertelsen K, Stuart G, et al. Longterm follow-up confirms a survival advantage of the paclitaxel–cisplatin regime over the cyclophosphamide-cisplatin combination in advanced ovarian cancer. *Int J Gynecol Cancer* 2003; **13**(Suppl 2): 144–148.

Pignata S, Scambia G, Savarese A, et al. Carboplatin and pegylated liposomal doxorubicin for advanced ovarian cancer: preliminary activity results of the MITO-2 phase III trial. *Oncology* 2009; **76**: 49–54.

Rebbeck TR, Lynch HT, Neuhausen SL, et al. Prophylactic oophorectomy in carriers of BRCA1 or BRCA2 mutations. *N Engl J Med* 2002; **346**: 1616–1622.

Russo A, Calo V, Bruno L, Rizzo S, Bazan V, Di Fede G. Hereditary ovarian cancer. *Crit Rev Oncol/Hematol* 2009; **69**: 28–44.

Rose P, Edwards R, Finkler N, et al. Canfosfamide (C, TLK286) plus carboplatin vs liposomal doxorubicin as 2nd line therapy of platinum resistance ovarian cancer: phase 3 study results. *Proc Am Soc Clin Oncol* 2007; **25**: LBA5529.

Rose PG, Nerenstone S, Brady MF, Clarke-Pearson D, Olt G, Rubin SC, et al. Secondary surgical cytoreduction for advanced ovarian carcinoma. *N Engl J Med* 2004; **351**: 2489–2497.

Rose PG, Blessing JA, Mayer AR, Homesley HD. Prolonged oral etoposide as second line therapy for platinum-resistant and platinum-sensitive ovarian carcinoma: a gynecologic oncology group study. *J Clin Oncol* 1998; **16**: 405–410.

Sehouli J, Alfaro V, Gonzalez Martin A. Trabectedin plus pegylated liposomal doxorubicin in the treatment of patients with partially platinum-sensitive ovarian cancer: current evidence and future perspectives. *Ann Oncol* 2012, **23**(3): 556–562.

Sehouli J, Oskay-Ozcelik G, Stengel D, et al. What is the best schedule of Topotecan? Weekly versus routine 5 days schedule in patients with platinum-resistant ovarian cancer–a randomized, multicenter trial of the North Eastern German Society of Gynaecological Oncology (TOWER). *Eur J Cancer Suppl* 2009; **7**(2): 450–451.

Sherman ME, Mink PJ, Curtis R, et al. Survival among women with borderline ovarian tumors and ovarian carcinoma: a population-based analysis. *Cancer* Mar 1 2004; **100**(5): 1045–1052.

Silverberg SG. Prognostic significance of pathologic features. *Curr Top Pathol* 1989; **78:** 85–109.

Tangjitgamol S, Manusirivithaya S, Laopaiboon M, Lumbiganon P. Interval debulking surgery for advanced epithelial ovarian cancer: a Cochrane systematic review. *Gynecol Oncol* 2009; **112**: 257–264.

The Cancer and Steroid Hormone Study of the Centers for Disease Control and the National Institute of Child Health and Human Development. Oral contraceptive use and risk of breast cancer. *New Engl J Med* 1986; **315**: 405–411.

Tingulstad S, Hagen B, Skjeldestad FE, Halvorsen T, Nustad K, Onsrud M. The risk of malignancy index to evaluate potential ovarian cancers in local hospitals. *Obstet Gynecol* 1999; **93**: 448–452.

Tinker AV, Gebski V, Fitzharris B, et al. Phase II trial of weekly docetaxel for patients with relapsed ovarian cancer who have previously received paclitaxel. *Gynecol Oncol* 2007; **104**(3): 647–653

Trimbos B, Timmers P, Pecorelli S, et al. Surgical staging and treatment of early ovarian cancer: Long-term analysis from a randomized trial. *J Natl Cancer Inst* 2010; **102**(13): 982–987.

Van Nagell Jr JR, Depriest PD, Ueland FR, et al. Ovarian cancer screening with annual transvaginal sonography: findings of 25,000 women screened. *Cancer* 2007; **109**: 1887–1896.

Vasey PA, Jayson GC, Gordon A, et al. Phase III randomized trial of docetaxel-carboplatin versus paclitaxel–carboplatin as first line chemotherapy for ovarian carcinoma. *J Natl Cancer Inst* 2004; **96**: 1682–1691.

Vasey P, Atkinson R, Osborne R, et al. SCOTROC 2A: Carboplatin followed by docetaxel or docetaxel-gemcitabine as first line chemotherapy for ovarian cancer. *Br J Cancer* 2006; **94**: 62–68.

Vernooij F, Heintz P, Witteveen E, van der Graaf Y. The outcomes of ovarian cancer treatment are better when provided by gynaecologic oncologists and in specialized hospitals: a systematic review. *Gynecol Oncol* 2007; **105**: 801–812.

Vergote I, Pecorelli S, Stuart G. Intergroup Study (EORTC 55971/NCIC OV13). A randomized phase III study comparing upfront debulking surgery versus neo-adjuvant chemotherapy in patients with stage IIIC or IV epithelial ovarian carcinoma. Available at http://www.cancer.gov/clinicaltrials/EORTC-55971 (accessed July 2008).

Vergote I, Trope CG, Amant F, et al. For the Gynecologic Cancer Intergroup study of the European organization for research and treatment of cancer: Gynaecological Cancer Group and the NCIC-Clinical Trials Group. Treatment options in Stage IIIc or IV ovarian cancer: neoadjuvant chemotherapy or primary surgery in stage IIIc or IV ovarian cancer. *N Engl J Med* 2010; **363**(10): 943–953.

Walker JL, Armstrong DK, Huang HQ, et al. Intraperitoneal catheter outcomes in a phase III trial of intravenous versus intraperitoneal chemotherapy in optimal stage III ovarian and primary peritoneal cancer: a gynecologic oncology group study. *Gynecol Oncol* 2006; **100**: 27–32.

Walker JL. Editorial: intraperitoneal chemotherapy for ovarian cancer: 2009 goals. *Gynecol Oncol* 2009; **112**: 439–440.

Welch S, Hirte H, Schilder RJ, et al. Phase II study of sorafenib (BAY43-90006) in combincation with gemcitabine in recurrent epithelial ovarian cancer: a PMH phase II consortium trial. *Proc Am Soc Clin Oncol* 2006; **24**(18s): 5084a.

Whittemore AS, Harris R, Itnyre J. Characteristics relating to ovarian cancer risk: collaborative analysis of 12 US case–control studies. IV. The pathogenesis of epithelial ovarian cancer. Collaborative Ovarian Cancer Group. *Am J Epidemiol* 1992; **136**: 1212–1220.

Winter WE, Maxell GL, Tian C, et al. Tumour residual after surgical cytoreduction in prediction of clinical outcome in stage IV epithelial ovarian cancer: a gynecologic oncology group study. *J Clin Oncol* 2008; **26**: 83–89.

Winter WE, Maxell GL, Tian C, et al. Prognostic factors for stage III epithelial ovarian cancer: a gynecologic oncology group study. *J Clin Oncol* 2007; **25**: 3621–3627.

Chapter 13

Ovarian Germ Cell Tumours

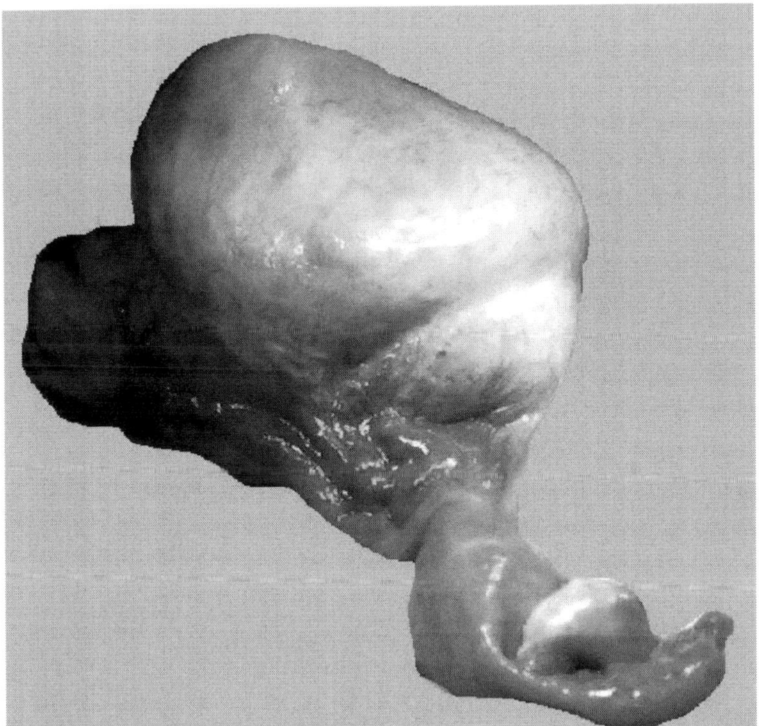

Gynaecologic Cancer: A Handbook for Students and Practitioners
Rushdan Noor, Eng Hseon Tay, and Jeffrey Low

ISBN 978-981-4463-06-5 (Hardcover), 978-981-4463-07-2 (eBook)
www.panstanford.com

Introduction

Malignant ovarian germ cell tumours are the rare type of ovarian cancer accounting for approximately 1–2% of ovarian malignancies. Malignant ovarian germ cell tumours are aggressive but curative because majorities are very chemosensitive. Unlike epithelial ovarian cancer, malignant ovarian germ cell tumours grow rapidly and usually present with symptoms secondary to capsular distension, haemorrhage or necrosis. This may account for why the majority is diagnosed at an early stage.

Epidemiology

Germ cell tumours account for 58% of all ovarian tumours in women younger than the age 20 years and 30% of these tumours are malignant.

According to report by Surveillance, Epidemiology, and Results (SEER) between 1973 and 2002, a total of 1262 cases of malignant ovarian germ cell tumours were identified:

(a) age-adjusted incidence was 0.330 per 100,000 women-year
(b) dysgerminoma (32.8%)
(c) immature teratoma (35.6%)
(d) mixed germ cell tumours (28.7%)

Except ovarian dysgerminoma, non-white women are more common than white and blacks. The peak age group at diagnosis was 15–19 years old.

Clinical Features

Median age group is 16–20 years old (range 6–46) and 15–20% of dysgerminoma is diagnosed during pregnancy and after delivery. Abdominal pain and palpable abdominal mass are presenting symptoms in 85% of cases. About 10% present as an acute abdomen due to twisted, haemorrhage or ruptured, especially in endodermal sinus tumour and mixed germ cell tumour. Other symptoms are abdominal distension (35%), fever (10–25%) and abnormal vaginal bleeding (10%). The duration of symptoms is usually short with a median duration of 2–4 weeks. Bilaterality is more common in dysgerminoma (10–15%) and rarely in others and ascites is a presenting sign in 20% of cases. Benign cystic teratoma is associated with 5–10% of malignant germ cell tumours. The stage of disease at presentation is (a) stage 1–2 (60–70%), (b) stage 3 (20–30%) and (c) stage IV (uncommon).

Lymph node metastasis and haematogenous spread are more common in malignant germ cell tumours than epithelial ovarian cancer. Peritoneal spread is similar to that in epithelial ovarian cancer. Some malignant germ cell tumours also excrete hormones leading to menstrual disturbances and isosexual precocity.

Compared to epithelial ovarian cancer, malignant germ cell tumours have following characteristics:

(1) lymphatic spread to lymph node is more common
(2) higher predilection to haematogenous spread to lung and liver
(3) 60–70% presented at stage 1 disease, 25–30% stage 3, while stage 2 and 4 are uncommon
(4) tumour more common on the right than left

Classification of Ovarian Germ Cell Tumours (WHO, 2003)

Table 13.1 WHO classification of ovarian germ cell tumour (2003)

Classification	Sub-classification
(A) Primitive germ cell tumours	(1) Dysgerminoma
	(2) Yolk sac tumour (Endodermal sinus tumour)
	(a) Polyvesicular vitelline tumour
	(b) Solid yolk sac
	(c) Grandular variant
	(d) Hepatoid variant
	(3) Embryonal carcinoma
	(4) Polyembryoma
	(5) Non gestational choriocarcinoma
	(6) Mixed germ cell tumour

(Continued)

Table 13.1 *(Continued)*

(B) Biphasic or triphasic teratoma	(1) Immature teratoma (2) Mature teratoma (a) Solid (b) Cystic (dermoid cyst) (c) Fetiform teratoma (homunculus)
(C) Monodermal teratoma and somatic-type tumour associated with biphasic or triphasic teratoma	(1) Thyroid group (2) Carcinoid group (3) Central nervous system tumour group (4) Carcinoma group (5) Melanocytic group (6) Sarcoma group (7) Sebaceous tumour group (8) Pituitary-type tumour group (9) Retinal anlage tumour group (10) Others

Tumour Markers in Malignant Ovarian Germ Cell Tumours

Elevation of α-fetoprotein and β-HCG is highly suggestive of ovarian germ cell tumours in young women presented with pelvic mass. Elevation of α-fetoprotein and β-HCG are found in almost all patients with an element of yolk sac and choriocarcinoma, respectively (Table 13.2). Both embryonal carcinoma and polyembryoma may produce α-fetoprotein and β-HCG. One third of immature teratoma produces α-fetoprotein. Lactic dehydrogenase (LDH) and placental alkaline phosphatase (PLAP) may be elevated in dysgerminoma.

Table 13.2 Serum tumour markers in malignant ovarian germ cell tumours

Histology	α-Fetoprotein	β-HCG
Dysgerminoma	None	±
Endodermal sinus tumour	+	None
Immature teratoma	±	None
Mixed germ cell tumour	±	±
Choriocarcinoma	None	+
Embryonal carcinoma	±	+
Polyembryoma	±	+

Pure dysgerminoma is commonly considered to have no tumour marker except in small percentage, which produces a low level of HCG. CA125 is also elevated in some patients with germ cell tumour.

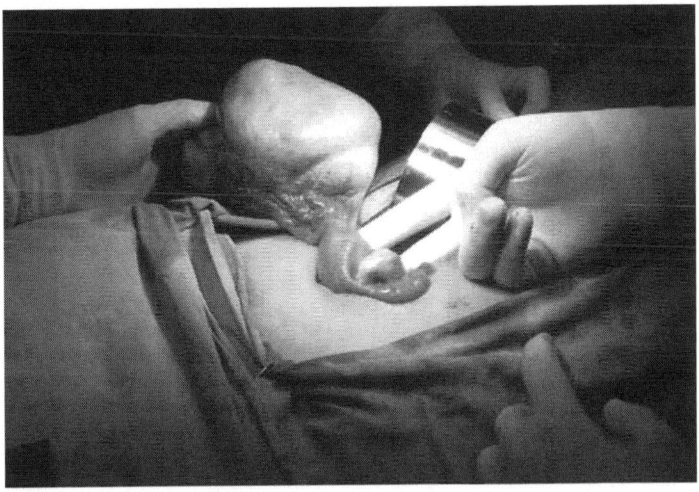

Figure 13.1 Ovarian germ cell tumour in young patients.

Dysgerminoma

Dysgerminoma is the most common malignant germ cell tumour of ovary and 75% cases of this tumour occur in patients in their third and fourth decade of life (Fig. 13.2). Dysgerminoma is also one of the most common ovarian neoplasms noted in pregnancy. Dysgerminoma is bilateral in 10–15% of cases and 10% of normal-looking contralateral ovary showed the presence of dysgerminoma microscopically. About 50% of primitive germ cell tumour of the ovary is dysgerminoma. It make up two thirds of all malignant ovarian neoplasms in women younger than 20 years. Gross appearances of dysgerminoma are solid, with a tan, flesh-like and pink coloured tumour. A key in the diagnosis of dysgerminomas is the use of OCT4 immunohistochemistry. Antibodies to OCT4 have been used as the basis for immunohistochemical staining. In 87% of cases, tyrosine kinase receptor c-kit is also overexpressed in the tumour. Five percent of dysgerminoma contain a syncytiotrophoblast cells producing HCG and small percentage of dysgerminoma can produce a low level of β-HCG related to the presence of multinucleated syncytiotrophoblastic giant cells.

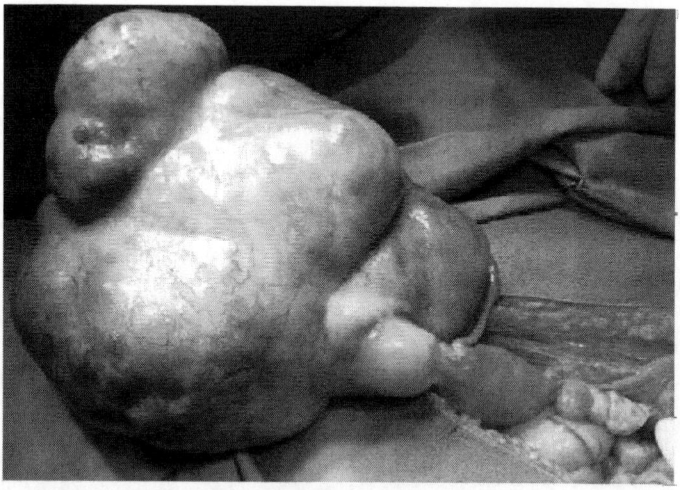

Figure 13.2 Ovarian dysgerminoma.

Dysgerminoma is more likely to be localized to the ovary, although bilaterality is more common and it spread late and do so primarily through the lymphatic system. Dysgerminoma is very chemosensitive and also sensitive to irradiation. Pelvic irradiation, however, is associated with sterility. This tumour is very responsive to cisplatin based chemotherapy (PVB/PEB) and even with stage 3 and 4 and measurable residual tumour, response rate was more than 90% and majority (>90%) are complete pathological responders (on second look). BEP (bleomycin, etoposide and cisplatin) is the regimen of choice as it is less toxic than PVB (cisplatin, vincristine and bleomycin). The other alternative chemotherapy regimens are VAC (vincristine, actinomycin D and cyclophosphamide) and MAC (methotrexate, actinomycin D and chlorambucin). Overall prognosis for patients with dysgerminoma is excellent; the five-year survival rate approaches 100% for patients with stage 1 disease and is 75–90% for patients with other stages of diseases. Poor prognostic factors are large tumour size, bilaterality, age less than 20 and more than 40 years and presence of other neoplastic germ cell elements. Recurrence rate in stage 1 disease without adjuvant therapy is 15–25%.

Yolk Sac Tumour (Endodermal Sinus Tumour)

Yolk sac tumour is also known as endodermal sinus tumour and is believed to originate from primordial germ cells that migrate from the extraembryonic yolk sac into the gonadal ridge at 6 weeks of embryonic life (Fig. 13.3). The most typical histological feature is a glomerular-like structure with central vessels surrounded by prominent large cuboidal cells called the Schiller-Duval body. Yolk sac tumour is the second most common malignant germ cell tumour of ovary and account 60% of ovarian malignancies among children. It accounts in 20% of primitive germ cell tumour and commonly presented at the age of 20–30 (median age 18–25). They are very rare in postmenopausal women. These tumours are mainly solid, rapid growing, aggressive and radioresistant. Before the advent of combination chemotherapy, these tumours were very fatal. Most of these tumours are unilateral, while bilateral in less than 5% of cases. They frequently invade the surrounding structures and exhibiting extensive spread within the abdominal cavity. Yolk sac tumour metastasizes early and mainly via lymphatic systems. Yolk sac tumours recapitulate primitive gut (glandular yolk sac tumour) and primitive liver (hepatoid yolk sac tumour).

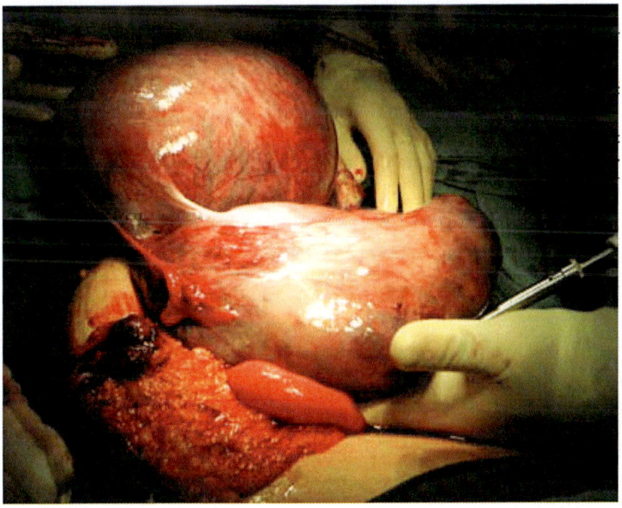

Figure 13.3 Endodermal sinus tumour of ovary diagnosed during pregnancy.

Yolk sac tumour has four subtypes:

(1) polyvesicular vitelline tumour
(2) solid yolk sac
(3) grandular variant
(4) hepatoid variant

All four subtypes may co-exist and the more mixture, the better the prognosis. Due to similarity in histologic features, yolk sac tumours occasionally difficult to differentiate with clear cell carcinoma and endometrioid carcinoma. Yolk sac tumour produces α-fetoprotein. All patients with yolk sac tumour will have raised α-fetoprotein level; however, many studies have shown no correlation between preoperative levels of α-fetoprotein and prognosis. The level of serum α-fetoprotein can reliably be used in monitoring of treatment and diagnosis of recurrence.

On immunohistochemistry, yolk sac tumours typically express α-fetoprotein and are consistently positive to cytokeratines. Placental-like alkaline phosphatase is found in 50% of cases.

The most common presenting symptom is abdominal pain in 55–80% of patients. Fever is present in 25% of cases. Approximately, 60–70% of patients presented at an early stage 1 and 2, 20–30% presented at stage 3 and rarely at stage 4.

Surgery and chemotherapy regimen for yolk sac tumour is similar to dysgerminoma. BEP regimen was found to have similar efficacy but less toxicity than PVB regimen. Three courses of BEP regimen are the current standard therapy, and four courses are recommended in case of bulky residual disease after surgery. The survival rate for patients with stage 1–2 disease is 60–100%, while in patients with stage 3–4 disease, their survival is 50–75% after adjuvant chemotherapy.

Mature Teratoma

Teratomas are germ cell tumours that are formed by cells derived from more than one of the three primitive embryonic layers, i.e. ectoderm, mesoderm and endoderm. Mature teratoma is a benign teratoma and it can be solid or cystic. Mature solid teratomas are rare, while mature cystic teratomas (dermoid cyst) are the most common ovarian germ cell tumours (Fig. 13.4). Bilaterality is seen in 12% of cases, and in 2/3 of cases, mature element consists of tissue differentiation derived from all three embryonic germ layers (Fig. 13.5). Each of these components can be benign or malignant. In matured cystic teratoma, ectodermal is a predominant element.

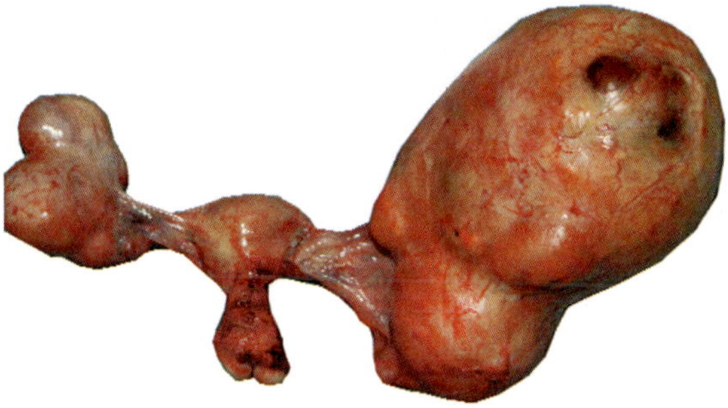

Figure 13.4 Bilateral benign cystic teratoma (mature teratoma).

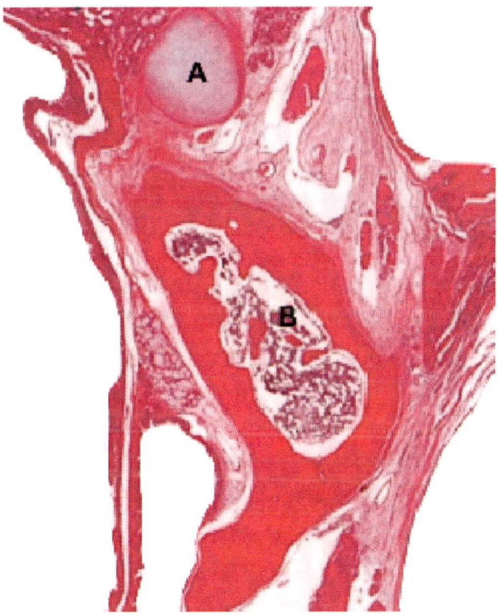

Figure 13.5 Histology of benign (mature) cystic teratoma. (A) Cartilage and (B) bone and marrow.

Matured cystic teratoma diagnosed after 40 years of age and with size larger than 10 cm should be thoroughly investigated for potential co-existing malignant transformation (incidence: 0.17–2%). Most important secondary tumour arising in a dermoid cyst is squamous cell carcinoma (>80% of cases), found in 1% of dermoid cyst. Other malignant tumours arising from a benign cystic teratoma are basal cell carcinoma, malignant melanoma, adenocarcinoma, sarcoma, etc. Prognosis of this malignant tumour is generally poor with a reported five-year survival rate of only 15–31%. Squamous cell carcinoma transformation carries better prognosis as compared to others. Squamous cell carcinoma antigen (SCC antigen) is raised in 81.3–86.5% of patients with SCC arising from a benign cystic teratoma while 60–70% of them have also raised CA125, CA19–9 and CEA (Chen et al.; Hackethal et al).

Treatment for malignant transformation is similar with malignant ovarian cancer, i.e. surgery followed by adjuvant chemotherapy in selected patients. Cisplatin-based chemotherapy is the chemotherapy of choice. Radiotherapy was found to be ineffective. Prognosis of patients with SCC transformation depends of stage at presentation, according to Chen et al. Five-year survival rates were 75.7% for stage 1, 33.8% for stage 2, 20.6% for stage 3 and 0% for stage 4.

Immature Teratomas

Immature teratoma contains primitive, immature or embryonal structures, and it may also have mature tissues (Fig. 13.6). Immature teratomas are more commonly unilateral, and bilaterality is only in less than 5% of cases. Immature teratoma constitutes 20% of primitive germ cell tumour. It is predominantly solid or predominantly cystic, predominantly solid tumours are more common. Solid components may consist of the nervous system, cartilage or bone, while the cystic component is often filled with serous/mucinous/sebaceous/hairs. Immature elements are almost always predominantly neuroectodermal (embryonal). The grading of immature teratoma is shown in Table 13.3.

The grading of immature teratoma by O'Conner and Norris is based on the amount of immature neural tissue contents: (a) low-grade immature teratoma and (b) high-grade (grades 2 and 3) immature teratoma.

Immature teratoma exhibits malignant behaviour and grows rapidly if the tumour is of high grade and spread by peritoneal transplantation and metastasized primarily through lymphatic channels. The treatment is similar to other malignant ovarian germ cell tumours. Extraovarian implants of mature glial tissue can occur anywhere, but it does not upstage the disease.

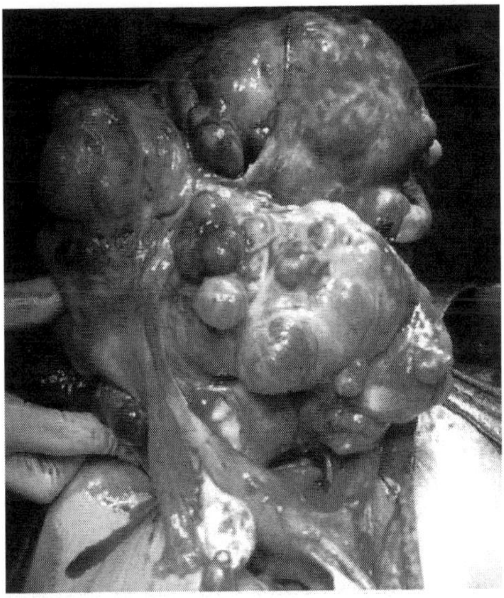

Figure 13.6 Immature teratoma.

Table 13.3 Grading of immature teratoma

(A) Thurlbeck and Scully grading system	
Grade 1	Cell well differentiated; rare small focci of embryonal tissue
Grade 2	Moderate quantities of embryonal tissue, atypia and mitosis +
Grade 3	Large quantities of embryonal tissue, atypia and mitosis +
(B) Norris grading system	
Grade 1	Some immaturity, neuroepithelium in low magnification 40 ×
Grade 2	Immaturity, neuroepithelium ≤3 low power field
Grade 3	Immaturity, neuroepithelium occupy ≥4 low magnification on single slide.

Growing Teratoma Syndrome

The growing teratoma syndrome (GTS) is a condition characterized by immature teratoma in the ovary with distance implantation/metastases of mature teratoma (benign). GTS was first described by Logothets et al. characterized by an enlarged neoplastic mass of non-seminomatous germ cell tumours following chemotherapy. The previously elevated tumour markers will become normal and GTS can occur in both non-seminomatous germ cell tumours of testis and ovary. The incidence of GTS in germ cell tumour of the testis is 1.9–7.6%, but it is less common in the ovary. Typically patients with GTS will initially diagnose as immature teratoma of any grade and treated with surgery followed by chemotherapy. GTS develops either during or after completion of chemotherapy. Patients with GTS present with increasing abdominal distension despite normalization of their tumour markers. Histologically, GTS is demonstrated as the presence of mature elements (mature teratoma) consisting of normal mature tissue elements such as normal skin elements, respiratory tract mucosa, mature cartilage, bone, and glial tissue. There will be no immature elements or malignant component found in any of the sections. Some gynaecologic literature described these phenomena as "chemotherapeutic retroconversion".

The underlying mechanism of GTS is not fully understood. There are three theories:

(a) Chemotherapy destroys only the immature malignant cells, leaving the mature benign teratomatous elements.
(b) Chemotherapy alters the cell kinetics toward transformation from a totipotent malignant germ cell toward a benign mature teratoma.
(c) An inherent and spontaneous differentiation of malignant cells into benign tissues. Chemotherapy just prolongs the course of the disease (patients survive long enough) to permit "spontaneous evolution" to occur.

GTS is always confused with recurrent immature teratoma. CT scans and colour Doppler may show multiple anechoic areas, calcification and absence of neovascularization. Treatment is by surgical resection, but chemotherapy and radiotherapy are ineffective and if the GTS is left untreated, some of its elements may transform into a malignant tumour. Some medical therapies have produced a response in patients with unresectable GTS such as interferon (Kattan; Tonkin) and bevacizumab (Mego).

Embryonal Carcinoma and Choriocarcinoma

Embryonal carcinoma and choriocarcinoma is very rare in the ovary as a pure carcinoma. The presentation of embryonal carcinoma is similar to endodermal sinus carcinoma and the patient's ages ranged between 4 and 28 years with median age of 14 years. Gross examination of embryonal carcinoma reveals a solid, haemorrhagic, necrotic tumour, resembling a larger for of yolk sac tumour. Embryonal carcinoma is the most aggressive cancer arising from the ovary. Most commonly it exists as one of the mixed germ cell tumours. Both embryonal carcinoma and choriocarcinoma produce HCG. They can result in endocrine changes such as sexual precocity and irregular menses. Embryonal carcinoma can be distinguished from choriocarcinoma by the absence of syncytiotrophoblastic and cytotrophoblastic cells. Treatment for embryonal carcinoma is similar to other ovarian carcinoma and the chemotherapy is BEP regimen.

Pure ovarian choriocarcinomas are rare but this tumour is aggressive and pose diagnostic and therapeutic challenges. The presence of malignant cytotrophoblasts and syncytiotrophoblasts, immunohistochemical staining with beta-hcg, and placental lactogen are diagnostic. There are extremely difficult to differentiate histologically between non-gestational and gestational choriocarcinomas. Currently, there is no definitive treatment modality has been established for this tumour due to extremely low incidence. Generally, pure ovarian choriocarcinoma is treated similar to other ovarian germ cell tumours including the choice of adjuvant chemotherapy (BEP regimen) (Lin et al., 2011).

Mixed Germ Cell Tumour

About 10% of primitive germ cell tumour is mixed germ cell tumour. The single most common combination is dysgerminoma and yolk sac tumour. If a dysgerminoma component is present, bilaterality is noted in 10% of cases. The prognosis depends on the proportion of the most malignant component.

Management

Surgery and Adjuvant Chemotherapy in Malignant Germ Cell Tumours

Treatment for malignant germ cell tumour of the ovary is similar to that for epithelial ovarian cancer. Surgical staging and abdominal exploration are similar to epithelial ovarian cancer. Surgery is the mainstay of treatment; however, since many of these patients are in their reproductive age group, fertility preserved surgery should be performed if possible. In general, biopsy of normal-looking contralateral ovary is not recommended. The risk of contralateral ovarian involvement is a very rare. Furthermore, routine biopsy will lead to adhesions and ovarian dysfunction. An exception to this is in dysgerminoma, where the biopsy of normal-looking contralateral ovary may be justifiable because microscopic tumour was noted in 5–10% of cases of apparent stage 1 disease.

In a retrospective study by Pecccatori, overall survival of 96% (mean follow-up time of 55 months) was obtained following fertility-preserved surgery done for 129 patients with malignant ovarian germ cell tumour.

The indication for adjuvant chemotherapy in malignant ovarian germ cell tumour is similar to epithelial ovarian cancer. Following are the indications of adjuvant chemotherapy in stage 1 malignant ovarian germ-cell tumour:

(1) stage 1C dysgerminoma as a pure or mixed germ cell tumour
(2) grade 2 and 3 immature teratoma
(3) embryonal tumour
(4) endodermal sinus tumour

The recommended number of cycle of the chemotherapy regimen in patients with ovarian malignant germ cell tumour is 3–4 cycles (three cycles for optimal cytoreduction and four cycles for patients with suboptimal cytoreduction). BEP (bleomycin, etoposide and cisplatin) is the most active chemotherapy regimen for ovarian malignancy germ cell tumour.

The recommended BEP regimen is as follows (3 courses, 21 days interval):

Cisplatin 20 mg/m^2 day 1 to 5
Etoposide 100 mg/m^2 day 1 to 5
Bleomycin 30 U weekly (Day 1, 8, 15)

Dimopoulos et al. suggested less toxic BEP regimen in their published prospective multi-centre study on FIGO stage 1–4 malignant ovarian germ cell tumour. Following are their proposed less toxic BEP regimen (21 days interval):

Cisplatin 40 mg/m^2 day 1 to 3
Etoposide 120 mg/m^2 day 1 to 3
Bleomycin 15 mg day 1 to 3

The other alternative chemotherapy regimen is PVB (cisplatin, vincristine and bleomycin) and VAC (vincristine, actinomycin D and cyclophospamide). The POMB-ACE (cisplatin, vincristine, methotrexate, bleomycin–actinomycin D, cyclophospamide, etoposide) was initially developed for the management of testicular cancer. Seven different cytotoxic drugs were given as soon as possible to decrease the risk of drug resistance. POMB and ACE were alternating every 2 weeks. POMB-ACE regimen was found to be effective and well tolerated in patients with aggressive and advanced ovarian malignant germ cell tumour (mainly non-dysgerminoma germ cell tumour).

Primary Surgery

The principles of surgery in ovarian germ cell tumours are similar to that for epithelial ovarian cancer. In general, the majority of ovarian germ cell tumours are unilateral except in dysgerminoma. Unilateral salpingoophorectomy can be safely performed in most patients with malignant ovarian germ cell tumour. The biopsy of the normal contralateral ovary is not recommended because unnecessary biopsy of normal-looking contralateral ovary may result in adhesion and ovarian failure. Chemotherapy is very effective in treating the germ cell tumour and there were reports of successful treatment with chemotherapy even without removal of both ovaries. If the tumour is confined to the ovary (apparent stage 1 disease), complete staging surgery should be performed and biopsy of the following structures is strongly recommended (apart from omentectomy and lymphadenectomy): (a) peritoneal surfaces (bilateral paracolic gutters, pouch of Douglas, lateral pelvic wall, utero-vesical reflection and subdiaphragmatic areas) and (b) suspicious adhesions.

Cytoreductive Surgery

The principle of cytoreductive surgery as primary treatment for ovarian germ cell tumour is similar to that for epithelial ovarian carcinoma, i.e. resection of as much tumour as is technically feasible and safe. Germ cell tumour that has been optimally resected has higher response rate to chemotherapy and longer progression free interval (Slayton; William et al.).

Germ cell tumour, especially dysgerminoma, is more chemosensitive than epithelial ovarian cancer; therefore, the role of aggressive resections of advanced and metastatic germ cell tumour, including tumour with bulky retroperitoneal nodes and extensive diaphragmatic diseases, is questionable. Even in extensive metastatic disease, it is not uncommon for the surgeon to be able to preserve a normal contralateral ovary. Secondary debulking is more justifiable in recurrent germ cell tumour as compared to recurrent epithelial ovarian cancer due to higher chemosensitivity of the former, especially those resectable isolated tumour in lung, liver, retroperitoneum or brain. Patients with recurrent germ cell tumour often have higher response rate to second line chemotherapy than epithelial ovarian cancer. Immature teratoma or in mixed germ cell tumour with immature teratoma component may develop growing teratoma syndrome following chemotherapy.

Chemotherapy in Advanced Disease

Treatment of ovarian germ cell was derived from the study and treatment of testicular cancer. In earlier time (1970's), VAC (vincristine, actinomycin-D and cyclophosphamide) regimen was used; however, long-term survival was less than 50%. PVB regimen (cisplatin, vincristine and bleomycin) was later introduced, PVB was found to be superior to VAC regimen in advanced disease (William; De Palo). However, toxicity is the main drawback of both VAC and PVB. Replacing vincristine (in PVB) with Etoposide (BEP) has reduced the neurologic toxicity, abdominal pain and constipation with equivalent efficacy and superiority in high-volume tumour (William; Gerhenson). BEP regimen is the regimen of choice since then. At least four cycles of BEP should be given in advanced germ cell tumour. Bleomycin is most important component and cisplatin is more superior to carboplatin.

Liver and brain metastases indicate poor prognosis with a survival rate of 50–60%. In platinum resistant/refractory cases (no response after PEB), likelihood of survival and cure following second line therapy is less than 5% whereas in platinum sensitive (complete remission after BEP), the survival rate is up to 50%. The POMB-ACE (cisplatin, vincristine, methotrexate, bleomycin –actinomycin D, cyclophospamide, etoposide) was initially developed for the management of testicular cancer. Seven different cytotoxic drugs were given as soon as possible to decrease the risk of drug resistance. POMB and ACE were alternating every 2 weeks. POMB-ACE regimen was found to be effective and well tolerated in patients with aggressive and advanced ovarian malignant germ cell tumour (mainly non-dysgerminoma germ cell tumour).

Chemotherapy for Recurrent Disease

Platinum-based chemotherapy (BEP) will cure almost all chemotherapy-naïve patients with dysgerminoma who develop relapse following surgery. Patients with recurrent dysgerminoma can be treated with second line chemotherapy such as VAC (vincristine, actinomycin D and cyclophosphamide) regimen. Similar treatment is offered to patients with recurrent non-dysgerminoma malignant ovarian germ cell tumour. However, in addition of VAC regimen, there are two other potential chemotherapy regimens, i.e. VIP (vindesine, ifosfamide, cisplatin) and TIP (cisplatin, ifosfamide, paclitaxel) regimens. TIP regimen is effective as salvage therapy in male germ cell tumours. Data in female is unknown. POMB-ACE regimen may be effective as a salvage therapy for patients with recurrent malignant ovarian germ cell tumour not responded to first or second line chemotherapy.

Late Effect of Therapy

Many of the late toxicities of therapy were extrapolated from treatment of male germ cell tumour. Infertility may be due to adhesion and unnecessary bilateral salpingo-ophorectomy/hysterectomy. Patients may also develop leukaemia-induced chemotherapy, mainly acute non-lymphoblastic leukaemia. Etoposide had been implicated to the development of leukaemia in 2.3% of patients who received more than 2000 mg/m^2 (total accumulating dose).

About 70% resume normal menses after oophorectomy followed by chemotherapy. The impact of chemotherapy on gonadal and reproductive function had been documented. In a case series analysis, 76% achieve at least one pregnancy following fertility-preserved surgery and chemotherapy treatment for malignant ovarian germ cell tumour.

The risk of cardiotoxicity in platinum-containing regimens, mainly hypertension, was in the range of 14–15%. Pulmonary fibrosis is a known side effect of bleomycin.

References

Bailey J, Church D. Management of germ cell tumours of the ovary. *Rev Gynaecol Pract*, 2005; **5**: 201–206.

Carlson RW, Siki BJ, Turbow MM, et al. Combination cisplatin, vinblastine, and bleomycin (PVB) for malignant germ-cell tumours of the ovary. *J Clin Oncol* 1983; **1**: 645–651.

Chen RJ, Chen KY, Chang TC, Sheu BC, Chow SN, Huang SC. Prognosis and treatment of squamous cell carcinoma from a mature cystic teratoma of the ovary. *J Formos Med Assoc* 2008; **107**(11): 857–868.

Cheng L, Thomas A, Roth LM, et al. OCT4: a novel biomarker for dysgerminoma of the ovary. *Am J Surg Pathol* 2004; **28**(10): 1341–1346.

Cicin I, Saip P, Guney N, et al. Yolk sac tumours of the ovary: Evaluation of clinicopathological features and prognostic factors. *Eur J Obstet Gynecol Reprod Biol* 2009; **146**: 210–214.

Dallenbach P, Bonnefoi H, Pelte MF, Vlastos G. Yolk sac tumours of ovary: an update. *EJSO* 2006; **32**: 1063–1075.

De Palo G, Zambetti M, Pilotti S, et al. Non-dysgerminomatous tumors of the ovary treated with cisplatin, vinblastine and bleomycin: long-term results. *Gynecol Oncol* 1992; **47**: 239–246.

Dimopoulos MA, Papadimitriou C, Hamilos G, et al. Treatment of ovarian germ cell tumors with a 3 day bleomycin, etoposide and cisplatin regimen: a prospective multicenter study. *Gynecol Oncol* 2004; **95**: 695–700.

Gershenson DM, Morris M, Cangir A, et al. Treatment of malignant germ cell tumors of the ovary with bleomycin, etoposide and cisplatin. *J Clin Oncol* 1990; **8**: 715–720.

Gorbatiy V, Spiess PE, Pisters LL. Review Article: The growing teratoma syndrome: *Curr Rev lit Indian J Urol* 2009; **25**(2): 186–189.

Hackethal A, Brueggmann D, Bohlmann M, Franke FE, Tinneberg HR, Munstedt K. Squamous cell carcinoma in mature cystic teratoma of the ovary: systematic review and analysis of published data. *Lancer Oncol* 2008; **9**: 1173–1180.

Hsieh TY, Cheng YM, Chang FM, Chou CY. Growing teratoma syndrome: An Asian woman with immature teratoma of left ovary after chemotherapy. *Taiwan J Obstet Gynecol* 2009; **48**(2): 186–189.

Kattan J, Droz JP, Culine S, Duvillard P, Theiellet A, Peillon C. The growing teratoma syndrome: A woman with non-seminomatous germ cell tumour of the ovary. *Gynecol Oncol* 1993; **49**: 395–399.

Khoo SK, Buntine DW, Massey PF, Jones IS. Endomermal Sinus tumour of the ovary: the place of alphafetoprotein detection, surgery and chemotherapy. *Aust Nz J Obstet Gynaecol* 1981; **21**(4): 217–225.

Kuwashima Y, Uehara T, Kurosumi M, et al. Cytologic distinction between clear cell carcinoma and yolk sac tumor of ovary. *Eur J Gynaecol Oncol* 1996; **17**(5): 345–350.

Lin Lv, Yang K, Peng Z, et al. Pure choriocarcinoma of the ovary: a case report. *J Gynecol Oncol* 2011, June 30; **22**(2): 135-139.

Mego M, Reckova M, Sycova-Mila Z, et al. Bevacizumab in a growing teratoma syndrome. Case report. *Ann Oncol* 2007; **18**: 962–963.

Murugaesu N, Schmid P, Dancey G, et al. Malignant ovarian germ cell tumors: identification of novel prognostic markers and long-term outcome after multimodality treatment. *J Clin Oncol* 2006; **24**(30): 4862–4866.

O'Brien ME, Perren T, Tan S, Fisher C, Wiltshaw E. The endodermal sinus tumour and clear cell ovarian cancer. *Ann Oncol* 1994; **5**(8): 753–756.

Pectasides D, Pecsides E, Kassanos D. Anti tumour treatment: germ cell tumors of the ovary. *Cancer Treat Rev* 2008; **34**: 427–441.

Peccatori F, Bonazzi C, Chiari S, Landoni F, Colombo N, Mangioni C. Surgical management of malignant ovarian germ-cell tumours: 10 years experience of 129 patients. *Obstet Gynecol* 1995; **86**(3): 367–372.

Sasaki H, Furusato M, Teshima S, et al. Prognostic significance of histopathological subtypes in stage I pure yolk sac tumour of the ovary. *Br J Cancer* 1994; **69**(3): 529–536.

Slayton RE, Park RC, Silverberg SG, Shingleton H, Creasman JA, Blessing JA. Vincristine, dactinomycin, and cyclophosphamide in the treatment of malignant germ cell tumors of the ovary. A Gynecologic Oncology Group Study (a final report). *Cancer* 1985; **56**(2): 243–248.

Tonkin KS, Rustin GJS, Wignall B, Paradinas F, Bennet M. Successful treatment of patients in whom germ cell tumour masses enlarged on chemotherapy while their serum tumour markers decreased. *Eur J Cancer Clin Oncol* 1989; **25**: 1739–1743.

William S, Blessing JA, Liao Y, Ball H, Hanjani P. Adjuvant therapy of ovarian germ cell tumors with cisplatin, etoposide, and bleomycin: a trial of the gynecologic oncology group. *J Clin Oncol* 1994; **12**(4): 701–706.

William SD, Blessing JA, Moore DH, Homesley HD, Adcock L. Cisplatin, vinblastine and bleomycin in advanced and recurrent ovarian germ cell tumors. A trial of the Gynecologic Oncology Group. *Ann Int Med* 1989; **111**(1): 22–27.

Chapter 14

Ovarian Sex Cord-Stromal Tumours

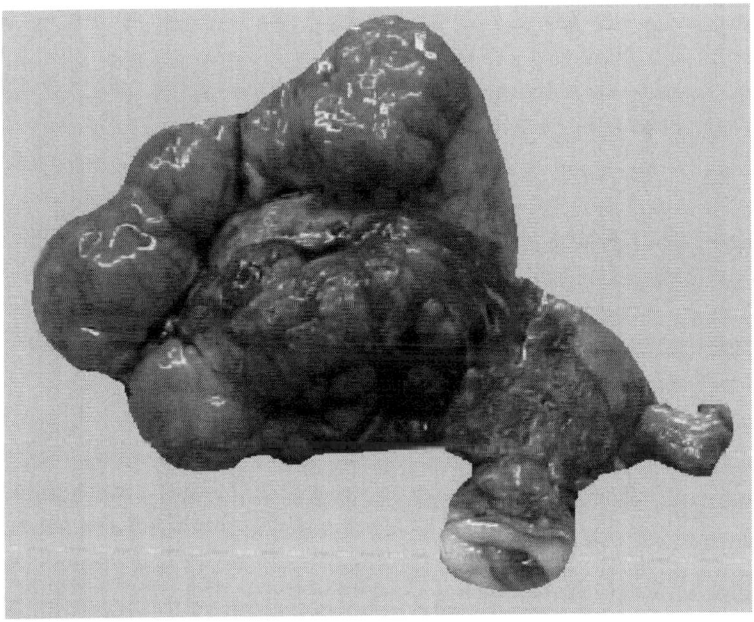

Gynaecologic Cancer: A Handbook for Students and Practitioners
Rushdan Noor, Eng Hseon Tay, and Jeffrey Low

ISBN 978-981-4463-06-5 (Hardcover), 978-981-4463-07-2 (eBook)
www.panstanford.com

Introduction

Sex cord-stromal tumour (SCST) originates from the cells in the ovarian matrix which are composed of granulosa cells, theca cells, Sertoli cells, Leydig cells and fibroblasts of stroma origin. Ovarian matrix supports the germ cells and is covered by epithelium. The cells in the matrix originate from the sex cords and mesenchymal of the embryonic gonad. Sex cord-stromal tumour of the ovary has many histological similarities to endometrioid carcinoma. It accounts for 7% of all malignant ovarian tumours and the majority are of low malignant potential (borderline). This tumour affects mainly women younger than 40 years. Many are steroid hormones-producing tumour, and therefore clinical manifestation is related to endocrinologic abnormalities. Oestrogen-producing tumour (granulosa cell tumour, theca cell and Sertoli cell tumour) may be manifested as the following depending on age:

(a) precocious puberty
(b) menometrorrhagia
(c) post-menopausal bleeding.

Early defeminization and virilization are manifested in androgen-producing tumour (Sertoli–Leydig cells and steroid cell tumours). Excessive oestrogen production can also be due to peripheral conversion of androgen to oestrogen.

The immunohistochemistry of SCSTs is as follows:

(a) Inhibin and calretinin are the most important markers.
(b) Sex cord-stromal tumours can also be positive to cytokeratin (CAM5.2, AE1/AE3), CD10, ER, PR, smooth muscle actin, desmin, S100 protein and WT-1.
(c) CD56 is a sensitive marker for these tumours and may also be useful in the diagnosis, especially in cases where inhibin or calretinin is negative.

The triad of immunohistochemistry for EMA, calretinin and inhibin is the most useful panel for the distinction of a carcinoma (EMA positive; inhibin and calretinin usually negative) from an SCST (EMA negative, inhibin and calretinin positive).

Classification of Sex Cord-Stromal Tumours

Ovarian sex cord-stromal sarcoma is classified into four main groups:

(1) Granulosa-stromal cells tumour

(2) Sertoli-stromal cell tumours
(3) Sex cord tumours of mixed or unclassified cell type
(4) Steroid cell tumours

The WHO classification of SCSTs is shown in Table 14.1.

Table 14.1 WHO classification of sex cord-stromal tumours

Classification	Sub-classification
Granulosa-stromal cells tumour	Granulosa cell tumour Adult type Juvenile type Tumour in the thecoma-fibroma group Thecoma: Typical, luteinized Fibroma: Cellular fibroma, fibrosarcoma Sclerosing stromal tumour Signet ring cell stromal tumour Unclassified
Sertoli-stromal cell tumours	Sertoli cell tumour Leydig cell tumour Sertoli–Leydig cell tumour
Sex cord tumours of mixed or unclassified cell type	Sex cord tumour with annular tubules Gynandroblastoma Sex cord-stromal tumour, unclassified
Steroid cell tumours	Stromal luteoma Leydig cell tumour Stromal luteoma Leydig cell tumour Hilus type Leydig cell tumours non-hilar type Leydig cell tumours, not otherwise specified Steroid cell tumours, not otherwise specified

Granulosa-Stromal Cells Tumour

Granulosa Cell Tumours

Granulosa cell tumour (GCT) was first described by Rokitansky in 1855. The WHO defines GCT as a neoplasm composed of a pure or at the least a 10% population of granulosa cells, often in a fibroatheromatous background. Granulosa cell tumour is the most common malignant SCSTs constituted 70% of all malignant SCSTs. Overall, GCT constituted to 5% of all ovarian malignancies and the annual incidence of GCT is 0.4 to 1.7 cases per 100,000 women. The peak age of GCT is perimenopausal age, average age: 52 year old. The case control study by Boyce that evaluated 72 patients with GCT found an association of this tumour with obesity, race (more common in non-white) and family history of ovarian and breast cancer. Parity and OCP were found to be protective as compared to general population. Almost all GCTs are hormonally active producing oestradiol. Granulosa cell tumours have been reported to be associated with endometrial hyperplasia (25% of cases) due to hyperstimulation of oestrogen and 13% of these patients develop well-differentiated endometrial adenocarcinoma. Spread of GCTs is local, direct extension or intraperitoneal seeding. The tumours may also spread haematogenously. Recurrent GCTs are classically occurred long after initial presentation. Recurrences may not be detected for more than 5 years after the initial diagnosis. The longest reported time period before recurrence was 37 years. The majority of GCTs (80–90%) presented at an early stage (stage 1). The treatments for GCTs are similar with other types of ovarian cancer. Fertility-preserving surgery in indicated in an early stage and if the patient wishes to preserve her fertility. If the uterus is preserved, endometrial biopsy should be performed.

Postoperatively, adjuvant chemotherapy is indicated in high-risk patients following primary surgical treatment. In stage 1 disease, adjuvant chemotherapy is indicated in large tumour, ruptured during surgery and high mitotic index. Platinum-based chemotherapy is the treatment of choice for adjuvant treatment as well as for recurrent GCTs. Among the chemotherapy regimen is BEP regimen. The other alternative is PVB (cisplatin, vinblastine, bleomycin) and CAP (cyclophosphamide/doxorubicin/cisplatin). Although platinum-based chemotherapy is clearly active, the efficacy of newer agents, such as gemcitabine, oxaliplatin is not known. Paclitaxel has been used in a patient with recurrent GCT with a good response (Brown et al.). For patients who previously treated with BEP, the VAC (vincristine, actinomycin-D/cyclophosphamide) regimen can be offered.

Radiotherapy has been used as an adjuvant therapy, treatment for inoperable disease and to treat recurrent GCTs but the results were conflicting. Hormonal treatment with anti-oestrogen (tamoxifen), gonadotropin releasing hormone and high dose progestogen have been tried for advanced recurrent disease with some response. Schmidt, et al. found that 94% of patients with GCT had a VEGF expression tumour. Tao evaluates the potential efficacy of anti-angiogenesis, i.e. bevacizumab in patients with recurrent GCT, the study reported response rate of 38%.

Five-year survival rates for stage 1 are 90–100%, 55–75% in stage 2 and 22–50% in stage 3. Ten-year survival rates are 84–95% for stage 1, 50–65% for stage 2 and 17–33% for stages 3 and 4.

Granulosa cell tumours are divided into two groups: (1) adult-type GCT and (2) juvenile-type GCT.

Adult-Type Granulosa Cell Tumour

The adult type constitutes 95% of all GCTs and occurs more often in postmenopausal women. The peak incidence is between 50 and 55 years old. The main presenting symptoms are abnormal vaginal bleeding, abdominal distension and pain. Prolonged ovarian stimulation by fertility drugs has been reported to have an association with the occurrence of GCTs in some patients (prevalence of 0.23% in fertility drug user). Oestrogen production by GCTs can lead to abnormal menses, post-menopausal bleeding, breast tenderness, uterine myohypertrophy, endometrial hyperplasia and even endometrial cancer. Occasionally, it can also produce progesterone leading to decidual reaction and rarely virilization can be one of the presenting signs. Majority of adult-type GCT is more than 12 cm size, while 10–15% is small and not palpable.

Gross appearances of GCTs are smooth or bosselated external surface. The cut section is either solid, partly solid and partly cystic, or rarely cystic. Solid areas may be hard and rubbery or soft in consistency and tend to be yellowish or gray in colour. Microscopic appearances of adult-type GCT may be characterized by a variety of growth patterns and more than one pattern is typically seen (microfollicular, macrofollicular, trabecular, insular, tubular, diffuse, gyriform, etc.). Microfollicular pattern is characterized by a well-known Call–Exner bodies. Call–Exner bodies are small round cavities usually containing eosinophilic material and surrounded by granulosa cells. Granulosa cell tumours are positive to inhibin and calretinin but negative for cytokeratin 7 and epithelial membrane antigen. The prognosis of this tumour is similar to epithelial borderline tumour.

Adult GCTs are tumours of low-grade malignancy characterized by slow growth and late recurrence even up to 37 years after initial diagnosis. About 80–90% of cases presented in stage 1 disease and bilaterality is only in less than 5% of cases. The overall 5-year survival rate is 90% and recurrence rate for stage 1 disease is 10%; mean interval for recurrence from primary surgery is 8.9 years.

The tumour markers for adult-type GCTs are as follows:

(a) **Oestradiol**: Elevated serum oestradiol is observed in 70% of patients with GCTs but the level is fluctuating and therefore is a not reliable marker of disease activity.
(b) **Inhibin**: Inhibin is a more reliable tumour marker than oestradiol.
(c) **Follicle-regulatory protein (FRP)**: Elevated levels of FRP have been detected in some patients with GCTs. The clinical importance of this marker is not yet known.
(d) **Mullerian-inhibitory substance**: This hormone may be a useful marker of GCTs activity.

Juvenile-Type Granulosa Cell Tumour

The juvenile type of GCTs is rare, accounting for about 5% of all GCTs. The tumour biology of juvenile type is different with adult type. About 90% of GCT is diagnosed in prepubertal and majority of tumours are found in women under the age of 30 years. The age groups are as follows: 44% of cases age less than 10, 78% age less than 20 year old and 3% age more than 30 years old.

In prepubertal girls, the presentation is related to excessive hormone production, e.g. precocious puberty, breast enlargement, pubic hair, leucorrhoea. In rare cases, patients may present with symptoms of hypercalcaemia due to secretion of parathyroid hormone-related protein by the tumour. Approximately, 15% of cases of sexual precocity are caused by ovarian tumours and in most cases are associated with GCTs. Both androgen and progesterone can also elevate in some cases. This tumour can also occur in infant and normally the prognosis is better. Bilaterality is seen in 5% of cases and 88% of cases presented at stage 1A.

Juvenile-type GCTs have been reported in association with Ollier's disease (enchondromatosis) and Maffucci's syndrome (haemangioma). Congenital form of juvenile GCT has been reported in leprechaunism (disease characterized by insulin resistance).

The gross appearances of juvenile-type GCTs are similar to adult type. The histologic characteristic of the juvenile type to distinguish the from adult type are

(a) rounded hyperchromatic nuclei
(b) moderate to abundant eosinophilic or luteinized cytoplasm
(c) mitotic rate higher than adult type
(d) rare Call–Exner bodies

The juvenile-type GCTs often exhibit strong and diffuse CD99 positivity and EMA overexpression is more common in juvenile-type GCTs as compared to adult-type GCTs.

The prognosis for stage 1 disease is good but for advanced stage, juvenile type is more aggressive with a higher incidence of recurrent, shorter disease-free interval and survival than adult type. Prognosis is better in younger age patients. Since a juvenile-type GCTs occur predominantly in prepubertal girls, and most of them are diagnosed at stage 1, conservative surgery is preferred. In advanced disease, combination chemotherapy with platinum-based agents is recommended. Use of palliation radiation therapy has been reported in case of recurrent disease. The tumour markers are similar to adult type and inhibin B has been shown to be a reliable marker for follow-up.

Tumour in the Thecoma-Fibroma Group

Thecoma (Theca Cell Tumour)

Thecoma is a benign tumour composed of plump spindle cells with obvious lipid-containing cytoplasm and resembling cells of the ovarian theca interna. Thecoma is the most hormonally active SCST. It occurs at any age but commonly over the age of 40. Thecoma constitutes 1% of all ovarian neoplasm and in more advanced age group than other sex cords stromal tumour (60–70 year old).

The tumour is bilateral in only 2% of cases. The size of tumour ranges from 1 cm to 40 cm in diameter. It is mainly a solid tumour and the cut surface is characteristically bright yellow to orange

(Fig. 14.1). The main symptoms are abnormal vaginal bleeding (60%) and abdominal mass. Thecoma is oestrogen-producing tumour and 37% of patients have endometrial hyperplasia. In almost 50% of cases, tumour is either non-functioning or androgenic. Androgenic thecomas are rare. Thecoma is a benign tumour; however, in a rare subtype, i.e. luteinized thecoma, it has been associated with sclerosing peritonitis. Luteinized thecoma is usually bilateral and mitotic count is usually elevated. There is no evidence to show that this tumour can metastasize.

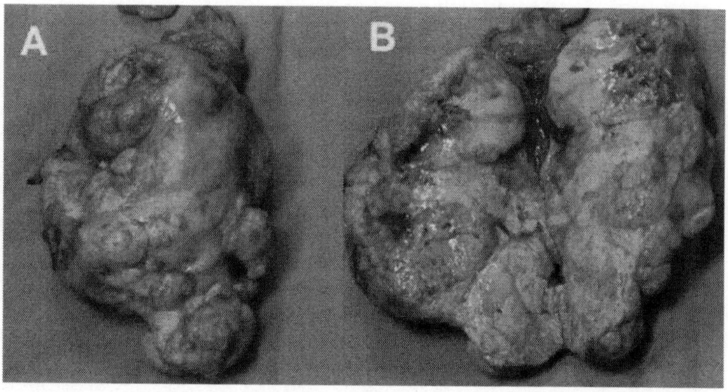

Figure 14.1 Ovarian thecoma. A: intact tumour, B: cross section of the same tumour.

Fibroma

Fibroma is the most common SCST, accounting for about two-thirds of neoplasm in this group. Fibroma constitutes 4% of all ovarian neoplasm and is a benign tumour (Fig. 14.2). It is bilateral in 5% of cases and it does not produce a hormone. It can occur at any age with the average age of 50. The fluid in the tumour can escape into the peritoneal cavity, especially when they are large and the patient may present with ascites. About 10–15% of fibromas of more than 10 cm in size are often associated with ascites. One percent develop hydrothorax to complete the syndromes called Meigs' syndrome. Meigs' syndrome comprises ovarian fibroma, ascites and hydrothorax, the condition is benign and is self-limiting after complete excision of the primary tumour. The other syndrome related to ovarian fibroma is known as Gorlin's syndrome. It is an inherited condition that predisposes the affected women to ovarian fibroma, basal cell nevi, etc. Histologically, fibroma demonstrating hypercellularity, pleomorphism, mild nuclear atypia and mitotic activity of less than 4 mitotic figures per 10 hpf are considered as low malignant potential. If the features are more than above, it is called fibrosarcoma, which is commonly large, highly vascular and aggressive.

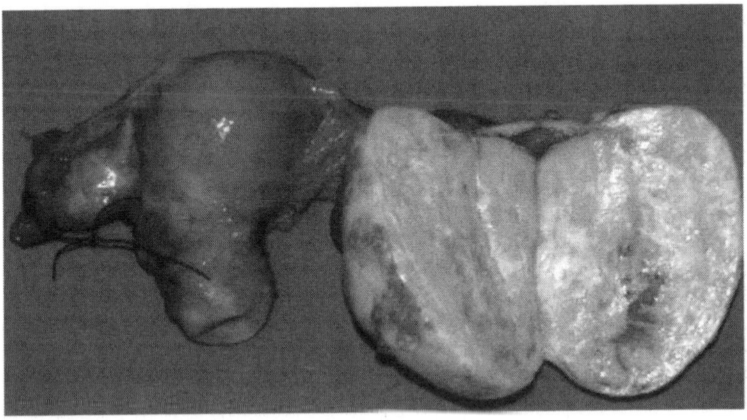

Figure 14.2 Right ovarian fibroma.

Sclerosing Stromal Tumour

Sclerosing stromal tumour (SST) of the ovary is a very rare SCST accounting less than 5% of this tumour. Sclerosing stromal tumour is a benign tumour and usually unilateral. About 80% of SSTs are diagnosed at the age of less than 30 years old. Sclerosing stromal tumour does not produce a hormone and it can be presented at any sizes up to 20 cm in diameter. The cut section of the tumour is solid and white with areas of oedema, cystic formation and yellowish discoloration. The prominent area of sclerosis in histology is the feature suggestive of SST.

Signet-Ring Stromal Tumour

Signet-ring stromal tumour is a benign tumour. Grossly, this tumour may be solid or mixed solid-cystic. Microscopically this tumour is composed of an admixture of spindle and round cells. Some of the round cells show a typical signet-ring appearance. These signet rings do not stain for lipid or mucin.

Sertoli-Stromal Cell Tumours

Sertoli-stromal cell tumours are tumours containing pure form or in various combination Sertoli cells, cells resembling rete epithelial cells, cells resembling fibroblasts, and Leydig cells in variable degree of differentiation. The morphologic characteristics are similar to the testes. Majority of Sertoli-stromal cell tumours are benign but 10–30% are clinically malignant.

Sertoli-stromal cell tumours are classified into three types:

(a) Sertoli cell tumour
(b) Leydig cell tumour
(c) Combination Sertoli–Leydig cell tumour

Sertoli Cell Tumour

Sertoli cell tumour is rare, less than 5% of all Sertoli-stromal cell tumours. Sertoli cell tumours typically occur in young patients with an average age of 27 years and two-thirds of tumours produce oestrogen and some may produce androgen as well. Some patients may present with precocious puberty, menstrual disorder and postmenopausal bleeding. Abdominal distension and pain are frequent complaints. Some produce rennin-causing refractory hypertension and hypocalaemia. The cut section of this tumour is solid tumour, lobulated and yellow in colour. Majority of Sertoli cell tumours is less than 10 cm in size and majority is benign. This tumour rarely shows features of malignancy and if so, it is very aggressive.

Sertoli–Leydig Cell Tumours

Sertoli–Leydig cell tumour is very rare, accounting less than 0.2% of all ovarian tumours. It contains both Sertoli and Leydig cell elements. The average age is 25 years old, 70–75% diagnosed before the age of 30. The most frequent complaints are menstrual problem, virilization and abdominal mass. Androgen production is more dominant (more than 50% of cases) with elevated serum testosterone. Hyperoestrogenic manifestations are observed in some due to peripheral conversion of androgen to oestrogen and rarely produced by the tumour itself. Frank virilization occurs in 35% of cases. Most frequent androgenic symptoms are amenorrhea, voice deepening, and hirsutism.

Sertoli–Leydig cell tumour has a tendency towards a familial occurrence. It had been reported to have an association with other conditions such as with other mesenchymal tumour, Ollier's disease and thyroid disease.

Elevated testosterone-to-androstenedione ratio generally suggests androgen-secreting ovarian tumour most likely Sertoli–Leydig cell tumour. This androgen production can be suppressed by GnRH analogue.

Sertoli–Leydig cell tumours can be well differentiated, moderately differentiated or poorly differentiated tumours. Well-differentiated Sertoli–Leydig cell tumours account for approximately 10% of tumours. The size of Sertoli–Leydig cell tumours ranges from 5–15 cm. The Large size may suggest moderately or poorly differentiated tumour. Majority of these tumours are solid; in a limited number of cases, they produced elevated alpha-fetoprotein (AFP) and inhibin. Increased AFP associated with a higher possibility of malignancy (45%). Overall, 13–18% of Sertoli–Leydig cell tumours are malignant. However, only 2–3% showed extra-ovarian spread at presentation. Abdominal cavity and retroperitoneal lymph nodes are the most common sites for recurrence.

Sertoli–Leydig Cell Tumour with Heterologous Elements

This tumour is different from other types purely based on histological grounds. The most common heterologous elements are gastrointestinal mucin-secreting epithelium. Approximately, 5% contain immature skeletal muscle and/or cartilage. Other rare heterologous elements are fat, carcinoid, smooth muscle, bone, endometrium, etc. This tumour is often mistaken for teratoma, and in poorly differentiated tumour it may mimic carcinosarcoma.

Retiform Variants

Retiform variants of Sertoli–Leydig tumour resemble rete testis. It occurs slightly in the younger age group with mean age of

15 years old. Retiform Sertoli–Leydig cell tumour may be confused with yolk sac tumour or serous adenocarcinoma.

Sex Cord-Stromal Tumours of Mixed or Unclassified Cell Types

Sex Cord Tumour with Annular Tubules

Sex cord tumour with annular tubules (SCTAT) was first described by Scully in 1970 and it representing 6% of SCSTs. Histologically, it is representative of an intermediate between Sertoli cell and GCTs. Microscopically it is characterized by simple and complex annular tubules with central hyaline bodies.

SCTATs can be clinically categorized into the following:

(a) **Peutz–Jeghers syndrome (PJS)-associated SCTATs** (almost all women with PJS have this tumour). This type of tumour accounts for about one third of ovarian SCTATs and is usually bilateral.

(b) **Non-PJS SCTATs**. Mean age group is 34 years, usually large solid tumour and unilateral.

It has a strong association with PJS, an autosomal dominant disorder; one-third of SCTAT occurred in patients with PJS. About 36% of SCTATS are observed in patients with PJS and mean age at presentation is 27 years. Fifteen percent of PJS-associated SCTATs also develop adenoma malignum of the cervix, which is very aggressive, and carry high mortality. Abnormal vaginal bleeding is the most common presenting symptoms. Interestingly, SCTATS can produce both oestrogen and progesterone. Approximately one-third of SCTATs are detected in women with PJS, PJS-tumour is small, multi-focal, bilateral and calcified. They are mostly benign. Malignant rate for non-PJS tumour is 20–25%. They are slow growing tumour and lymphatic metastases invariably ipsilateral. Tumour markers for this tumour that has potential role for monitoring purposes are serum inhibin and mullerian inhibiting substance (MIS).

Gynandroblastoma

Gynandroblastoma is an extremely rare tumour; only less than 20 cases have been reported worldwide and occur in a wide age range. The age range is from 16 to 65 years with the average age of 30 years old. Gynandroblastoma is a well-differentiated tumour and contain testicular elements. Microscopically, it shows admixture of well-differentiated Sertoli cell (testicular elements) and granulosa cell components (ovarian element). The ovarian elements are seen as nests of mature granulosa cells in which Call–Exner bodies may be found. This tumour is more commonly androgenic but hyperoestrogenic or no endocrine manifestation can be encountered. Patients may be presented with amenorrhea, hirsutism and clitorimegaly: manifestations of elevated level of serum testosterone. Gynandroblastoma is considered as tumour of low malignant potential.

Steroid Cell Tumours

Steroid cell tumours are tumours composed entirely or predominantly of cells resembling steroid hormone-secreting cells. Steroid cell tumours constitute 0.1% of all ovarian neoplasms. The predominant components of tumours are steroid hormone-secreting cells (Lutein cells, Leydig's cells or adrenocortical cells). They can be sub-classified into three types:

(a) stromal luteoma
(b) Leydig cell tumour
(c) steroid cell tumours, not otherwise specified (mixture component)

A steroid cell tumour, not otherwise specified, is the most common type of steroid cell tumours. Typically the tumour is solid with an average diameter 8.4 cm and bilateral in 5% of cases. In 60% of cases, the tumour histologically shows benign features.

Stromal Luteoma

Stromal luteoma is a small tumour less than 3 cm and usually unilateral. It constitutes 25% of steroid cell tumours. It arises from luteinized stromal cells. The average age is more than 65 years old and 80% of cases are postmenopausal. The primary presenting complaint is abnormal vaginal bleeding (postmenopausal bleeding). This tumour is predominantly oestrogenic; however, 12% of cases presented with hyperandrogenism. About 20% of tumours are non-functioning/quiescent.

Leydig Cell Tumours

Leydig cell tumours account for 15–20% of steroid cell tumours. Sternberg subdivided this tumour into two groups according to the location: (a) hilar type (located at the hilus of the ovary, can extend to stroma) and (b) non-hilar type (located in the stroma, very rare). The tumour is unilateral in almost all cases. It is typically small-size tumour (mean 2.7 cm) but can reach up to 15 cm. The mean age at diagnosis is 58 years old (37–86 years old). The clinical manifestation of this tumour is related to hyperandrogenic state and overt sign of virilization is observed in 80% of cases. The on-set of virilization is longer than in Sertoli–Leydig cell tumour, up to 7 years. Elevation of serum testosterone is the biochemical feature of this tumour. Oestrogenic manifestation may occasionally be observed in a patient with this tumour, e.g. irregular menses and post-menopausal bleeding. Leydig cell tumour is essentially a benign tumour.

Steroid Cell Tumours, Not Otherwise Specified

This is the most common type of steroid cell tumours. It lacks of characteristic of the above two tumours. The natural history and biology are different from others. The average age is 45 years (10–15 earlier than others). The tumour can occur in early childhood till the ninth decade of life. About 80% of cases are diagnosed at stage 1 disease and the main clinical signs and symptoms are related to hyperandrogenism in 40% of cases, while oestrogen excess is seen in 10–15% of cases, some show cortisol excess. Approximately, 10–15% of patients with this tumour are asymptomatic. The tumour can be benign or malignant, 17% of malignant tumour reported to be associated with Cushing's syndrome. Therefore, presence of Cushing's syndrome should raise the suspicion of malignancy. The serum testosterone and androstenedione are invariably elevated. The malignancy rate is higher and 43% developed extra-ovarian spread during primary surgery or follow-up for 3 years. All malignant tumours are larger size tumour of more than 7 cm in size. About 78% of tumours sized more than 7 cm are malignant. The tumour markers other than steroid hormones are not elevated.

Treatment of Ovarian Sex Cord-Stromal Tumours

Definitive treatment depends on the following factors:

(1) surgical stage
(2) histologic subtype
(3) age and desire for procreation
(4) prognostic factors

Operative Management

The approach of management is similar with any other ovarian malignancy. Sex cord-stromal tumours that can be treated with simple surgical excision (e.g. salpingoophorectomy) without adjuvant therapy include

(a) thecoma
(b) fibroma
(c) gynandroblastomas
(d) stromal luteomas
(e) Leydig's cell, Sertoli cell
(f) well differentiated Sertoli–Leydig cell tumours

In sex cord tumour with annular tubules associated with PJS, assessment of the endocervix is essential due to possibilities of adenoma malignum of the cervix.

Nodal metastasis in ovarian SCSTs is rare and therefore, routine lymphadenectomy may not be necessary. Brown et al. evaluated the patterns of metastasis in ovarian sex-cord stromal tumours, they found that in 58 patients underwent routine lymphadenectomy, none have positive lymph nodes and in 117 patients with recurrent disease, only 5.1% had lymph node involvement. Lymphatic spread is in SCST is not as common as in other ovarian cancers.

Sex cord-stromal tumours that require proper surgical staging, including peritoneal biopsy, omentectomy and lymph nodes sampling are

(a) granulosa cell tumour
(b) moderately and poorly differentiated Sertoli–Leydig cell tumour

(c) non-PJS SCST with annular tubules
(d) unspecified steroid cell tumours

In young patients, fertility-preserving surgery is justifiable in selected patients similar to germ cell tumours. Thorough endometrial evaluation should be done in any of the above tumours when uterine conservation is decided. The role of secondary tumour debulking remains controversial but may be acceptable (for palliation) in germ cell tumour and sex cord tumour with annular tubules (those not associated with PJS) as this tumour is more indolent (slow growing).

Post-Operative Management

(1) Granulosa cell tumour: See respective topics.
(2) Sertoli–Leydig cell tumour
  (a) The effectiveness of radiation therapy is unknown.
  (b) VAC and PAC regimen has been reported to be useful.
(3) Sex cord tumour with annular tubules
  (a) Experience is scant because of rarity.
  (b) Complete response to PEB regimes has been reported in recurrent SCTAT.

References

Boyce EA, Costaggini I, Vitonis A, et al. The epidemiology of granulosa cell tumors: a case control study. *Gynecol Oncol* 2009; **115**: 221–225.

Brown J, Shvartsman HS, Deavers MT, et al. The activity of taxanes compared with bleomycin, etoposide and cisplatin in the treatment of sex cord-stromal tumours. *Gynecol Oncol* 2003; **97**: 489–496.

Brown J, Sood AK, Deavers MT, et al. Patterns of metastasis in sex cord-stromal tumours of the ovary: can routine staging lymphadenectomy be omitted? *Gynecol Oncol* 2009; **113**: 86–90.

Esheba GE. Ovary, Sex Cord Stromal Tumours. e-medicine article 2009. Web URL: http://emedicine.medscape.com/article/1627984.

Manchana T, Ittwut C, Mutirangura A, Kavanagh JJ. Targeted therapies for rare gynaecological cancers. Lancet Oncology, published online April 1, 2010, DOI: 10.1016/S1470-2045(09)70368–73687.

Pectasides D, Pectaside E, Psyrri A. Granulosa cell tumor of ovary. *Cancer Treat Rev* 2008; **34**: 1–12.

Sivasankaran S, Itam P, Coker LA, Sanchez J, et al. Juvenile Granulosa cell ovarian tumour: a case report and review of literature. *J Pediatr Adolesc Gynecol* 2009; **22**: e114–e117.

Tao X, Sood AK, Deavers MT, et al. Anti-angiogenesis therapy with bevacizumab for patients with ovarian granulosa cell tumors. *Gynecol Oncol* 2009; **114**: 431–436.

Wilkinson N, Osborn S, Young RH. Sex cord-stromal tumours of the ovary: a review highlighting recent advances. *Diagn Histopathol* 2008; 14: **8**: 388–400.

Chapter 15

Gestational Trophoblastic Diseases

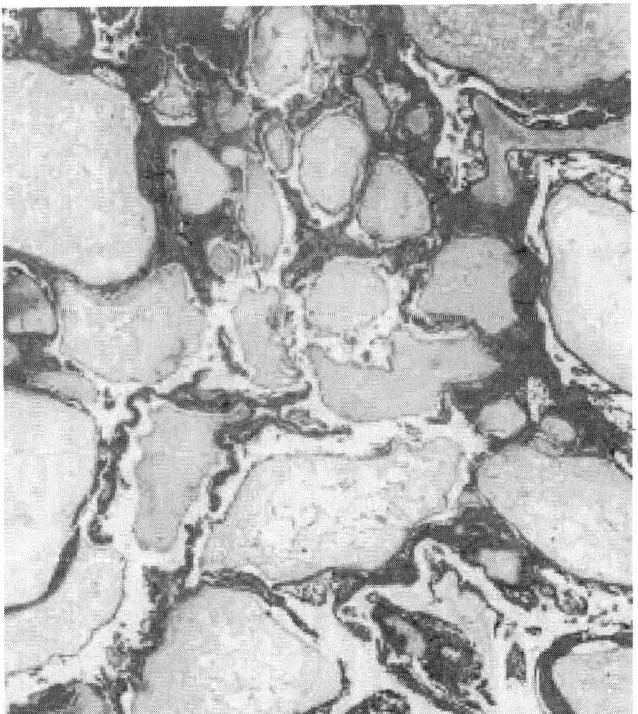

Gynaecologic Cancer: A Handbook for Students and Practitioners
Rushdan Noor, Eng Hseon Tay, and Jeffrey Low

ISBN 978-981-4463-06-5 (Hardcover), 978-981-4463-07-2 (eBook)
www.panstanford.com

Introduction

Gestational trophoblastic disease (GTD) was probably first described by Hippocrates around 400 BC. However, only in 1895, GTD was found to be associated with pregnancy. Gestational trophoblastic disease is a group of interrelated tumours originating from the placenta. Gestational trophoblastic disease consists of a spectrum of pregnancy-related disorders ranging from benign hydatidiform mole, clinically malignant conditions like the invasive mole and metastatic mole, to neoplastic conditions such as choriocarcinoma, placental-site trophoblastic tumour and epithelioid trophoblastic tumour (ETT).

Epidemiology

The incidence of GTD varies dramatically in different regions. The incidence is higher in Asia and Latin America than in Western countries. Incidence in South Asia ranges from 3.2–9.9 per 1000 pregnancies as compared to 0.6–1.1 per 1000 pregnancies in Europe and North America. The incidence of molar pregnancy in Taiwan was 1 in 125 pregnancies, while in United States, 1 in 1500 pregnancies. In United States, hydatidiform moles are observed in approximately 1 in 600 therapeutic abortions and 1 in 1500 pregnancies. The high incidence in some populations was attributed to socioeconomic and nutritional factors. Incidence of molar pregnancy in certain Asian countries shows a decreasing trend probably related to the change in socio-economic status, lifestyle and diet.

Risk Factors for Gestational Trophoblastic Disease

Following are the risk factors for GTD:

(a) Women older than 40 year have 5–10-fold higher risk of hydatidiform mole.
(b) Almost one-third of pregnancies in women older than 50 results in molar gestation.
(c) Young women are also at higher risk of hydatidiform mole.
(d) Use of the oral contraceptive pills is associated with an increased risk of GTD with relative risks ranging from 1.1 to 2.6.

(e) Low intake of dietary carotene and animal fat (case control studies).
(f) History of molar pregnancy (risk of 1–2% in women with one previous history of molar pregnancy, after 2 molar pregnancy, the risk of third molar pregnancy is 15–20%). The risk is not decreased by a change of partner.
(g) Recent genetic studies also showed that hydatidiform mole can also be associated with mutation of NLRP7 gene, which could explain the recurrent type of this condition.

There is no relation between paternal age, smoking, alcohol intake, blood group and infection with the risk of GTD. The actual incidence of choriocarcinoma and placental-site trophoblastic tumour is less well known. These diseases can arise after any form of pregnancy either full term, miscarriage or ectopic pregnancy. In UK, the incidence of choriocarcinoma is thought to be approximately one in 50,000 deliveries, while 0.2% of reported gestational trophoblastic neoplasms (GTNs) were a placental-site trophoblastic tumour.

Classification of Gestational Trophoblastic Disease

There are various classifications of GTD. The WHO classification is the most commonly used in many textbooks and literature. Table 15.1 shows four different types of classifications of GTD.

Table 15.1 Classification of gestational trophoblastic diseases

Type of classification	Sub-classification

(1) WHO classification of gestational trophoblastic disease (GTD), 2003.	Hydatidiform mole
	    Complete mole, Partial mole
	Invasive hydatidiform mole
	Choriocarcinoma
	Placental site trophoblastic tumour
	Trophoblastic lesions, miscellaneous
	    Exaggerated placental site
	    Placental site nodules and plaques
	Unclassified trophoblastic lesion

(*Continued*)

Table 15.1 (*Continued*)

Type of classification	Sub-classification
(2) Histological classification of GTD	Complete mole, Partial mole Invasive mole Metastatic mole Choriocarcinoma Placental-site trophoblastic tumour Epithelioid trophoblastic tumour
(3) Patho-biological classification of Gestational trophoblastic diseases (modified WHO classification 2003), Shih IM 2007, *Lancet Oncol* 2007; **8**: 642–650	***Benign trophoblastic lesions*** Exaggerated placental reaction Placenta-site nodule ***Hydatidiform mole (abnormally formed placentas)*** Complete mole, Partial mole, Invasive mole ***Trophoblastic neoplasia*** Choriocarcinoma Placental-site trophoblastic tumour Epithelioid trophoblastic tumour
(4) Classification based on present or absent of villi	***With villi*** Hydatidiform mole (complete mole, partial mole) Invasive mole Persistent mole Cholangiocarcinoma ***Without villi*** Placental site nodules and plaques Placental site trophoblastic tumour Epithelioid trophoblastic tumour Choriocarcinoma

Pathogenesis of Gestational Trophoblastic Disease

Hydatidiform Mole

All GTDs are derived from the placenta. The hydatidiform mole usually arises when an ovum without maternal chromosomes is fertilized by single sperm that then duplicates its DNA resulting in a 46XX in which all chromosomes are derived from paternal (Androgenic diploid-monospermic). In approximately 10% of cases, complete hydatidiform moles are 46XY when the empty ovum is fertilized by 2 sperms (Androgenic diploid: dispermic).

Partial hydatidiform moles are almost always triploid resulting from fertilization of a healthy ovum by two sperms (biparental triploid). The zygot of partial mole is therefore, becomes triploid containing 69, XXY, XXX and rarely XYY.

Immunostaining is helpful in differentiating hydropic abortion, complete mole (Fig. 15.1) and partial mole. Ki-67 proliferating marker is positive in >65% of molar pregnancies as compared to only <25% in hydropic abortion. Gene p57 (KIP2) is expressed by maternal allel and is visible on histology as nuclear staining of cytotrophoblast and villous mesenchyme in placenta of all gestations apart from androgenetic complete mole. Therefore, in complete mole, since all the DNA is derived from paternal, p57 staining is negative (in cytotrophoblasts and villous stromal cells). On the other hand, since the partial mole contains maternal DNA, p57 is positive.

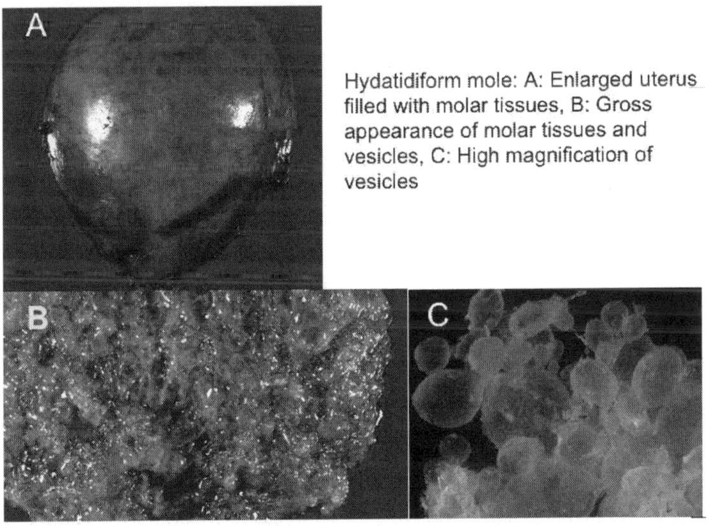

Figure 15.1 Complete hydatidiform mole.

Hydatidiform moles and choriocarcinoma arise from villous trophoblast, while placental-site trophoblastic tumours from interstitial trophoblast. The differences between complete mole and partial mole are shown in Table 15.2. When the foetus is identified with partial moles, they are often growth retarded and multiple congenital anomalies. Neoplastic sequelae occur in less than 5% of patients with partial moles compared with approximately 20% after evacuation of complete hydatidiform mole.

Table 15.2 Comparison between complete and partial hydatidiform mole

Features	Complete mole	Partial mole
Foetal or embryonic tissue	Absent	Present
Hydatidiform swelling of chorionic villi	Diffuse	Focal
Trophoblastic hyperplasia	Diffuse	Focal
Scalloping of chorionic villi	Diffuse	Focal
Trophoblastic stromal inclusion	Absent	Present
Implantation-site trophoblast	Marked atypia	Mild atypia
Karyotype	46, XX (mainly) 46, XY (10%) Chromosome entirely from paternal Mitochondrial DNA is maternal origin	Triploid (90%) Diploid
Uterine size	50% larger than gestational age	Often small for gestational age
Theca lutein cysts	15–25% of cases	Rare
Medical complication	<25%	Rare
Postmolar malignancy sequelae	6–32%	<5%

Presentations of Hydatidiform Mole

The presentation of hydatidiform mole has changed dramatically over the past 30 years, mainly as a result of early recognition through ultrasound and hCG measurement (see Table 15.3).

Table 15.3 Changing in clinical presentation of complete hydatidiform mole: New England Trophoblastic Disease Center (Berkowitz and Goldstein)

Symptoms/signs	1965–1975 (N = 306)	1988–1993 (N = 74)
Vaginal bleeding	97%	84%
Anaemia (Hb < 10g/dl)	54%	5%
Uterine size > date	51%	28%
Preeclampsia	27%	1%
Hyperemesis	26%	8%
Hyperthyroidism	7%	0
Respiratory distress	2%	0

Presentations of Complete Hydatidiform Mole

Patients may be asymptomatic when the diagnosis is made in first trimester during regular antenatal check-up. Vaginal bleeding is a presenting symptom in 89–97% of cases. The prune-juice like fluid (blood undergone oxidation) leak from the uterine cavity is not an uncommon symptom. Anaemia is currently less common due to early detection of molar pregnancy (current figure is 5% as compared to 54% previously). Patients may present with theca lutein cysts (usually with size of more than 6 cm). Following is the information regarding theca lutein cyst in hydatidiform mole:

(a) It is detected in 15–25% of patients.
(b) Theca lutein cyst is generally 6–12 cm in size but it can enlarge up to 20 cm.
(c) It is detected in patients with high serum hCG.
(d) It usually resolves over 8 weeks.
(e) The risk of torsion is 2.3%.

The uterus is larger than the period of gestation in 28% of complete HM and less than 10% in partial mole. In complete hydatidiform mole, 8% of patients presented with excessive vomiting requiring antiemetic and intravenous fluid replacement. Pre-eclampsia is observed only in 1% of patients with complete hydatidiform mole. Hyperthyroidism is presented in patients with very high level of serum hCG, mainly in complete hydatidiform mole. The incidence of hyperthyroidism is approximately 7%. Pulmonary insufficiency observed in 0–2% of cases. Normally resolve within 72 hours. Pulmonary insufficiency in molar pregnancy may be attributed to the following factors: (a) Molar tissue embolization, (b) Cardiovascular complications of thyroid storm, (c) Cardiovascular complications of Pre-eclampsia and (d) Cardiovascular complications of fluid replacement.

Presentations of Partial Mole

Diagnosis of a partial moles often been made following evacuation of the uterus for suspected missed miscarriage. Patients with partial mole may have all similar presentations (theca-lutein cyst, hyperemesis, hyperthyroidism, etc.) with complete hydatidiform mole but at a lower rate.

Diagnosis of Hydatidiform Mole

The diagnosis of hydatidiform mole is confirmed by histological examination. Ultrasound is an important diagnostic tool to detect hydatidiform mole with reasonable accuracy, especially during the late first trimester and second trimester. With the introduction of high-resolution transvaginal ultrasound scans, the majority of patients with hydatidiform mole are diagnosed during the first trimester. The diagnosis of HM during the first trimester may be more difficult because many features of normal and molar placenta were found to be similar during the earliest weeks (5–6 weeks). The most challenging task is to differentiate between hydropic abortions and trisomy with HM, which often required immunostaining as well as cytogenetic analysis. The diagnosis of partial hydatidiform mole is even more difficult in first trimester.

Ultrasound scans is the most useful diagnostic tool to detect hydatidiform mole during the late first trimester (9–12 weeks) and second trimester of pregnancy. The combination of ultrasound and serum β-hCG significantly improved the diagnostic accuracy. Ultrasound features of complete hydatidiform mole are as follows (accuracy rate 58%): (a) Enlarged uterus with no foetal parts, (b) Placenta tissue demonstrating the classical "snowstorm" appearance representing a hyperechoic endometrial echo complex, containing multiple hypoechoic and anechoic spaces (placental lakes resulting from stasis of blood between the hydropic villi) and (c) Presence of bilateral theca lutein cysts.

Sonographic features of the partial moles are as follows (accuracy rate 17%):

(a) focal cystic changes in the placenta
(b) increased placental echogenicity
(c) increased ratio of transverse:anterioposterior diameter of gestational sac >1.5 (may be part of manifestation of embryopathy)
(d) presence of the foetal part or growth-retarded foetus with multiple congenital anomalies associated with a focally hydropic placenta

The differential diagnosis of hydatidiform mole is hydropic degeneration of missed miscarriage, incomplete miscarriage, degenerated leiomyoma, adenomyosis and uterine malignancy.

Human Chorionic Gonadotropin in Gestational Trophoblastic Disease

Human chorionic gonadotropin (HCG) is a glycoprotein produced by syncytiotrophoblasts. Human chorionic gonadotropin comprises α subunit and β subunit. The α subunit shared with other members of the glycoprotein hormones, including thyroid-stimulating hormone and luteinising hormone. Both subunits are joined by non-covalent bonds. In normal pregnancy, most hormone HCG is intact and hyperglycosylated during the first trimester. In GTD, there is a higher proportion of β-HCG compared with normal pregnancy. There is also a presence of various subtypes of β-HCG such as free β-HCG, nicked free-β, β-core and carboxyl-terminal fragment. Human chorionic gonadotropin assays are used to detect all forms of HCG and not only those found in healthy pregnancy; however, most commercial assays fail to or variably detect all form of β-HCG. Every HCG assay is susceptible to false positive and false negative results. False positive results may be due to cross-reacting to heterophilic antibodies. However, these antibodies do not pass into the urine. These heterophilic antibodies are also known as phantom HCG or pseudohypergonadotropinemia. False negative results can also occur in a patient with too high level of hormone HCG. When HCG level is too high, there are not enough antibodies in the solution to bind the HCG molecules and hence much of them is being washed away without being measured. In this case, serum should be diluted first prior to testing. Almost 50% of patients with complete hydatidiform mole have serum HCG level of more than 100,000 IU/L. However, only 7% of the partial moles have HCG of more than 100,000 IU/l.

Hyperglycosylated HCG is a variant of regular HCG with double size of sugar units boosting the size of HCG from 36,700 to more than 40,000 molecular weight. It acts as an autocrine growth factor or cytokine to promote cytotrophoblast cell invasion and malignancy as occurs in implantation of pregnancy and in all invasion cases by trophoblast cells. The aggressiveness of GTN can be assessed based on the level of hyperglycosylated HCG. Lower level associated with less invasive disease and chemorefractory. The GTD with low or absence hyperglycosylated HCG is known as quiescent GTD. Hyperglycosylated HCG not only can measure the behaviour of trophoblast disease but also can guide in terms of timing to commence chemotherapy (high level will respond well to chemotherapy). Some centre adopting the policy of allowing patients to wait without treatment until their HCG level reaches certain level, e.g. >3000 IU/L before treating with chemotherapy. Poor response to chemotherapy is most likely in patients with slow rising in total HCG, doubling rate of 2–6 weeks and <40% hyperglycosylated HCG from total HCG (Cole Muller).

Management of Hydatidiform Mole

Patients with hydatidiform mole must be treated with uterine evacuation after thorough assessment and stabilization. Pre-evacuation investigations should include a complete blood count, clotting profiles, renal and liver function test, blood type, serum HCG and chest X-ray. Patients with medical complications must be referred to physician and anaesthetist before evacuation.

Suction evacuation is the preferred method of treatment. Medical induction using oxytocic or prostaglanding is not recommended due to potential bleeding and high risk of neoplastic sequelae, including tumour embolization. Sharp curettage should follow suction, and Rhogam is given in Rhesus-negative patients. Evacuation of the uterus could also be guided by ultrasound scan to ensure that the entire tissues are removed from the uterine cavity.

Hysterectomy may be indicated in selected patients who are not keen on preserving their fertility, mainly in perimenopausal age and patients with massive life-threatening haemorrhage. In some studies, hysterectomy decreases the overall risk of post-molar GTN to 3.5% as compared 20% risk of postmolar GTN following suction evacuation, this in mainly in older women who have higher risk of malignant sequelae (Goedhals et al., 2010; Tsukamoto et al., 1985). The rate of hysterectomy in a patient with GTD is 1 in 150 caes. Routine hysterectomy is not recommended due to potential risk of operative procedures, molar embolization and study have shown that hysterectomy does not prevent invasive disease (Pisal et al.). Even, after hysterectomy, the patients must still required close follow up especially in elderly women as the risk of post hysterectomy GTD is 8–20% (Davidson et al., 1997).

The role of prophylactic chemotherapy in a high-risk group is controversial as many will receive unnecessary chemotherapy. Chemoprophylaxis has been shown to significantly reduce the rate of GTN in a high-risk group from 31% to 10–15% (50% reduction). However, with this policy almost 50% of patients will receive chemotherapy unnecessarily. Chemoprophylaxis may be helpful in a patient with poor compliant or in a centre where monitoring of serum HCG is unavailable. Chemoprophylaxis does not significantly influence the occurrence of persistent tumour in patients with low-risk hydatidiform mole.

Following uterine evacuation, the patient must be followed up closely to ensure remission and to identify the patients with persistent disease. The follow-up schedule varies in different institutions; it is recommended that the patient be followed up 1–2 weekly until their serum HCG becomes undetectable and subsequently monthly for 6 months. The patient is then seen every 3–6 monthly for the total duration of 24 months. In some Institution, once serum HCG returns to normal, monitoring was continued with urine HCG. The patient must be counsel on contraception for at least 6 months after HCG level return to normal. Intrauterine device (IUCD) is not recommended until serum HCG normalizes. Intrauterine device insertion may lead to uterine perforation, bleeding and infection if the residual disease is presents. The use of combined oral contraceptive pills (COC) by a patient with GTD following treatment is controversial, the literature search done by Gaffield ME and colleagues have reported that the incidence of postmolar trophoblastic disease was lower among COC users compared with non-users in six studies, but higher among COC users in three studies. Five studies reported shorter human chorionic gonadotropin (hCG) regression duration among COC users compared with other methods. They conclude that the risk of postmolar trophoblastic disease does not increase among women using COCs following molar pregnancy evacuation as compared with a use of other contraceptive methods (including IUCD) or no method (Gaffield et al.).

Natural History of Molar Pregnancy and Prognostic Factors

Following molar evaluation, more than 80% of patients will achieve complete remission, while approximately 15% will progress to local invasive disease and 4% to metastatic disease.

The patient with complete hydatidiform mole is at higher risk of developing GTN if they have the following features:

(a) serum HCG >100,000 mIU/mL at presentation
(b) excessive uterine enlargement
(c) theca lutein cyst >6 cm in diameter

Other risk factors for post-molar GTN are age more than 40 and patients with recurrent molar pregnancy. In a high-risk group (presence of high risk factors), the risk of local invasion and metastases is 31% and 9%, respectively, while the patient in a low-risk group has a risk of 3.4% and 0.6%, respectively (Berkowitz and Goldstein).

In partial mole, the risk of progression to non-metastatic GTN was 6.6% (out of 240 patients in New England Trophoblastic Center), while based on data collection from 9 centres with the total of 1, 125 cases of partial mole, the risk of persistent trophoblastic disease was 3.5% and the risk of metastatic GTN was 0.6%.

Gestational Trophoblastic Neoplasm

The term gestational trophoblastic neoplasia encompasses a group of interrelated but distinct tumours that include choriocarcinoma, placental-site trophoblastic tumour and ETT. Gestational trophoblastic neoplasia is genetically related to foetal tissues and therefore, represents semiallografts in patients. Choriocarcinoma is the most common GTN. The term GTN is also designated to the patient who presented with plateauing or increasing level of serum HCG despite complete evacuation of hydatidiform mole.

Similar to hydatidiform mole, GTN is more common in Southeast Asia than in the West. The incidence of GTN in India and Indonesia is 15–19 per 1000 pregnancies and that in the West is 0.2–0.7 per 1000 pregnancies. Patients with GTN required treatment with chemotherapy.

Following is the indications for chemotherapy in a patient with an initial diagnosis of hydatidiform mole (UK guideline):

(a) Plateauing or rising HCG concentration after evacuation. Plateauing HCG concentration is defined as four or more equivalent values of HCG for at least 3 weeks (day 1, 7, 14 and 21) and rising as 2 consecutive increases in HCG concentration of 10% or more for at least 2 weeks (days 1, 7 and 14).

(b) Heavy vaginal bleeding or evidence of gastrointestinal or intraperitoneal haemorrhage.

(c) Serum HCG concentration of 20,000 IU/L or more, 4 weeks or more after evacuation.

(d) Raised HCG concentration 6 months after evacuation, even when still showing decreasing trend.

Choriocarcinoma is malignant hCG-producing epithelial tumours with characteristic biphasic architecture recapitulating cytotrophoblast-like cells and multi-nucleate, pleomorphic syncytiotrophoblast-like regions. In some patients, metastatic spread of choriocarcinoma is manifested following term delivery; this could be explained by the presence of intraplacental choriocarcinoma. Choriocarcinoma is a highly malignant epithelial tumour that can be associated with any type of gestational event, mainly with complete hydatidiform mole. Overexpression of p53 protein has been detected in choriocarcinoma. The other genes that are potentially involved in choriocarcinoma are NECC1, EGFR, DOC-2/hDab2, etc.

Placental site trophoblastic tumour (PSTT) is the rarest malignant GTD arises from trophoblastic tissue at the placental insertion site and can complicate any form of pregnancy. It was first described in 1976 and was initially thought to be benign.

Placental site trophoblastic tumour is characterized by the absence of villi with a proliferation of intermediate trophoblast cells. Placental site trophoblastic tumour arises from intermediate trophoblast, unlike choriocarcinoma, which arise from villous trophoblast. This tumour leads to fewer hemorrhagic lesions and necrosis. The production of hCG is lower in PSTT due to the lower ratio of syncytiotrophoblast cells in PSTT as compared to choriocarcinoma. Placental site trophoblastic tumour is also known to produce placental lactogen (hPL) and 95% of cases follow full term pregnancy, immunostaining for hPL is helpful in the diagnosis of this disease. Placental site trophoblastic tumour is known to usually develop in patients at reproductive age with median age of 31 years. Metastasis occurred in about 16–54% of patients at initial diagnosis. Lymphatic spread in PSTT is more common than other GTN with the overall incidence of at least 6%. Para-oartic lymph nodes are the most common site of nodal metastases, which carry poor prognosis.

Epithelioid trophoblastic tumour (ETT) defers from PSTT as in ETT, neoplastic cytotrophoblast differentiates into chorionic-type extravillous (intermediate) trophoblastic cells in the chorion leave. Majority of PSTT and ETT are thought to behave like benign tumour and only 15–25% of cases showed malignant behaviour such as local invasion and distant metastasis.

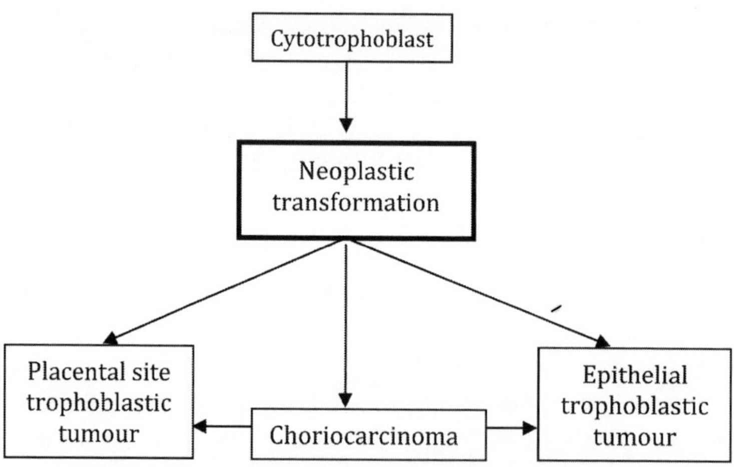

Figure 15.2 The proposed model for pathogenesis of GTN.

The exact pathogenesis of GTN is still unclear but new model of its pathogenesis has been proposed recently as shown in the Fig. 15.2. According to this model, choriocarcinoma, PSTT and EST are derived from common cytotrophoblast stem cell which subsequent underwent a malignant transformation. Choriocarcinoma is the most primitive trophoblastic tumour, whereas PSTT and ETT are relatively more differentiated. This model explains why some patients have mixed histological features (Shih).

Invasive GTN can perforate the uterus and erode uterine vessel leading to vaginal bleeding.

The most common site for metastatic GTN is lung (80%), vagina (5–16%), brain (10%) and pelvis (4–7%). Liver and abdominal metastases accounted for 1–4% and 2–4%, respectively (Evan Jr). Except for vaginal metastasis, it is rare to have other metastatic diseases in the absence of lung metastases.

Metastatic Gestational Trophoblastic Neoplasm

Metastatic GTN is seen in 4% after evacuation for complete hydatidiform mole. Metastasis to the lung can lead to pulmonary hypertension and respiratory failure. The mortality rate for respiratory failure in this case is approaching 100%. Typical lung lesions are rounded, soft tissue density measuring up to 3 cm in diameter usually less than 10 and may rarely cavitate. Approximately, 40% of patients with lung metastases are not detected on the plain chest radiograph.

Gestational trophoblastic neoplasia is often highly vascular and is the commonest cause of uterine vascular malformations. These vascular malformations persist in up to 15% of patients despite complete response to chemotherapy. Bleeding is control either by uterine artery ligation, surgery, hysterectomy or less invasive technique using vascular embolization (uterine artery embolization). Chemotherapy may also cause bleeding at the metastatic site.

Majority of patients with brain metastasis presented with symptoms of increased intracranial pressure. The majorities of lesions are multiple, occur at the grey-white matter junction, and are most commonly located in the parietal lobe.

Majority of patients with liver metastasis is asymptomatic. The most common site of vaginal metastasis is a fornices and suburethral region. They are very vascular and may bleed heavily after biopsy.

Patients with lung and vaginal metastases should also undergo CT/MRI brain (Fig. 15.3). If the imaging does not show any brain metastasis while there is clinical suspicion, cerebrospinal (CSF) can be aspirated to measure the HCG level. In brain metastasis, the serum HCG: CSF HCG is >60 IU/L in 60% of cases. Other rare sites of metastatic disease are kidneys, spine, gastrointestinal tract and skin. Metastatic disease to the neonate was also reported when choriocarcinoma is concurrent with a normal pregnancy.

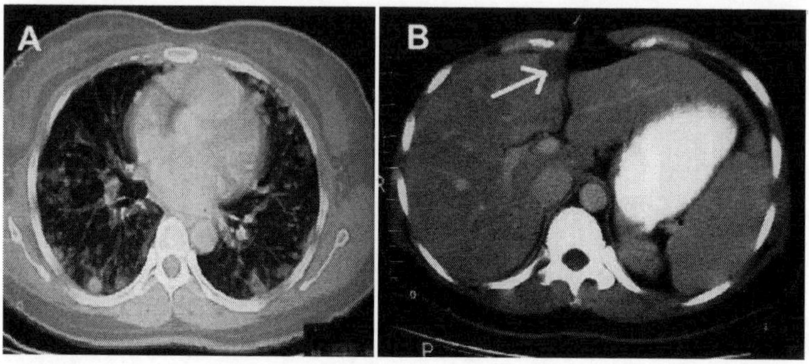

Figure 15.3 Choriocarcinoma. A: multiple pulmonary metastases, B: liver nodule (arrow).

Staging and Prognostic Scoring in Gestational Trophoblastic Neoplasm

There are many staging and prognostic scoring system. Despite the fact that anatomical and clinical classifications as well as prognostic scoring systems have been in use for many years, there is still no agreement on which is the best for GTN. The FIGO Committee on Gynecology Oncology, in collaboration with various international societies and agencies, has updated the most recent staging for gynaecological cancer. The current staging and prognostic scoring system approved by FIGO committee 2009 is shown in Tables 15.4 and 15.5.

Table 15.4 FIGO anatomical staging of GTN

Stage I	Disease confined to the uterus
Stage II	GTN extends outside of the uterus, but is limited to the genital structures (adnexa, vagina, broad ligament)
Stage III	GTN extends to the lungs, with or without known genital tract involvement
Stage IV	All other metastatic sites

Source: FIGO Committee on Gynecologic Oncology. *Intl J Gynecol Obstet* 2009; **105**: 3–4.

Note: To stage and allot a risk factor score (see Table 15.5), a patient's diagnosis is allocated to a stage as presented by a Roman numeral I, II, III and IV. This is then separated by a colon from the sum of all the actual risk factor scores expressed in Arabic numeral, e.g. Stage II: 4, Stage IV: 9. This stage and score will be allotted for each patient. Stage I is also includes all patients with persistently elevated HCG level (persistent trophoblastic disease).

Table 15.5 Modified WHO prognostic scoring system as adopted by FIGO

Score	0	1	2	4
Age	<40	≥40	—	—
Antecedent pregnancy	mole	abortion	term	—
Interval months from index pregnancy	<4	4–6	7–12	>12
Pretreatment serum HCG (IU/L)	$<10^3$	10^3–10^4	10^4–10^5	$>10^5$
Largest tumour size (including uterus)	<3 cm	3–4 cm	≥5 cm	—
Site of metastases	lung	Spleen, kidney	gastrointestinal	Liver, brain
Number of metastases	—	1–4	5–8	>8
Previous failed chemotherapy	—	—	Single drug	≥2 drugs

Note: To stage and allot a risk factor score, a patient's diagnosis is allocated to a stage as presented by a Roman numeral I, II, III and IV (refer Table 15.4). This is then separated by a colon from the sum of all the actual risk factor scores expressed in Arabic numeral, e.g. Stage II: 4, Stage IV: 9. This stage and score will be allotted for each patient. Stage I is also includes all patients with persistently elevated HCG level (persistent trophoblastic disease).

Prognostic scoring is helpful in predicting the likelihood of drug resistance and to assist in selecting appropriate chemotherapy. Based on the modified WHO scoring system, patients with GTN are divided into low-risk group (WHO score 0–4), medium risk group (WHO score 5–7) and high-risk group (WHO score >7). There is increasing number of institutions that have omitted the medium risk group and divided the patients with GTN into a low-risk groups (WHO prognostic score <7) and high-risk group (WHO prognostic score ≥7).

Treatment of Low-Risk Gestational Trophoblastic Neoplasm

Patients with low-risk GTN are those with the WHO prognostic scoring <7 and they can be in stage I, II or III disease. Single agent methotrexate (MTX) is the treatment of choice for the low-risk patients. Actinomycin D is the second choice and in fact, both cytotoxic drugs have achieved excellent and comparable remission rates in both non-metastatic as well as low-risk metastatic GTN. There are various regimens and one of the most common regimens used in UK is 50 mg methotrexate intramuscular injection on days 1, 3, 5 and 7 with 7.5–15 mg oral folinic acid 30 hours after methotrexate on days 2, 4, 6 and 8 repeated every 2 weeks (8 days regimen). Unlike actinomycin D, this regimen does not induce hair loss; thus it has been widely used. Patients who develop methotrexate resistance can be switched to actinomycin D provided the serum HCG is ≤300IU/L. Patients with serum HCG >300 IU/L may not respond well to single agent and are therefore recommended for multi-agent chemotherapy. In New England Trophoblastic Center, single-agent MTX chemotherapy achieved complete remission in 90.2% of patients with stage I GTN and 68.2% in low-risk stage II and III GTN (Berkowitz).

Several protocols using MTX and actinomycin D have been used effectively but at present there is no strong evidence to show any one regimen is superior to others. In some centres, patients with low-risk GTN were given single agent chemotherapy in the form of sequential MTX and actinomycin. Osborne and colleagues have presented the phase III trial comparing single agent MTX 30 mg/m^2 versus pulsed actinomycin 1.25 mg/m^2 in patients with low-risk GTN; the remission rate with MTX was 53% compared to 69% in actinomycin D. There are also studies showed that both MTX and actinomycin D has a similar efficacy. At present single agent MTX is perhaps still considered the drug of choice, especially in low resource setting because of the easier administration (MTX can be given via intramuscular injection, while actinomycin can be given via intravenous infusion/bolus).

Kang and colleagues have compared the efficacy of weekly intramuscular methotrexate 50 mg/m^2 without dose escalation versus 8 days MTX regimen in low-risk GTN, and they have reported that weekly MTX is as effective as 8 days regimen (primary remission rate of 70.8% versus 69.5%, $p > 0.99$). They also found that weekly MTX regimen was associated with less toxicity, better tolerability and more convenient for patients. Patients with low-risk metastatic GTN was also responded to single-agent chemotherapy either with MTX or actinomycin. The complete response rate was ranging from 47–60% (Hertz; Soper; McNeish; Khan).

Patients should be monitored by serial serum HCG 1–2 weekly to assess the response; 2–3 more courses will be given for consolidation after HCG return to normal level (<2 IU/L). Additional chemotherapy given after the first normal HCG level reduced recurrence rate to less than 5% (Mutch).

Patients with low-risk GTN who develops resistance to single agent chemotherapy can be treated with combination chemotherapy either with EMA-CO (etoposide, MTX, actinomycin D, cyclophosphamide and Oncovin) or MAC (MTX, actinomycin D and Cyclophosphamide). Berkowitz RS preferred MAC regimen because etoposide in EMA-CO regimen is associated with an increased risk of second tumour, including 1% risk of leukaemia (Berkowitz and Goldstein). Ngan et al. recommended a single agent actinomycin given to patients who developed resistance to single agent MTX in low-risk GTN provided their serum HCG is <100 IU/L. Patients with serum HCG >100 IU/L should be treated with multi-agent chemotherapy. Approximately, 25% of patients with low-risk GTN will require second line chemotherapy either due to resistance to single agent chemotherapy or drug toxicities; however, the overall cure rate is still high (almost 100% cure rate) after second-line chemotherapy.

Hysterectomy may be considered in perimenopausal women presented with stage I GTN and patients who developed resistance to both single agent and multi-agent chemotherapy.

Hysterectomy performed early during the course of disease was associated with fewer numbers of a chemotherapy cycle needed. However, the risk of performing a hysterectomy must be weighed and should not be done routinely. Early hysterectomy does not appear to improve the outcome in women with high-risk metastatic disease.

Treatment for High-Risk and Metastatic Gestational Trophoblastic Neoplasm

Patients with high-risk GTN should be treated with primary multi-agent chemotherapy, and the most popular choice is EMA-CO regimen. Patient in Fig. 15.4 is high risk choriocarcinoma and had complete response to EMA-CO regimen. MAC is less effective in this group of patients. EMA-CO induced complete remission in about 80% of the cases and overall survival rates of 90%. The major side effects of EMA-CO regimen are mucositis, pleuritis, alopecia, liver derangement, myelosuppression and vincristine-related peripheral neuropathy. If a patient is noted to have CNS metastases, the dose of MTX should be increased to 1 g/m^2 given as an intravenous infusion. The other multi-agent chemotherapy for high-risk GTN is CHAMOMA (cyclophospamide, hydroxyurea, actinomycin MTX, vincristine, melphalan and doxorubicin), CHAMOC (cyclophosphamide, hydroxyurea, actinomycin-D, MTX and vincristine) and MEA (MTX, etoposide, actinomycin).

The relapse rate in high-risk GTN is 7–10%. Patients who developed resistance to EMA-CO regimen may be treated with second line multi-agent chemotherapy as listed above. Patients with EMA-CO resistance tumour can also be treated with EMA-EP regimen (modification of EMA-CO). Despite recurrent disease, the overall five-year survival rate in high-risk GTN is approaching 85%.

Patients with liver and brain metastasis are those who have the poorest prognosis. They are also known as ultra high-risk GTN. The long-term survival for a patient with liver metastases was 27%, 70% with brain metastases and only 10% in patients with both metastases. Intensive early treatment for high-risk GTN improves the survival and reduced recurrence rate. In New England Trophoblastic Disease Center, 80% of patients with stage IV GTN achieved complete sustained remission with relapse rate of less than 10% following aggressive approach. Patients with brain metastases may require multi-modality treatment comprises chemotherapy, radiotherapy or surgery. Whole brain irradiation can be given concurrently with initiation of chemotherapy if the metastases are multiple. Surgery can be performed to excise localized brain lesion. Brain's metastases can also be treated with combined chemotherapy using a higher dose of MTX (1 g/m^2) to improve the penetration of drug into the CNS. Some suggested adding intrathecal MTX with the CO component in the EMA-CO regimen. The other active chemotherapy regimens for patients with relapse of high-risk GTN are TP/TE (paclitaxel, cisplatin/paclitaxel, etoposide), BEP (bleomycin, etoposide, cisplatin) and VIP (vincristine, ifosfamide and cisplatin).

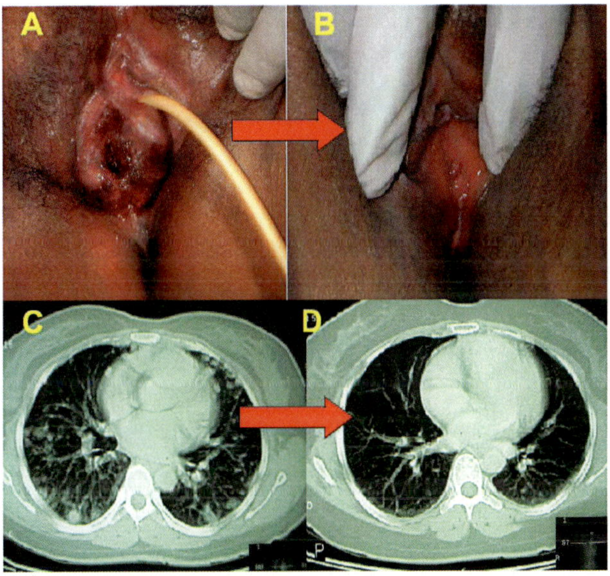

Figure 15.4 Choriocarcinoma is a very chemosensitive tumour. A: periurethral nodule before chemotherapy and B: complete disappearance of nodule after chemotherapy, C: multiple lung nodules before and D: complete response after chemotherapy.

Treatment of Placental Site Trophoblastic Tumour

Placental site trophoblastic tumour is a very rare GTN. Placental site trophoblastic tumour has the following features: (1) slow-growing tumour (2) produces less HCG (3) late metastases and (4) more commonly involves lymph nodes. A serum β-hCG level in PSTT does not correlate with the burden and malignant behaviour of this tumour thus appears to have no predictive value.

Management of PSTT is different from that for choriocarcinoma. Most patients with PSTT required hysterectomy. Ovarian preservation is safe as the risk of ovarian micrometastasis is only 3% in PSTT. If the lesion is localized and the patient is keen on preserving her fertility, local resection can be done hysteroscopically. Patients with metastatic PSTT should be treated with combined chemotherapy such as EMA-EP, EMA-CO, MAE (MTX, actinomycin D, etoposide) or TP–TE regimen. Patients with resistance chemotherapy can be treated with CEC regimen (cyclophosphamide, etoposide, cisplatin) (Hassadia et al.). Patients with stage I PSTT had a 10 year overall survival of 90% and did not benefit from postoperative chemotherapy. Outcome for a patient who had a recurrent or refractory disease was poor with five-year survivals of 22%. Multivariate analysis showed that the only significantly independent predictor of overall survival and recurrence-free survival was time since antecedent pregnancy (cut-off point of 48 months since antecedent pregnancy) (Schmid et al.). Treatment for ETT is similar to PSTT.

Post Chemotherapy Follow-Up

Patients treated with chemotherapy should be followed up closely similar with other gynaecological cancers. Studies have shown that 80% of recurrent GTN occurs within 18 months of primary treatment. Patients are advised not to get pregnant until 12 months after completion of chemotherapy. EMA-CO regimen does not lead to significant complications during subsequent pregnancy, including increasing rate of congenital malformation. Monitoring of patients with GTN can be done by urine HCG and the duration of follow-up is similar with other gynaecological malignancies. In the United Kingdom, a patient with GTN is followed up weekly for the first 6 week, then 2 weekly for up to 12 months; the interval of follow-up is longer on subsequent year. After 5 years, the patient will be followed up every 6 months. The follow-up is for life. A long-term follow-up study of 15279 patient years by Rustin et al. found no significant increase in the incidence of second tumours after MTX therapy; however, 26 patients receiving combination chemotherapy for GTN developed second cancer.

Chemotherapy Regimen for Gestational Trophoblastic Neoplasm[1]

(1) Single Agent Methotrexate

Drugs	Route	Dose (mg/m^2)	Infusion time	Days
Methotrexate	IV or IM	30–50 mg/m^2	1 hour	1, 3, 5 and 7
Folinic Acid 24 hours after each dose of MTX	IM or Oral	6–12 mg or 0.1 mg/kg	Bolus	2, 4, 6 and 8

Note: Chemotherapy is given till HCG levels come down to normal then 2–3 further courses are given.
There should be an interval of 7 days between the last day of folinic acid and the first day of the next course.

(2) EMA-CO Regimen

Drugs	Route	Dose (mg/m^2)	Infusion time	Days
EMA				
Etoposide	IV	100	30 minutes	1, 2
Actinomycin D	IV	0.5 mg	Bolus	1, 2
Methotrexate	IV	100	1 hour	1
Methotrexate[a]	IV	200	12 hours	
Folinic acid (24 hours post MTX X 4 doses)	Oral or IV	15 mg	12 hourly	2–3
CO				
Vincristine	IV	1.0	Bolus	8
Cyclophosphamide	IV	600	30 minutes	8

[a]MTX 200 mg/m^2, 12 hours infusion is commenced following 1 hour infusion
Notes: (a) Cycles are repeated on day 15 until HCG level return to normal. This is followed by another 2 cycles.
(b) Subcutaneous filgrastim may be administered in selected patients with significant neutropenia. It must be started 24–48 hours after day 2 chemotherapy and then last dose should be at least 24 hours before CO.

[1]The chemotherapy regimens listed above are just examples; each centre has their own regimens and protocols.

(3) EMA-EP Regimen (Berkowitz RS)

Drugs	Route	Dose (mg/m^2)	Infusion rate	Days
EMA				
Etoposide	IV	100	30 mins–1 hour	1, 2
Methotrexate	IV	100	1 hour	1
Methotrexate[a]	IV	1000	12	1
Actinomycin D	IV	0.5	Bolus	2
Folicin acid	IV, Oral, IM	15–30 mg	12 hourly	
EP				
Etoposide	IV	100	30 mins–1hour	8
Cisplatin	IV	60	12 hours	8

[a]Some institutions give 200 mg/m^2.

(4) BEP Regimen (Bleomycin, Etoposide, Cisplatin)

(Benedet JL, Pecorelli S, Ngan HYS, et al. *CPG Gynae Cancer,* FIGO and IGCS, 3rd edition)

Etoposide: 100 mg IV in 500 mL normal saline over 1 hour, days 1, 2, 3, 4.

Cisplatin: 100 mg/m^2 day 1, IV continuous infusion for 24 hours with normal saline × 6 at 250 mL/hour; add 20 meq KCL and 2 mg $MgSO_4$ to each of last 2 litres.

Bleomycin: 10 unit/m^2 per day for 3 days; day 2, 3 and 4; IV continuous infusion for 96 hours.

(5) TP-TE Regimen for Relapsed Gestational Trophoblastic Neoplasm

Drugs	Route and dose
Day 1 (TP)	
Paclitaxel	3 hours intravenous infusion/135 mg/m^2
Cisplatin	3 hours intravenous infusion/60 mg/m^2
Day 15 (TE)	
Paclitaxel	3 hours intravenous infusion/135 mg/m^2
Etoposide	1 hour intravenous infusion/150 mg/m^2

References

Abrao RA, de Andrade JM, Tiezzi DG, et al. Treatment for low risk gestational trophoblastic disease: Comparison of single-agent methotrexate, dactinomycin and combination regimens. *Gynecol Oncol* 2008; **108**: 149–153.

Alhamdan D, Bignardi T. Recognising gestational trophoblastic disease. *Best Pract Res Clin Obstet Gynaecol* 2009; **23**: 565–573.

Allen SD, Lim AK, Seckl MJ, Blunt DM, Mitchell AW. Review: Radiology of gestational trophoblastic neoplasia. *Clin Radiol* 2006; **61**: 301–313.

Bagshawe KD, Dent J, Webb J. Hydatidiform mole in England and Wales 1973–1983. *Lancet* 1986; **328**: 673–667.

Bandy LC, Clarke-Pearson DL, Hammond CB. Malignant potential of gestational trophoblastic disease at the extremes of reproductive life. *Obstet Gynecol* 1984; **64**: 395–399.

Benedet JL, Pecorelli S, Ngan HYS, Hacker NF. Staging Classifications and Clinical Practise Guidelines for Gynaecological Cancers. A Collaboration between FIGO and IGCS. Third Edition, 2006.

Berkowitz RS, Goldstein DP. Chorionic tumors. *N Engl J Med* 1996; **335**: 1740–1748.

Berkowitz RS, Cramer DW, Bernstein MR, et al. Risk factors for complete molar pregnancy from case-control study. *Am J Obstet Gynecol* 1985; **152**: 1016–1020.

Berkowitz RA, Goldstein DP. Current management of gestational trophoblastic disease. *Gynecol Oncol* 2009; **112**: 654–662.

Berkowitz RS, Goldstein DP, Bernstein MR. Ten years experiences with methotrexate and folinic acid as primary therapy for gestational trophoblastic disease. *Gynecol Oncol* 1986; **23**: 111–118.

Bracken MB. Incidence and aetiology of hydatidiform mole: an epidemiology review. *Br J Obstet Gynaecol* 1987; **94**: 1123–1135.

Cole LA, Muller CY. Hyperglycosylated hCG in the management of quiescent and chemorefractory gestational trophoblastic diseases. *Gynecol Oncol* 2010; **116**: 3–9.

Cole LA, Dai D, Leslie KK, et al. Gestational trophoblastic disease: Pathophysiology of hyperglycosylated HCG-regulated neoplasia. *Gynecol Oncol* 2006; **102**: 144–149.

Curry SL, Blessing JA, DiSaia PJ, et al. A prospective randomized comparison of methotrexate, dactinomycin and chlorambucil versus methotrexate, dactinomycin, cyclophosphamide, doxorubicin, melpalan, hydroxyurea and vincristine in poor prognosis metastatic gestational trophoblastic disease: a gynecologic oncology group Study. *Obstet Gynecol* 1989; **73**: 357–362.

DuBeshter B, Berkowitz RS, Goldstein DP, et al. Metastatic gestational trophoblastic disease: experience at the New England Trophoblastic Disease Center, 1965–1985. *Obstet Gynecol* 1987; **9**: 390–395.

El-Helw L, Hancock BW. Treatment of metastatic gestational trophoblastic neoplasia. *Lancet Oncol* 2007; **8**: 715–724.

Evan AC Jr, Soper JT, Hammond CB. Clinical features of molar pregnancies and gestational trophoblastic tumour. In: Gestational trophoblastic disease. (Hancock BW, Newlands ES, Berkowitz RS, Cole LA, eds.) Gestational trophoblastic disease 2nd edition. Sheffield: *Intl Soc Study Trophoblastic Dis.* 2003.

Gaffield ME, Kapp N, Curtis KM. Combined oral contraceptive and intrauterine devise use among women with gestational trophoblastic disease. *Contraception* 2009; **80**(4): 363–371.

Garret LA, Garner EI, Feltmate CM, et al. Subsequent pregnancy outcomes in patients with molar pregnancy and persistent gestational trophoblastic neoplasia. *J Reprod Med* 2008; **53**: 481–86.

Goedhals J, Botha MC, Theron M. Case report. Complete hydatidifom mole in a 57 year old woman. *SAJOG* 2010; **16**(1): 22–23.

Goldstein DP, Berkowitz RS. Prophylactic chemotherapy of complete molar pregnancy. *Semin Oncol* 1995; **22**: 157–160.

Gordon AN, Gershenson DM, Copeland LJ, et al. High risk metastatic gestational trophoblastic disease: further stratification into two clinical entities. *Gynecol Oncol* 1989; **34**: 54–56.

Hammond CB, Weed Jr JC, Currie JL. The role of operation in the current therapy of gestational trophoblastic disease. *Am J Obstet Gynecol* 1980; **136**: 844–858.

Hassadia A, Gillespie A, Tidy J, et al. Placental site trophoblastic tumour: Clinical features and management. *Gynecol Oncol* 2005; **99**: 603–607.

Hertz R, Lewis J Jr, Lipsett MB. Five years experiences with the chemotherapy of metastatic choriocarcinoma and related trophoblastic tumour in women. *Am J Obstet Gynecol* 1961; **82**: 631–640.

Kang WD, Choi HS, Kim SM. Weekly methotrexate (50 mg/m^2) without dose escalation as a primary regimen for low risk gestational trophoblastic neoplasia. *Gynecol Oncol* 2010; **117**: 477–480.

Khan F, Everard J, Ahmed S, et al. Low risk persistent gestational trophoblastic disease treated with low dose methotrexate: efficacy, acute and long-term effects. *Br J Cancer* 2003; **89**: 2197–2201.

Lan C, Li Y, He J, Liu J. Placental site trophoblastic tumor: lymphatic spread and possible target markers. *Gynecol Oncol* 2010; **116**: 430–437.

McNeich IA, Strickland S, Holden L, et al. Low risk persistent gestational trophoblastic disease: outcome after initial treatment with low dose methotrexate and folinic acid from 1992 to 2000. *J Clin Oncol* 2002; **20**: 1838–1844.

Montz FJ, Schlaerth JB, Morrow CP. The natural history of theca lutein cysts. *Obstet Gynecol* 1988; **72**: 247–251.

Mutch DG, Soper JT, Babcock CJ, et al. Recurrent gestational trophoblastic disease: experience of the Southeastern Regional Trophoblastic Disease Center. *Cancer* 1990; **66**: 978–982.

Ngan HYS, Chan KKL, Tam KF. Gestational trophoblastic disease. *Curr Obstet Gynaecol* 2006; **16**: 93–99.

Osborne R, Filiaci V, Schink J, et al. A randomized phase III trial comparing weekly parenteral methotrexate and pulsed dactinomycin as primary management of low risk gestational trophoblastic neoplasia: a gynecologic oncology group study. *Gynecol Oncol* 2008; **108**:s2.

Parazzini F, La Vecchia C, Mangili G, et al. Dietary factors and risk of trophoblastic disease. *Am J Obstet Gynecol* 1988; **158**: 93–99.

Parazzini F, Mangili G, La Vecchia C, et al. Risk factors for gestational trophoblastic disease: a separate analysis of complete and partial hydatidiform moles. *Obstet Gynecol* 1991; **78**: 1039–1045.

Pisal N, North C, Tidy J, Hancock B. Role of hysterectomy in management of gestational trophoblastic disease. *Gynecol Oncol* 2002; **87**: 190–192.

Rustin GJ, Newlands ES, Begent RH, et al. Weekly alternating etoposide, methotrexate and actinomycin/vincristine and cyclophosphamide chemotherapy for the treatment of CNS metastases of choriocarcinoma. *J Clin Oncol* 1989; **7**: 900–903.

Rustin GJS, Newlands ES, Lutz JM, et al. Combination but not single agent methotrexate chemotherapy for gestational trophoblastic tumours (GTT) increases the incidence of second tumours. *J Clin Oncol* 1996; **14**: 2769–2773.

Sasaki Y, Ladner DG, Cole LA. Hyperglycosylated hCG the source of pregnancy failure. *Fertilit Steril* 2008; **89**: 1786–1871.

Schlaerth JB, Morrow CP, Montz FJ, d'Abling G. Initial management of hydatidiform mole. *Am J Obstet Gynecol* 1988; **158**: 1299–1306.

Scmid P, Nagai Y, Agarwal R, et al. Prognostic markers and long-term outcome of placental-site trophoblastic tumours: a retrospective observational study. *Lancet* 2009; **374**: 48–55.

Sebire NJ, Foskett M, Fisher RA, et al. Risk of partial and complete hydatidiform molar pregnancy in relation to maternal age. *BJOG* 2002; **109**: 99–102.

Sebire NJ, Fisher RA, Foskett M, et al. Risk of recurrent hydatidiform mole and subsequent pregnancy outcome following complete or partial hydatidiform molar pregnancy. *BJOG* 2003; **110**: 22–26.

Seckl M, Sebire NJ, Berkowitz RS. Gestational trophoblastic disease. *The Lancet* 2010, Published online DOI: 10.1016/S0140-6736(10) 60280-2.

Sebire NJ, Lindsay I, Fisher RA. Recent advances in gestational trophoblastic neoplasia. *Curr Diagn Pathol* 2007; **13**: 210–221.

Shih IM. Gestational trophoblastic neoplasia—pathogenesis and potential therapeutic targets. *Lancet Oncol* 2007; **8**: 642–650.

Schmid P, Nagai Y, Agarwal R, et al. Prognostic markers and long-term outcome of placental-site trophoblastic tumours: a retrospective observational study. *Lancet* 2009; **374**: 48–55.

Soper JT, Clarke-Pearson DL, Berchuck A, et al. 5 days methotrexate for women with metastatic gestational trophoblastic disease. *Gynecol Oncol* 1994; **54**: 76–79.

Soper JT. Staging and evaluation of gestational trophoblastic disease. *Clin Obstet Gynecol* 2003; **46**: 570–578.

Soper JT, Mutch DG, Schink JC. Diagnosis and treatment of gestational trophoblastic disease: ACOG Practice Bulletin No. 53. *Gynecol Oncol* 2004; **93**: 575–585.

Tse KY, Chan KK, Tam KF, Ngan HYS. Gestational trophoblastic disease. *Obstet, Gynaecol Rep Med* 2008; **19**(4): 89–97.

Tsukamoto N, Iwasaka T, Kashimura Y, et al. Gestational trophoblastic disease in women aged 50 or more. *Gynecol Oncol* 1985; **20**: 53–61.

Chapter 16

Breast Cancer for Gynaecologic Oncologist

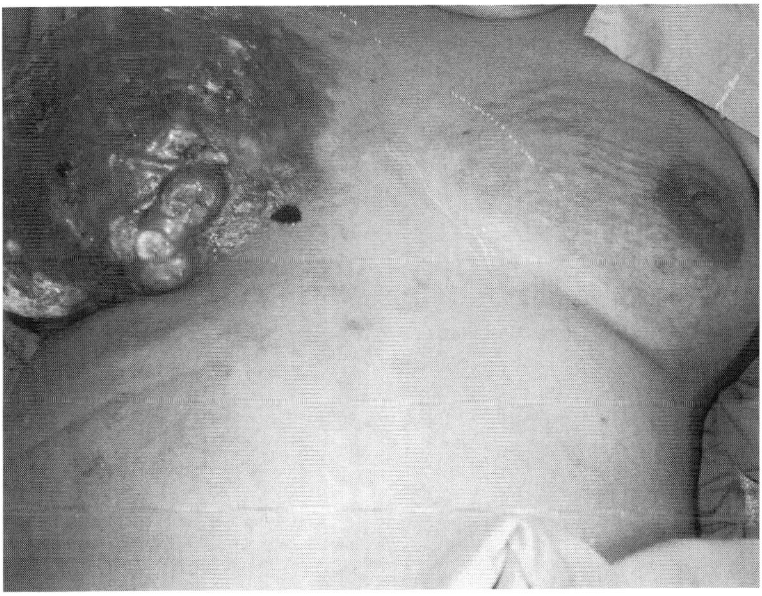

Gynaecologic Cancer: A Handbook for Students and Practitioners
Rushdan Noor, Eng Hseon Tay, and Jeffrey Low

ISBN 978-981-4463-06-5 (Hardcover), 978-981-4463-07-2 (eBook)
www.panstanford.com

Basic Anatomy of the Breast

The breast is bounded by the clavicle superiorly, the sternum medially, the lateral border of the latissimus muscle laterally and the inframammary fold inferiorly. Fibrous bands known as suspensory ligaments of Cooper divide the breast parenchyma into 12–20 separate lobes of glandular tissue. Each lobe is formed by several groups of lobules. Each lobule is composed of grape-like clusters of acini known as alveoli, the hollow sacs that make and hold breast milk. The lobules are arranged around ducts that funnel milk to the nipples. About 15–20 ducts come together near the areola to form a distended cavity (ampullae) that stores the milk before it reaches the nipple surface. Montgomery's glands are small sebaceous glands that are located around each areola. They release a lubricant that protects the nipples during nursing. Most of the lymphatic drainage from breast goes to axillary lymph nodes. Axillary lymph nodes are referred to by levels, which are defined by their relation to pectoralis minor muscle. Level 1 axillary nodes are lateral, level 2 nodes are behind and level 3 nodes are medial to the pectoralis minor muscle. The lymphatic drainage from medial part of the breast is also drained to internal mammary nodes. The arterial blood supplies to the breasts are from external mammary artery and perforators of the internal mammary artery. Venous drainage follows arterial blood supply.

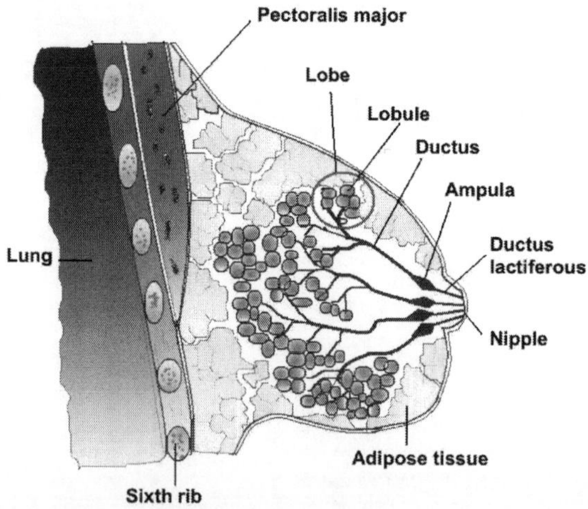

Figure 16.1 Anatomy of the breast.

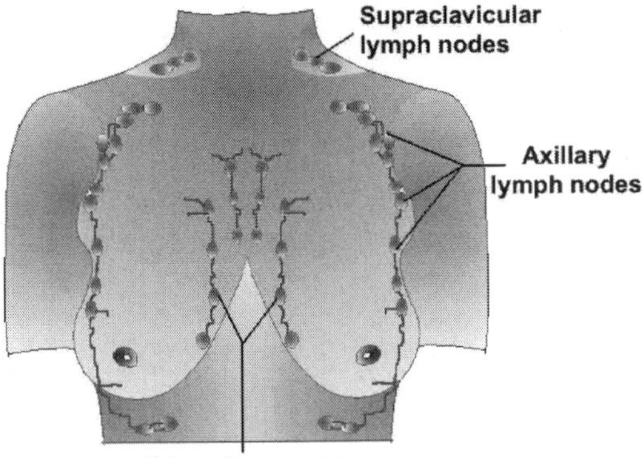

Figure 16.2 Lymphatic drainage of the breast.

Introduction to Breast Cancer

The breast cancer is the most common cancer in women and the leading cause of cancer death among women. The WHO estimated 508,000 women died in 2011 due to breast cancer. Although the breast cancer is more common in less developed countries, 58% of all breast cancer deaths occur in developing countries (WHO Global Burden of Disease, 2013). According to GLOBOCAN 2008, breast cancer is the second most common cancer overall with 1.4 million new cases reported in 2008 or 10.9% of total new cancer cases worldwide. The age-standardized incidence of breast cancer was 39.0 per 100,000 population and cumulative risk of 4.1% (GLOBOCAN 2008). Breast cancer survival rate is highest (80%) in developed countries and lowest (40%) in low-income countries due to lack of early detection programmes, the higher proportion of women presented with late-stage disease and lack of adequate diagnosis as well as treatment facilities.

The American Cancer Society estimated 1.4 million new cases of invasive breast cancer worldwide in 2008. Incidence rate of breast cancer varied from 3.9 cases per 100,000 in Mozambique to 101.1 cases per 100,000 in the United States. Incidence rate in Asian and Pacific Islander is approximately 89 in 100,000 populations. The highest incidence rate is reported in westernized countries. Over the past 25 years, the incidence rate of breast cancer have risen globally probably due to increased in detection via screening, change in reproductive patterns, dietary changes and lack in physical activity. The lifetime risk of breast cancer is 1 in 12 women. Breast cancer is the most common single cause of all deaths in women aged 35–54. The cause of breast cancer in unknown and majority of women have no risk factors. Survival rates for breast cancer have improved significantly because of progress in our understanding of the disease, more efficient and less toxic treatments, increased public awareness and improved screening.

Aetiology of Breast Cancer

The exact aetiology of breast cancer is unknown. Current understanding of breast tumorigenesis is that invasive cancers arise through a series of molecular alterations at the cellular level. Molecular alterations at the cellular level lead to outgrowth and spread of breast epithelial cells.

Based on genomic profiling, there are four subclasses of breast cancers (each has distinct clinical behaviour):

(a) **Luminal A** (ER+ and/or PR+, HER2–): Most common and good prognosis
(b) **Luminal B** (ER+ and/or PR+, HER2+): Poorer outcome than Luminal A
(c) **Basal-Like** (Triple negative, cytokeratin 5/6+ and/or EGFR+): Aggressive subtype, high grade and risk at younger age (<40)
(d) **HER 2 positive** (ER negative): Less common, highly aggressive, risk at younger age (<40)

Breast Cancer Risks

Several risk factors for breast cancer have been well documented; however, the majority (75%) of women presenting with breast cancer did not have identifiable risk factors.

Reproductive Factors/Endogenous Hormones

(*IARC, 2008, Lacey et al., 2009*)

The breast shows dramatic changes during different stages of life. The age incidence curves are similar to endometrial and ovarian cancer. Development of breast cancer is related to interaction between female hormones, exogenous factors and lifestyle.

Risk factors for breast cancer

- frequent cyclical hormone exposure during the years of active ovulation
- greater number of menstrual cycle before first full term pregnancy (late age of first term pregnancy (>30 years old)
- shorter menstrual cycle (more time in luteal phase)
- oestrogens and progesterone induce more cell division than oestrogen alone (oestrogen-augmented-by-progesterone hypothesis).
- early menarche (<12 years old)
- late menopause

Protective factors for breast cancer:

- reverse of above factors
- pre-menopausal obesity
- early oophorectomy
- moderate physical exercise

Pregnancy and Lactation

Early age at first delivery reduced the risk of breast cancer. Long-term lactation slightly reduced the risk in young women. However, lactation does not reduce the risk in post-menopausal women.

Family History and Other Gynaecological Cancer

Having family history of breast and gynaecological cancer is the most widely recognized breast cancer risk.

The relative risk (RR) of breast cancer related to the family history

(a) two or more relatives (mother, sister): RR > 5
(b) one first-degree relative: RR > 2
(c) family history of ovarian cancer in women <50 years old: RR > 2

The lifetime risk may increase up to 50% in familiar type of breast cancer. Mutation of p53 and BRCA 1 gene has been identified in hereditary breast cancer. BRCA1 gene is estimated to account for about 45% of families with several cases of breast cancer and 67% if age of onset is less than 45. Almost 100% of families with a breast-ovarian carcinoma syndrome have BRCA 1 mutations. Without genetic predisposition, a woman with history of breast cancer in her first-degree relative has a RR of 1.5 to 3.0. Women with ovarian cancer have three- to four-fold increased risk of developing breast cancer and women with breast cancer have two-fold risk of ovarian cancer.

Oral Contraceptive Pills

The evidence of the association of oral contraceptive pills (OCPs) and breast cancer is based on the review of the following studies:

(a) Cancer and Steroid Hormone Study (CASH)
(b) Swedish Study
(c) UK National Case-Control Study
(d) Australian Case-Control Study
(e) WHO study

Overall, there is no increased risk of breast cancer if OCP was ever used less than 5 years. If OCP is taken in early age (younger than 36 years old), estimated RR is 1.43 after 4–8 years' use and 1.74 after more than 8 years' total OCP use. Any increase in risk of breast cancer with long-term OCP may be counterbalanced by a reduced risk of endometrial and ovarian cancer. Furthermore, the risks appear to decrease with age and time from OCP discontinuation. Breast cancer risk returns to that of the average population after approximately 10 years following cessation of oral contraceptives. Long-term use of progestogen-only pills (long-term) reduces the risk by 35–40%.

Hormone Replacement Therapy

Women's Health Initiative (WHI), large multi-centre trial in the United States involving 16,608 post-menopausal women randomized into two groups, placebo versus combined HRT (conjugated equine oestrogen 0.625 mg and medroxyprogesterone acetate 2.5 mg). After 5.2 years of follow-up study of WHI trial, there were 26% increase in the risk of invasive breast cancer, more abnormal mammogram reports and increased breast density with HRT usage compared to placebo. The risk is greater in women taking combination oestrogen plus progestogen formulations compared to the oestrogen-only formulation (HR 0.77 for unopposed oestrogen versus placebo). In women with breast cancer, HABITS trial from Stockholm involving 447 breast cancer survivors, HRT group was found to have over twice the risk of breast cancer recurrence compared to controls. Results were similar regardless of oestrogen receptor status and tamoxifen use. HRT was found to be more strongly associated with hormone-receptor-positive cancers than negative.

Personal History

History of breast cancer carries an increased cancer risk to contralateral breast with relative risk (RR) of 3–4. Women with BRCA 1/BRCA 2 mutation have an increased risk of breast cancer with RR of more than 4. Breast biopsy with atypical hyperplasia carries a RR of 4–5 for breast cancer, while biopsy with LCIS (lobular carcinoma in situ) or DCIS (ductal carcinoma in situ) carry a RR of 8–10 for breast cancer. Danaei et al. evaluated the role of personal lifestyle factors and the risk of breast cancer; following is their report:

(a) About 21% of all breast cancer deaths worldwide are attributable to obesity, sedentary lifestyle and alcohol.
(b) Obesity, RR 1.5–2.
(c) Sedentary lifestyle, RR 1.3–1.5.
(d) Alcohol consumption (moderate drinker ≥ 2 drinks/day), RR 1.5.
(e) Diet increased in animal fat have been associated with an increased risk for breast cancer.

An increased rate of breast cancer has been observed in survivors of the atomic bomb explosion in Japan with the peak latency period of 15–20 years. Patients with Hodgkin's lymphoma who are treated with mantle irradiation, particularly younger than 20 years old, have an increased incidence of breast cancer.

Risk Assessment of Breast Cancer

Using various risk factors and developing a multivariate analysis, risk of breast cancer can be calculated and predicted. Some risk assessment tools use the information from the family tree, personal and family profiles as well as BRCA status in order to predict the absolute risk of developing breast cancer.

There are two types of risk assessment tools for breast cancer prediction:

(a) the assessment tool to calculate absolute risk of developing breast cancer over time
(b) the assessment tool to determine the likelihood that an individual is a carrier of BRCA 1, BRCA 2 or unknown gene mutation.

Gail Model is one of the risk assessment tools to predict the risk for developing breast cancer over time. Gail's model was originally developed in 1989 and originally intended to improve screening guidelines. **Gail Model 2** (a revised Gail Model 1) is now being extensively used in clinical practice. Example, the US FDA approved modified Gail model as the basis for eligibility for the prophylactic use of tamoxifen. Tamoxifen is approved for women aged 35 years and older who have five years Gail's risk of breast cancer of ≥1.67%. This model, however, may be less accurate in populations that differ from the population on which it was built. A new, CARE Model is being developed using data from a large case control study (CARE: Women's Contraceptive and Reproductive Experiences).

Examples of risk assessment tools to determine the likelihood of carrier for genetic mutations are:

(a) BRCAPRO model
(b) BOADCEA (Breast and Ovarian Analysis of Disease Incidence and Carrier Estimation Algorithm)
(c) Ontario Family History Assessment Tool (FTAT)

To date, these assessment tools are yet to receive an endorsement because of insufficient data regarding their applicability in asymptomatic and cancer-free women.

Breast Cancer and Genetic Factors

Generally, 20–30% of women with breast cancer have at least one relative with a history of breast cancer. Only 5–10% of women with breast cancer have an identifiable hereditary predisposition. The most important genetic mutations are tumour suppressor BRCA 1 and BRCA 2 mutations accounting for the majority of autosomal dominant inherited breast cancer. BRCA 1 gene is located on chromosome 17, while BRCA 2 is located on chromosome 13. The incidence of BRCA gene mutations in general breast cancer population is unknown but estimated to be around 3–8% and 15–20% of familiar breast cancer patients have BRCA 1 and BRCA 2 mutations, respectively. Women with BRCA 1 or BRCA 2 mutations have a lifetime risk of 50–80% for developing ovarian cancer.

Breast cancers that are associated with BRCA 1 mutation are more likely high grade, oestrogen receptor negative (ER–), progesterone receptor negative (PR–) and HER 2 negative, while breast cancers associated with BRCA 2 mutation are more likely high grade, ER+, PR+ and HER 2 negative. BRCA 2 mutation is also a risk factor for male breast cancer. Other genetic mutations associated with breast cancers are TP53 (in Li–Fraumeni syndrome) and PTEN (in Cowden disease). Several laboratory methods have been adopted to detect BRCA 1 and BRCA 2 mutations. However, currently this technology misses 8–10% of abnormalities.

Women with high possibility of BRCA 1 and/or BRCA 2 mutation may be referred to genetic clinic for genetic counselling. They may be offered a genetic testing to confirm the mutation.

Genetic testing is controversial; the guideline from the American Society of Clinical Oncology (ASCO) recommend that cancer predisposition testing be offered only in the following situations:

(a) A person has a strong family history of cancer or early onset of disease.
(b) The test can be adequately interpreted.
(c) The results will influence the medical management of the patient or family member.

The potential risks of genetic testing for BRCA 1 and BRCA 2 are

(a) false interpretation of the test leading to under-treatment or over-treatment
(b) psychological problem, i.e. anxiety and depression
(c) cost: the test is expensive (more than USD 3500)
(d) insurability is the most important concern among women

For more information regarding genetic counseling and genetic testing, please refer to Chapter 2 and 12.

Screening for Breast Cancer

Early detection is the main aim of the breast cancer–screening program. Early-stage and smaller tumours are more treatable and therefore have the better prognosis. The most widely recommended method for screening for early detection of breast cancer is screening mammography.

Breast Self-Examination and Clinical Breast Examination

The role of breast self-examination (BSE) and clinical breast examination (CBE) is controversial because BSE and CBE have not been found to reduce breast cancer mortality. However, a meta-analysis reported women who performed BSE were more likely to have smaller tumours and less likely to have axillary node involvement. Another study found that BSE resulted in additional imaging procedures and biopsies. American Cancer Society recommends starting monthly BSE beginning at the age of 20 and 3-yearly CBE. The 2009 USPSTF guidelines recommend against teaching women how to perform BSE. The other major problem with BSE is that it is rarely performed well, only 2–3% of women do a correct examination a year after instruction has been provided.

Mammography

Mammography is currently the best available population-based method to detect early breast cancer. According to a Cochrane database systematic review by Gotzsche analyzing randomized controlled trials involving 600,000 women, regular mammographic screening significantly reduced the breast cancer mortality by 19% (RR: 0.81, 95% CI 0.74–0.87). The benefits of mammography estimated by USPSTF (US Preventive Services Task Force) are as follows:

(a) for women age 50–74: 30% reduction in risk of death
(b) for women age 40–49: 17% reduction in risk of death

A recent study by Cady et al. demonstrated that in a large cohort of women followed up for a median of 12.5 years, 74.8% of all breast cancer deaths occurred in women not participating in regular mammography screening. The study concluded that the most effective method of avoiding death from breast cancer is for women to participate in regular screening mammography. The sensitivity of mammography is 67.8%, while specificity is 75%. Mammography combined with clinical breast examination slightly improves sensitivity to 77.4%. Mammography will detect lesions 1–2 years before it will be detected by clinical examination.

Recent advances in mammography include the development of digital mammography and computer-aided diagnosis systems (CAD). Digital mammography allows the image to be recorded and stored. Digital mammography was approved by FDA since 2000. Cost-effective analyses by Lindfors et al. have shown that these systems increased the effectiveness of mammographic screening by 29% with a comparable increase in screening cost. The National Comprehensive Cancer Network (NCCN) 2009 has recently updated their clinical guidelines for the screening of high-risk women for breast cancer, including the addition of annual screening with Magnetic Resonance Imaging (MRI) to annual screening mammograms for women in the highest risk categories. For women with average risk, NCCN's guidelines advise 1–3 yearly clinical breast examination from the age of 20. Subsequently, after the age of 40, annual clinical breast examination and annual mammogram are recommended. Based on epidemiologic evidence that pre-menopausal familial breast cancer often presents at similar ages among affected family members, it is recommended unaffected family members to begin imaging screening 5–10 years prior to the youngest age at which her first-degree relative was diagnosed with breast cancer. American College of Obstetrician and Gynecologist (ACOG) recommends screening mammogram and clinical breast examination to begin from 40 years old 1–2 yearly until 50 years old. Women above 50 years old should undergo screening annually. However, in November 2009, USPSTF updated their guideline and does not recommend routine screening mammograms before age of 50 years old instead the decision to do screening mammogram in women age 40–49 should be individualized. The USPSTF recommends stopping screening at the age of 74 because there is insufficient evidence to suggest the benefits of screening in women age 75 and above. Breast ultrasound has become a widely available and useful adjunct to mammography in diagnosis of breast abnormalities. Ultrasound alone, however, is a poor screening tool for breast cancer due to failure to detect microcalcifications and poor specificity (34%).

Reporting of Mammogram

The American College of Radiology established the radiologic interpretation of mammogram known as BI–RADS system (Breast Imaging and Data System):

- BI–RADS 1: Normal
- BI–RADS 2: Benign, repeat study in 1 year
- BI–RADS 3: Likely to be benign, repeat mammogram in 6 months
- BI–RADS 4: Suspicious, consider biopsy
- BI–RADS 5: Highly suspicious for malignancy, biopsy recommended

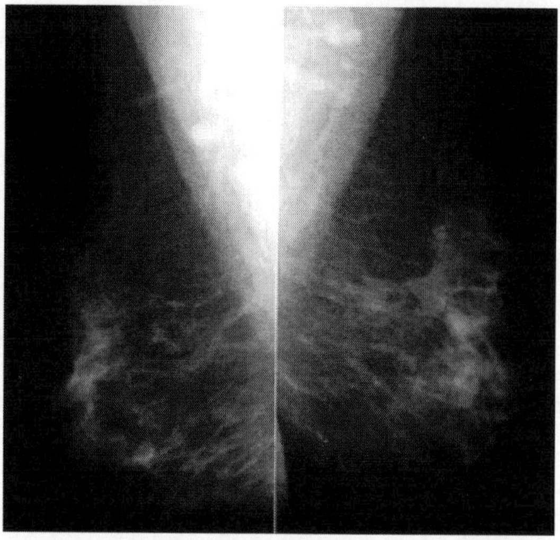

Figure 16.3 Mammograph.

Magnetic Resonance Imaging

Magnetic resonance imaging (MRI) (combination of T-1, T-2 and 3D contrast-enhanced techniques) when combined with mammogram and clinical breast examination produce sensitivity of 99% in detecting breast cancer in high-risk and younger women. The disadvantages of MRI as screening tool for breast cancer are high cost and low specificity (26%). American Cancer Society (2007) recommended MRI (annual screening) only be used as screening for breast cancer in the following groups of women:

(a) BRCA mutation
(b) Lifetime risk approximately 20–25% or greater as defined by BRCAPRO or other risk models
(c) Radiation to the chest when aged 10–30 years.
(d) Li–Fraumeni syndrome and first-degree relatives
(e) Cowden and Bannayan–Riley–Ruvalcaba syndromes and first-degree relatives
(f) Optional for women with history of lobular carcinoma in situ, atypical ductal hyperplasia and women with personal history of breast cancer, cancer including DCIS

The ACS does not recommend MRI screening in women who have lifetime risk of less than 15%. The advantages of MRI compared with conventional imaging techniques to detect breast cancer include the following: (a) Improved staging and treatment planning, (b) Enhanced evaluation of enhanced breast, (c) Improved screening in high-risk patients and (d) Better detection of recurrence.

Evaluation of Patients with Breast Cyst and Solid Breast Lump

Breast Cyst

Cystic mass can be further evaluated by ultrasound to determine whether a cyst is simple or complex. Simple cyst can be managed conservatively. Complex cyst (intracystic mass, thickened wall or septa) warranted biopsy. Breast cyst can be aspirated using fine needle aspiration. Benign cyst contains clear or yellowish fluid. The biopsy is indicated if the cyst contains bloody fluid. Less than 1% of breast cancers are cystic. The indications for breast biopsy are (a) Persistent cyst despite aspiration, (b) Blood-stained fluid aspirated and (c) Complex cyst.

Solid Breast Lump

The decision to observe a patient with solid breast mass that appeared to be benign should be made only after careful clinical and radiological examinations. Mammography is important to screen contralateral breast apart from evaluating the radiologic appearance of the mass. Fine needle aspiration cytology (FNAC) is acceptable but false negative rate can be from 3–27% Currently image-guided core biopsies have replaced conventional excisional or incisional biopsy. Core biopsy is better than FNAC. When the procedure is performed with a large core needle (8–11G) and vacuum assistance (mammotome biopsy), a mass up to 2–3 cm can be excised. This will avoid second operation. Image guided breast biopsy may be performed with ultrasound, stereotactic or MRI guidance.

Evaluation of Non-Palpable Mammographic Abnormalities

Up to 80% of patients with non-palpable mammographic lesions are candidates for stereotactic core biopsy. Stereotactic core biopsy is unsuitable if the mass is close to the chest wall or immediately behind the nipple, diffuse lesions and in patients who are unable to lie prone on the stereotactic table. False negative rate for stereotactic biopsy is less than 2%. Ultrasound guided core biopsy is another alternative. Ultrasound guided or stereotactic fine needle aspiration is less invasive than core biopsy, but it can only provide cytologic diagnosis and not histologic diagnosis. Under good cytopathologist, this technique can be very helpful. The specificity of all types of needle biopsies is very high ranging from 95% to 100%.

The other imaging modality for evaluation of non-palpable mammographic abnormalities or as a primary diagnostic test is MRI. Breast MRI is currently used in at least the following conditions: (a) to search for an occult primary tumour in the setting of known metastasis, (b) to evaluate the extent of disease, (c) to assess lesions in implant-augmented breasts and (d) for screening of high-risk women with dense breasts and with equivocal findings on mammogram or ultrasound.

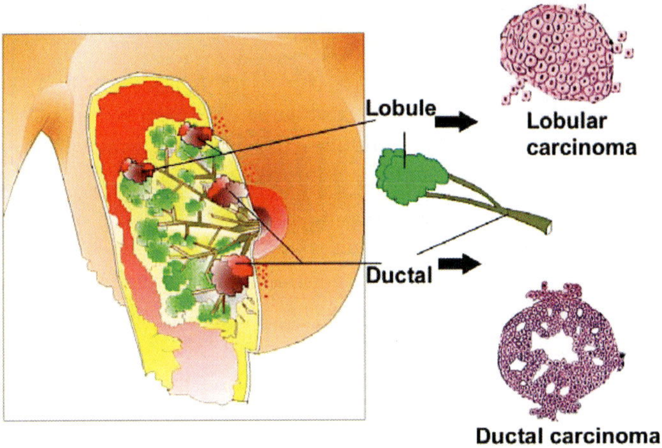

Figure 16.4 The origin of breast cancer. Cancer arising from cells lining the lobule is known as lobular carcinoma, while cancer arising from cells lining the duct system is known as ductal carcinoma.

Ductal Carcinoma in situ

Ductal carcinoma in situ (CIS) is considered as an early stage of breast cancer and often detected by mammogram. It is a non-invasive breast cancer, with good prognosis, and is curable. DCIS is divided into comedo and non-comedo subtypes (papillary, micropapillary, solid and cribriform). Subtype comedo characterized by high nuclear grade, ER–, HER2+ and poorer prognosis as compared to non-comedo subtype. Most lesions represent a combination of at least two of these subtypes.

Approximately, 2% of DCIS has co-existing microinvasion. The standard treatment of DCIS is a surgical treatment (lumpectomy, mastectomy) with or without adjuvant radiotherapy/hormonal therapy. Indications for adjuvant treatment are patients who undergo lumpectomy and comedo subtype. Tamoxifen is the only hormonal therapy currently approved for adjuvant therapy in patients treated with breast-conserving surgery and radiation for DCIS. The other potential hormonal therapy under evaluation is the aromatase inhibitor (anastrozole). If DCIS recurs after primary surgery, 50% of cases will have coexisting invasive cancer.

Lobular Carcinoma in situ

Lobular carcinoma in situ (LCIS) is not considered as cancer, but it signifies an increased risk of breast cancer. Women with LCIS have 1% risk per year of developing an invasive breast cancer (20% risk in 20 years). The peak incidence is in women aged 40–50 years. In contrast to DCIS, LCIS is difficult to detect on clinical examination or mammography. The diagnosis is often incidental finding on histologic examinations. Treatment options for LCIS include surgery, chemoprevention with SERM or close observation (no treatment).

Mammary Paget Disease

Mammary Paget disease (MPD) is considered as a rare form of breast cancer that appears as a moist rash on the nipple and may spread out onto the areola. MPD is more common in older women (mean age 57 years) and constitutes 1–4% of all breast cancers. Paget's cells are large, pale epithelial cells with a hyperchromatic, atypical nucleus, dispersed between the keratinocytes as a single or cluster of cells. The presenting symptoms of MPD are itching, tingling, burning or pain. It is associated with underlying breast cancer in 75% of cases. The standard treatment for MPD is surgery and comprises mastectomy with axillary node dissection. Breast-conserving surgery can achieve satisfactory results but recurrence rate is higher.

Invasive Carcinoma of Breast

Invasive carcinoma of breast is originates from epithelial cells of ductal systems (ductal carcinoma) or lobular systems (lobular carcinoma). Infiltrating ductal carcinoma is the most common invasive carcinoma of breast accounting 75% of breast cancers. Infiltrating lobular carcinoma constituted less than 15% of cases and the prognosis is comparable to ductal carcinoma. Other histological types of breast cancers are medullary carcinoma, mucinous carcinoma, tubular carcinoma, papillary carcinoma and metaplastic breast cancer. All these histotypes were rare. The tumours with oestrogen and progesterone receptor positive have a better prognosis and respond to hormonal treatment. Tumour with HER2 (Human epidermal Growth Factor Receptor) positive is associated with an increased incidence of recurrence and shortened overall survival. HER2 is overexpressed in 20–30% of breast cancers.

Recurrence rate of breast cancer can be calculated based on the so-called recurrence score (RS). RS is derived from an assay of 21 genes (16 cancer genes and 5 reference genes) using reverse transcriptase polymerase chain reaction. The total score will be calculated and if the recurrence score higher than 30, the patient is considered to have high risk of recurrence (low risk if RS < 18). Oncotype DX assay is using this method, and it has been approved by FDA for women with early stage, ER positive and nodes negative. Low score will benefit adjuvant hormonal treatment.

Prognostic Factors of Invasive Carcinoma of Breast

There are various factors that determine the rate of recurrence and overall prognosis in breast cancer. It is known that the number of axillary lymph node involvement correlates with prognosis. Survival of breast cancer is directly related to the number of involved lymph nodes. Patients with no lymph node involvement will have 10-year survivals of 70% and five-year recurrence rates of 19%. With 1–3 lymph nodes involved, five-year recurrence rate increases to 30–40% and with 4–9 lymph nodes involved; 5-year recurrence rates are 44–70%. The recurrence rate increase to 72–82% if more than 10 lymph nodes involved.

The risk of recurrence is also correlated with the tumour size, larger tumour size, especially more than 5 cm carries a higher risk of recurrence. Patients with positive or close tumour margins following surgical treatment are at increased risk of recurrence. Patients who underwent lumpectomy (breast-preserving surgery) without subsequent radiotherapy are also at a higher risk of recurrence.

Presence of lymphatic/vascular invasion is associated with poorer prognosis. Younger age group, women under age 60—particularly those under age 35 at the time of their original breast cancer diagnosis, has a higher risk of recurrence. The other important prognostic factor is histologic types and inflammatory breast cancer is known to carry poorer prognosis compared to others.

The status of oestrogen and progesterone receptor is known prognostic factor. Hormone receptor–positive tumour has a better prognosis and is responsive to hormonal therapy compared to receptor negative tumour. HER2/neu over-expression (positive) was associated with more aggressive tumour and worse prognosis. HER2-positive patients responded to certain anticancer drugs, e.g. doxorubicin, HER2-targeted therapies, e.g. trastuzumab and tyrosine kinase inhibitor (lapatinib). HER2 testing must be performed by validated immunohistochemistry and if necessary undergoing HER2 gene amplification method. This is because 20% of current HER2 testing is inaccurate.

Presentation

Most patients with breast cancer are asymptomatic. If patients are presented with a breast lump, following symptoms may suggest cancer: (a) Change in breast size and shape, (b) Skin dimpling, (c) Axillary lump and (d) Recent nipple inversion. Blood-stained discharge from the nipple is also a warning sign of underlying malignancy. In late-stage disease, following symptoms correlate with the site of metastatic diseases:

(a) breathing difficulties
(b) bone pain
(c) jaundice
(d) significant loss of weight and appetite
(e) abdominal distension
(f) altered cognitive function
(g) localizing neurological signs
(h) symptoms of hypercalcaemia

The physical signs to look for when examining the breasts are

(a) lump or contour change (irregular, hard, fixation to skin or muscle, etc.)
(b) skin tethering
(c) nipple inversion
(d) ulceration

(e) dilated veins
(f) presence of lesions suspected Paget's disease.
(g) oedema or peau d'orange (Fig. 16.5)

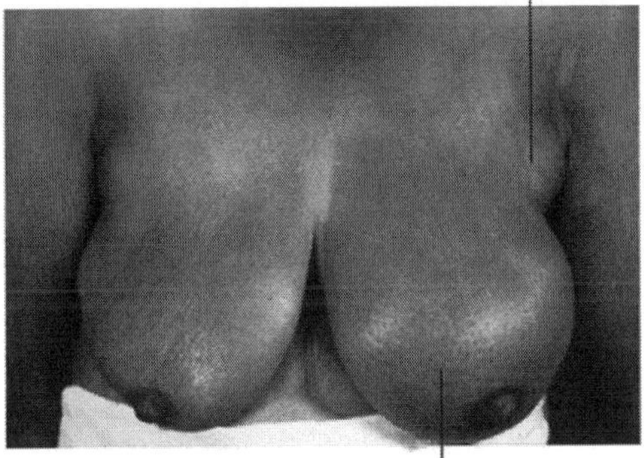

Figure 16.5 Clinical features of breast cancer.

Evaluation of Patients with Breast Cancer

Patients with a breast lump or having radiologic breast abnormalities must undergo thorough evaluation. The common approach is through so-called triple assessment involving clinical examination, imaging and biopsy. Biopsy is a diagnostic test, and once the diagnosis is made, the patient and her family members must be invited to attend the counselling session. Subsequent evaluation is to determine the extent of the disease and to judge the most appropriate treatment to offer. Evaluation is also to judge whether surgery is required and if so, to plan the most appropriate surgery Imaging techniques such as Chest X-ray, mammography, Ultrasound, CT scan, MRI and Bone scan are indicated in selected patients with confirmed breast cancer. Not all patients need to undergo all this imaging evaluation. The purpose of these imaging techniques is to assess the extent of disease, to study the characteristic of the tumour and to plan and determine the most appropriate surgical treatment. MRI is useful in detailing architectural abnormalities of the breast and can help detecting lesions as small as 2–3 mm. A study by Wasif et al. found that MRI was more accurate than ultrasonography and mammography for determination of the size of the cancer mass in the breast. PET scan is the most sensitive and specific of all the imaging modalities for breast disease; however, it is very expensive and not widely available. At present, its main use is helping to detect recurrences in scarred breasts, in multi-focal disease, detecting axillary nodes involvement and in equivocal findings of distance metastases uncharacterized by other imaging modalities. The role of PET scan is expanding with time.

Blood testing is also important to determine the patients general health and evidence of organ involvement in breast cancer. Following are the relevant blood investigations for assessment of breast cancer:

(a) **Liver involvement**: levels of bilirubin, alkaline phosphatase, alanine and aspartate transaminase, albumin, etc.
(b) **Bone involvement**: hypercalcaemia, levels of alkaline phosphatise isoenzymes
(c) **Tumour markers**: CA15-3, CA72-4, CEA
(d) **Bone marrow involvement**: full blood count, full blood picture, bone marrow aspiration.

Staging of Breast Cancer

Staging of breast cancer is mandatory before deciding on definitive treatment for a newly diagnosed breast cancer. With proper staging, appropriate plan for surgical treatment can be made for patients with operable disease. The American Joint Committee on Cancer (AJCC) Breast Cancer staging system is the most widely used system. This system is based on tumour size (T), the status of regional lymph nodes (N) and the presence of distant metastasis (M).

Table 16.1 TNM staging system for breast cancer

Tumour (T)	
Stage Tx:	Tumour not accessible
Stage T0:	No primary tumour
Stage Tis:	Carcinoma in situ
Stage T1a:	Tumour diameter greater than 0.1 cm but not greater than 0.5 cm

Stage T1b:	Tumour diameter greater than 0.5 cm but not greater than 1 cm
Stage T1c:	Tumour diameter greater than 1 cm but not greater than 2 cm
Stage T2:	Tumour diameter greater than 2 cm but not greater than 5 cm
Stage T3:	Tumour larger than 5 cm
Stage T4a:	Involvement of chest wall
Stage T4b:	Involvement of skin
Stage T4c:	Stage T4a and T4b
Stage T4d:	Inflammatory cancer
Nodes (N)	
Stage Nx:	Node not assessable
Stage N0:	No regional lymph node metastases
Stage N1:	Palpable ipsilateral axillary lymph nodes
Stage N2:	Fixed ipsilateral axillary lymph nodes
Stage N3:	Ipsilateral internal mammary nodes
Metastasis (M)	
Stage Mx:	Metastasis not assessable
Stage M0:	Stage M0: No evidence of metastasis
Stage M1:	Distant metastasis, including ipsilateral supraclavicular nodes

Treatment for Breast Cancer

Surgical Treatment

The primary treatment for breast cancer is surgery. The goals of breast surgery are:

(a) curative: to excise the tumour with good margin and to remove all involved lymph nodes
(b) to obtain information regarding the characteristic of primary tumour and the extent of nodal involvement
(c) to obtain information regarding prognostic factors and to plan for appropriate treatment after surgery in order to reduce recurrence and mortality rate

Types of Surgical Treatment for Breast Cancer

(a) Lumpectomy

Lumpectomy is a complete surgical resection of a primary tumour with a goal of achieving at least 1 cm negative margin with preservation of the breast. A patient with free margin of less than 2 mm is often required re-excision. The landmark study NSABP-B6 involving 2163 patients had found that lumpectomy followed by radiotherapy to be as effective as modified radical mastectomy. (NSABP: National Surgical Adjuvant Breast Project). Lumpectomy must be followed by adjuvant radiotherapy. The meta-analysis conducted by Early Breast Cancer Trialist's Collaborative Group comparing breast-conserving surgery (BCS) versus BCD plus radiotherapy demonstrated that the addition of radiotherapy reduced the risk of local recurrence by 75% and resulted in a disease-free survival advantage as well as the reduction in the risk of dying in both nodes negative and positive patients. Lumpectomy is contraindicated in multi-centric disease, large primary tumour, repeated positive margin and inability to undergo radiation therapy.

(b) Mastectomy

Total mastectomy is the complete removal of all breast tissue (superior border: clavicle, medial border: sternum, lateral border: anterior axillary line) with en bloc resection of the fascia of pectoralis major muscle. There are at least two variants of total mastectomy, i.e. skin-sparing total mastectomy (SSM) and nipple sparing total mastectomy (NSM). SSM and SSM are for patients who elect to have immediate reconstructive surgery. Radical mastectomy is total mastectomy plus en bloc resection of pectoralis major, minor and axillary lymph node dissection till level 3. Modified radical mastectomy is total mastectomy plus axillary lymph node dissection (level 1 and 2). Complications of total mastectomy are local recurrence, wound infection, seroma, skin flap necrosis, haematoma, pain, lymphaedema and fibrosis.

(c) Axillary lymph node dissection

Axillary lymph nodes are grouped into level 1, level 2 and level 3. Level 1 nodes are lateral to pectoralis minor muscle. Level 2 are beneath the muscle, and level 3 are medial to the muscle. Axillary lymph node dissection for breast cancer is a complete en bloc removal of the level 1 and 2 lymph nodes. Level 3 are not removed, unless suspected to have involved with cancer. Potential complications are lymphoedema (25%), shoulder dysfunction, wound infection, seroma, nerve injury, numbness, pain, etc.). Sentinel lymph node dissection will identify patients who do not require axillary node dissection in early breast cancer. Lymphatic mapping may be performed with radioisotope (technetium 99 sulphur colloid) alone or radioisotope plus blue dye. One to three lymph nodes are removed, and immediate axillary lymph node dissection will be performed if a sentinel node is unequivocally positive for nodal metastasis.

(d) Reconstructive breast surgery

Reconstructive surgery is performed after mastectomy in order to restore a breast to near normal shape, appearance and size. Breast reconstructive surgery may be performed in the immediate or the delayed setting. Immediate reconstruction usually provides better cosmetic results. Delayed reconstructive surgery is performed for patients who very likely required adjuvant radiotherapy or if the reconstructive surgeon is unavailable. There are at least three types of reconstructive surgery, i.e. (a) implant-based method (b) tissue flap and (c) combination of the flap and implant. Example of tissue flap breast reconstruction is the latissimus dorsi flap, transverse rectus abdominus myocutaneous flap (TRAM) and deep inferior epigastric perforator flap (DIEP). Together with reconstructive breast surgery, prosthetic or false areolar-nipple complex can be created using skin adhesive/graft and tattooing. Implants are made of silicone shells and filled with silicone gel or saline. Gradual inflation of the implant is done over few weeks through a port that is connected to the implant. Complications related to reconstruction include infection, implant rupture, capsular contracture, flap necrosis, flap rejection, asymmetry and scarring.

Radiotherapy

Radiotherapy has become the standard treatment after breast-conserving surgery, high-grade non-invasive cancer and following some mastectomy. The purpose of radiotherapy is to eradicate a residual disease and, therefore, improve the local control of the cancer. Radiotherapy following surgery can reduce the local recurrence rates up to 75% (for tumours of more than 4 cm).

The specific areas that can be treated with radiotherapy are

- remaining breast tissue
- chest wall (after mastectomy)
- axilla
- supraclavicular area
- internal mammary chain

Radiotherapy to the chest wall provides significant benefit in women with tumour larger than 5 cm, four or more positive axillary lymph nodes and tumour infiltrating the pectoralis major muscle. Radiotherapy to axillary is indicated in women with positive axillary lymph nodes when at the same time, full axillary clearance has not been performed. Radiation therapy to the supraclavicular area is recommended in patients with four or more positive axillary lymph nodes. Whole breast radiotherapy comprises external beam radiotherapy delivered to the breast at a dose of 50–55 Gy over 5–6 weeks with or without booster dose.

Post-mastectomy radiation therapy is indicated in patients with (American Society of Clinical Oncology guideline)

- positive margin
- primary tumour larger than 5 cm
- involvement of four or more lymph nodes
- undergoing breast-preserving surgery

Partial breast irradiation is employed to deliver a larger fraction within a shorter time of the period while maintaining low risk of side effects.

Systemic Therapy

Studies have shown that in some women with early breast cancer who receive adjuvant systemic therapy (hormonal or chemotherapy), has better outcomes in terms of longer survival and fewer recurrences.

Chemotherapy for Breast Cancer

For breast cancer, chemotherapy is used in three main conditions:

(1) adjuvant therapy after surgery or radiotherapy
(2) neoadjuvant chemotherapy before surgery
(3) advanced or metastatic breast cancer

Indications for adjuvant chemotherapy following surgery are

(1) lymph node involvement
(2) tumour is larger than 2 cm in diameter.
(3) grade 3 tumour
(4) lymphvascular space invasion
(5) oestrogen-negative tumour

Chemotherapy regimens (given in 4–6 cycles) are

(1) FAC (5-fluorouracil, doxorubicin, cyclophosphamide)
(2) FEC (5-fluorouracil, epirubicin, cyclophosphamide)
(3) CMF (cyclophosphamide, methotrexate, 5-fluorouracil
(4) AC (doxorubicin, cyclophosphamide)
(5) FEC + taxane
(6) TAC (docetaxel, doxorubicin, cyclophosphamide)

Chemotherapy regimens for advanced and metastatic breast cancer are similar. FAC and FEC regimens were found to be more superior to CMF in both adjuvants as well as metastatic disease setting. Taxane-based chemotherapy may be considered if the patient develops progression of disease despite first line treatment. Docetaxel is probably more active than paclitaxel in metastatic disease. Taxanes can be used as a single agent or in combination.

Hormonal Therapy for Breast Cancer

Hormonal therapy is indicated in all patients with ER and PR positive including hormone responsive or hormone uncertain. Hormonal therapy is benefited for both pre and post-menopausal women with ER positive tumour. The currently available hormonal therapies are anti-oestrogen (Tamoxifen, toremifen, fulvestrant) and Aromatase inhibitors (anastrazole, letrozole, exemestane, formestane). Tamoxifen is a selective oestrogen receptor modulator (SERM), which binds to and inhibits oestrogen receptor signalling in the breast. Aromatase inhibitors inhibit aromatase enzyme found in body fat, adrenal gland and breast tissues which responsible for converting other steroid hormones into oestrogen. In an analysis of 55 trials evaluating tamoxifen versus placebo in the adjuvant treatment of breast cancer, 5 years of Tamoxifen therapy results in a 47% reduction in recurrence and a 22% reduction in mortality. Pre-menopausal women should be given anti-oestrogen, i.e. tamoxifen 20 mg daily for 5 years. As the aromatase inhibitors have no effect on ovarian oestrogen production, it is not useful in pre-menopausal women. In post-menopausal women, both tamoxifen and aromatase inhibitors are beneficial and aromatase inhibitor, e.g. letrozole can be considered if a patient has a contraindication to tamoxifen. Letrozole can be used for women who have already received standard adjuvant tamoxifen as an extended adjuvant for another 5 years, particularly in patients with node positive (improve overall survival in Canadian lead MA.17 trial). Several large randomized trials, including BIG1-98 and ATAC (Arimidex, Tamoxifen, alone or in combination) have shown aromatase inhibitor (anastrozole) to be superior to tamoxifen with regard to disease-free survival in post-menopausal women with early-stage breast cancer. In ATAC trial, anastrozole (Arimidex) was also found to be associated with fewer side effects than tamoxifen and more tolerable.

Targeted Therapy for Breast Cancer

Human Epidermal Growth Factor Receptor (HER 2) Inhibitor

Approximately, 25% of breast cancer patients have a tumour that is HER 2 positive. HER stands for human epidermal growth factor receptor. Tumour with HER 2 positive is more aggressive and required adjuvant treatment. HER 2 proteins are expressed on the surface of normal cell. HER 2 gene is found in the DNA (chromosome 17) of a cell, and this gene will encode HER 2 proteins. HER 2 protein is important in transmitting the growth signals from outside to inside the cell. In HER 2 positive breast cancer, the cancer cells have an abnormally high number and deformed HER 2 genes and proteins. Anti HER2 has been developed in the form of monoclonal antibody. One of the HER 2 receptor inhibitor is Trastuzumab. Trastuzumab is monoclonal antibodies against HER 2 protein. Trastuzumab will bind to HER2 receptor, deactivated and interrupting the growth signal leading to slow progression or cancer cell death. Trastuzumab (Herceptin) is approved for the adjuvant treatment of HER 2 positive patients. It is also found to have an important role in metastatic breast cancer. HER2 testing is mandatory in all newly diagnosed breast cancers and accurate results are critical. Immunohistochemistry is the method of choice to detect HER2. HER 2 score is dependent on the percentage of cells staining and the intensity and completeness of membrane staining. A score of 3+ is deemed positive and the patient qualifies for trastuzumab therapy. A score of 2+ requires FISH (fluorescent in situ hybridization) test to confirm the positivity. The FDA has approved Trastuzumab to be used as adjuvant treatment in the following conditions: (1) HER 2, 3+ by Immunohistochemistry and overexpressed by FISH and (2) High risk of recurrence.

The FDA and NCCN guidelines have approved trastuzumab for use in adjuvant setting as part of a treatment regimen containing doxorubicin, cyclophosphamide and paclitaxel for patients with HER-2-positive and node-positive. NCCN guidelines recommend adding 1 year of trastuzumab to standard adjuvant chemotherapy. Trastuzumab can also be incorporated with adjuvant radiotherapy and hormonal therapy.

Following are the other indications of trastuzumab:

(1) HER 2 positive metastatic breast cancer either in the first line setting in combination with paclitaxel or as monotherapy for patients who received at least one prior chemotherapy (Approved by FDA)

(2) Neoadjuvant therapy for locally advanced breast cancer or inflammatory breast cancer. Phase 3 Neoadjuvant Herceptin (NOAH) trial evaluated the role of trastuzumab in locally advanced breast cancer with HER 2 positive; chemotherapy was given with or without trastuzumab and pathological complete response rate was significantly better in the trastuzumab arm (43% versus 23%, $p = 0.02$) (Gianni, et al.).

Lapatinib

Lapatinib in an orally available dual kinase inhibitor of EGFR and ERBB2. Lapatinib has various modes of action, including inhibiting intracellular signalling mediated by the insulin growth factors 1 receptor in trastuzumab resistant cancer cells. Lapatinib is approved by FDA for patients affected by HER 2 positive breast cancer pre-treated with trastuzumab, anthracyclines and taxanes. The approval was based on phase 3 trial by Geyer et al. Patients with metastatic breast cancer and HER 2 positive were given capecitabine alone or capecitabine plus lapatinib. The second arm was found to have a significant reduction in risk of progression and longer time to progression.

Anti-Angiogenesis

Bevacizumab is antiangiogenesis that has been evaluated in the management of metastatic breast cancer. Phase 3 trial known as RIBBON-2 showed improved progression-free survival with a combination of bevacizumab plus standard chemotherapy versus chemotherapy alone as a second-line treatment of metastatic breast cancer (Brufsky, et al.).

Locally Advanced Breast Cancer

Locally advanced breast cancer is defined as primary tumour of larger than 5 cm (Stage T3 and above). The intention to treat locally advanced breast cancer (LABC) is still to cure. In some LABC, the tumour is still resectable but in unresectable tumours, neoadjuvant chemotherapy is the treatment of choice. The indications for neoadjuvant chemotherapy are: (a) Inoperable locally advanced breast cancer and (b) Operable but large tumour. Appropriate regimens for neoadjuvant chemotherapy are FAC/FEC, AC, CMF and taxane-based regimens. Patients with LABC who achieve good tumour reduction with neoadjuvant therapy are good candidates for subsequent breast-conserving surgery. Reconstructive breast surgery is not recommended for LABC and inflammatory breast cancer patients because it may compromise their oncologic care.

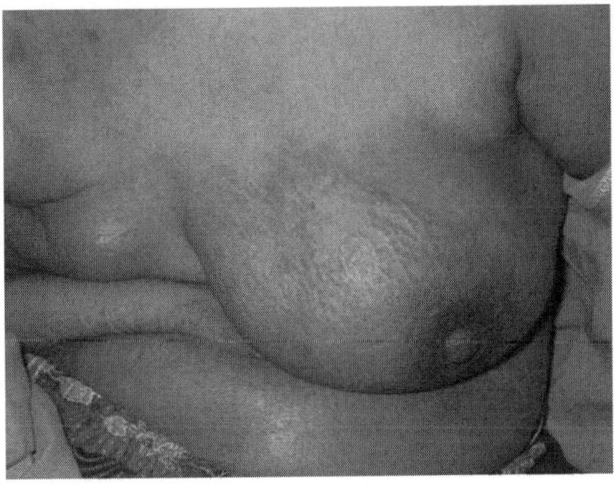

Figure 16.6 Recurrent breast cancer on the opposite breast. The patient had past history of right mastectomy.

Prevention of Breast Cancer

Lifestyle changes: There is increasing evidence that lifestyle changes may alter an individual's breast cancer risk.

Physical activity: Women who exercise regularly 3–4 times a week may have a reduced incidence of breast cancer, when compared with women who do not exercise.

Avoid alcohol consumption: Women who consumed 2.3–4.5 bottles of beer, 2.5–5.6 glasses of wine per day, or 2–4 shots of liquor per day had a 41% higher risk of developing invasive breast cancer. Avoid alcohol consumption is therefore, will reduce the risk of breast cancer.

Low intake of animal fat: A reduced incidence of breast cancer has been observed in countries where the diet is typically low in animal fat.

Avoid smoking: Avoiding smoking and breast-feeding may have protective effect on breast cancer risk, although there is no concrete scientific evidence.

Chemoprevention: NSABP-BCPT (National Surgical Adjuvant Breast and Bowel Project—Breast Cancer Prevention Trial) evaluated the role of tamoxifen as chemoprevention in high-risk women. Women who had a risk of developing breast cancer equivalent to that of women 60 years of age qualified as participants in this double-blind randomized trial. This study has shown that tamoxifen prophylaxis leads to 30–50% reduction in the risk of ductal carcinoma in situ and invasive breast cancer in all age groups. There was, however, no survival advantage. FDA has approved tamoxifen for use in women at high risk of breast cancer (1.66% chance of getting breast cancer in the next 5 years based on Gail's model). The problem with long-term tamoxifen is side effects. Raloxifene is a good alternative and in CORE trial (Continuing Outcomes Relevant to Evista trial) has reported the 59% risk reduction of breast cancer in post-menopausal women taking raloxifene as compared to placebo. The STAR trial (Study of Tamoxifen and Raloxifene Trial) compared tamoxifen (20 mg/day) versus raloxifene (60 mg/day) by post-menopausal women and women older than 35 years but at increased risk of breast cancer by Gail's model. The authors concluded that raloxifene is as effective as tamoxifen in reducing the risk of invasive breast cancer. There was, however, no statistically significant difference in non-invasive breast cancer.

Current Recommendations of Chemoprevention

(1) For women with increased risk of breast cancer, offer tamoxifen (20 mg daily for 5 years) to reduce the risk of invasive ER positive breast cancer.

(2) In post-menopausal women, raloxifene (60 mg daily for 5 years) may be an alternative to tamoxifen.

(3) Aromatase inhibitors (e.g. anastrazole, exemestane, letrozole), fenretinide, or other SERMs are not recommended outside of a clinical trial.

References

Anderson BO, et al. Guideline implementation for breast healthcare in low-income and middle-income countries: overview of the Breast Health Global Initiative Global Summit 2007. *Cancer* 2008; **113**: 2221–2243.

Andreetta C, Minisini AM, Miscoria M, Puglisi F. First line chemotherapy with or without biologic agents for metastatic breast cancer. *Crit Rev Oncol/Hematol* 2010, doi:10.1916/j.critrevonc. 2010.01.007.

A randomized trial of Letrozole in postmenopausal women after five years of Tamoxifen therapy for early-stage breast cancer *NEMJ* 2003; **349**: 1793–1802.

Berg WA, Gutierrez L, Ness Aiver MS, et al. Diagnostic accuracy of mammography, clinical examination, US, and MR imaging in preoperative assessment of breast cancer. *Radiology* Dec 2004; **233**(3): 830–849.

Boccardo F, et al. Switching to Anastrozole Versus Continued Tamoxifen Treatment of Early Breast Cancer: Preliminary Results of the Italian Tamoxifen Anastrozole Trial. *JCO* 2005; **23**(22): 5138–5147.

Bonneterre J, et al. Anastrozole is superior to Tamoxifen as first-line therapy in hormone receptor positive advanced breast carcinoma. *Cancer* 2001; **92**: 9.

Brufsky A, Bondarenko IN, Smirnov V, et al. RIBBON-2: a randomized, double-blind, placebo-controlled phase III trial evaluation the efficacy and safety of bevacizumab in combination with chemotherapy for second-line treatment of HER2-negative metastatic breast cancer. In: *Program and Abstracts of the 32nd Annual San Antonio Breast Cancer Symposium*: 2009 (Abstract 42).

Cady B, Webb M, Michaelson J, Smith Bl. Death from breast cancer occurs predominantly in women not participating in mammographic screening. Abstract No. 24, Proc. ASCO Breast Cancer Symposium. San Francisco; October 2009. http://www.asco.org/ASCOv2/Meetings/Abstract.05?&vmview=abst_detail_view&confI D = 70 & abstractI D = 40559 (accessed 02.05.2010).

Coleman MP, et al. Cancer survival in five continents: a worldwide population-based study (CONCORD). *Lancet Oncol* 2008; **9**: 730–756.

Danaei G, et al. Causes of cancer in the world: comparative risk assessment of nine behavioral and environmental risk factors. *Lancet* 2005; **366**: 1784–1793.

Dang CM, Zaghiyan K, Karlan SR, Phillips EH. Increased use of MRI for breast cancer surveillance and staging is not associated with increased rate of mastectomy. *Am Surg* Oct 2009; **75**(10): 937–940.

Gail MH, Anderson WF, Garcia-Closas M, Sherman ME. Absolute risk models for subtypes of breast cancer. *J Natl Cancer Inst* 2007; **99**(22): 1657–1659.

Gail MH, Brinton LA, Byar DP, et al. Projecting individualized probabilities of developing breast cancer for white females who are being examined annually. *J Natl Cancer Inst* 1989; **81**: 1879–1886.

Gail MH, Costantino JP, Pee D, et al. Projecting individualized absolute invasive breast cancer risk in African American Women. *J Natl Cancer Inst* 2007; **99**(23): 1782–1792.

Geyer CE, Forster J, Lindquist D, et al. Lapatinib plus capecitabine for HER 2 positive advanced breast cancer. *N Engl J Med* 2006; **355**(26): 2733–2743.

Gianni L, Semiglazov V, Manikhas GM, et al. Neoadjuvant trastuzumab in locally advanced breast cancer (NOAH): antitumor and safety analysis. *J Clin Oncol* 2007; **25**: 18S (abstract 532).

Goldhirsch, et al. Progress and promise: highlights of the international expert consensus on the primary therapy of early breast cancer. *Ann Oncol* 2007; **18**: 1133–1144.

Goss PE, Ingle JN, Martino S, et al. Efficacy of letrozole extended adjuvant therapy according to estrogen receptor and progesterone receptor status of the primary tumor: National Cancer Institute of Canada Clinical Trials Group MA.17. *J Clin Oncol* 2007; **25**(15): 1957–1959.

Goss PE, et al. Randomized trial of letrozole following tamoxifen as extended adjuvant therapy in receptorpositive breast cancer: updated findings from NCIC CTG MA.17. *J Natl Cancer Inst* 2005; **97**(17): 1262–1271.

Goss PE, Ingle JN, Martino S, et al. Randomized trial of Letrozole following tamoxifen as extended adjuvant therapy in receptor positive breast cancer: Updated finding from NCIC CTG MA.17. *J NCI* 2005; **97**(17): 1262–1271.

Gotzsche PC, Nielsen M. Screening for breast cancer with mammography. *Cochrane Database Syst Rev* 2009; (4). Art. No. CD001877.

Greif JM. Mammographic screening for breast cancer: an invited review of the benefits and costs. *Breast* 2010, doi: 10.1016/j.breast.2010.03.017.

Harvey V, et al. Phase III trial comparing three doses of docetaxel for second-line treatment of advanced breast cancer. *JCO* Nov 1 2006; **23**(31): 4963–69.

Howell A, Cuzick J, Baum M, et al. Results of the ATAC (Arimidex, Tamoxifen, Alone or in Combination) trial after completion of 5 years adjuvant treatment for breast cancer. *Lancet* 2005; **365**: 60–62.

IARC. World cancer report 2008. Lyon, International Agency for Research on Cancer.

Jakesz R, et al. Switching of postmenopausal women with endocrine responsive early breast cancer to anastrozole after 2 years' Adjuvant tamoxifen: combined results of ABCSG trial 8 and ARNO95 trial. *Lancet* Aug 2005; **366**: 455–462.

Jassem J, et al. Doxorubicin and paclitaxel versus fluorouracil, doxorubicin and cyclophosphamide as first-line therapy for women with metastatic breast cancer: final results of a randomized phase III Multicenter trial. *JCO* Mar 15 2001; **19**(6): 1707–1715.

Jones SE, et al. Randomized Phase III Study of Docetaxel Compared With Paclitaxel in Metastatic Breast Cancer. *JCO* Aug 20 2005; **23**(24): 5542–5551.

Kaufmann M, et al. Improved overall survival in postmenopausal women with early breast cancer after anastrozole initiated after treatment with tamoxifen compared with continued tamoxifen: the ARNO 95 Study. *JCO* 2007; **25**(19): 2664–2670.

Keshtgar M, Davidson T, Pigott K, Falzon M, Jones A. Review: Current status and advances in management of early breast cancer. *Intl J Surg* 2010; **8**: 199–202.

Laey JV, et al. Breast cancer epidemiology according to recognized breast cancer risk factors in the Prostate, Lung, Colorectal and Ovarian (PLCO) Cancer Screening Trial Cohort. *BMC Cancer* 2009; **9**: 84.

Lehman CD, Smith RA. The role of MRI in breast cancer screening. *J Natl Compr Cancer Netw* 2009; **7**: 1109–1115.

Lindfors KK, McGahan MC, Rosenquist CJ, et al. Computer-aided detection of breast cancer: a cost-effectiveness study. *Radiology* 2006; **239**: 710–717.

Mouridsen H, et al. Phase III study of Letrozole versus Tamoxifen as first-line therapy of advanced breast cancer in postmenopausal women: analysis of survival and update of efficacy from the International Letrozole Breast Cancer Group. *JCO* 2003 June 1, **21**(11) 2102–2109.

NCCN Practice Guidelines. Invasive Breast Cancer. 2010.

Paridaens R, et al. Paclitaxel versus doxetaxel as first-line single agent chemotherapy for metastatic breast cancer: a European Organisation for Research and Treatment of Cancer randomized study with cross-over. *JCO* 2000 Feb, **18**(4): 724–733.

Patani N, Mokbel K. Herceptin and breast cancer: an overview for surgeons. *Surg Oncol* 2010; **19**: e11–e21.

Response of the American College of Obstetricians and Gynecologists to New Breast Cancer Screening Recommendations from the U.S. Preventive Services Task Force. American Congress of Obstetricians and Gynecologists. Available at http://www.acog.org/from_home/Misc/uspstfResponse.cfm. Accessed December 2009; 17.

Rockhill B, Spiegelman D, Byrne C, Hunter DJ, Colditz GA. Validation of the Gail et al. model of breast cancer risk prediction and implications for chemoprevention. *J Natl Cancer Inst* 2001; **93**(5): 358–366.

Saslow D, Boetes C, Burke W, Harms S, Leach MO, Lehman CD. American Cancer Society guidelines for breast screening with MRI as an adjunct to mammography. *CA Cancer J Clin* Mar–Apr 2007; **57**(2): 75–89.

Screening for breast cancer: U.S. Preventive Services Task Force recommendation statement. *Ann Int Med* Nov 17 2009; **151**(10): 716–726, W-236.

Smith RA, Cokkinides V, Brawley OW. Cancer screening in the United State, 2008: a review of current American Cancer Society guidelines and cancer screening issues. *CA Cancer J Clin* 2008; **58**(3): 161–179.

Swart R, Stopeck A. Next generation of targeted therapies in breast cancer. *Biol Ther Breast Cancer* 2008; **9**(2): 3–10.

The Adjuvant Breast Cancer Trials Collaborative Group Polychemotherapy for Early Breast Cancer: Results From the International Adjuvant Breast Cancer Chemotherapy Randomized Trial. *J Natl Cancer Inst* 2007; **99**: 506–515.

The ATAC (Arimidex, Tamoxifen Alone or in Combination) Trialists' Group* Anastrozole alone or in combination with tamoxifen versus Tamoxifen alone for adjuvant treatment of postmenopausal women With early breast cancer: first results of the ATAC_uppressio trial. *Lancet* 2002; **359**: 2131–2139.

The ATAC Trialists' Group Results of the ATAC (Arimidex, Tamoxifen, Alone or in Combination) trial after completion of 5 years' adjuvant treatment for breast cancer. *Lancet* 2005; **365**: 60–62.

The French Epirubicin Study Group. Epirubicin-Based Chemotherapy in Metastatic Breast Cancer Patients: Role of Dose-Intensity and Duration of Treatment. *JCO* 2000; **18**(17): 3115–3124.

Veronesi U, Cascinelli N, Mariani MD, et al. Twenty year follow up of a randomized study comparing breast-conserving surgery with radical mastectomy for early breast cancer. *NEJM* 2002; **347**: 1227–1232.

Veronesi U, Cascinelli N, Mariani MD, et al. Early Breast Cancer Trialist's Collaborative Group. Radiotherapy after breast conserving surgery in small breast carcinoma: long term results of a randomized trial. *Ann Oncol* 2001; **12**: 997–1003.

Visvanathan K, Chlebowski RT, Hurley P, et al. American society of clinical oncology clinical practice guideline update on the use of pharmacologic interventions including tamoxifen, raloxifen, and aromatase inhibition for breast cancer risk reduction. *J Clin Oncol* 2009; **27**(19): 3235–3258.

Vogel VG, Costantino JP, Wickerham DL, et al. National Surgical Adjuvant Breast and Bowel Project (NSABP): effects of tamoxifen vs raloxifene on the risk of developing invasive breast cancer and other disease outcomes: the NSABP Study of Tamoxifen (STAR) P-2 trial. *JAMA* 2006; **295**: 2727–2741.

Wasif N, Garreau J, Terando A, Kirsch D, Mund DF, Giuliano AE. MRI versus ultrasonography and mammography for preoperative assessment of breast cancer. *Am Surg* Oct 2009; **75**(10): 970–975.

Weir L, Worsley D, Bernstein V. The value of FDG positron emission tomography in the management of patients with breast cancer. *Breast J* May–Jun 2005; **11**(3): 204–209.

Chapter 17

Gynaecologic Cancer during Pregnancy

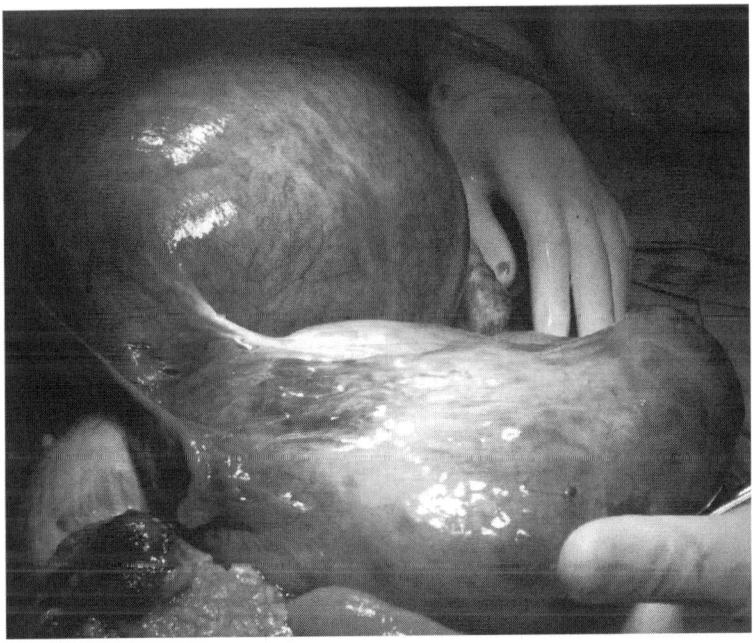

Gynaecologic Cancer: A Handbook for Students and Practitioners
Rushdan Noor, Eng Hseon Tay, and Jeffrey Low

ISBN 978-981-4463-06-5 (Hardcover), 978-981-4463-07-2 (eBook)
www.panstanford.com

Introduction

Cancer in pregnancy is an uncommon problem diagnosed in about 1 in 1000 term pregnancies. The incidence is expected to increase with the rising trend of postponing pregnancy to later in life. Generally maternal prognosis is similar to that in the non-pregnancy state, provided a delay in treatment is avoided and standard treatment is aimed for. Pregnancy does not accelerate the cancer.

Breast cancer is the most common cancer during pregnancy, constituting 46% of cases (incidence 1:3000–10,000) followed by haematological malignancies in approximately 18–25% of cases. Cervical cancer is the second most common women cancer diagnosed during pregnancy. (incidence: 1.2:10,000). Pregnancy-associated malignancies present significant challenge as a result of the dilemma between optimum maternal treatment and foetal well-being. Due to the small number of cases and lack of large studies, there are no evidence-based guidelines for the management of cancer during pregnancy.

Radiation Exposure during Pregnancy

Staging imaging tests should be limited to those with the lowest exposure to radiation. Abdominal plain X-ray, isotope scans and computed tomography scans should be avoided. Magnetic resonance imaging (MRI), chest X-ray and ultrasound scan are acceptable for staging purposes. The use of iodinated contrast media together with imaging technique is controversial; the most important potential harmful effect of iodinated contrast media during pregnancy is depression of foetal thyroid function caused by free iodide in the contrast solution. If this contrast medium has to be given, neonatal thyroid function should be checked during the first week after delivery. Nuclear medicine studies using a radionuclide bounded to a chemical agent is one of the imaging studies that may be indicated in patients with cancer. Radionucleic substances may affect the foetus, depending on the placental permeability, foetal distribution, tissue affinity, dose, half-life and type of radiation emitted. Foetal can also be exposed to radiation from radionucleic substances deposited in the urine of the maternal urinary bladder. The ventilation-perfusion scan for a suspected pulmonary embolus is among the most common nuclear medicine studies obtained in pregnant women.

Sentinel node mapping is perhaps second most important nuclear medicine studies in pregnancy indicated for patients with breast cancer. Generally, the standard dose of radioisotope used in sentinel node mapping will deliver a negligible amount of radiation to the foetus. Weighing the risks and benefits of this procedure, sentinel node mapping is not an absolute contraindication in pregnancy.

PET scans using standard F18-FDG-PET examination results in a dose exposure of a 6-month-old foetus of 5–6 mSv, which is still acceptable in many indications. However, consultation from a nuclear medicine physician must first be obtained.

The cells are more radiosensitive if they have a high division rate, a long dividing future and a low differentiation level, which are the characteristic of foetal tissue. Gonad is the most radiosensitive organ in the human's body. Radiation-induced biological effects are directly related to the stage of gestation: the earlier the stage, the more detrimental the expected effects. The potential effects of radiation to the fetus and the absorbed fetal radiation are shown in Tables 17.1, 17.2 and 17.3.

Table 17.1 Potential effects of radiation in relation to gestational age (Pavlidis et al.)

Stage of pregnancy	Period of gestation	Potential adverse effect
Pre-implantation/ immediate post-implantation	From conception till day 9–10	Lethal, if not lethal the foetus will recover completely ("all or none")
Early organogenesis	2–6 weeks	Teratogenesis, growth retardation
Late organogenesis/ early foetal period	12–16 weeks	Mental and growth retardation, microcephaly
Late foetal stage	From 20–25 weeks till birth	Sterility, malignancies, genetic defects

Table 17.2 Radiation dose and foetal effects (Pavidis et al.)

Dose (rad)	Effect on foetus
<10	No deterministic effects, only minor risk of stochastic effects
10–15	Increased risk
250	Malformation in most
>3000	Miscarriage

Table 17.3 Absorbed foetal radiation during radiological examination (minimum and maximum predicted exposure)

Investigation	Foetal dose exposure (rad)
Abdominal X-ray	0.2–2.0
Abdominal CT scan	0.8–5.0
Chest X-ray	<0.001
Chest CT	<0.05
Pelvic X-ray	0.3–0.8
Pelvic CT	2.5–7.9
Skull X-ray	<0.001
IVP	0.3–1.2
Lumbar spine X-ray	0.3–2.0
Barium enema	1.6–8.0
Lung ventilation with Tc 99 m	0.002–0.16
Lung perfusion with Tc 99 m	0.01–0.07
Bone scintigraphy	0.13–0.33

Note: 1 rad = 1 centigray (0.01 Gy); 1 Gy = 100 rad.

There are two categories of radiation-related effects in human:

(1) **"Deterministic effects"** occur short after a considerable amount of radiation once a certain threshold is exceeded. The relation of foetal effects and radiation exposure is conclusive. Example of these effects is to the unborn foetus, e.g. foetal death, microcephaly, physical deformities, etc.

(2) **"Stochastic effects"** are probabilistic effects, since they may or may not occur in any given exposed individual. It generally manifest many years later and cannot definitely be associated with radiation exposure (e.g. cancer development or genetic alteration in the future).

Radiotherapy during Pregnancy

The first 8 weeks of organogenesis are the most susceptible to the teratogenic effects of radiation. Permanent sterility dose for ovaries is 250–600 rad (cGy) and 350–600 rad for testis. Radiation therapy given below the diaphragm depressed fertility in both sexes in 25% of cases. Potential risk to genetic mutation in offspring is very minimal (animal study: 100/10,000 livebirth/100 rad).

Radiation therapy for breast cancer in pregnancy (breast and chest wall irradiation) will expose the foetus to 0.1–0.3% of total dose, i.e. 5–15 rad if the total treatment dose is 5000 rad (Muirhead et al.). Effects on the radiation-exposed foetus are miscarriage, microcephaly, intrauterine death, intra-uterine growth restriction, mental retardation, long-term risk of cancer in later life and germ cell abnormality to the foetus leading to infertility or genetic abnormality in next generation. A study by Tralins has reported that one in four women undergoing breast and chest irradiation can achieve full lactation. Breast and chest wall irradiation is not contraindicated in pregnancy. Pelvic radiotherapy is an absolute contraindication in pregnancy if the foetus is to be salvage. The absorbed fetal radiation dose during cancer treatment in pregnancy is shown in Table 17.4.

Table 17.4 Absorbed fetal radiation dose during treatment of cancer in pregnancy (rad)

Technique of radiotherapy	Absorbed foetal dose (rad)
External beam radiotherapy for cervical cancer (shielding not possible)	4500–5000
Mantle field radiotherapy for Hodgkin's lymphoma (with and without shielding)	2–17
Chest wall radiotherapy for breast cancer at 16 weeks (with shielding)	14–18

Chemotherapy and Targeted Therapy during Pregnancy

Valid data on transplacental transport of chemotherapy are lacking but a fraction of chemotherapy may crosses the placenta and reaches the foetus based on the reported incidences of congenital malformations, neonatal alopecia, neonatal haematopoietic suppression, etc. The most vulnerable phase is the phase of organogenesis, which expands from 10 days until 8 weeks after conception. Overall, taking into account a background risk of foetal malformation of 3%, the use of cytotoxic drugs during the organogenesis is associated with a risk of 17% (6% risk if excluding folate antagonist) (Cardonick). Cardonic and Iacobucci have reported the risk of in utero exposure to chemotherapy to 375 foetuses. Among foetal and neonatal complications they have reported were intrauterine death (5%), prematurity (5%), neonatal death (1%) and neonatal transient myelosuppression (4%). Folic acid antagonists, including methotrexate carry the highest risk of foetal malformation. Methotrexate is associated with the neural tube defects and clefting abnormalities.

It is recommended to wait until 14-week pregnancy before initiating chemotherapy because after organogenesis, the eye, genitals, haematopoietic and central nervous system remains vulnerable.

Anti-tumour antibiotics such as doxorubicin and epirubicin can be used in pregnancy without risking foetal development. Alkylating agents such as cyclophosphamide, cisplatin and carboplatin are also relatively safe in pregnancy. Cisplatin is more preferred to carboplatin because carboplatin results in more bone marrow toxicity and is less protein bound, possibly resulting in more transplacental transfer. Vinca alkaloids are also relatively safe in pregnancy as it has been use for a long time in many reported cases.

Physiologic changes during pregnancy such as an increase in glomerular filtration rate will results in more rapid clearance, particularly of drugs that are excreted by the kidney. Metabolisation of drugs in the liver is also increased and can influence the presence of active drugs. GFR increased in pregnancy-enhanced renal clearance of chemotherapeutic drugs but in pregnancy, protein binding is lower and this may increase the effective dose. These two factors will cancel the effect of each other.

Since haematological toxicity can impose the risk of infection and bleeding complications to the mother and the foetus during delivery, the last chemotherapy must be given no later than 3–4 weeks before expected date of delivery. Women with no obstetrics complications and are allowed carrying their pregnancy until term must not be given chemotherapy after 35–36 week gestation. The placenta eliminates the drugs for the foetus, whereas if born just after treatment the newborn baby may not be able to metabolize the agents, leading to toxicity. The long-term complication of chemotherapy following in utero exposure to chemotherapy is still unknown. Aviles and Neri have reported a long-term follow-up (median follow-up of 18 years) of 84 cases of in utero exposure to chemotherapy administered for haematological malignancies. All cases were found to have normal development.

Experiences with targeted therapy during pregnancy are still limited. Reported cases of using trastuzumab in pregnant women with breast cancer revealed a possible association of this drug with oligohydramnios and anhydramnios. This condition was thought to be due to foetal renal insufficiencies.

Management of Gynaecological Cancer during Pregnancy

There are two general principles of managing cancer during pregnancy:

(1) Management depends upon the stage of disease, gestational age, and the wishes of the patient and her family.
(2) Given the moral, ethical, and emotional issues that surround this situation, the treating physician (gynaecologic oncologist), social workers, perinatologists, and maternal-foetal specialists should support the patient and help guide the decision-making process.

Following are the guidelines of cancer management during pregnancy based on the gestational age:

(1) Gestational age 0–20 weeks: Treat and ignore the pregnancy.
(2) Gestational age 20–32 weeks: Delay treatment and delivery or treat and delay delivery.
(3) Gestational age >32 weeks: Delivery and treat at the same time (e.g. deliver by caesarean section and proceed with radical hysterectomy) or delivery followed by treatment.

Breast Cancer

The incidence of breast cancer during pregnancy is 10–30 cases per 100,000 term pregnancies. Breast cancer diagnosed during pregnancy was found to have tendencies of more unfavourable prognosis due to late diagnosis rather than related to tumour biological behaviour. Foetal radiation exposure to a mammogram is less than 0.5 μGy (0.5 rad) thus far below the threshold dose. Ultrasound is more sensitive than a mammogram (high false negative) during pregnancy due to physiological changes to the breast (more density). CT scan is best avoided during pregnancy, while the use of MRI must be cautioned due to potential risk of heating and contrast media (gadolinium). Bone scan may be acceptable in patients with breast cancer during pregnancy provided after detail discussion between oncologist and nuclear medicine physician.

Surgical treatment is similar to non-pregnant women. Since radiotherapy to the breast and chest wall is not an absolute contraindication during pregnancy, breast-preserving surgery can be considered in patients with early breast cancer. Proper shielding can reduce foetal exposure to below a threshold dose. Higher fraction of radiation exposure will occur late in pregnancy due to foetal growth. Radiotherapy should not be given during last 4–6 weeks of pregnancy. Chemotherapy is a more common adjuvant treatment given during pregnancy and radiotherapy is often postponed to after delivery. The indications for adjuvant treatment are similar to non-pregnant patients. FAC regimen (5-Fluorouracil, doxorubicin and cyclophosphamide) are well tolerated and currently a preferred regimen for breast cancer patients in pregnancy. However, the CMF regime containing Methotrexate should be avoided during pregnancy. Tamoxifen is best avoided during pregnancy due to reported cases of genital abnormalities (e.g. ambiguous genitalia) and Goldenhar's syndrome (Cullin).

Cervical Cancer

Cervical cancer is one of the most common malignancies diagnosed during pregnancy with the incidence of 10–50 cases in 100,000 term pregnancies. Treatment for cervical cancer in pregnancy is similar to that in non-pregnant women. The risks of vaginal delivery in patients with cervical cancer during pregnancy are:

(1) dissemination of malignant cells into lymphatics or vascular channels
(2) haemorrhage
(3) cervical laceration
(4) tumour implantation at episiotomy sites

Surgical treatment is feasible in more than 80% of cervical cancer diagnosed during pregnancy. Generally, if gestational age <20 weeks, radical hysterectomy and pelvic lymphadenectomy with the foetus in situ is an acceptable approach (Fig. 17.1). In selected cases where the cancer is non-aggressive histotype (e.g. verrucous carcinoma, well differentiated, etc.) and the patient desires to preserve her pregnancy, delaying treatment until 30–32 weeks may be justifiable. Pelvic radiation will lead to spontaneous miscarriage usually within 24–34 days.

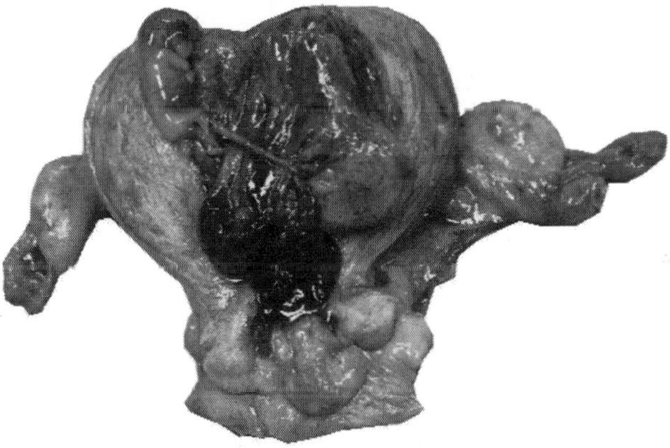

Figure 17.1 Radical hysterectomy specimen with foetus in utero. The patient was diagnosed as adenocarcinoma of cervix during her first trimester.

Gestational age between 20 and 28 weeks poses a major decision dilemma. There are at least three options:

(1) delaying treatment (6–12 weeks), delivery at 32–34 weeks
(2) neoadjuvant chemotherapy followed by classical caesarean section and radical hysterectomy
(3) immediate treatment in case of aggressive tumour

A patient with cervical cancer diagnosed after 28 weeks is best managed by delaying the treatment till 32–34-week gestation and deliver the baby via classical caesarean section and treatment (Fig. 17.2). Patients who opted for delaying their treatment must be thoroughly followed up and have serial imaging study preferably MRI to assess the progress of the disease.

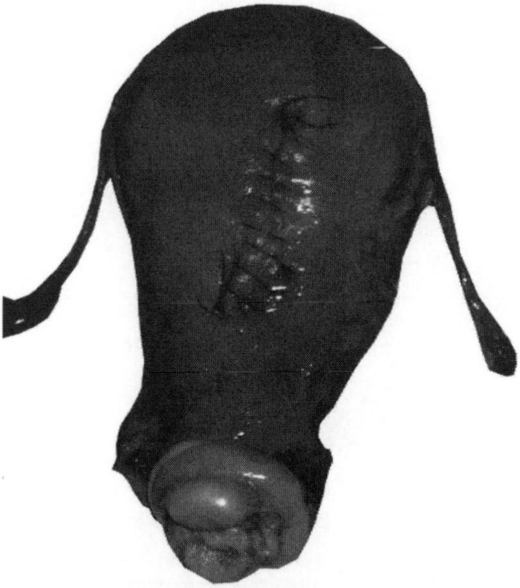

Figure 17.2 Adenocarcinoma of cervix diagnosed at 28 weeks gestation. Pregnancy was allowed to progress until 32 weeks with close monitoring. Subsequently classical caesarean section followed by radical hysterectomy and pelvic lymphadenectomy was performed.

Fertility-preserving surgery is feasible in selected cases. Conization and radical trachelectomy have been described in several case reports. Large cervical conization can be offered to a patient with stage 1A1 cervical cancer. The risks of cervical conization during pregnancy are excessive bleeding (5–15%), miscarriage (25%), pre-term delivery and persistent disease (up to 50%). To minimize the risk of miscarriage and bleeding, the optimal time for cervical conization is between 14 and 20 weeks. In patients with inoperable cervical cancer, the principles of treatment are still the same. If the disease diagnosed during the late second trimester, delaying treatment up to 4 weeks is safe, delivery should be by caesarean section followed by radiotherapy/chemoradiation. There was a case report of treating cervical cancer diagnosed during pregnancy with chemotherapy from 14-week gestation until 38 weeks and subsequently delivered by caesarean section. Neoadjuvant chemotherapy followed by surgery has been reported in the literature.

Ovarian Cancer

The prevalence of ovarian mass in pregnancy varies between 0.19% and 8.8%, while the prevalence of malignancy among ovarian masses diagnosed in pregnancy varies from 0–6.8% (Bignardi).

Surgical management of ovarian masses in pregnancy is indicated in the following conditions:

(1) suspicious of malignancy
(2) large ovarian cyst >8 cm
(3) complicated ovarian cyst, i.e. torsion, infected, etc.
(4) the cyst posing the risk of obstructed labour

Between 1% and 6% of adnexal masses found during pregnancy were malignant tumours. Bigger-size cysts are more likely to undergo torsion, infected, rupture and also malignancy (8.7% versus 0.85%, cut-off point of 8 cm diameter). Approximately 60% of ovarian torsion occurred between the 10th and 17th weeks of gestation and only 5.9% occurred after 20 weeks (Yen).

The incidence of ovarian cancer in pregnancy is 1–2 in 10,000 pregnancies. Majority (80%) of ovarian cancer diagnosed during pregnancy were at an early stage. Epithelial ovarian cancer is the most common type (49–75%) followed by germ cell tumours (39%).

Tumour markers such as CA125, β-HCG, α-fetoprotein and inhibin are normally raised in pregnancy. CA125 reaches the highest level at first and third trimester generally not more than 80 U/mL (8% of women can have up to 140 U/mL). α-Fetoprotein reaches it peak level at 30-week gestation (100–200 ng/mL) and β-HCG reaches its peak value at 16–18 weeks (100,000 IU/L). Carcinoembryonic antigen (CEA) is more stable and does not elevate in normal pregnancy.

Treatment of ovarian cancer in pregnancy is also similar to that in non-pregnant women (Fig. 17.3). Before 20-week gestation, surgery is performed followed by chemotherapy in high-risk patients. Fertility-preserving surgery is indicated similar to non-pregnant patients. Platinum-based regimen is the first line and preferably begins with single agent platinum during pregnancy and added paclitaxel after delivery. Dose of carboplatin is based on body

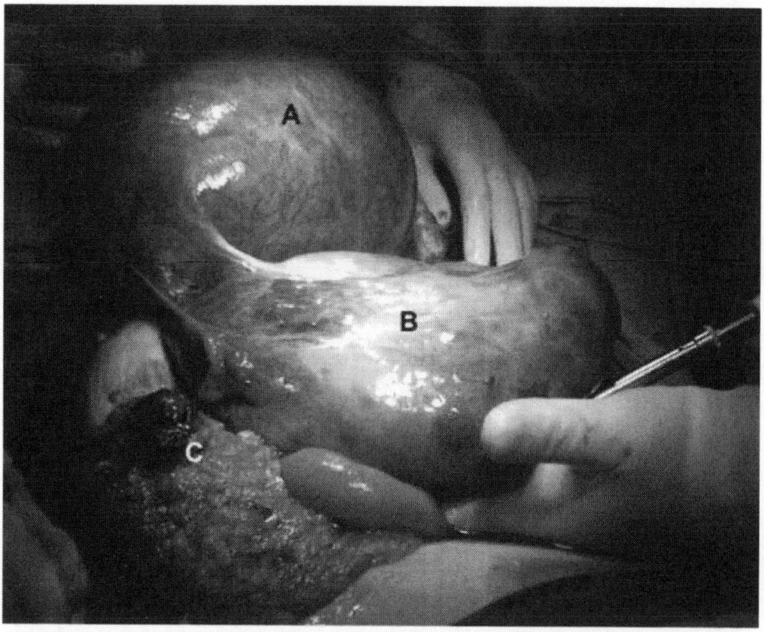

Figure 17.3 Ovarian cancer diagnosed during pregnancy. A: gravid uterus, B: left ovarian tumour (endodermal sinus tumour) and C: omental nodule.

surface area instead of AUC. The drug-free interval must be at least 3–4 weeks before delivery to minimize the risks of neonatal infection and haematological complications. Breastfeeding is not recommended when the patients are on chemotherapy. There was a case report of a patient with stage 3C epithelial ovarian cancer treated with bilateral salpingoophorectomy, tumour debulking and omentectomy at 15-week gestation followed by six cycles of chemotherapy. Subsequently, she had re-laparotomy, caesarean section and hysterectomy at 36 weeks (Ferrandina).

Vulvar Cancer

Vulvar cancer in pregnancy is extremely rare because the majority of patients were diagnosed after their reproductive age. Less than 50 cases had been reported worldwide. Vulvectomy and groin node dissection can be performed during pregnancy but the risk of bleeding is more than in non-pregnant. Generally delaying treatment carries poorer outcome.

Carcinoma of Endometrium

Carcinoma of endometrium is extremely rare during pregnancy but has been reported in less than 30 publications. Pregnancy is a natural treatment/prevention of endometrial cancer due to a high level of progesterone. Endometrial cancer related to pregnancy is defined as any endometrial cancer diagnosed during pregnancy or during the puerperium. Most cases are detected after evacuation of the uterus for miscarriages or bleeding after delivery. Majority of cases is localized disease and well-differentiated tumour.

Choriocarcinoma

Choriocarcinoma diagnosed during pregnancy is also extremely rare with a reported incidence of 1 in 160,000 deliveries. Choriocarcinoma can co-exist with normal pregnancy. Majority of patients presented with postpartum haemorrhage after delivery of normal-term baby.

Following is the hypothesis of how choriocarcinoma can occur during pregnancy:

(1) choriocarcinoma developed from placenta in recent pregnancy
(2) choriocarcinoma developed from the placenta in previous pregnancy with spontaneous regression of primary tumour after metastasis
(3) malignant changes in chorionic remnant from previous pregnancy
(4) multiple pregnancy with one pregnancy undergoing malignant change to choriocarcinoma

References

Amant F, Brepoels L, Halaska MJ, Mina Mhallem G, Calsteren KV. Gynaecologic cancer complicating pregnancy: an overview. *Best Pract Res Clin Obstet Gynaecol* 2010; **24**: 61–79.

Amant F, Calsteren KV, Vergote I, Ottevanger N. Gynecologic oncology in pregnancy. *Crit Rev Oncol/Hematol* 2008; **67**: 187–195.

Aviles A, Neri N. Hematological malignancies and pregnancy: a final report of 84 children who received chemotherapy in utero. *Clin Lymphoma* 2001; **2**: 173–177.

Azim Jr HA, Peccatori FA, Pavlidis N. Tumour Review: treatment of the pregnancy mother with cancer: a systematic review on the use of cytotoxic endocrine, targeted agents and immunotherapy during pregnancy. Part 1: Solid tumors. *Cancer Treat Rev* 2010; **36**: 101–109.

Bader AA, Petru E, Winter R. Long term follow up after neoadjuvant chemotherapy for high risk cervical cancer during pregnancy. *Gynecol Oncol* 2007; **105**: 269–272.

Bignardi T, Condous G. The management of ovarian pathology in pregnancy. *Best Pract Res Clin Obstet Gynaecol* 2009; **23**: 539–548.

Caluwaerts S, Van Calsteren K, Mertens L, et al. Neoadjuvant chemotherapy followed by radical hysterectomy for invasive cervical cancer diagnosed during pregnancy: report of a case and review of the literature. *Int J Gynecol Cancer* 2006; **16**: 905–908.

Cardonick E, Iacobucci A. Use of chemotherapy during human pregnancy. *Lancet Oncol* 2004; **5**: 283–291.

Ferrandina G, Distefano M, Testa A, et al. Management of an advanced ovarian cancer at 15 weeks of gestation: case report and literature review. *Gynecol Oncol* 2005; **97**: 693–696.

Kal HB, Struikmans H. Radiotherapy during pregnancy: fact and fiction. *Lancet Oncol* 2005; **6**: 328–333.

Marret H, Lhomme C, Lecuru F, et al. Review: Guidelines for the management of ovarian cancer during pregnancy. *Euro J Obstet Gynecol Reprod Biol* 2010; **149**: 18–21.

Mi Lee S, Kang JH, Oh SY, et al. A successfully treated case of primary tubal choriocarcinoma coexistent with viable intrauterine pregnancy. *Gynecol Oncol* 2005; **97**: 671–673.

Muirhead CR, Cox R, Stather JW, MacGibbon BH, Edwards AA, Laylock RGE. Estimates of late radiation risks to the UK population. *NRPB* 1983; **4**: 15–157.

Neumann G, Rasmussen KL, Petersen LK. Cervical adenosquamous carcinoma: tumor implantation in an episiotomy scar. *Obstet Gynecol* 2007; **110**: 467–469.

Palaia I, Pernice M, Graziano M, et al. Neoadjuvant chemotherapy plus radical surgery in locally advanced cervical cancer during pregnancy: a case report. *Am J Obstet Gynecol* 2007; **197**: e5–e6.

Pavlidis NA. Coexistence of pregnancy and malignancy. *Oncologist* 2002; **7**: 279–287.

Plante M, Lau S, Brydon L, et al. Neoadjuvant chemotherapy followed by vaginal radical trachelectomy in bulky stage 1B1 cervical cancer: case report. *Gynecol Oncol* 2006; **101**: 367–370.

Robova H, Pluta M, Hreborcak M, et al. High dose density chemotherapy followed by simple trachelectomy: full-term pregnancy. *Int J Gynecol Cancer* 2008; **18**: 1367–1371.

Shah AH, Shafi MI. Problem-based learning in Obstetrics. Cancer in pregnancy. *Obstet, Gynaecol Reprod Med* 2008; **18**(10): 279–284.

Sivanesaratnam V. Review: Gynaecological malignancies in pregnancy. *Rev Gynaecol Pract* 2004; **4**: 162–168.

Tralins AH. Lactation after conservative breast surgery combined with radiation therapy. *Am J Clin Oncol* 1995; **18**: 40–43.

Ungar L, Smith JR, Palfalvi L, Del Priore G. Abdominal radical trachelectomy during pregnancy to preserve pregnancy and fertility. *Obstet Gynecol* 2006; **108**: 811–814.

Vaccarello L, Apte SM, Copeland LJ, et al. Case report: Endometrial carcinoma associated with pregnancy: a Report of three cases and review of the literature. *Gynecol Oncol* 1999; **74**: 118–122.

Van Calsteren K, Vergote I, Amant F. Cervical neoplasia during pregnancy: diagnosis, management and prognosis. *Best Pract Res Clin Obstet Gynecol* 2005; **19**: 611–614.

Van Calsteren K, Heyns L, De Smet F, et al. Cancer during pregnancy; an analysis of 215 patients emphasizing the obstetrical and neonatal outcome. *J Clin Oncol* 2010; **28**(4): 683–689.

Yen CF, Lin SL, Murk W, et al. Risk analysis of torsion and malignancy for adnexal masses during pregnancy. *Fertil Steril* 2008; Mar 20 (Epub ahead of print).

Chapter 18

Tumour Markers in Gynaecologic Cancers

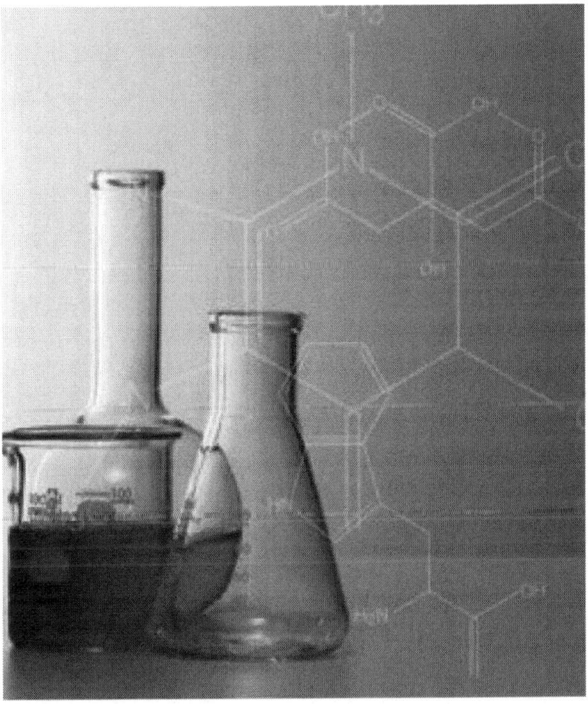

Gynaecologic Cancer: A Handbook for Students and Practitioners
Rushdan Noor, Eng Hseon Tay, and Jeffrey Low

ISBN 978-981-4463-06-5 (Hardcover), 978-981-4463-07-2 (eBook)
www.panstanford.com

Introduction

Tumour markers are a spectrum of molecules of widely divergent characteristics but sharing an association with malignancy that facilitates their application in the clinical detection (diagnosis, screening) and management (monitoring, prognosis) of cancer patients.

The characteristics of an ideal tumour marker are

(1) tumour specific (high sensitivity and specificity)
(2) produced in a sufficient amount to be able to be detected even in minimal disease
(3) quantitatively reflects tumour burden

Tumour markers are generally not diagnostic (except in gestational trophoblastic disease) although they can provide information that may contribute to the diagnostic process. No tumour markers are specific to malignancy and that normal tumour markers result never necessarily excludes malignancy or recurrence. Following the development of monoclonal antibodies, many new tumour markers have been discovered during the past 2 decades. The use of tumour markers not only depends on its sensitivity and specificity, but also on its ability to influence decisions between alternatives plans for patient management.

Sensitivity is the percentage of test results, which are correctly positive in the presence of a tumour. The greater the sensitivity, the fewer the false-negatives. Specificity is the percentage of normal persons or persons with a benign condition for whom a negative result is obtained. The greater the specificity, the lower the false positives. The ideal tumour marker should have high sensitivity and specificity. It should also have high positive predictive value.

There are at least five types of tumour markers:

(1) cell surface antigens
(2) cytoplasmic proteins
(3) enzymes
(4) hormone
(5) proteomics

Tumour markers can be classified into three classes:

(1) **Class I**: Antigens unique to a neoplasm not shared by other tumours of same histological type.

(2) **Class II**: Antigens expressed by many or most tumours of a specific histological type and of other histological type. Class II tumour markers are not expressed by normal adult tissue.
(3) **Class III**: Antigens expressed by both cancer and normal adult tissue.

Tumour Markers in Ovarian and Fallopian Tube Cancer

Cancer Antigen 125 (CA125)

A serum value of 35 U/mL, representing 1% of healthy female and accepted as upper normal limits. The level of CA125 is lower in post-menopausal and post-hysterectomy women. CA125 of more than 35 U/mL in seen in about 85% of women with epithelial ovarian cancer (EOC). The level of CA125 also depends on the stage; in stage 1 disease, 50% of women have CA125 more than 35 U/mL, while in advanced stage, more than 90% have the elevation. CA125 is less often elevated in mucinous, clear cell and borderline tumour. It is more often elevated in Serous Cystadenocarcinoma. The other conditions with elevated CA125 are (a) pancreatic, breast, colon and lung malignancies, (b) pregnancy (16% of women in first trimester), (c) endometriosis and (d) menstruation. CA125 is also found to be increased in 0.2% of healthy blood donors and 1% of healthy women. It lacks specificity as a screening if used in isolation. CA125 plus pelvic ultrasound achieve 99.9% specificity, 27% positive predictive value and 78.6% sensitivity. The value of this screening test is higher in post-menopausal women. In post-menopausal women with palpable adnexal mass undergoing diagnostic laparoscopy, CA125 more than 35 U/mL has a sensitivity of 78%, specificity 95% and PPV of 82%. Combination of CA125 plus CA19-9 was found to have higher sensitivity (93%). In stage 1 disease, pre-operative CA125 value correlate well with prognosis. The risk of dying is six-fold, if elevated. The levels of CA125 can transiently be elevated post-operatively due to inflammation induced by surgery; therefore, it is advisable to start measuring CA125 after 4 weeks of surgery.

CA125 levels also reflect progression or regression of disease in more than 90% of a patient with ovarian cancer if elevated pre-operatively. About 12–38% of patients have an active disease on second look laparotomy despite CA125 being less than 35 U/mL. Hence, the trend of CA125 is more important than absolute value or cut-off point. CA125 level prior to third course has been used successfully to assess response to therapy. CA125 declining in exponential regression pattern is more useful in assessing response. The correlation between serum CA125 and clinical course in ovarian cancer is shown in Fig. 18.1.

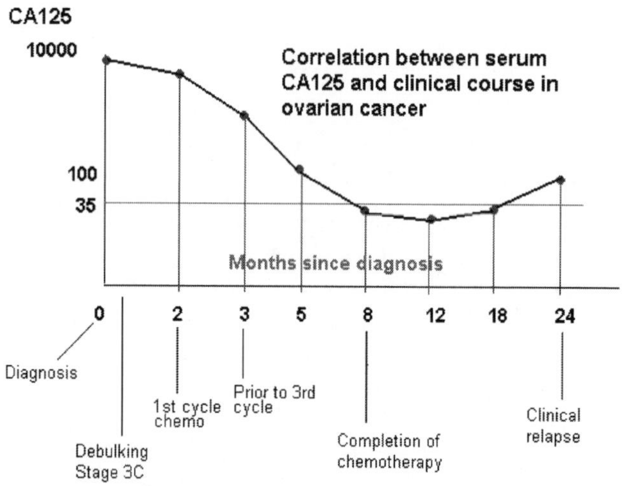

Figure 18.1 Correlation between serum CA125 and clinical course in ovarian cancer.

Kang et al. found that the nadir level of CA125 has an independent prognostic role in patients with advanced EOC. Additional facts about CA125 are as follows:

(a) About 50% of women with stage 1 and 2 ovarian cancer have CA125 more than 65 U/mL.

(b) A single reading is not strong; it needs at least annual measurement.

(c) For women younger than 50 years, CA125 of more than 35 U/mL has a specificity of 97%.

(d) Specificity is increased to 99.8% if the cut-off point level is set at 95 U/mL.

Serum Biomarkers in Screening of Epithelial Ovarian Cancer

CA125 has been extensively evaluated in attempts to develop a screening model of EOC. Fixed serum thresholds for CA125 (>35 U/mL) have limited utility as a screening tool as only 50–60% of women with stage 1 EOC will have elevated serum levels, thereby limiting its sensitivity for detecting ovarian cancer when it is still confined to the ovary. The specificity of CA125 is also limited by the facts that the markers are also elevated in many other conditions, including benign lesions. To improve the effectiveness of serum level of CA125 as a screening test, combined tests or multi-modality tests are currently being extensively evaluated.

At present, there are many ongoing studies that are evaluating the role of multi-modality tests for screening, prediction and diagnosis of EOC. Following are some of them:

(1) Jacob et al. evaluated the role of CA125 and transabdominal ultrasound (TAS) scan as a screening test involving 21,959 post-menopausal women. Transabdominal ultrasound was performed if CA125 ≥ 30 U/mL. Women with abnormal TAS will be subjected to laparotomy. Results: PPV: 26.8%, Specificity 99.9%, sensitivity 78.6% at 1 year, 57.9% at 2 years. However, there was no advantage in terms of overall survival (Jacob et al., 1993)

(2) Ongoing trial known as NIH PLCO Screening Trial had accrued its full complement of 152,000 patients. Screening was performed by physical examination, CA125 level and transvaginal ultrasound scans. Since women will be followed up for at least 17 years, final results (ovarian cancer mortality) are not yet available.

(3) The United Kingdom Collaborative Trial of Ovarian Cancer Screening (UKCTOCS) has completed recruiting more than 200,000 post-menopausal women age 50–74 years old. Screening methods were annual ultrasound or annual CA125 followed by ultrasound compared to control group (no intervention). The primary endpoint was ovarian cancer mortality. Preliminary results: Screening sensitivity was

similar but specificity was slightly higher for multi-modality using CA125 followed by ultrasound scan (99.8% versus 98.2%, p value <0.0001).The sensitivity and positive predictive value for multi-modality were 89.5% and 35.1%, respectively. The effect of screening on mortality is still unavailable.

(4) Apart from a combination of CA125 and ultrasonography, studies were also done to evaluate the role of combinations of biomarkers, e.g. combination of CA125 with leptin, prolactin, osteopontin, insulin-like growth factor II and macrophage migration inhibitory factor (Visitin et al.). Although the specificity and sensitivity of the test were better than CA125 alone, the PPV was only 6.5%, which does not support using this test for screening of the general population.

Serum Biomarkers in the Evaluation of Women with Pelvic Masses

Approximately, 200,000 women will undergo surgery for pelvic mass and 13–21% of them will be diagnosed as EOC. The ability to predict the nature of pelvic tumour pre-operatively will be very helpful not only to the counselling of patients but also assisting care providers to plan an appropriate pre-operative and operative care. Patients with a high possibility of malignancy will be referred to a centre with gynaecologic oncologist.

Risk of malignancy index (RMI) is a scoring system based on the level of CA125, ultrasound findings and menopausal status. The score will provide a prediction regarding the nature of ovarian cyst/tumour either benign or malignant (refer Table 18.1). Risk of malignancy index score of 200 or greater gives a sensitivity of 85% and specificity of 97% for ovarian cancer. Subsequent studies evaluating the role of RMI have reported sensitivity and specificity ranging from 71–88.5% and 74.3–97%, respectively.

Using 200 as cut-off score, the patient will be referred to a centre with gynae oncologist or general gynaecologist with special interest in gynae oncology if RMI is >200. This cut-off score can also be used to triage patients during surgery (in apparent early stage) either to undergo frozen section or not. As the specificity of RMI is very high, low score is very reassuring and therefore, frozen section is not warranted.

Table 18.1 Risk of malignancy index

Criteria	Score awarded	Score
Menopausal status		**A** (1 or 3)
Pre-menopausal	1	
Post-menopausal	3	
Ultrasound features	None of these features, score 0	**B** (0, 1 or 3)
Multi-loculated	One feature, score 1	
Solid areas	More than one features, score 3	
Bilaterality		
Ascites		
Metastasis		
Serum CA125 concentration (IU/mL)	Absolute concentration of CA125	**C**
Risk of malignancy index (RMI) = A X B X C		

Source: *J Clin Pathol* 2004; **57**(11): 1232.

The other method to predict patients with ovarian cancer who presented with pelvic mass is OVA1 test, which was approved by FDA in September 2009. OVA1 uses a blood sample to test for levels of five proteins that altered in ovarian cancer. The test combines five separate results into a single numerical score between 0 and 10 to indicate the likelihood of pelvic mass to be ovarian cancer. OVA1 is intended for women age >18 undergoing surgery for pelvic mass. The accuracy was 92% when combined with radiological test. OVA1 test, however, has high false positive test (64%). Five proteins involved in OVA1 test are apolipoprotein A1 (decrease in cancer), beta 2 microglobulin (increased in cancer), CA125 (increase), prealbumin (decrease) and transferrin (decrease in cancer).

Human epididymis protein (HE4) is a potential biomarker for EOC. Human epididymis protein has been shown to be overexpressed by EOC and circulate in the serum. There is a subset of ovarian cancers that do not express CA125 but do express HE4. Human epididymis protein has a greater specificity than CA125 in a pre-menopausal age group due to its lack of overexpression in patients with benign gynaecologic disease. The prospective study by Moore et al. have found that by combining CA125 and HE4 testings, they achieved a sensitivity for detecting invasive EOC of 76.4% and specificity of 95%, which was higher than either test alone.

Biomarkers for Monitoring the Disease Status in Epithelial Ovarian Cancer

Biomarkers can also be used to monitor the response to treatment and follow up patients during and after treatment. Two serum biomarkers have been approved by FDA for monitoring patients with EOC, i.e. CA125 and HE4. Approximately, 90% of patients with EOC have an elevation of either CA125 or HE4.

CA125 alone has been used to monitor the response to treatment and the progress of disease. Human epididymis protein has been shown to be elevated in over half of the EOC where CA125 was not a marker.

Carcinoembryonic Antigen

Carcinoembryonic antigen (CEA) is an oncofoetal antigen. Carcinoembryonic antigen is also elevated in colon and pancreatic cancer. It can also be elevated in endometroid and Brenner tumour of the ovary. There was a reported case of high CEA levels in clear cell and serous tumour of the ovary. Carcinoembryonic antigen can also be raised in benign disease of liver, GIT, lung and in smokers. Overall, CEA is elevated in 25–50% of a patient with ovarian cancer. Carcinoembryonic antigen is also frequently present in patients with secondary cancer of the ovary when the primary cancer is from breast and gastrointestinal tracts.

Alpha-Fetoprotein

Alpha-fetoprotein (AFP) is an oncofoetal glycoprotein produced by foetal yolk sac, liver and upper GIT. Alpha-fetoprotein is elevated in pregnancy and liver, pancreatic, gastric and colonic tumour. During pregnancy, AFP is a major component of foetal plasma, reaching a peak concentration of 3 mg/mL at 12 weeks of gestation.

Alpha-fetoprotein is elevated in

(a) endodermal sinus tumour (100%)
(b) immature teratoma (62%)
(c) dysgerminoma (12%)

Alpha-fetoprotein (AFP) is a reliable tumour marker in endodermal sinus tumour and embryonal carcinoma. It accurately predicts the presence of yolk sac elements in mixed germ cell tumour. On rare occasions, AFP is also elevated in EOC.

Human Chorionic Gonadotrophin

Human chorionic gonadotrophin (HCG) is a glycoprotein hormone. In pregnancy, HCG is produced by a syncytiotrophoblast. Human chorionic gonadotrophin is an ideal tumour marker in gestational trophoblastic neoplasm (GTN) and in GTN, there is a close correlation of HCG and tumour burden.

Lysophosphatidic Acid

Lysophosphatidic Acid (LPA) is bioactive phospholipids. Lysophosphatidic acid is mitogenic and growth factors that stimulate proliferation of cancer cells. It is an important growth factor present in ascitic fluid of ovarian cancer. Lysophosphatidic acid is significantly higher in the ascitic fluid of ovarian cancer patients than other cancers. The serum level of LPA is also elevated in ovarian cancer in higher proportion than CA125. Lysophosphatidic acid is a potential tumour marker for ovarian cancer and other gynaecological malignancies.

Inhibin and Activins

Inhibin and activins have been isolated in ovarian follicles fluid. Inhibin is elevated in Granulosa cell tumour and other Sex cord-stromal tumour. It can also be elevated in EOC, particularly mucinous carcinoma.

New Tumour Markers in Ovarian Cancer

As 20% of ovarian cancers express little or no CA125, many other serum tumour markers have been evaluated in combination with CA125 to improve the sensitivity, specificity and positive predictive value of the test. Ovarian carcinoma antigen (OCA): **NB/70K** has a sensitivity equal to that of CA125 but is less specific.

Macrophage colony-stimulating factor (**MCS-F**), which is secreted by the ovarian carcinoma cell line, is elevated in ascites and blood in 70% of women with ovarian cancer. It is also elevated in 40% of ovarian cancer patients with normal CA125.

OVX-1 is useful only if used in combination with other tumour markers such as CA125. A study suggested that OVX-1 is increased in the serum of a major proportion of patients with stage 1 ovarian cancer who have serum CA125 concentrations within normal limits.

Lysophosphatidic acid (**LPA**) stimulates proliferation of ovarian cancer cell in vitro. Lysophosphatidic acid has been shown to be a multi-functional signalling molecule in fibroblast and other cells. Lysophosphatidic acid has been found in the ascitic fluid of patients with ovarian cancer and is associated with the ovarian cancer cell proliferation. Further studies are needed to determine the role of these markers.

Topoisomerase II expression was detected in a sample of ovarian cancer by immunohistochemistry and may be clinically relevant biomarker for survival in patients with advanced EOC.

L1 (CAM) expression represents a novel diagnostic marker in serous ovarian neoplasms that shows characteristics of tumour progression. L1 expression is also associated with a chemotherapy response.

Human epididymal protein 4 or HE4. HE4 test in combination with CA-125 can improve the sensitivity and specificity of CA125 alone in identification and monitoring of ovarian cancer.

Zhang et al. developed a biomarker panel based on proteomic data with sensitivity 74% and specificity of 97% to detect stage 1 and 2 ovarian cancer.

There are at least three classes of potential candidates of biomarkers. These three major classes are the major proteins related to normal ovarian physiology, which are altered in their expression in cancer:

(1) hormonal control of cellular proliferation/ovarian physiology (PAEP-glycodelin and Inhibin)
(2) extracellular mucins/epithelial cell signalling (CA125, MUC-1)
(3) control of proteolysis/coagulation/fibronolytic pathways (MMP-7, SLPI, HE-4, PAI-1 and Plau-R)

Tumour Markers in Cervical Cancer

To date, there is no serology marker for screening of cervical cancer. Many potential tumour markers have been investigated for the purpose of assessing prognosis, monitoring treatment response and detecting recurrence:

(a) squamous cell carcinoma antigen (SCC)
(b) CEA/CA125
(c) tissue polypeptide antigen (TPA)
(d) CYFRA 21-1

Squamous Cell Carcinoma Antigen

Squamous cell carcinoma antigen is a sub-fraction of a tumour-associated antigen known as TA-4. It is belongs to the family of serine protease inhibitors. Elevated SCC is observed in 52–85% of women with primary squamous cell carcinoma of the cervix. Higher incidence of elevation in well differentiated tumour (78%) than poorly differentiated one (38%). It may have some prognostic significance and can be useful to monitor response and occurrence of relapse. Elevation also seen in other squamous cell carcinoma, e.g. head, neck, oesophagus, lung. Squamous cell carcinoma antigens are also elevated in several non-malignant conditions such as pemphigus and renal failure. The levels of SCC antigen of more than 10 ng/mL were associated with enlarged lymph nodes at CT scan. In several studies, a pre-treatment level of SCC antigen was correlated with prognosis and response to treatment. Scambia et al. reported that at multivariate analysis SCC levels more than 5 ng/mL were related to a poor chemoresponsiveness in 102 patients with locally advanced cervical carcinoma. Strauss et al. found that pre-operative serum SCC more than 3 ng/mL was an independent poor prognostic factor for both recurrence-free survival and overall survival in 129 patients with stage 1A2-2B SCC cervix who underwent radical surgery. Study by Esajas et al. reported that recurrence of early-stage cervical cancer (treated with surgical treatment) was preceded by raised SCC antigen (sensitivity of 74%). Squamous cell carcinoma antigen is more sensitive than CYFRA 21-1 for squamous cell carcinoma of cervix in most series.

In summary, although SCC antigen is not suitable for screening or diagnosis of cervical cancer, serum SCC antigen levels correlate with tumour stage, tumour size, residual tumour after treatment, recurrent or progression disease, and survival. Squamous cell carcinoma antigen shows a strong correlation with the clinical course and is suitable for monitoring disease after primary treatment, and may therefore be useful in the management of patients.

CA125 in Cervical Cancer

Serum CA125 is elevated only in 13–21% of cervical squamous cell carcinoma. It is a better tumour marker than SCC in adenocarcinoma of the cervix. Elevated CA125 levels are detectable in 20–75% of patients with cervical adenocarcinoma. Elevated CA125 was associated with poorer prognosis and more advanced disease in adenocarcinoma of the cervix. Patients with adenocarcinoma of the cervix were also noted to have elevated CA19-9 and CEA. Pre-treatment level of CA125 and SCC antigens were also correlates with survival in some studies. Carcinoembryonic antigen is less useful in cervical cancer (sensitivity 15%, specificity 90%). Recently, SCC Antigen was found to be useful independent predictor of response in women undergoing neoadjuvant chemotherapy.

CYFRA 211-1

Cytokeratins are intermediate filament structural proteins found in the cytoskeleton of epithelial tissue. The release of cytokeratins into circulation likely occurs by numerous mechanisms such as cellular apoptosis, abnormal mitosis, or spill-over from proliferating cells. CYFRA 21-1 measures serum fragments of cytokeratin 19. CYFRA 21-1 has been tested as a serum tumour marker of lung cancer, oesophageal cancer, head and neck cancer, anal canal cancer and gynaecological cancers. Elevated CYFRA 21-1 levels have been found in 42–63% of patients with squamous cell carcinoma of the cervix. Serum CYFRA 21-1 was less sensitive than SCC antigen for both early and advanced disease. Puthucode-Easwaran et al. reported that CYFRA 21-1 assay was a significant predictor of lymph-vascular space invasion and lymph node metastases. Pre-treatment of CYFRA 21-1 was associated with survival according to study done by Molina.

Other Markers in Cervical Cancer

Sawada et al. have reported an elevation of Immunosuppressive acidic protein (IAP) in 43% of patients with cervical cancer. Immunosuppressive acidic protein is a sub-fraction of the acute-phase reactant α-1-acidic glycoprotein first identified in gastric cancer.

Vascular endothelial growth factor (VEGF) was found to be elevated in pre-invasive stage of cervical cancer (50% in CIN 3). Vascular endothelial growth factor was also elevated in higher proportion in invasive cervical carcinoma and in patients with persistent disease. Clinical relevance of serum VEGF assay is still investigational.

Tumour Markers in Endometrial Cancer

There is no established tumour marker in endometrial cancer as CA125 in ovarian cancer. CA125 level is elevated in 10–20% early-stage endometrial cancer and 63–67% in advanced stage. Beck et al. demonstrated that CA125 level was elevated in 15% of stage 1, 33% in stage 2 and 62% in stage 3 uterine cancers. Elevated level of CA125 was noted in approximately 60% of patients with recurrent endometrial malignancy. There have been a number of studies evaluating individual serum tumour markers in endometrial cancer such as CEA, CA72.4, CA19-9, CA15.3 and M-CSF and were shown to be elevated in only 20–30% of patients. Human epididymis protein serum level had been evaluated by Moore RG as a potential serum tumour marker for endometrial cancer. The combination of serum HE4 and CA125 raised the sensitivity of detection compared to that of CA125 alone. Human epididymis protein was found to be better (higher sensitivity) than CA125 as an individual tumour marker in stage 1 disease. Recent report indicated that CA125 monitoring did not add to clinical findings and imaging in the follow-up of women with endometrial cancer.

References

Bailey J, Tailor A, Naik R, et al. Risk of malignancy index for referral of ovarian cancer cases to a tertiary center: does it identify the correct cases? *Int J Gynecol Cancer* 2006; **16**(Supp. 1): 30–34.

Beck EP, Wagner M, Anselmino L, Xu F, Bast Jr RC, Jaeger W. Is OVX1a suitable marker for endometrial cancer? *Gynecol Oncol* 1997; **65**(2): 291–296.

Brown AK, Miller MC, Robison K, et al. Differential expression of CA125 and a novel serum tumour marker HE4 in epithelial ovarian cancer. *J Clin Oncol* 2009; **26**(20 Suppl; abstr 5533).

Cherchi PL, Dessole S, Ruiu GA, Ambrosini G, Farina M, Capobianco G, et al. The value of serum CA 125 and association CA 125/CA 19-9 in endometrial carcinoma. *Eur J Gynaecol Oncol* 1999; **20**(4): 315–317.

Drapkin R, con Horsten H, Lin Y, et al. Human epididymis protein 4 (HE-4) is a secreted glycoprotein that is overexpressed by serous and endometrioid ovarian carcinomas. *Cancer Res* 2005; **65**(6): 2162–2169.

Duffy MJ, Bonfrer JM, Kulpa J, et al. CA125 in ovarian cancer: European Group on Tumor Markers guidelines for clinical use. *Int J Gynecol Cancer* 2005; **15**(5): 679–691.

El-Shalakany A, Abou-Talib Y, Shalaby HS, Sallam M. Preoperative serum inhibin levels in patients with ovarian tumours. *J Obstet Gynaecol Res* 2004; **30**(2): 155–161.

Enakpene CA, Omigbodum Ao, Goecke TW, et al. Preoperative evaluation and triage of women with suspicious adnexal masses using risk of malignancy index. *J Obstet Gynaecol Res* 2009; **35**(1): 131–138.

Esajas MD, Duk JM, de Bruijn HWA, et al. Clinical value of routine serum squamous cell carcinoma antigen in follow up of patients with early stage cervical cancer. *J Clin Oncol* 2001; **19**: 3960–3966.

Gadducci A, Scambia G, Benedetti Panici P, et al. The prognostic relevance of pretreatment serum immunosuppressive acidic protein (IAP) in patients with squamous cell carcinoma of the uterine cervix: a comparison with squamous cell carcinoma antigen (SCC). *Cancer J* 1994; **7**: 241–252.

Gadducci A, Tana R, Cosio S, Genazzani AR. The serum assay of tumour markers in prognostic evaluation, treatment monitoring and follow up of patients with cervical cancer: A review of the literature. *Critical Rev in Onco/Hemato* 2008; **66**: 10–20.

Geomini P, Kruitwagen R, Bremer GL, Cnossen J, Mol BW. The accuracy of risk scores in predicting ovarian malignancy: a systematic review. *Obstet Gynecol* 2009; **113**(2 Pt 1): 384–394.

Hareyama H, Sakuragi N, Makinoda S, Fujimoto S. Serum and tissue measurements of CA72-4 in patients with endometrial carcinoma. *J Clin Pathol* 1996; **49**(12): 967–970.

Havrilesky LJ, Whitehead CM, Rubatt JM, et al. Evaluation of biomarker panels for early stage ovarian cancer detection and monitoring for disease recurrence. *Gynecol Oncol* 2008; **110**: 374–382.

Hellstrom I, Raycraft J, Hayden-Ledbetter M, et al. The HE4 (WFDC2) protein is a biomarker for ovarian carcinoma. *Cancer Res* 2003; **63**(13): 3695–3700.

Jacob I, Oram D, Fairbanks J, Turner J, Frost C. A risk of malignancy index incorporating CA125, ultrasound and menopausal status for the accurate preoperative diagnosis of ovarian cancer. *Br J Obstet Gynaecol* 1990; **97**(10): 922–929.

Kang S, Seo SS, Park SY. Nadir CA125 level is an independent prognostic factor in advanced epithelial ovarian cancer. *J Surg Oncol* 2009; **100**(30): 244–247.

Molina R, Filella X, Auge JM, et al. CYFRA 21-1 in patients with cervical cancer: comparison with SCC and CEA. *Anticancer Res* 2005; **25**: 1765–1771.

Moore RG, Maclaughlan S, Bast RC. Current state of biomarker development for clinical application in epithelial ovarian cancer. *Gynecol Oncol* 2010; **116**: 240–245.

Robertson DM, Stephenson T, Pruysers E, et al. Inhibins/activins as diagnostic markers for ovarian cancer. *Mol Cell Endocrinol* 2002; **191**(1): 97–103.

Moore RG, Brown AK, Miller MC, et al. The use of multiple novel tumour biomarkers for the detection of ovarian carcinoma in patients with a pelvic mass. *Gynecol Oncol* 2007; **108**: 402–408.

Moore RG, Brown AK, Miller CM, et al. A novel multiple biomarker assay for the detection of ovarian carcinoma. *J Clin Oncol* 2006; **24**: 5023.

Seppala M, Taylor RN, Koistinen H, et al. Glycodelin: a major lipocalin protein of the reproductive axis with diverse actions in cell recognition and differentiation. *Endocr Rev* 2002; **23**(4): 401–430.

Moore RG, Brown AK, Miller MC, et al. Utility of a novel serum tumor biomarker HE4 in patients with endometrioid adenocarcinoma of the uterus. *Gynecol Oncol* 2008: **110**; 196–201.

Olt G, Soper J, Ramakrishnan S, Xu F, Berchuck A, Clarke-Pearson D, et al. Preoperative evaluation of macrophage colony-stimulating factor levels in patients with endometrial cancer. *Am J Obstet Gynecol* 1996; **174**(4): 1316–1319.

Puthucode Easwaran S, Naik R, Athavale R, et al. Comparison of pretreatment CYFRA 21-1 and ACC antigen assay in primary cervical carcinoma—a preliminary report. *J Obstet Gynaecol* 2005; **25**: 486–488.

Sawada M, Okudaira Y, Matsui Y, Shimizu Y. Immunosuppressive acidic protein in patients with gynecologic cancer. *Cancer* 1984; **54**: 652–656.

Scambia G, Benedett PP, Foti E, et al. Multiple tumour marker assays in advanced cervical cancer: relationship to chemotherapy response and clinical outcome. *Eur J Cancer* 1996; **32A**: 259–263.

Strauss HG, Laban C, Lautenschlager C, et al. SCC antigen in the serum as an independent prognostic factor in operable squamous cell carcinoma of the cervix. *Eur J Cancer* 2002; **38**; 1987–1991.

Takeshima N, Shimizu Y, Umezawa S, Hirai Y, Chen JT, Fujimoto I, et al. Combined assay of serum levels of CA125 and CA19-9 in endometrial carcinoma. *Gynecol Oncol* 1994; **54**(3): 321–326.

Van Trappen O, Steele D, Lowe DG, et al. Expression of vascular endothelial growth factor (VEGF)-C and VEGF-D, and their receptor VEGFR-3, during different grades of cervical carcinogenesis. *J Pathol* 2003; **201**: 544–554.

Visintin I, Feng Z, Longton G, et al. Diagnostic markers for early detection of ovarian cancer. *Clin Cancer Res* 2008; **14**(4): 1065–1072.

Zhang Z, Yu Y, Zu F, et al. Combining multiple serum tumour markers improves detection of stage 1 epithelial ovarian cancer. *Gynecol Oncol* 2007; **107**(3): 526–531.

Chapter 19

Diagnostic Imaging in Gynaecologic Oncology

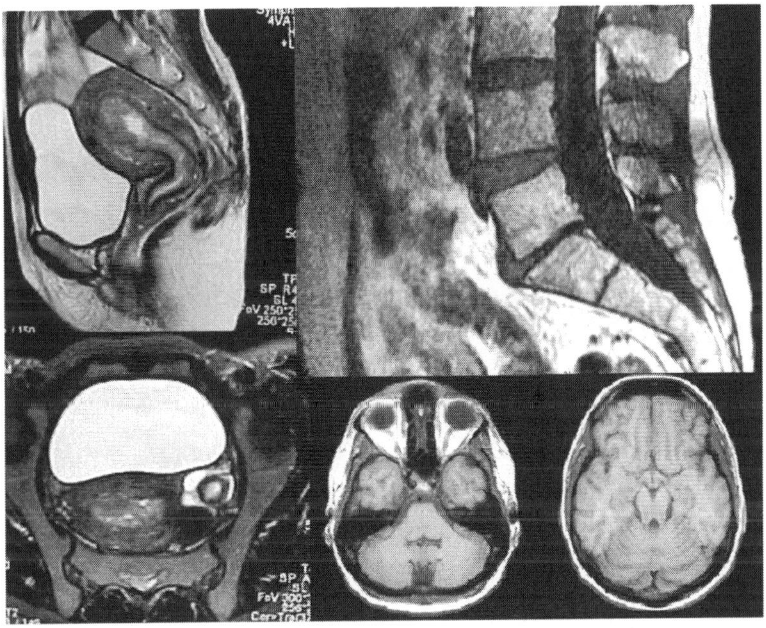

Gynaecologic Cancer: A Handbook for Students and Practitioners
Rushdan Noor, Eng Hseon Tay, and Jeffrey Low

ISBN 978-981-4463-06-5 (Hardcover), 978-981-4463-07-2 (eBook)
www.panstanford.com

Introduction

Imaging plays an important role in the management of gynaecologic oncology. There are many imaging modalities available in assisting the clinician to diagnose, treat and monitor the patients with cancer. In the last decade, there has been a significant advancement of diagnostic imaging modalities to provide best care for patients with gynaecologic cancer.

The four most important imaging modalities in gynaecologic oncology are

(1) ultrasound/Doppler
(2) computed tomography (CT scan)
(3) magnetic resonance imaging (MRI)
(4) positron emission tomography (F-FDG PET)

The indications for imaging technique are

(1) tumour detection
(2) tumour diagnosis with image-guide biopsy
(3) tumour staging
(4) monitoring of response to treatment
(5) to differentiate between tumour recurrence with post-radiation/post-operative changes

Imaging Study: Technique, Description and Normal Anatomy

Ultrasound

In gynaecologic oncology, there are two types of ultrasound: (a) transvaginal ultrasound (TVS) and (b) transabdominal scan (TAS). The other rarely used ultrasound technique in gynaecology is transrectal ultrasound.

The tissue density demonstrated by ultrasound is described as echogenicity, i.e. hypoechoic, isoechoic and hyperechoic. Tumour can appear hypo/hyper/iso/mixed echogenicity depending on tissue composition but most tumours appear hypoechoic. Hysterosonography involves the instillation of fluid in the uterine cavity during TVS to visualize intra-uterine lesions. Transrectal ultrasound scan (TRUS) is using high-frequency 5 MHz transducer, mainly to have better visualization of the cervix. Transrectal ultrasound scan is capable in demonstrating the cervix better by eliminating bowel gas interference. This technique can also help in the assessment of the parametrium, i.e. the upper part of the parametrium is generally hypoechoic due to uterine venous plexus, while lower part is usually hyperechoic due to predominantly fibrillar connective tissue.

Ultrasound Features of Normal Uterus and Ovary

All gynaecologists should be familiar with the ultrasonographic features of the normal uterus and ovary. Following are the ultrasound features of the normal uterus:

(a) Endometrial thickness: Measure distance from anterior endometrium-myometrium to posterior endometrium-myometrium junction
(b) Proliferative phase endometrium ET: 3–5 mm
(c) Secretory phase ET: 6–12 mm
(d) Post-menopausal ET (not on HRT): 2–3 mm
(e) Post-menopausal ET > 5 mm is considered abnormal.

Ultrasound features of normal ovary are shown below:

(a) Volume: 0.523 × length × width × height
(b) Normal ovarian volume: 9.8 ± 5.8 cc
(c) Ovarian volume at menopause: 2.9 ± 2.2 cc

Computed Tomography (CT Scan)

Tomography is derived from the Greek "tomos", which means "slices", and "graphein", which means "to write". It is also called computed axial tomography (CAT scan). CT scan is a medical imaging device consisting X-ray tube and detector capable in producing two-dimensional tomographic images in a large series. The X-ray tube transmitted X-ray around the body of the patient in a single axis of rotation where three-dimensional reconstructed images can be derived from these large series of images. CT scan studies of the pelvis required contrast opacification of the distal small bowel, colon and bladder. Diluted oral contrast 500–1000 mL is given 1 hour prior to study. Another 200 mL of diluted contrast may be given via enema to opacified the recto-sigmoid. **Spiral CT** is a specialized CT scan technique: (a) required mechanical power injector to administer intravenous contrast agents at a rate of 2 mL per second and (b) scanning progress from caudad to cephalad. Spiral CT is a technique that allows images to be acquired during various vascular phases, including the venous, capillary and arterial phase of enhancement following intravenous contrast administration. It provides a better delineation of uterine anatomy (myometrium, endometrium, cervix and parametrium) and major pelvic vessels. It is capable in creating 3D images. The tissue density is described as low attenuation (hypodense) or high attenuation (hyperdense), while tumour necrosis usually demonstrated low attenuation (hypodense) appearance.

In CT scan evaluation, an intravenous Iodinated contrast is given for the following reasons:

(a) opacification of normal organs such as the bladder and uterus
(b) pattern of tumour opacification
(c) differentiation of contrast-filled blood vessels from adjacent lymph nodes
(d) better visualization of the endometrial cavity and myometrium
(e) to delineate tumour boundaries excluding local invasion into a contiguous normal adjacent structure.

Magnetic Resonance Imaging

Magnetic resonance imaging is a non-ionizing radiation equipment with a powerful magnetic field capable in manipulating the nuclear magnetization of water contents from body tissues by aligning the hydrogen atoms. The MRI scanner is a tube surrounded by a giant circular magnet. The magnetic field will align the protons of hydrogen atoms, which is then exposed to a beam of radio waves. Spinning of the proton in the body will produce the signal, and this signal will be picking up by the receiver. Receiver will transfer the signal into a computer to produce an image. Oral contrast may be given, and antiperistalsis (i.m. Glucagon 1 mg) is recommended 4 to 6 hours prior to study to optimize image quality.

Intravenous MR contrast, i.e. gadolinium chelates (0.1 mmol/kg) is given to

(a) demonstrate abnormal tissue pathology or masses
(b) delineate the boundary of tumour excluding local invasion and highlight tumour interface
(c) opacify vessels
(d) highlight tumour interface
(e) assess lymph nodes status
(f) detect fistula
(g) identify metastases

In MRI, image is described as low signal intensity (hypointense), medium signal intensity (isointense) and high signal intensity (hyperintense). Water content of the lesion will produce low signal intensity on T1-weighted image and high signal intensity on T2-weighted image. The cortical bone shows a low signal intensity, while fatty tissue show high signal intensity on both T1- and T2-weighted images except in a fat saturation image. The endometrium shows a higher signal intensity than fat and the myometrium has medium signal intensity (innermost myometrium: low signal intensity).

MRI is more superior to ultrasound and CT scan in delineating the primary tumour site and description of T-staging, including site, dimension and extent of the disease. MRI is also superior to CT in the work-up of uterine and cervical cancer. Apart from that, MRI is useful to differentiate between radiation fibrosis and recurrent tumour.

MRI is contraindicated in patients with non-MR-friendly foreign body implants such as pacemaker, cochlear implants and vascular clips.

Advantages of Magnetic Resonance Imaging

Following are the advantages of MRI:

(a) superior soft tissue resolution
(b) no ionizing radiation
(c) fast (no need breath-holding)
(d) multi-planar capability

(e) can be used in patients with known hypersensitivity reaction to CT scan contrast media.

Disadvantages of MRI

Following are the disadvantages of MRI:

(a) prone to movement artifact
(b) gadolinium may cause renal fibrosis
(c) claustrophobia

Imaging in Cervical Carcinoma

CT Scan and Cervical Cancer

CT scan is an important imaging technique in diagnosis, staging and monitoring of disease in cervical cancer (Fig. 19.1). Based on the recommendation by FIGO cervical cancer is staged clinically. Clinical staging is obtained by physical examination, colposcopy, biopsies, CXR, cystoscopy, IVU and barium enema. However, FIGO clinical staging is flawed when compared to surgical staging with error rate of 17–67% mainly due to the difficulty in assessing the parametrium. Intravenous urogram has limited role if kidney is not functioning. Therefore, CT scan with/without contrast is better in assessing exact side of ureteral obstruction even in the absence of renal function. Currently, CT scan with contrast has replace IVU in assessing urinary system in many oncology centres. The overall accuracy of conventional CT scan in the staging of cervical cancer is 63–88%.

In staging of cervical cancer, CT scan imaging should be performed with intravenous contrast injection. The primary goal of CT scan evaluation is to differentiate tumour confined to the cervix from that has invaded the parametrium. The accuracy of CT scan in the assessment of parametrium involvement is 55–80% and the accuracy increases to 92% in stage IIIB to IVB. The overall accuracy of CT scan in assessment of lymph node status is 77–85%, with sensitivity of 44% and specificity of 93%.

In recurrent cervical cancer, CT scan is helpful in assessing central pelvic recurrent, bladder and rectal extension. The major limitation of CT scan is inability to differentiate accurately between tumour recurrence and post-radiation/post-surgical fibrosis.

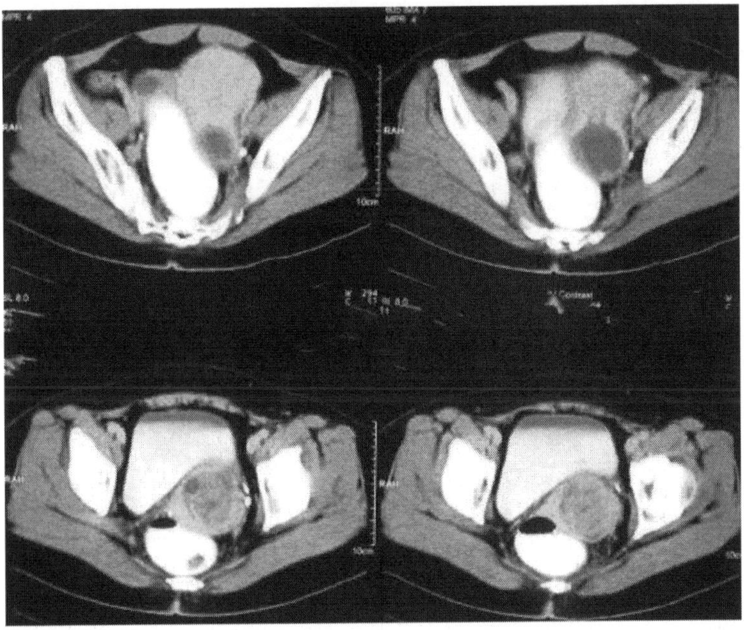

Figure 19.1 Huge cervical cancer shown on CT scan.

Magnetic Resonance Imaging in Cervical Cancer

In cervical cancer, the two areas in which MRI is superior to CT scan are local disease staging and evaluation for local recurrence. The overall accuracy of MRI staging in cervical cancer is 76 to 89%, with improvement in the technique and better contrast media, the accuracy of more than 90% can be achieved. The sensitivity and specificity of evaluating FIGO stage 1B and above is more than 90%. Understaging was reported in 5–15% of cases, while overstaging was reported in 9–14% of cases.

The accuracy for assessing parametrium is 83–96%. The negative predictive value of parametrial involvement is 95%, while positive predictive value for parametrial involvement is 67%. Therefore, MRI is very useful in selecting the appropriate candidates for surgery. The MRI has an accuracy of 87–100% in assessing the bladder invasion. In assessing lymph node metastasis, MRI and CT scan have comparable sensitivity and specificity. Currently, with the introduction of ultrasmall superparamagnetic iron oxide particles contrast (lymph node specific contrast) given intravenously, the negative predictive value of MRI can be as high as 96–100% for nodes greater than 3 mm.

Pre-treatment MRI has been shown to help minimize costs. The use of MRI findings to guide treatment decisions in women with cervical cancer greater than 2 cm in diameter resulted in a decrease in the number of diagnostic tests ordered and decreased in the number of invasive procedures performed.

Following are the general indications for MRI in patients with cervical cancer:

(a) tumour that is endocervical or predominantly infiltrative and cannot be accurately assessed clinically
(b) patients not suitable for CT scan
(c) tumour in pregnant patients or with concomitant uterine lesions
(d) suspected recurrent cervical cancer

In recurrent cervical cancer, MRI is the most successful modality for differentiating recurrent tumour from post-treatment (radiation, surgery or chemotherapy) fibrosis. Old post-radiation fibrosis is low SI compared to tumour recurrence, which is intermediate to high SI.

Imaging in Endometrial Carcinoma

Ultrasound Scan in Endometrial Carcinoma

Transvaginal ultrasound is superior to transabdominal ultrasound. Transvaginal ultrasound has a sensitivity of 77–100% in evaluating myometrial invasion. Post-menopausal women who presented with vaginal bleeding and endometrial thickness (ET) of more than 5 mm should be offered endometrial biopsy. Study had shown that with cut-off point ET 5 mm, the sensitivity and specificity are 91–98% and 60%, respectively, with negative predictive value of 100% for the detection of endometrial pathology (in symptomatic patients). Doppler ultrasound has limited role in endometrial carcinoma.

CT Scan in Endometrial Carcinoma

The CT scan assessment of endometrial carcinoma requires good bowel opacification. Oral, intravenous and rectal contrasts are necessary in all cases. Endometrial tumour is seen as hypodense mass relative to normal myometrium. The greatest clinical impact of CT scan in endometrial cancer is in confirming parametrial and sidewall extension in stage III and in detecting pelvic lymphadenopathy. The accuracy of CT scan in stage III and IV is 83–86%. The limitation of CT includes a tendency to understage endometrial carcinoma because of failure to detect microscopic parametrial, lymph node, bowel, or bladder invasion.

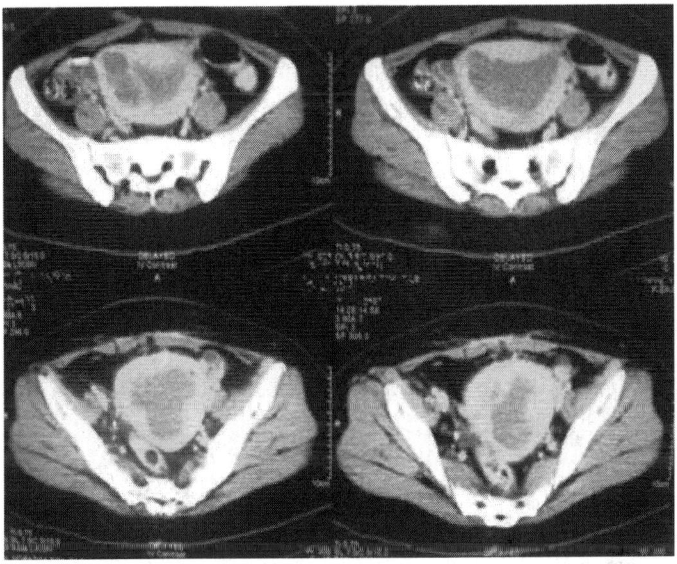

Figure 19.2 Carcinoma of endometrium. CT scan showed an enlarged uterus with hydrometra and tumour occupying the uterine cavity.

Magnetic Resonance in Endometrial Carcinoma

The MRI feature of endometrial carcinoma is isointense on unenhanced image. In an enhanced image, endometrial carcinoma appears variable or heterogeneous in intensity. The overall accuracy of MRI in staging endometrial carcinoma is 70–92%. The contrast enhanced MRI improves the diagnostic accuracy. A dynamic contrast enhanced MRI is the best technique to detect myometrial invasion with an accuracy of 85–93%. MRI can be useful in assessment of myometrial invasion. The sensitivity and specificity of MRI in detecting deep myometrial invasion range from 33–89% and from 88–100%, respectively. MRI is also an accurate method to detect cervical involvement in endometrial cancer with sensitivity between 50–72% and specificity of 90–100%. The accuracy is more than 83%. Generally, contrast enhanced MRI is better than TVS and CT scan in assessing myometrial invasion.

Imaging in Gestational Trophoblastic Disease

Ultrasound in Gestational Trophoblastic Disease

The typical ultrasound feature of complete hydatidiform mole is multiple small cystic lesions within the uterine cavity known as "snow storm appearance". The cystic spaces represent hydropic villi. Ultrasound is also useful to detect persistent or recurrent gestational trophoblastic disease (GTD). The Doppler study may improve the accuracy and it shows abnormal vascularity and high diastolic blood flow.

CT Scan in Gestational Trophoblastic Disease

In GTD, CT scan demonstrates an enlarged uterus. With contrast, uterine enhancement is heterogeneous with a focal enlargement or irregular hypodense region in myometrium. Using a dynamic CT, dilated uterine artery can be visualized. CT scan is also useful in assessment of extra-uterine manifestation of GTD (Fig. 19.3). CT scan can detect a local regional spread manifesting as enhancing soft tissue density in the parametrium and obliteration of pelvic fat or muscle planes.

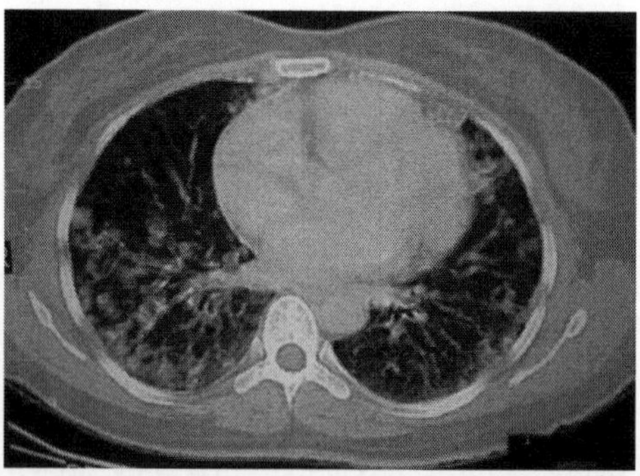

Figure 19.3 Multiple lung nodules in choriocarcinoma (CT scan).

Magnetic Resonance Imaging in GTD

Gestational trophoblastic neoplasm shows high signal intensity mass on MRI. MRI can also demonstrate an enlarged uterine artery and hypervascular in broad ligament.

Imaging in Carcinoma of Ovary

Ultrasound Scan and Doppler in Ovarian Carcinoma

Colour and duplex ultrasound scanning is a potential tool to differentiate between benign and malignant ovarian tumour. Malignant tumour has neovascularization with thin vessel wall lacking in muscle and easily distensible. It shows low resistance index. The cut-off point for resistance index is 0.4 to 0.5 to differentiate between benign and potentially malignant lesions. The Doppler can also assess the distribution of the blood vessel; distribution of a blood vessel in malignancy is in central, within papillary and septate. With ultrasound scan, the morphologic criteria (septation, papillary projection, irregular wall, solid and size more than 9 cm) have a sensitivity of 82–100% and specificity of 60–95% in detecting malignant ovarian tumour. The sensitivity of colour Doppler is only 37% if using RI cut-off point of 0.4. With combined approach of morphologic and Doppler study, the sensitivity and specificity increase to 88–97% and 97–100%, respectively.

CT Scan in Ovarian Carcinoma

CT scan is commonly used to determine the extent of cytoreductive surgery required to optimize the subsequent chemotherapeutic response. The accuracy of CT scan in differentiating malignant and benign is more than 92%. CT scan is able to detect peritoneal implant as small as 5 mm (detected in 50% of cases). The limitation of conventional CT scans in staging ovarian cancer is inability to reliably detect mesenteric or bowel surface tumour implants <1 cm in size. The overall staging accuracy of CT scan in ovarian cancer is 70–80%. CT scans has a sensitivity of 51–84% and specificity of 81–93% in detecting recurrent and persistent disease. CT scans can also be used to assess operability of recurrent disease, if multiple lymph nodes involvement, liver secondaries and pulmonary/pleural secondaries present, re-exploratory laparotomy may not be justifiable. Various CT scan features of ovarian carcinoma are shown in Figs. 19.4, 19.5 and 19.6.

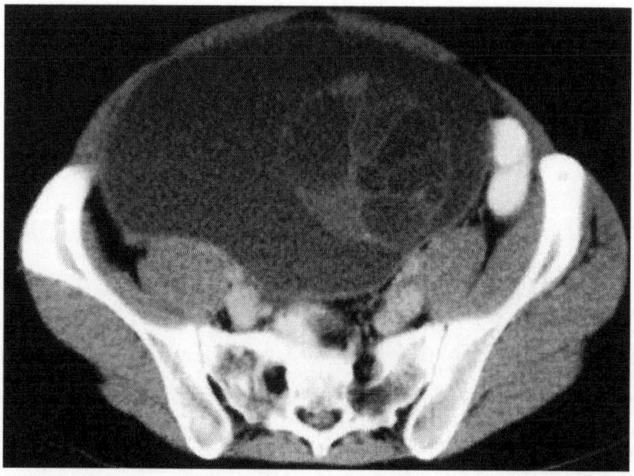

Figure 19.4 Solid-cystic ovarian tumour. Histology confirmed mucinous borderline tumour.

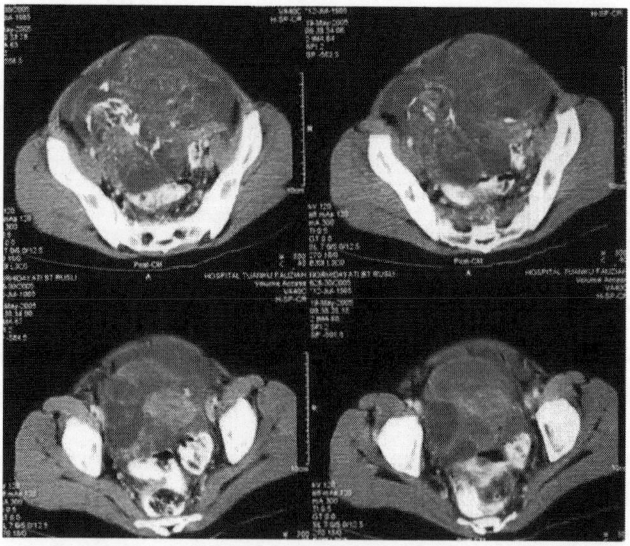

Figure 19.5 CT scan of the pelvis showed predominantly solid ovarian tumour with high vascularity. Histology reported malignant mixed germ cell tumour of the ovary.

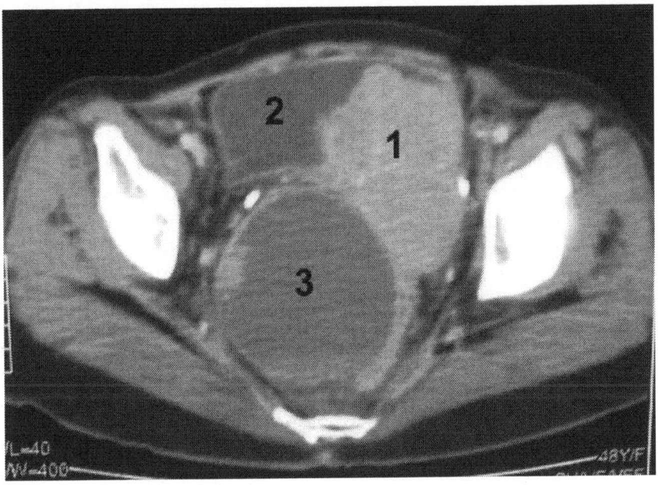

Figure 19.6 CT scan of the pelvis showed recurrent ovarian cancer infiltrating (1) the bladder (2). The recurrent tumour is also appearing as predominantly cystic lesion (3) posterior to the bladder.

MRI in Ovarian Carcinoma

The role of MRI in ovarian carcinoma is still evolving. MRI has a positive predictive value and negative predictive value of 83.3% and 66.7%, respectively, in detecting malignant lesions of the ovaries. (Nam et al.). In terms of detecting malignant lesions outside the pelvis, the sensitivity of MRI is 94%, specificity 71.4%, positive predictive value of 94% and negative predictive value of 71%. The overall accuracy of MRI in staging ovarian cancer is 75–78%. MRI is also useful in assessing spread of tumour to adjacent structures.

Imaging in Vulvar Cancer

Ultrasound Scan in Vulvar Cancer

The high-resolution and high-frequency ultrasound is useful in assessing regional lymph nodes. Using this ultrasound, as small as 5 mm of a groin node can be detected, and this can facilitate fine-needle aspiration for cytology (FNAC). On ultrasound, lymph nodes with metastatic disease tend to be more than 1 cm and rounded in shape with a ratio of long/short axis diameter of the node less than 2 and irregular margin. Cytology of groin nodes has a specificity of 100% but a sensitivity of only 58%; however, when combined with ultrasound guided FNAC, the sensitivity can approach 100%.

CT Scan in Vulvar Cancer

Among all gynaecological cancer, CT scan has the least impact on the clinical management of vulvar cancer. CT scan is expected to have been superseded by MRI and in many centres, CT scan is not routinely done. However, in a centre without the facility of MRI, CT scan still plays an important role similar to other gynaecological cancers.

MRI in Vulvar Cancer

MRI is more accurate in assessing the characteristic of groin nodes as compared to CT scan. It can produce cross-sectional images of lymph node and allow assessment of the depth of the nodes from the skin surface. This information is important for radiotherapy planning. Accurate localization of lymph nodes is also important to guide surgical excision. The most useful observations on MRI for identifying metastatic lymph nodes are contour irregularity and cystic change. A new contrast medium (given intravenously) known as ultra-small-iron-oxide-particle (USIOP) is currently available to improve the accuracy of MRI (MRI lymphography) in assessing lymph nodes. Lymph node with metastatic disease does not accumulate the iron oxide and therefore, show no significant change in signal intensity on post-contrast T2- and T2*-weighted images.

Lymphoscintigraphy and Sentinel Node Detection in Vulvar Cancer

Sentinel node is defined as the first node in the lymphatic chain or basin that receives primary lymphatic flow from the lesion. If the sentinel node is negative for metastatic disease, the remaining lymph nodes should also be negative. In early vulvar cancer, groin node dissection may not be necessary if they are negative for metastatic disease. Routine groin node dissection may result in considerable morbidity.

In sentinel node detection's procedures, radioactive tracer (commonly Technetium 99 m) is injected into the lesion or around the lesion, this radioactive will be taken up by the sentinel node. Handheld gamma probe is used to identify this sentinel node and subsequently the node will be removed for histological confirmation. Radioactive tracer can also be combined with blue-dye techniques to improve the detection rate.

Following are the drawbacks of sentinel node detection:

(a) It requires radioactive substances.
(b) Metastasis to the deep inguinal or femoral nodes has been found without evidence of superficial node involvement.
(c) If only superficial groin nodes removed, the incidence of groin recurrence is higher.

Positron Emission Tomography in Gynaecologic Malignancies

CT scan and MRI are imaging techniques mainly guided by altered normal anatomical planes to diagnose. Therefore, they have the limitations in detecting morphologically small tumours in anatomically normal organ and lymph nodes. CT scan and MRI are also difficult to differentiate between disease recurrences from post-therapeutic changes.

Positron emission tomography scan is a functional imaging modality that can overcome the limitation of CT scan and MRI. PET scan is a scintigraphic technique using radioactive tracer (^{18}fluorine) 2-fluoro-deoxy-D-glucose (FDG). This technique generates three-dimensional images of the body through the detection of so-called annihilation photons that is a result of radionuclide decay. FDG will be taken up by metabolically active tumour cells and utilized through a glycolysis process. The rate of FDG uptake and glycolysis in tumour cells is much faster than normal cell, and depending on aggressiveness of the tumours and time of image acquisition. Generally, F-FDG PET scan imaging diagnoses, stages and restages many cancers with accuracies ranging from 80–90%. The US Food and Drug Administration (FDA) has approved F-FDG PET scan for all cancers. Positron emission tomography has a potential capability of detecting tumour cell prior to morphologic changes. Currently, there is a growing body of evidence supporting the use of F-FDG PET/CT in gynaecological malignancies. Apart from staging and diagnostic purposes, FDG-PET images may now be incorporated into radiotherapy planning in order to refine the delineation of dose according to metabolically active sites of disease.

F-FDG Pet Scan in Cervical Cancer

The data and support on the role of F-FDG PET scan in local staging of cervical cancer are growing. The sensitivity of F-FDG PET scan in detecting nodal involvement is relatively low ranging from 38% to 72%. However, their specificity is high up to 99.7%. The sensitivity is higher if the cut-off point for lymph node size is higher (>0.5 cm). Narayan et al. analyzed the role of pre-treatment F-FDG PET scan. The results demonstrated that nodal status on F-FDG PET scan was the major predictor of the outcome and was superior than FIGO staging. F-FDG PET scans is also useful in addition to conventional imaging study in the depiction of distant metastases. Yen et al. found that F-FDG PET scan provides an important added value over conventional imaging in 73.8% of patients with recurrent cervical cancer. F-FDG PET/CT (incorporating F-FDG PET and CT scan) was also very accurate in diagnosis of recurrent cervical cancer with sensitivity and specificity of more than 90%. FFDG PET/CT scan can resolve the false-positive F-FDG PET results due to hypermetabolic activity of benign/inflammatory lesions and physiological variants. F-FDG PET/CT is also able to detect local recurrence and regional/distant metastasis missed by F-FDG PET alone.

F-FDG Pet Scan in Endometrial Cancer

Study on F-FDG PET scan in endometrial cancer is still lacking and less than cervical cancer. Kitajima et al. showed that F-FDG PET scan is useful in detecting lymph node status pre-operatively with sensitivity and specificity of 53.3% and 99.6%, respectively. F-FDG PET scan is also potentially useful in detecting tumour recurrence.

F-FDG PET Scan in Ovarian Cancer

F-FDG PET scans can improve the accuracy of pre-surgical diagnosis of patients with inconclusive ultrasound scan findings and showed higher concordance over CT scan with final surgical staging. Study also had shown that F-FDG PET/CT was more accurate (92%) than ultrasound (83%), CT scan and MRI (75%) in discriminating malignant/borderline from benign tumour. (Nam et al.). F-FDG PET scan is also useful in diagnosis of pelvic malignancy and detecting peritoneal seeding and peritoneal carcinomatosis. F-FDG PET scan when combined with CT (F-FDG PET/CT) will have higher sensitivity and specificity in detecting peritoneal disease, detection of residual viable disease after surgery and also identifying patients at an earlier stage not responding to chemotherapy. Studies on the role of F-FDG PET/CT in detection of recurrent disease were very promising with sensitivity of 88.2–94.5% and specificity of 71.4–100% (Nanni et al., 2005; Thrall et al., 2005).

References

Kinkel K, Kaji Y, Yu KK, et al. Radiologic staging in patients with endometrial cancer: a meta analysis. *Radiology* 1999; **212**(3): 711–718.

De la Pena MJ, Fernandez VMD, Rodriguez MR, et al. Current imaging modalities in the diagnosis of cervical cancer. *Gynecol Oncol* 2008; **110**: S49–S54.

Manfredi R, Mirk P, Maresca G, et al. Local-regional staging of endometrial carcinoma; role of MR imaging in surgical planning. *Radiology* 2004; **231**(2): 372–378.

Musto A, Rampin L, Nanni C, Marzola MC, Fanti S, Rubello D. Present and future of PET and PET/SCAN in gynaecologic malignancies. *Eur J Radiol* 2010, doi:10.1016/j.ejrad.12.035.

Nagar H, Dobbs S, McClelland R, et al. The diagnostic accuracy of magnetic resonance imaging in detecting cervical involvement in endometrial cancer. *Gynecol Oncol* 2006; **103**: 431–434.

Nakao Y, Yokoyama M, Hara K, et al. MR imaging in endometrial carcinoma as a diagnostic tool for the absence of myometrial invasion. *Gynecol Oncol* 2006; **102**(2): 343–347.

Nam EJ, Yun MJ, Oh YT, et al. Diagnosis and staging of primary ovarian cancer: correlation between F-FDG PET/CT, Doppler US and CT or MRI. *Gynecol Oncol* 2010; **116**: 389–394; 19: 912–918.

Nanni C, Rubello D, Farsad M, et al. 18F-FDG PET/CT in the evaluation of recurrent ovarian cancer: a prospective study on forty-one patients. *Eur J Surg Oncol* 2005; **31**: 792–797.

Narayan K, Fisher RJ, Bernshaw D. Patterns of failure and prognostic factor analyses in locally advanced cervical cancer patients staged by positron emission tomography and treated with curative intent. *Int J Gynecol Cancer* 2009; **19**: 912–918.

Rockall AG, Sohaib SA, Harisinghani MG, et al. Diagnostic performance of nanoparticle-enhanced magnetic resonance imaging in the diagnosis of lymph node metastases in patients with endometrial and cervical cancer. *J Clin Oncol* 2005; **23**: 2813–2821.

Rockall AG, Meroni R, Sohaib SA, et al. Evaluation of endometrial carcinoma on magnetic resonance imaging. *Int J Gynecol Cancer* 2007; **17**(1): 188–196.

Rockall AG, Ghosh S, Alexander Sefre F, et al. Can MRI rule out bladder and rectal invasion in cervical cancer to help select patients for limited EUA? *Gynecol Oncol* 2006; **101**: 244–249.

Sironi S, Buda A, Picchio M, et al. Lymph node metastasis in patients with clinical early-stage cervical cancer: detection with integrated FDG F-FDG PET/CT. *Radiology* 2006; **238**: 272–279.

Thrall MM, DeLoia JA, Gallion H, Avril N. Clinical use of combined positron emission tomography and computed tomography (FDG-PET/CT) in recurrent ovarian cancer. *Gynecol Oncol* 2007; **105**: 17–22.

Undurraga M, F-FDG PETignat P, Pelte MF, Jacob S, Dubuisson JB, Loubeyre P. Magnetic resonance imaging to identify risk of lymph node metastasis in patients with endometrial cancer. International. *J Gynecol Obstet* 2009; **104**: 233–235.

Vasconcelos C, Felix A, Cunha TM. Preoperative assessment of deep myometrial and cervical invasion in endometrial carcinoma: comparison of magnetic resonance imaging and histopathologic evaluation. *J Obstet Gynaecol* 2007; **27**(1): 65–70.

Yen TC, Lai CH, Ma SY, et al. Comparative benefits and limitations of (18)F-FDG PET and CT-MRI in documented or suspected recurrent cervical cancer. *Eur J Nucl Med Mol Imaging* 2006; **33**: 1399–407.

Chapter 20

Peri-Operative Care for Gynaecologic Cancer Patients

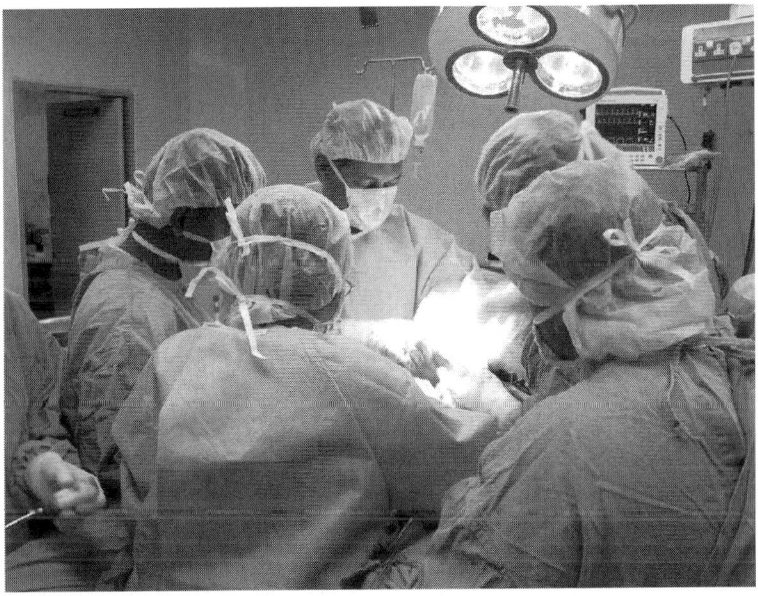

Gynaecologic Cancer: A Handbook for Students and Practitioners
Rushdan Noor, Eng Hseon Tay, and Jeffrey Low

ISBN 978-981-4463-06-5 (Hardcover), 978-981-4463-07-2 (eBook)
www.panstanford.com

Introduction

Surgery is one of the most important modalities of treatment for gynaecological cancer patients. The objectives of surgery in cancer patients are (a) tumour resection with good surgical margin to achieve a cure, (b) to obtain tissue for diagnosis, (c) to analyse histological risk factors in order to select of the best treatment and (d) symptomatic relief.

Surgical treatment for patients with gynaecological cancer often requires a specialized skill because of not only the complexity of the surgery but also patient-related factors such as age and the presence of co-morbid conditions. Surgery in gynaecological cancer carries a higher risk of complications because the primary tumour is arising from the pelvis, where many vital organs and structures are located and at risk of injuries such as bladder, ureter, rectum and pelvic vessels. One of the most important measures to ensure that cancer patients receive an optimal surgical treatment with good oncological outcomes is to provide adequate peri-operative care. Peri-operative care in a cancer patient is very critical because unlike non-cancer patients, patients with cancer are often older and have nutritional problems. They also have the higher possibility of suffering from medical illnesses. Cancer patients may also have undergone chemotherapy or radiotherapy prior to surgery, which will further complicate the surgery. Thromboembolism, immunosuppression and infection are more common in cancer patients.

Peri-Operative Morbidity and Mortality Risk Prediction

The most universally accepted classification system to predict peri-operative morbidity and mortality is American Society of Anaesthesiologists (ASA) physical status classification system, which was introduced in 1963. This classification is based on the patient's functional status and co-morbid condition. American Society of Anaesthesiologists class I and II correspond to low risk, class III as moderate risk and class IV and V as high risk (see Table 20.1).

Table 20.1 American Society of Anesthesiologists physical status classification: non-emergency surgery

Classification	Description	Examples	Post-op mortality
Class I	Normal, healthy patient	Uterine fibroid in a healthy women	0.08%
Class II	Patient with mild to moderate systemic disorder related to the condition to be treated or to some other, unrelated process	Moderate obesity, extremes of age, diet-controlled diabetes, mild hypertension, chronic obstructive pulmonary disease	0.27%
Class III	Patient with severe systemic disease that limits activity but is not incapacitating	Morbid obesity, severely limiting heart disease, angina pectoris, healed myocardial infarction, insulin-dependent diabetes, moderate to severe pulmonary insufficiency	1.80%
Class IV	Patient with incapacitating systemic disease that is life threatening	Organic heart disease with signs of cardiac insufficiency, unstable angina, refractory arrhythmia, advanced pulmonary, renal, hepatic or endocrine disease	7.80%
Class V	Moribund patient not expected to survive 24 hours without an operation	Ruptured aortic aneurysm with profound shock, massive pulmonary embolus, major cerebral trauma with increasing intra-cranial pressure	9.40%

Source: Dripps RD, Echenhoff JE, Vandom D. *Introduction to Anesthesia: The Principles of Safe Practice*. WB Saunders Co, Philadelphia, 1988, p. 17.

The most important parameter in pre-operative assessment is a cardiovascular and pulmonary function. Many studies have shown that patients in the elderly age group of more than 70 years often have ASA class III and IV due to co-existing medical problems, although age alone is not an independent risk factor. Patients with ASA class III and IV have a higher risk of post-operative complications and longer hospital stay as compared to ASA class I and II. A study by Giannice et al. on elderly gynaecological oncology patients older than 70 years found that patients with ASA class III and IV have significantly higher rate of post-operative morbidity than ASA class I and II (48% vs. 28%). Severe post-operative complications were significantly more in patients with ASA class III and IV (17% vs. 5%; $p < 0.005$), while mortality rate in this group of patients was 2–4%.

Peri-Operative Care to Optimize High-Risk Surgical Patients Undergoing Gynaecological Cancer Surgery

Peri-operative care for a cancer patient must begin from the pre-operative period. Proper counselling and good communication between surgical team and patients will prevent post-operative misunderstanding and dissatisfaction.

Informed Consent and Counselling

Post-operative misunderstanding can often be prevented by educating a woman and her family pre-operatively. A thorough and well-documented consent helps to ensure that the patient's expectations for her surgery, recovery, and final outcome are realistic and appropriate. The surgical team should discuss the planned procedure with the woman, and encourage her to include family or friends. The discussion is not limited to one encounter; a second appointment is scheduled before hospitalization and the woman is encouraged to write down any questions arising between the initial and subsequent encounter. Women should be approached in an open, direct, and detailed fashion; statements such as "don't worry, I am competent enough to take care of this" and "everything will be fine" may later lead to serious allegations if complications arise during or after surgery; no surgical outcome can be guaranteed.

Peri-Operative Care in Gynaecological Cancer Patients History and Physical Examination

A thorough history and physical examination are extremely important as in most instances, the majority of risk factors have been discovered through good history and complete physical examination. Recent myocardial infarction (MI) (<6 months), unstable angina, symptomatic cardiac arrhythmias, recent stroke, pulmonary problem, uncontrolled diabetes and renal insufficiencies are very important high risk factors. A patient who smokes carries a higher risk of cardiovascular, pulmonary complications and surgical site infection. Patients on aspirin should stop the medication at least a week prior to surgery in order to reduce the risk of bleeding.

Physical examination can also provide the information on the extent of the disease in terms of operability. Hard and fixed pelvi-abdominal mass supported with the signs of bowel or bladder invasion as well as ureteric dilatation on imaging technique always indicates difficult surgery with potentially high risk of operative morbidity.

Pre-Operative Investigations

Basic blood investigations and urinalysis are mandatory in all patients. Chest X-ray, ECG and coagulation profiles almost always required by all women undergoing major gynaecological oncology surgery. Specific investigations such as the echocardiogram and lung function test are indicated in selected patients.

Optimization of Co-Morbid Illnesses

Endocrine-Related Conditions

The most relevant endocrine disorders in the peri-operative period are hypothyroidism, hyperthryroidism, diabetes mellitus, pheo-chromocytoma, and adrenal insufficiency (in particular, iatrogenic adrenocortical insufficiency secondary to steroid use within the preceding 6 months). All of these conditions should be stabilized and normalized before an elective surgery, whether by hormone replacement, by adrenergic blockade, or by the administration of stress-dose steroids.

Diabetes is a very common disease and can potentially impose a higher risk of cardiovascular complication (due to angiopathy) and sepsis. Compared with their non-diabetic counterparts, cancer patients with pre-existing diabetes are 50% more likely to die after surgery. A study showed that with good control of diabetes, exercise therapy and preventive medical management, the risk of cardiovascular and microvascular complications can be reduced significantly in a diabetic patients. The objectives of peri-operative management of diabetes are to avoid major disturbance to glucose haemostasis such as hypoglycaemia, hyperglycaemia and ketoacidosis.

A patient undergoing surgery following chemotherapy should be thoroughly evaluated with regard to not only the effect of antineoplastic drugs to their blood count but also the use of steroid during and after chemotherapy. The patient requires parenteral steroid treatment intra-operatively.

Thyroid storm in hyperthyroidism can be triggered by intubation, surgery and infection. To avoid this, a thyrotoxic patient should be stabilized with beta blocker and antithyroid medication prior to surgery. A patient with a previous history of long-term steroid therapy is predisposed to adrenal insufficiency. The major surgical risk of adrenal insufficiency is cardiovascular collapse. The patient should be given hydrocortisone prior to the induction of anaesthesia and then 8-hourly after operation.

Cardiac Disease

Cardiac patients should be referred to a cardiologist for full cardiac assessment and optimization before undergoing surgery. Significant cardiovascular risk factors include angina pectoris, dyspnoea and evidence of right-side or left-side heart failure, any cardiac rhythm other than sinus rhythm, more than five ectopic ventricular beats per minute, aortic stenosis with left ventricular hypertrophy, mitral regurgitation, and previous MI. The risk of intra-operative or post-operative MI is much higher in patients who have suffered heart muscle damage within the preceding 6 months. In large retrospective reviews, 37% of patients experienced re-infarction when they underwent operation within 3 months of an infarction; however, the incidence of re-infarction decreased to 16% when the operation was performed between 3 and 6 months after the first infarction and to 4.5% when the operation was performed more than 6 months afterward. A number of trials have indicated that peri-operative beta blockade can reduce the risk of peri-operative cardiac complications in patients with known or suspected CAD, who are undergoing major non-cardiac procedures. Risk of developing peri-operative cardiac complications can be predicted by Goldman multi-factorial cardiac risk index (MCRI). MCRI is base on nine independent parameters, namely, MI within 6 months, age >70, emergency operation, poor general medical conditions, signs of congestive heart failure, significant aortic stenosis, arrythmia, 5 or more PVC's per minute and intraperitoneal/intrathoracic/aortic surgery.

Respiratory Disease

The incidence of a post-operative pulmonary complications after laparotomy was reported to be 14% but in patients with high risk factors such as a COPD, prolonged procedures and other co-morbid problem, the risk increased to 47%. Patients with respiratory disease should be referred to a respiratory physician, and they may benefits from the pre-operative optimizing program such us smoking cessation, use of bronchodilators, chest physiotherapy and antibiotics. Cardiorespiratory function may also be impaired by pleural effusions, or ascites in patients with ovarian carcinoma. Both pleural effusions and ascites should be drained pre-operatively if they are clinically significant and symptomatic. Peri-operative pulmonary complications are reduced by pre-operative optimisation of respiratory status, education and preparation for post-operative physiotherapy.

Renal Disease

Thirty percent of the elderly surgical patients have a pre-existing renal disturbance causing peri-operative stress-related decompensation. Approximately, 20% of peri-operative deaths in elderly patients are caused by acute renal failure. To prevent renal failure, it is important to ensure adequate hydration. A patient with cancer is also predisposed to acute kidney injury secondary to hypovolaemia. Acute kidney injury occurring after surgery has been demonstrated to be associated with a significant increase in patient morbidity and mortality. Acute kidney injury is best considered as a rapid reduction in kidney function resulting in a rise in serum creatinine ≥ 25 μmol/L or a 1.5-fold increase from the baseline value. Treatment of hypovolaemia in surgical patients with acute kidney injury should follow similar principles to those outlined for patients with normal renal function.

Haematological Disorders

A patient with cancer often has haematological abnormalities due to bone marrow infiltration, malnutrition or treatment-related complications (e.g. chemotherapy, radiotherapy). Anaemia may be due to bleeding, bone marrow infiltration, bone marrow suppression or prior chemotherapy. Anaemia must be corrected before surgery. Leucopenia with neutrophil count of $<1.0 \times 10^9$/L is an indication to defer surgery. Thrombocytopenia may be due to chemotherapy or heparin treatment and must be corrected especially if the level is less than 100,000/μL. Both hypercoagulable and hypocoagulable state are equally hazardous and should be recognized and treated early before surgery. Coagulation profile should be done prior to surgery and corrected. Hypercoagalable state can be due to disease such as polycytaemia rubra vera, blood dyscrasia and paraneoplastic phenomena. It can also be due to physiological state such as dehydration, and this can be easily overcome by providing an adequate hydration before, during and after surgery. Thromboprophylaxis either in a form of drug such as heparin or by using the mechanical method such as TED stocking and pneumatic compression is mandatory in a cancer patients undergoing major pelvic and abdominal surgery. Thromboprophylaxis must be continued after operation.

Peri-Operative Thromboprophylaxis

Patients with cancer are known to have a higher risk of thromboembolism. Factors that contribute to higher risk of thromboembolism in cancer patients are

(a) venous stasis from immobilization
(b) elevated levels of coagulation factors

(c) activation of the coagulation system by tumour-induced platelet aggregation
(d) elaboration of procoagulants by tumour-associated macrophages.
(e) tumour cell production of procoagulants.
(f) treatment related to cancer such as surgery and chemotherapy.
(g) use of central venous catheters

The risk of fatal pulmonary embolism is 0.5–1% in major abdominal surgery. Approximately, 66% of deaths occur within 30 minutes. The incidence of deep vein thrombosis (DVT) in major gynaecologic malignancy surgery is 17% and 85% of cases occur in the calf vein. In the majority of cases, DVT involving calf vein will resolve spontaneously. Thromboprophylaxis with heparin (both unfractionated heparin [UFH] and low-molecular-weight heparin [LMWH]) given to the patient after major abdominal and pelvic surgery was associated with 15% reduction in the risk of DVT. The risk levels of thromboembolism and recommended thromboprophylaxis are shown in Table 20.2.

There are various methods of reducing the risk of thromboembolism (thromboprophylaxis):

(a) adequate hydration and early ambulation
(b) external pneumatic calf compression–used intra-operatively and 5 days after operation; no benefit if used for a shorter period; proper use of external pneumatic calf compression may result in up to 65% reduction in the risk of thromboembolism
(c) Unfractionated heparin: 10% risk of thrombocytopenia due to anti-platelet antibody production
(d) Low-molecular-weight heparin has at least similar efficacy with unfractionated heparin but associated with less risk of bleeding complication and thrombocytopenia; low-molecular-weight heparin has better bioavailability, longer half-life and more predictable anticoagulant response than UFH; a patient on LMWH does not require laboratory monitoring.

Patients with risk of bleeding should be offered mechanical thromboprophylaxis such as intermittent pneumatic compression or venous foot pumps and/or graduated compression stockings and consider switching to an anticoagulant when the bleeding risk decreases.

Table 20.2 Risk levels of thromboembolism and recommended thromboprophylaxis in hospital patients

Risk level	Surgical parameter	Approximate DVT risk without prophylaxis (%)	Suggested thromboprophylactic options
LOW	Minor surgery in mobile patients Medical patients who are fully mobile	<10%	None specific Early and aggressive ambulation
MODERATE	Most general, open gynaecologic or urologic surgery patients Medical patients, bed rest or sick	10–40%	LMWH (at recommended dose), LDUH bd or tid, Fondaparinux
HIGH	Hip or knee arthroplasty, hip fracture surgery Major trauma, spinal cord surgery	40–80%	LMWH (at recommended dose), fondaparinux, oral vitamin K antagonist (INR 2–3)

Source: Adapted from 2008 American College of Chest Physicians (ACCP) Consensus Conference (Hirsh et al.).
Abbreviations: DVT, deep vein thrombosis; LMWH: low-molecular-weight heparin, LDUH, low-dose unfractionated heparin.

In PEGASUS trial, fondaparinux was associated with a significant reduction in the risk of thromboembolism compared with dalteparin (4.7% vs. 7.7%; p = 0.02), leading to a relative risk reduction of 38.6% (Agnelli et al.). Studies have also shown that cancer patients may benefit from a longer duration of prophylaxis for up to 1 month after surgery. In the ENOXACAN II trial, patients undergoing abdominal or pelvic surgery who received enoxaparin for 30 days after surgery had a 60% reduction in venous thromboembolism compared with those who received the standard duration of

6–10 days (Bergqvist et al.). A prospective study by RISTOS project has reported that 40% of symptomatic venous thromboembolism events occurred more than 3 weeks after surgery and 46% of deaths were due to fatal pulmonary embolism (Agnelli et al.).

The absolute contraindications to antithrombotic or anticoagulant therapy are active bleeding, severe bleeding diathesis or platelet count less than 20,000/μL, neurosurgery, ocular surgery or intra-cranial bleeding within the past 10 days. Patients with renal insufficiency (creatinine clearance < 30 mL/min) should not receive fondaparinux. Patients with the venous thromboembolism (VTE) diagnosed prior to surgery may be offered insertion of inferior vena cava umbrella or filter. Insertion of IVC filters (IVCF) is done 7–10 days prior to surgery and removed few days after the surgery. Fulwell and colleagues have reported that pre-operative IVCF placement in women with proven VTE and gynaecological cancer is safe. Filter related complications are low. Women at higher risk of developing recurrent VTE may benefit from permanent IVCF placement. However, larger studies need to be conducted.

Peri-Operative Nutritional Support for Cancer Patients

Poor nutritional status is a known risk factor for higher rate of the operative complications in cancer patients, particularly patients with advanced ovarian cancer who often suffered from malnutrition.

Poor nutrition or malnutrition among cancer patients is attributed to the following factors:

(a) wasting of host tissue
(b) gradual loss of protein stores
(c) impaired nutrient use
(d) decreased nutrient intake and absorption

A loss of more than 15% body weight during the previous 6 months is associated with an increased incidence of post-operative complications, including delayed wound healing, decreased immunologic competence, and inability to meet the metabolic demand for the respiratory effort. Peripheral oedema and signs of specific vitamin deficiencies are suggestive of severe malnutrition. Serum Albumin is one of the important parameters for nutritional status and also a very important predictor for operative morbidity and mortality. A study showed that a decrease in serum albumin concentration from greater than 4.6 g/dl to less than 2.1 g/dl was associated with an increase in mortality from less than 1% to 29% and an increase in morbidity rate from 10% to 65%. Hypoalbuminaemia is also a specific risk factor for a poor wound healing and anastomotic breakdown.

Patients with severe malnutrition should be referred to a dietician and receive nutritional therapy before and after the surgery. Patients with poor bowel functions and unable to consume food orally for more than 5 days should be subjected for parenteral nutrition. A trial done by the Veterans Affairs Total Parenteral Nutrition Cooperative Study Group concluded that pre-operative nutritional intervention was necessary is severely malnourished patients; they found that this intervention could decrease the operative risk in a patient with malnutrition, especially those who lost more than 15% of their body weight. A study by Wu et al., which evaluated the role of peri-operative parenteral nutrition for gastric cancer patients, found that TPN use, peri-operatively or post-operatively is helpful in reducing the morbidity and mortality of these patients.

Following are the NICE guidelines on peri-operative nutritional support (supported by British Consensus Guidelines on Intravenous Fluid Therapy for Adult Surgical Patient 2008):

(a) Patients who are significantly malnourished and are due to undergo major abdominal surgery should be considered for pre-operative nutritional support.
(b) Oral intake should be resumed as soon as possible after surgery. Following colorectal and some other abdominal surgery, oral intake is usually possible within 24 hours. The patient should be monitored carefully for any signs of nausea and vomiting.
(c) Post-operatively, only malnourished patients should receive enteral tube feeding within 48 hours of surgery.
(d) Parenteral nutrition should be reserved for malnourished patients who cannot be fed via the intestine pre-operatively, and for patients who remain unable to eat or receive enteral feeds 5 days after abdominal surgery.

Peri-Operative Fluid and Electrolyte Management

Optimization of fluid status and correction electrolyte imbalance are very important factors to ensure smooth running of the operative procedures and minimized operative and post-operative complications. The total body water contributes 50–70% of total body weight. Two-thirds of water is in the intra-cellular compartment, one third in interstitial, while the remaining is in the intra-vascular compartment. It is known that fat contains little water; the lean individual has a greater proportion of water to total body weight than the obese person. Furthermore, total body water as a percentage of total body weight decreases steadily and significantly with increasing age.

Cancer patients often have poor oral intake and fasting before surgery; they may be further deprived of not only nutrition but also fluid and electrolytes. Fluid and electrolytes imbalance had been associated with various physical problems that could further complicate the anaesthesia and surgery. Poor oral intake causes depletion of potassium, sodium and water. Patients with poor oral intake require 3 L water daily in a form of dextrose saline with KCL supplement (1 mmol/kg/day). Hyponatraemia normally due to altered physiologic states that affects the measurement rather than actual sodium loss such as in overhydration, elevated serum lipid and immunoglobulins as well as extreme hyperglycaemia. True sodium loss is due to diuretics, diarrhoea, hypotonic fluid replacement, SIADH, and others. Hypokalaemia is due to diarrhoea, intestinal fistula, ileo conduit, vomiting, diuretic, alkalosis, and others. Refractory hypokalaemia not responding to potassium replacement may be due to hypomagnesaemia (Mg is required by the membrane pump in renal tubule for K retention). Calcium is transported mainly via albumin; alkalosis increases albumin binding and reduces free calcium. Low albumin level causes reduction in total calcium. Hypocalcaemia can also be due to malnutrition, pancreatitis and hypomagnesaemia.

Following are some of the recommendations from British Consensus Guidelines on Intravenous Fluid Therapy for Adult Surgical Patient 2008:

(1) To meet maintenance requirements, adult patients should receive sodium 50–100 mmol/day, potassium 40–80 mmol/

day in 1.5–2.5 L of water by the oral, enteral or parenteral route (or a combination of routes). Additional amount should only be given to correct the deficit or continuing losses.

(2) In patients without disorders of gastric emptying undergoing elective surgery, clear non-particulate oral fluids should not be withheld for more than 2 hours prior to the induction of anaesthesia.

(3) In the absence of disorders of gastric emptying or diabetes, pre-operative administration of carbohydrate rich beverages 2–3 hours before induction of anaesthesia may improve patient well being and facilitate recovery from surgery. It should be considered in the routine pre-operative preparation for elective surgery.

(4) Routine use of pre-operative mechanical bowel preparation is not beneficial and may complicate intra- and post-operative management of fluid and electrolytes balance.

(5) When mechanical bowel preparation is used, fluid and electrolyte derangements commonly occur and should be corrected by simultaneous fluid therapy with Hartmann's or Ringer lactate type solution.

(6) In high-risk surgical patients, pre-operative treatment with intravenous fluid and inotropes should be aimed at achieving pre-determined goals for cardiac output and oxygen delivery as this may improve survival.

(7) In patients undergoing some forms of orthopaedic and abdominal surgery, intra-operative treatment with intravenous fluid to achieve an optimal value of stroke volume should be used where possible as this may reduce post-operative complication rates and duration of hospital stay.

(8) Hypovolaemia due predominantly to blood loss should be treated with either a balanced crystalloid solution or a suitable colloid until packed red cells is available.

(9) When patients leave the theatre for the ward, HDU or ICU their volume status should be assessed. The volume and type of fluids given peri-operatively should be reviewed and compared with fluid losses in theatre, including urine and insensible losses.

(10) In patients who are euvolaemic and haemodynamically stable a return to oral fluid administration should be achieved as soon as possible.

(11) In high-risk patients undergoing major abdominal surgery, post-operative treatment with intravenous fluid and low-dose dopexamine should be considered, in order to achieve a pre-determined value for systemic oxygen delivery, as this may reduce post-operative complication rates and duration of hospital stay.

Table 20.3 Daily requirement for calories and minerals

Nutrient and mineral	Daily requirement
Calorie	20–30 kcal/kg/day
Potassium	1 mmol/kg/day (1 gm = 13 mmol)
Sodium	1–2 mmol/kg/day
Calcium	0.1–0.15 mmol/kg/day
Magnesium	0.05–0.15 mmol/kg/day
Chloride	1.3–2.0 mmol/kg/day

Example of calculating total calorie need based on type of activity (Harris-Benedict Equation):
Total calorie need = BMR × Activity factor × Injury factor
$BMR = 665.1 + 9.56W + 1.85H - 4.68A$,
where W = weight in kg, H = height in cm, A = age in year.
Activity factor, e.g. 1.2 if confined to bed; injury factor, e.g., 1.4 for cancer, elective surgery.

Bowel Preparation

Bowel preparation, especially mechanical methods should not become a routine procedure because improper use of mechanical bowel preparation may result in dehydration and electrolytes imbalances. Unless corrected pre-operatively, these fluid and electrolyte imbalances may complicate intra- and post-operative fluid management.

The primary goals of bowel preparation are

(a) reduction in the bacterial flora inhabiting the GIT and, therefore, reduction in the risk of bacteraemia and post-operative infection
(b) removal of solid faecal materials from the colon.

The stomach has fewer bacteria colonies due to acidity with pH of 3.0. H2 antagonist can increase the bacteria colonies due to increased in pH. The small intestine is relatively sterile due to rapid movement, acidity and bile content. The colon has higher number of bacterial colonies due to (a) less motility, (b) less bile and (c) higher pH.

Bowel preparation consists of

(a) mechanical bowel preparation using oral polyethylene glycol electrolyte agents, enema, etc; polyethylene glycol or PEG is often preferred for patients with kidney, heart and liver conditions because they do not cause mineral or fluid changes that can lead to dehydration
(b) parenteral antibiotics (e.g. metronidazole and cephalosporin) given prior to the induction of anaesthesia; addition of antibiotics reduced the incidence of wound infection from 15% to 5% in colorectal surgery.

The actual role of bowel preparation before surgery is still unclear. Various studies showed conflicting results; a study by Slim et al. reported that mechanical bowel preparation might increase the risk of the anastomotic leak (Slim et al.). A multi-centre randomized trial by Contant et al. evaluating the role of mechanical bowel preparation for elective colorectal surgery had concluded that there was no difference in the rate of the anastomotic leak between both study and control group. Patients who had mechanical bowel preparation had fewer abscesses after anastomic leakage. Combined metanalyses had shown that there was no evidence that mechanical or antibiotic bowel preparation significantly improves the patient's surgical outcome (Ellis).

Following are the recommendations from British Consensus Guidelines on Intravenous Fluid Therapy for Adult Surgical Patient 2008, regarding bowel preparation:

(1) Routine use of preoperative mechanical bowel preparation is not beneficial and may complicate intra- and post-operative management of fluid and electrolyte balance. Its used should, therefore, be avoided whenever possible.
(2) Where mechanical bowel preparation is used, fluid and electrolyte derangement commonly occurs and should be corrected by simultaneous intravenous fluid therapy with Hartmann's or Ringer–Lactate solutions.

Pain Management

Pain management is extremely important because various physical and psychological problems are potentially arising from poor pain control. Pain is unpleasant and causes psychological stress to a patient; poor pain control also associated with higher risk of physical complications such as chest infections, thromboembolism and delayed recovery. Good post-operative pain control is best given by pain team; therefore, all hospitals must have pain team leads by Anaesthetist that is specifically trained in pain control. Pain team will be responsible in assessment of a patient pre-operatively, providing counselling, deciding the best pain control techniques and management of pain post-operatively.

Among pain control techniques available are the following:

(1) Patient-controlled analgesia (PCA): Patient-controlled analgesia is the standard technique for the management of moderate or severe post-operative pain. In PCA, pain control drugs that commonly used are low-dose morphine and fentanyl. Regular paracetamol and NSAIDs can be used simultaneously if the PCA does not provide adequate pain control.

(2) Epidural analgesia can provide an excellent pain management after major surgery; usually a combined local anaesthetic and opiate infusion is used. Local anaesthetic will provide blockade of small nerve fibres (pain and temperature) but maintain fine sensation and motor power, while the opiate augments the analgesic effect at a spinal level.

(3) Other pain control techniques include as fentanyl patch, non-opiate drugs (clonidine, tramadol) continuous nerve blocks and novel drugs used with epidural.

References

Agnelli G, Bergqvist D, Cohen AT, et al. Randomized clinical trial of postoperative fondaparinux versus perioperative dalteparin for prevention of venous thromboembolism in high risk abdominal surgery. *Br J Surg* 2005; **92**(10): 1212–1220.

Agnelli G, Bolis G, Capussotti I, et al. A clinical outcome-based prospective study on venous thromboembolism after cancer surgery: the @ ISTOS project. *Ann Surg* 2006; **243**(1): 89–95.

Auerbach AD, Goldman L. ß-Blockers and reduction of cardiac events in noncardiac surgery. *JAMA* 2002; **287**: 1435–1444.

Barone BB, Stein KB, Yeh BC, et al. Postoperative mortality in cancer patients with pre-existing diabetes. Systematic review and meta-analysis. *Diab Care*, 2010; **33**(4): 931–939.

Bergqvist D, Agnelli G, Cohen AT, et al. Duration of prophylaxis against venous thromboembolism with enoxaparin after surgery for cancer. *N Engl J Med* 2002; **346**(13): 975–980.

Contant CME, Hop WCJ, Van't Sant HP, et al. Mechanical bowel preparation for elective colorectal surgery: a multicentre randomised trial. *Lancet* 2007; **370**: 2112–2117.

Dean MM, et al. Predictors of complications and hospital stay in Gynecologic Cancer surgery. *Obstet Gynecol* 2001; **97**(5): 721–724.

Dripps RD, Echenhoff JE, Vandom D: *Introduction to Anesthesia: The Principles of Safe Practice*. WB Saunders Co, Philadelphia, 1988, p 17.

Efficacy and safety of enoxaparin versus unfractionated heparin for prevention of deep vein thrombosis in elective cancer surgery: a double-blind randomized multicentre trial with venographc assessment. ENOXACAN Study Group. *Br J Surg* 1997; **84**(8): 1099–1103.

Ellis CN. Bowel preparation before elective colorectal surgery: what is the evidence. *Semin Colon Rectal Surg* 2010; **21**(3): 144–147.

Fuchtner C, Manetta A, Walker JL, Emma D, Berman M, Di Saia PJ. Radical hysterectomy in the elderly patient: analysis of morbidity. *Am J Obstet Gynecol* 1992; **166**: 593–597.

Fulwell L, Taylor-Clarke M, Chatterjee J, et al. P1013 Morbidity and mortality associated with the use of inferior vena caval filters prior to major gynaecological oncology surgery in patients with venous thromboembolism: experience at the Hammersmith Hospital, London, UK. Poster presentations/*International Journal of Gynecology & Obstetrics* 107S2 (2009) S413–S729.

Gibbs J, Cull W, Henderson W, et al. Preoperative serum albumin level as a predictor of operative mortality and morbidity: results from the National VA Surgical Risk Study. *Arch Surg* 1999; **134**: 36–42.

Hirsh J, Guyatt G, Albers GW, Harrington R, Schunemann HJ. The American College of Chest Physicians. Antithrombotic and thrombolytic therapy:

American College of Chest Physicians evidence-based clinical practise guidelines (8th ed.) *Chest* 2008; **133**(6 Suppl): 110S–112S.

Kerridge RK. Perioperative patient management. *Best Pract Res Clin O&G* 2006; **20**(1): 23–40.

Kirschner CV, De Serto TM, Isaacs JK. Surgical treatment of the elderly patient with gynecologic cancer. *Surg Gynecol Obstet* 1990; **170**: 379–384.

Lee AYY. The roles of anticoagulants in patients with cancer. *Thromb Res* 2010; **125**(Suppl 2): S8–S11.

Pereire EDB, Fernendez ALG, Ancoa HDS. Prospective assessment of the risk of postoperative pulmonary complications in patients submitted to upper abdominal surgery. *Sao Paulo Med J* 1999; **117**: 151–160.

McLeod RS, Geerts WH, Sniderman KW, et al. Subcutaneous heparin versus low molecular weight heparin as thromboprophylaxis in patients undergoing colorectal surgery: results of the Canadian colorectal DVT prophylaxis trial: a randomized, double blind trial. *Ann Surg* 2001; **233**(3): 438–444.

Moore J, McLeod A. Anaesthesia for gynaecological oncology surgery. *Curr Anaesth Crit Care* 2009; **20**: 8–12.

National Collaborating Centre for Acute Care. Nutrition support in adults Oral nutrition support, enteral tube feeding and parenteral nutrition. London: National Collaborating Centre for Acute Care, 2006.

Powell-Tuck J, Gosling P, Lobo DN. British Consensus Guidelines on Intravenous Fluid Therapy for Adult Surgical Patients. *GIFTASUP* (2008).

Raffaella Giannice, et al. Perioperative morbidity and mortality in elderly gynecological oncological patients (70 Years) by the American Society of Anesthesiologists Physical Status Classes. *Ann Surg Oncol* **11**(2): 219–225.

Selzman CG, Miller SA, Zimmerman MA, et al. The case for beta-adrenergic blockade as prophylaxis against perioperative cardiovascular morbidity and mortality. *Arch Surg* 2001; **136**: 286–290.

Slim K, Vicaut E, Panis Y, et al. Metanalysis of randomized clinical trials of colorectal surgery with or without mechanical bowel preparation. *Br J Surg* 2004; **91**: 1125–1130.

Sorensen LT, Karlsmark T, Gottrup F. Abstinence from smoking reduces incisional wound infection: a randomized controlled trial. *Ann Surg* 2003; **238**: 1–5.

Tarhan S, Moffitt EA, Taylor WF, et al. Myocardial infarction after general anesthesia. *Anesth Analg* 1977; **56**: 455–461.

The Veterans Affairs Total Parenteral Nutrition Cooperative Study Group Perioperative total parenteral nutrition in surgical patients. *N Engl J Med* 1991; **325**: 525–532.

Wu MH, Lim MT, Chen WJ. Effective of perioperative parenteral nutritional support for gastric cancer patients undergoing gastrectomy. *Hepatogastroenterology* 2008; **55**(82–83): 799–802.

Chapter 21

Basic Anatomy and Principles of Surgery in Gynaecologic Oncology

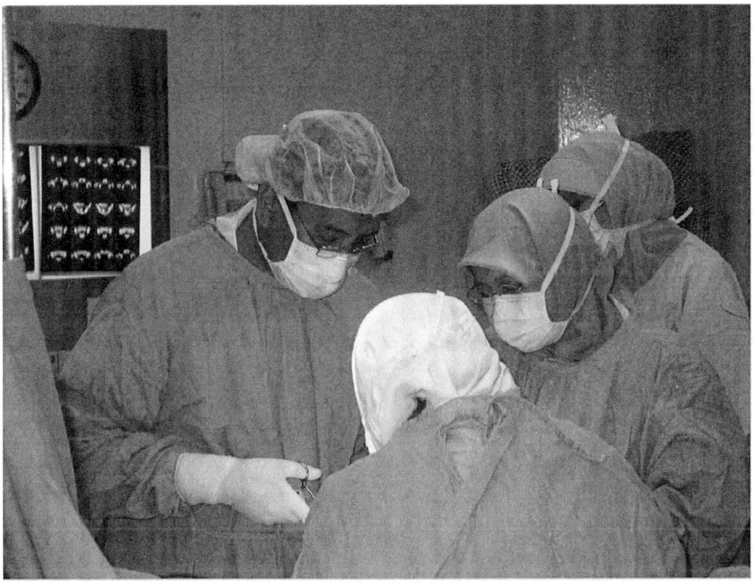

Gynaecologic Cancer: A Handbook for Students and Practitioners
Rushdan Noor, Eng Hseon Tay, and Jeffrey Low

ISBN 978-981-4463-06-5 (Hardcover), 978-981-4463-07-2 (eBook)
www.panstanford.com

Basic Anatomy of the Pelvis

Pelvic can be divided into a true and false pelvis. The dividing border between the true and false pelvis is an oblique line that extends from the sacral promontory along the anterior aspect of S1 to the symphysis pubis. True pelvis is below this line and is smaller than the false pelvis. The reproductive organs, bladder, pelvic ureters, small bowel loops and rectum lie within the true pelvis. Pelvic cavity is divided into the anterior and posterior compartment by broad ligaments and uterus. Adnexal triangle is a useful anatomic landmark because major pelvic vessels and ureter lies beneath this triangle (Fig. 21.2). Adnexal triangle is bounded anteriorly by the round ligament, posteriorly by the infundibulopelvic ligament and laterally by peritoneal reflection on the psoas muscle. The structures within the women's pelvis are shown in Fig. 21.1.

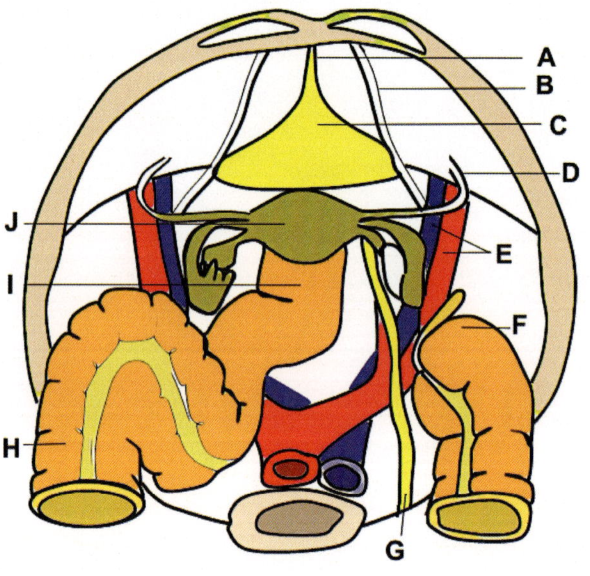

Figure 21.1 Structures within the women pelvis. A: median umbilical ligament and urachus, B: medial umbilical ligament, C: bladder, D: round ligament, E: external iliac artery and vein, F: caecum, G: ureter, H: sigmoid colon, I: rectum, J: uterus, fallopian tubes and ovaries.

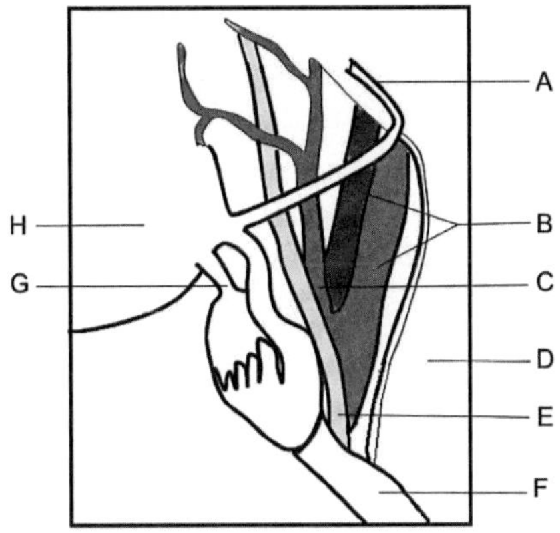

Figure 21.2 Adnexal triangle; boundaries and the structures underneath: A: round ligament, B: external iliac vein and artery, C: internal iliac artery, D: pelvic side wall, E: ureter, F: infundibulo-pelvic ligament, G: ovarian ligament and H: uterus.

Pelvic Ligaments

Broad ligament is formed by two layers of a peritoneum and extend laterally to the pelvic sidewall. Broad ligaments divide the true pelvis into anterior and posterior compartments. The **round ligament** extends from the anterolateral aspect of the uterine fundus and entering the inguinal canal, finally terminating in the labia majora. The **cardinal ligament** or transcervical ligament extends from the cervix and upper vagina to merge with the fascia of the obturator internal muscle. It forms the base of the broad ligament and is the most important support of the uterus and upper vagina. The **uterosacral ligament** extends posteriorly from the posterior-lateral aspect of the cervix and upper part of the vagina to the lateral aspect of the rectum and anterior body of the sacrum at the second and third sacral vertebra.

Pelvic Spaces

Pelvic space is the extra-peritoneal and avascular compartment that commonly used as a guide by the pelvic surgeon to identify the anatomy of the pelvic structures (Fig. 21.3). By developing the spaces, the surgeon will be able to identify the pelvic anatomy accurately and assist them in performing a complex pelvic surgery such as radical hysterectomy and pelvic lymphadenectomy with minimal blood loss. Many disease processes involve the pelvic peritoneum and required the surgeon to enter the retroperitoneal spaces to identify the vital retroperitoneal structures such as ureters and blood vessels and keep them away from any potential injuries.

Following are the most important pelvic spaces (see Fig. 21.3):

(a) **Paravesical space** (medial border: Bladder and vagina, lateral border: obliterated umbilical artery and obturator fossa)
(b) **Pararectal space** (medial border: rectum, lateral border: internal iliac artery)
(c) **Vesicovaginal space** (vesicocervical space: between bladder and cervix, vesicovaginal space: between bladder and vagina)
(d) **Rectovaginal space** (space between the vagina anteriorly and rectum posteriorly)

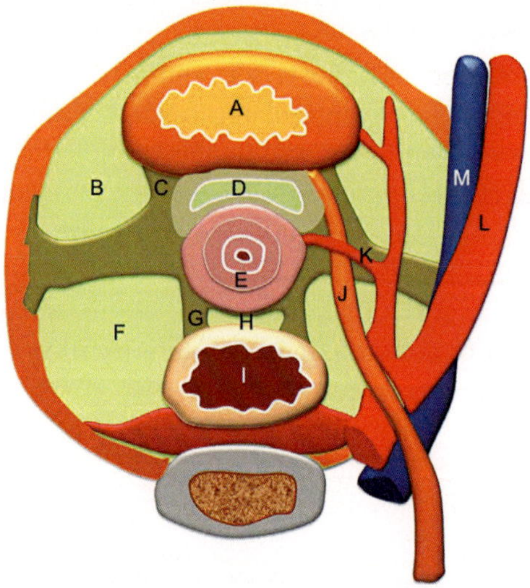

Figure 21.3 Pelvic ligaments and spaces. A: bladder, B: paravesical space, C: vesicouterine ligament, D: vesicovaginal space, E: cervix, F: pararectal space, G: uterosacral ligament, H: rectovaginal space, I: rectum, J: ureter, K: uterine artery, L: external iliac artery and M: external iliac vein.

Internal Iliac Artery

The internal iliac artery is a branch of common iliac artery. Internal iliac artery is important because it supplies the walls and viscera of the pelvis, the buttock, the reproductive organs and the medial compartment of the thigh. Internal iliac artery is divided into anterior division and posterior division (Fig. 21.4). Anterior division comprises obturator artery, inferior gluteal artery, umbilical artery, uterine artery, vaginal artery, inferior vesical artery, middle rectal artery and internal pudendal artery. Posterior division of internal iliac artery gives rise to the superior gluteal, iliolumbar and lateral sacral arteries.

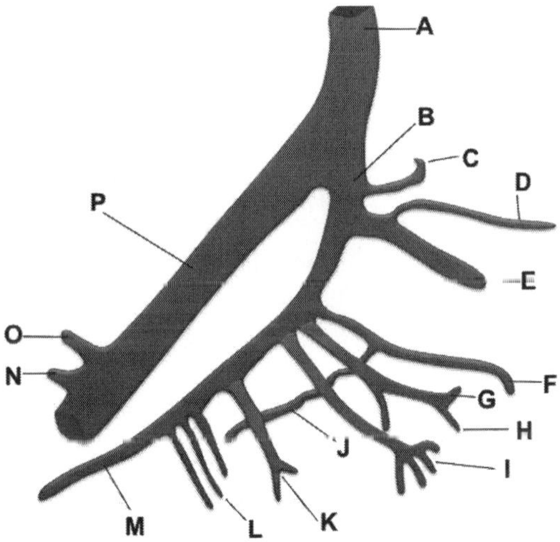

Figure 21.4 Arterial supply to the pelvis. A: common iliac, B: internal iliac, C: ilio-lumbar, D: lateral sacral, E: superior gluteal, F: inferior gluteal, G: middle rectal, H: internal pudendal, I: inf vesical, J: obturator, K: uterine, L: superior vesical, M: obliterated umbilical artery, N: inferior epigastric, O: deep circumflex iliac, P: external iliac.

Ureter

Ureter is one of the most important structures in the pelvis. There are two segments of the ureter, known as the abdominal ureter and pelvic ureter.

Table 21.1 The course of ureter

	The description of the course of ureter
Abdominal ureter	At ureteropelvic junction, ureters lie dorsal to the renal vein and artery. Abdominal ureter descends almost straight down to the pelvic brim, resting on the fascia of the psoas muscle about 5 cm from the midline and cross over the genitofemoral nerve near the pelvic brim.
Pelvic ureter	Pelvic ureter enters the pelvis by crossing at or just proximal to the bifurcation of the common iliac artery. On the left, the ureter, as it enters the pelvis, passes under the proximal sigmoid colon and on the right side, passes under the caecum and terminal ileum. The ovarian vessels cross over the ureter at the pelvic brim. As the ureter enters the true pelvis, it runs parallel to anterior division of internal iliac artery, and it becomes attached to the lateral pelvic wall peritoneum. Ureter and peritoneum separated as it reached the posterior leaf of broad ligament and uterosacral ligament. Then it runs under the uterine artery and enters the ureteric tunnel in the cardinal ligament. Ureter then runs toward the bladder, passing over the anterolateral vaginal fornix as it traverses the bladder pillar and then enters the bladder at the inferolateral portion. The ureters are 5–6 cm apart at the point of entry into the bladder wall. It takes a 1.5 cm course through the bladder wall and then enters the bladder mucosa at the sides of the trigone about 2.5 cm apart.
Sites where the ureter is narrow and vulnerable to kinking and stricture.	At the uteropelvis junction, the large renal pelvis tapers to a diameter of 2–3 mm. Distal to this, the ureter widens to a diameter of 10 mm until it reaches the pelvic brim. Here, the ureter narrows again to approximately 4–6 mm as it crosses over the common iliac vessels. At the UVJ, the ureter narrows to 1–5 mm as it enters the bladder.

Following are characteristic of the ureter:

(a) It is the most superficial structure in the pelvis and 25 cm long.
(b) It shows peristalsis.
(c) It adheres to the posterior surface of the peritoneum.
(d) It passes around the pelvic brim 1 cm short of the ischial spine and then swings medially.
(e) It enters the bladder at the level of the pubic tubercle on a plain abdominal X-ray.
(f) The most vulnerable sites to kink are at pelviureteric junction, at pelvic brim and ureterovesical junction.
(g) The blood supply to the ureter is through the ureteric branches from renal, ovarian artery, common iliac artery, vesical artery, vaginal artery and occasional small branches from the aorta. Middle third of the ureter is the least blood supplied.

The course of the ureter from kidney to the bladder is described in Table 21.1.

Pelvic Lymph Nodes

Lymphatics are the main pathway for the distant spread of gynaecologic tumours (Fig. 21.5). Pelvic nodes are the most common sites of occult metastases of cervical and uterine tumours, it has been suggested that systematic lymphadenectomy may have a therapeutic role in selected clinical conditions. Lymphadenectomy is performed for staging and therapeutic purposes. Well-defined boundaries of dissection should be set, and a sufficient number of nodes should be removed if the best prognostic information and the maximum therapeutic benefit are to be gained. A pathologic study on patterns of lymphatic spread has shown that the nodes primarily draining the cervix are those located at the iliac bifurcation, over the obturator nerve. More than 37% of nodal metastases are sized less than 2 mm, and that 50% of enlarged nodes are not metastatic. The cut off point for an enlarged lymph node is 1 cm in the largest diameter. Table 21.2 showed numbers of pelvic lymph nodes removed from patients with gynaecologic malignancy.

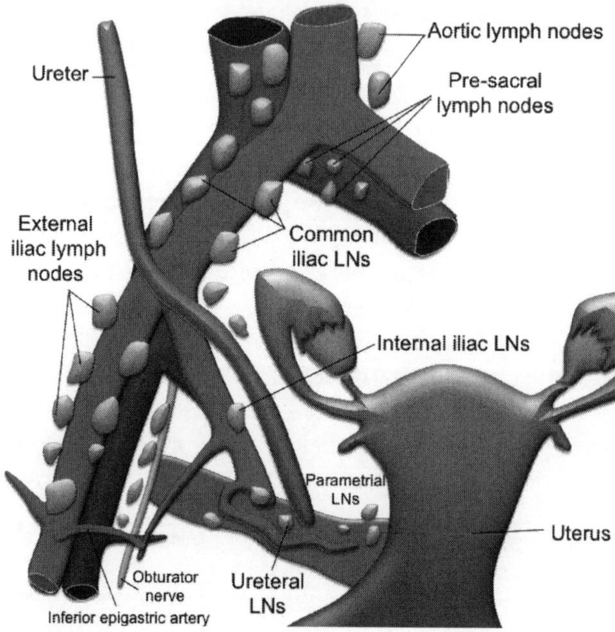

Figure 21.5 Pelvic lymph nodes.

Table 21.2 Number of lymph nodes removed from each pelvic node group in 631 patients

Node group	Median	Range
Common iliac	8	5–14
Deep common iliac	4	2–10
External iliac	10	5–15
Obturator		
Superficial	12	8–20
Deep	4	2–8
Internal iliac	7	4–9
Parametrial	3	1–11
Pre-sacral	4	2–10

References: Benedetti-Panici P, Scambia G, Baiocchi G, et al. Anatomical study of para-aortic and pelvic lymph nodes in gynecologic malignancies. *Obstet Gynecol* 1992; **79**: 498.

Pelvic Nerve

The uterus, vagina, urinary bladder and rectum are innervated by sympathetic and parasympathetic nerve (Table 21.3). The sympathetic nerve fibres originate from T11-L2, which forms the superior hypogastric plexus, while parasympathetic fibres originate from S2, 3 and 4 and form the inferior hypogastric plexus to innervate the uterus and the urinary bladder (Fig. 21.6).

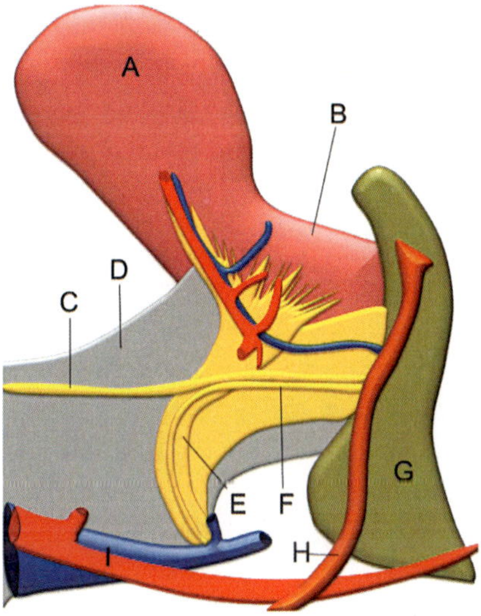

Figure 21.6 Pelvic nerve supplying the uterus and bladder. A: uterus, B: vagina, C: hypogastric nerve, D: cardinal ligament, E: pelvic splanchnic nerve, F: bladder branch from the inferior hypogastric plexus, G: bladder, H: ureter, I: Internal iliac artery. Adapted from Fujii S. *Gynecol Oncol* 2008; **111**: S33–S41.

Table 21.3 Nerve supply to pelvic organs

Nerve roots	Nerves	Organs
S2, 3, 4 (parasympathetic)	Pudendal nerve; inguinal nerve; genitofemoral nerve; posterior femoral nerve; pelvic and parasympathetic nerves; pelvic splanchnic nerve	Perineum, vulva, lower and upper vagina, cervix and lower uterus, posterior urethra, trigone, lower ureter, rectosigmoid colon

(*Continued*)

Table 21.3 (*Continued*)

Nerve roots	Nerves	Organs
T11-12 (sympathetic)	Hypogastric plexus	Uterine fundus, proximal third fallopian tube, broad ligament, upper bladder, caecum, appendix and terminal large bowel
T9-10 (sympathetic)	Aortic plexus; superior mesenteric plexus; renal plexus	Distal fallopian tube; upper ureter; ovaries

The pelvic nerve is often transected and injured during radical hysterectomy leading to bladder and rectal dysfunction.

Following are the sites of pelvic nerve injuries occurred during radical hysterectomy:

(a) hypogastric nerves during the resection of the uterosacral ligament at the posterior pelvic wall
(b) pelvic splanchnic nerve (parasympathetic) during lymphadenectomy medial to the internal iliac vein and around the deep uterine vein and during the division of the deep uterine vein in the cardinal ligaments
(c) vesical branches of the pelvic plexus during resection of the vesicouterine ligament
(d) inferior hypogastric plexus during the resection of the uterosacral and rectovaginal ligaments
(e) superior hypogastric plexus during pre-sacral and periaortic lymph node dissection

Introduction to Anatomy of Vulva

Vulva

The vulva includes mons pubis, labia minora, labia majora, clitoris, vestibule, glands (Bartholin's glands, Skene's glands and minor vestibular glands) and perineal body. The other term for vulva is pudendum. Following are the borders of the vulva:

- Superior: anterior abdominal wall and mons pubis
- Lateral: labio-crural fold at a medial thigh

- Posterior: anus

The mons pubis is the superior border of the vulva described as directly anterosuperior to the pubic symphysis. This area is covered by skin where sexual hair development occurs at the time of puberty.

The labia majora form the lateral boundaries of the vulva. They are composed of folds of adipose and fibrous tissue. The labia majora correspond to the scrotum in male. Labia majora fuse anteriorly into the mons pubis and posteriorly they terminate 3–4 cm in front of the anus where they are united by the posterior commissure or fourchette. The labia majora are covered by skin consisting of stratified squamous epithelium. It contains sweat and sebaceous glands and many nerve endings.

The labia minora, or nymphae, consist of two folds of connective tissue which has little or no adipose tissue. Labia minora is situated between the labia majora and extending from the clitoris to the fourchette. Labia minora is divided into two parts anteriorly; one part passes over the clitoris to form the prepuce, while the other part joins beneath the clitoris to form a frenulum. Posteriorly, labia minora blend with the medial surfaces of the labia majora. The skin and mucosa covering the labia minora are rich in sebaceous glands, sweat glands and many nerve endings.

The clitoris is situated at the middle and upper part of the labia minora. The clitoris is an erective structure, homologous with the penis. Although much smaller than the man's penis, the clitoris has as many nerve endings as the penis and is formed from the same tissue during development. The clitoris is made up of two crura, which attach to the periosteum of the ischiopubic rami. It has two small muscles called ischiocarvernosa, which are inserted into the crura of the clitoris. The average length of the clitoris is 1.5–2.0 cm and about 1 cm width in adult female. Clitoris is innervated by the terminal branch of the pudendal nerve known as dorsal nerve of the clitoris.

The vestibule is the area (triangular shape) between the labia minora and behind the gland of clitoris and extends to the fourchette posteriorly. The vestibule is where the urethral meatus and vaginal orifices are found. It also gives rise to the opening of the glands, i.e. Skene's glands and Bartholin's glands bilaterally. It is lined by non-keratinized squamous epithelium. The squamous cells in the epithelium are well glycogenated and resemble the vaginal or cervical squamous cells. The structures found in the vestibule include the Bartholin's glands (Major vestibular glands), the minor vestibular glands, Skene's glands (periurethral gland), the opening of the urethra and vaginal orifice. The external urethral orifice is a sagittal cleft situated about 2.5 cm behind the clitoris. The total length of female urethra is from 3.5 to 5.0 cm.

The hymen is a thin mucous membrane partially covered the vaginal orifice. In other words, the opening of the vaginal orifice is actually a cleft between the hymen. The hymen has many shapes and when stretched, the posterior part is the broadest. It can be absent or form a complete septum across the vaginal opening and this condition is known as imperforate hymen. When the hymen is ruptured, the remaining part will form rounded elevations known as carunculae hymenales. The shallow depression between the hymen and the frenulum of the labia is called navicular fossa.

The other structure found in the vulva is the vestibular bulbs or bulbus vestibuli. The vestibular bulbs are two masses of erectile tissue that lie deep to the bulbocavernosus muscles bilaterally, on each side of the vagina orifice. Each mass measures approximately 2.5 cm in length and is united to each other anteriorly by a median band known as pars intermedia. Their posterior end is in contact with the Bartholin's gland. The deeper surface of vestibular bulb is in contact with fascia of pelvic diaphragm, while superficially they are covered by the bulbocavernosus.

Skene's glands, or periurethral glands, are glands that secrete the mucous for lubrication at the opening of the urethra. The duct of this gland is about 0.5 to 1.5 cm long and located in the floor of the terminal end of the urethra and open just within or external to the meatus.

Bartholin's glands (or greater vestibular glands) are two small mucus-secreting glands situated within a subcutaneous tissue of the posterior labia majora, have ducts that open onto the posterolateral portion of the vestibule. Bartholin's glands are homologous of bulbo-urethral glands in male. There are two Bartholin's glands, one on each side of the vaginal orifice in contact with the posterior end of each lateral mass of the bulb of the vestibule. It has a 2 cm duct opening immediately lateral to the hymen and medial to the posterior part of labia minora. It secretes mucus for lubrication of the vagina.

The minor vestibular glands are small glands corresponding to the penile glands of Littre in male. These glands are located within the vestibule and lined by a single layer of columnar cells secreting a mucin.

The other glands located in the vulva are apocrine glands, sebaceous glands and sweat glands. Sweat glands are primarily involved in heat regulation.

Blood Supply and Innervation of the Vulva

The main blood supply to a vulva is from the **internal pudendal artery** (terminal branch of anterior division of internal iliac artery) and **external pudendal artery** from a femoral artery. Internal pudendal artery supplies ischiocavernosus, bulbocavercosus muscle, perineal body, urethra and clitoris. External pudendal artery supplies labia majora and their deep structures.

The main sensory supply to the vulva is via the pudendal nerves. The pudendal nerve also provides motor innervation to all the muscles of the perineum, including the levator ani muscle, voluntary urinary and bowel sphincters. The mons pubis and upper labia majora are supplied by **ilioinguinal nerve (L1)**, **genitofemoral nerve (L1-2)** and also from the perineal branches of the posterior cutaneous nerves of the thigh, while lower vagina, labia, clitoris, perineal body and their supporting structures are supplied by the **pudendal nerve (S2-3).**

Lymphatic Supply of the Vulva

Lymphatic drainage of the vulva is mainly to superficial inguinal lymph nodes (10 nodes in a triangle below, along the saphenous vein) (Fig. 21.7). Some part of clitoris and middle structures drain to the pelvic lymph nodes (obturator and iliac nodes). Generally, the lymphatic drainage of one side of the vulva does not cross the midline. The midline is defined as 1 cm within an imaginary line from the clitoris to the anus. There are two groups of inguinal lymph nodes:

(a) Superficial inguinal lymph nodes (subcutaneous lymph nodes situated between Camper's fascia and cribriform fascia). They are further subdivided into oblique and vertical groups.

(b) Deep inguinal lymph nodes (within the cribriform fascia and medial to the femoral vein and runs towards the femoral canal).

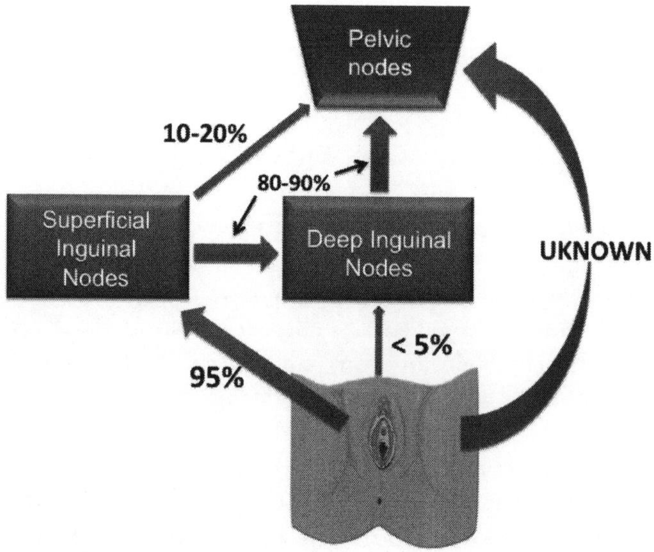

Figure 21.7 Lymphatic drainage of the each side of vulva.

Superficial inguinal lymph nodes drain into the deep inguinal lymph nodes and subsequently into the external iliac lymph nodes. Direct spread of the cancer to the deep inguinal nodes without metastasis to the superficial group has been documented, although it is uncommon, representing less than 5% of cases. Furthermore, 10–20% of lymphatic flow from the superficial inguinal group travels directly to the pelvis without passage through the deep inguinal group.

The lymphatic vessels draining the midline structures of the vulva decussate and drain to the bilateral groin nodes. The lymphatic vessels of the anterior vulva also drain directly into the deep nodes, accounting for the direct metastasis of cancer to the deep nodes without involving the superficial nodes in less than 5% of patients.

Some part of clitoris and middle structures drain to pelvic lymph node (obturator, iliac nodes). Approximately 10–20% of lymphatic flow from the superficial inguinal group travels directly to the pelvis without passing through the deep inguinal group.

Peritoneal Cavity

The peritoneum is a common site of tumour spread in gynaecologic malignancy in particularly ovarian carcinoma. The peritoneal surface consists of a single layer of the epithelium known as mesothelium. Peritoneum is divided into a parietal and visceral peritoneum. The peritoneum lining the abdominal wall is called the parietal peritoneum, while peritoneum covering the visceral is called visceral peritoneum. Parietal and visceral peritoneum is separated with each other by space known as peritoneal cavity, which is filled with peritoneal fluid. The peritoneal cavity is divided into two separated sacs known as the greater sac and the lesser sac. The lesser sac is also known as omental bursa, lies posterior to the stomach, lesser omentum and liver (Fig. 21.8). The rest of the peritoneal cavity is the greater sac. The greater sac and the lesser sac communicate through the omentum foramen also known as epiploic foramen or foramen of Winslow (Fig. 21.9).

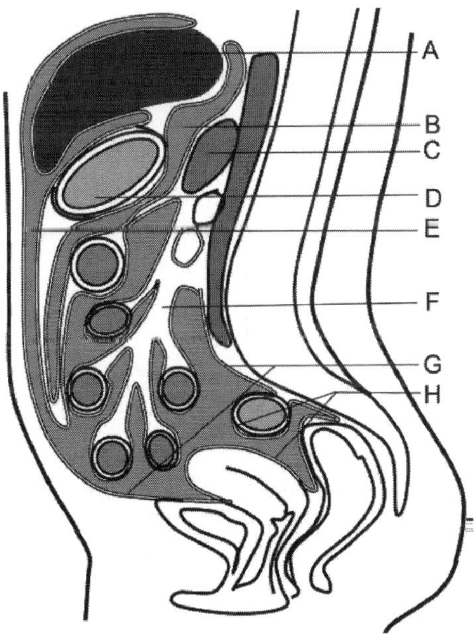

Figure 21.8 Peritoneum and peritoneal cavity. A: liver, B: lesser sac, C: pancreas, D: stomach, E: greater sac, F: mesentery, G: parietal peritoneum, H: visceral peritoneum.

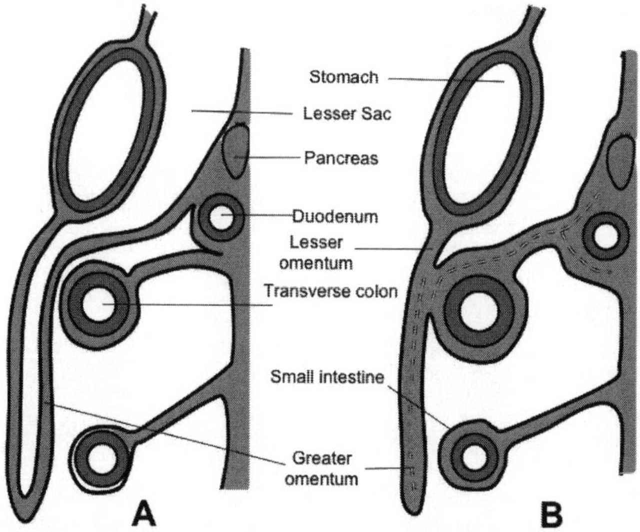

Figure 21.9 Greater and lesser omentum. The relationship between the greater omentum, stomach, colon and lesser sac in newborn (A) and in adult (B). In B, the leaves of the greater omentum have fused with each other and with the transverse mesocolon. The portion of the greater omentum between transverse colon and stomach is also known as gastrocolic ligament.

Omentum

The omentum is a highly vascular, fatty tissue approximately 14 inches in length and 10 inches wide that hangs like an apron over the intestines and lower abdomen. Scientists are now discovering that omentum is a physiologically dynamic tissue. It contains angiogenic factors that stimulate the growth of new blood vessels and rich in lymphatic vessels and tissue that are critical in removing metabolic waste and excess fluid. Evidence suggests that omental tissue contains stem cell-omnipotent master cells that can differentiate into a variety of cell types. Omentum is also a rich source of the biological material that enhances tissue growth, including angiogenic factors, key neurotransmitters, nerve growth factors, and agents involved in inflammatory and immune processes. Omentum is divided into the greater omentum and the lesser omentum.

The greater omentum has following features:

(a) It is also known as great omentum, gastrocolic omentum and epiploon.
(b) It is a largest peritoneal fold.
(c) It is made of four layers of the mesothelium.
(d) These individual layers may be easily demonstrated in the young, but in the adult, they are more or less inseparably blended.
(e) The left border of the greater omentum is continuous with the gastrolienal ligament.
(f) The right border extends as far as the commencement of the duodenum.
(g) Between its two anterior layers, a short distance from the greater curvature of the stomach, is the anastomosis between the right and left gastroepiploic vessels.

The lesser omentum is also known as small omentum or gastrohepatic omentum. It extends from the lesser curvature of the stomach and the first part of the duodenum to the liver (porta hepatis). At the right border of the omentum, the two layers are continuous and form a free margin which constitutes the anterior boundary of the epiploic foramen.

Blood Supply to the Bowel

The main blood supply to large and small bowels is from superior and inferior mesenteric artery. Arterial blood supply to the distal small intestines and right side of the colon (including promixal 2/3 of the transverse colon) is from the branches of superior mesenteric artery, i.e. ileal branch, ileo-colic, right colic and middle colic artery. The left colon, rectum and upper anal canal are supplied by branches of the inferior mesenteric artery, i.e. left colic, sigmoid arteries and superior rectal artery (Fig. 21.10).

Bowel Injury and Basic Bowel Surgery

Bowel involvement is not uncommon in gynaecological malignancy, mainly in advanced ovarian carcinoma. Bowel injuries can occur during entering into the abdomen or during resection of the tumour that closely attached to the bowel. One of the most common causes of bowel injury is a laceration during entrance into the peritoneal cavity, especially to the small bowel due to adhesion from previous surgery. Injury to the bowel can be classified as superficial (serosal injury), minor (small breach of the mucosa) and major injury (breaching of the mucosa in multiple adjacent sites or significant loss of tissue). Most of the superficial bowel injury can be handled without any intervention, unless if the muscle layer is divided down to the mucosa. In this case, it should be treated similar to minor type of injury. Minor bowel injury should be treated by closing the defect with a single layer of interrupted serosubmucosal suture using 3/0 absorbable sutures such as vicryl. The suturing involves placing sutures 4–5 mm apart and 4–5 mm from the cut edge of the bowel through the serosa, muscle layers and submucosa, leaving the mucosa intact. Most of the major small bowel injury is treated with bowel resection and end-to-end anastomosis. The suturing method is similar to what has been described in minor bowel injury. Major injury to the large bowel is more complicated and the patient may require colostomy or ileostomy to divert the faecal content.

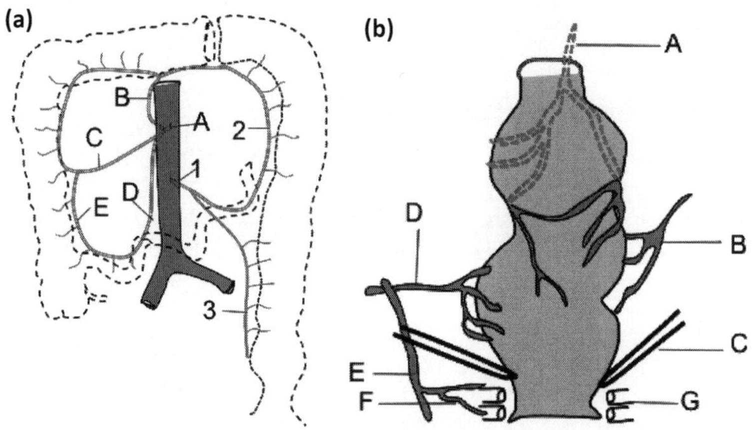

Figure 21.10 (a) Blood supply to the colon. A: sub-mesenteric, B: middle colic, C: right colic, D: ileal branch, E: ileo-colic; 1: inf mesenteric, 2: left colic, 3: sup. rectal. (b) Blood supply of the rectum. A: superior rectal artery, B: left medial rectal artery, C: levator ani muscle, D: right medial rectal artery, E: internal pudendal artery, F: inferior rectal artery.

Small and Large Bowel Resection and Anastomosis

Figures 21.11 and 21.12 showed the techniques of small and recto-sigmoid resection and re-anastomosis.

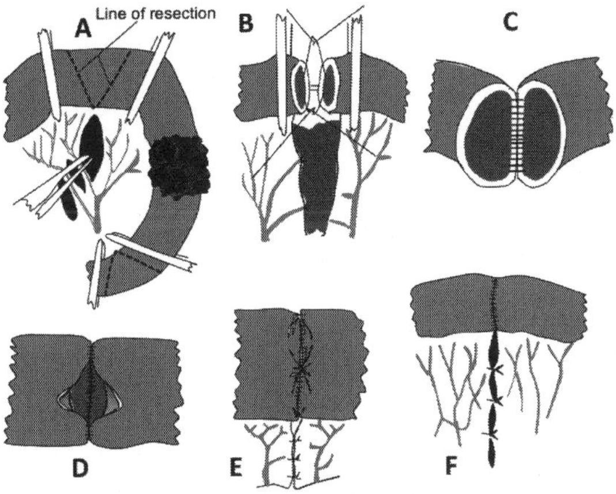

Figure 21.11 Small bowel resection and end-to-end anastomosis. Closure is done in two layers using absorbable suture sized 3/0, continuous suturing for first layer and interrupted suturing for second layer.

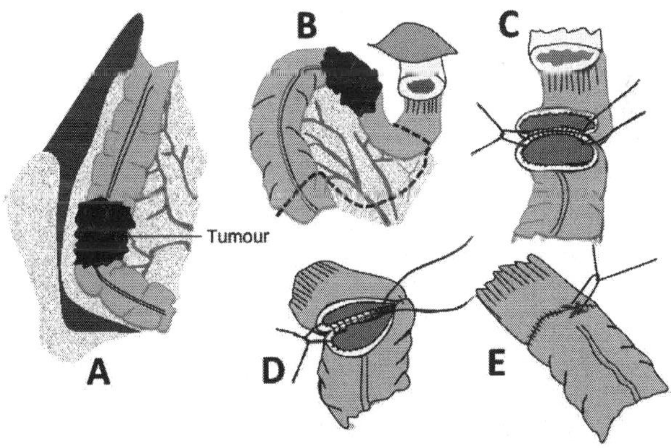

Figure 21.12 Resection of recto-sigmoid and end-to-end anastomosis. A: mobilization of the sigmoid and descending colon, B: resection of the recto-sigmoid, C, D, E: re-anastomosis. Re-anastomosis of the bowel is done in two layers using absorbable suture size 3/0. The first layer uses continuous suturing; interrupted suturing for second layer (serosal).

Urinary Tract Injuries and Repair

The overall incidence of urological injuries during pelvic surgery is approximately 0.4–1%. The most important urinary tract injury is the injury to the ureter. There are at least five types of ureteric injuries, i.e. due to ligation, crushing, laceration, stretching and devascularization. The viability of the ureter can be assessed by looking at few features such as blanching, blood flowing through the vessels supplying the ureter, ureteral peristalsis and any changes in the colour of the ureter. If the viability of the ureter is in doubt, segmental resection, and end-to-end anastomosis should be done. In call cases of ureteric injury, stenting must be done and the stent is left in situ for few weeks. The repair is done using fine sutures such as 5/0 vicryl. If the distal ureter is injured and required resection, the distal end can be reimplanted into the bladder (ureteroneocystostomy). There are various methods of uretero-neocystostomy and one of the most commonly performed is Boari–Ockerbald procedure as shown in Fig. 21.13. Resection and re-anastomosis of a ureter are shown in Fig. 21.14.

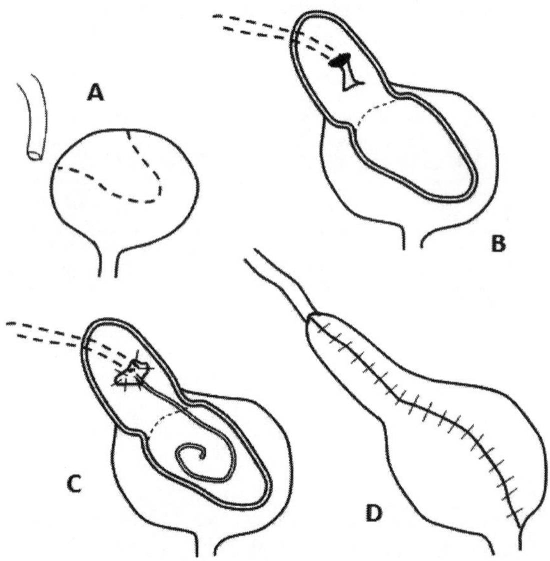

Figure 21.13 Boari–Ockerbald procedure (Boari flap). Transected ureter is drawn through the tunnel (B) and anastomosed to the urothelium and the stent is inserted (C). Psoas hitch may be performed to reduce the tension.

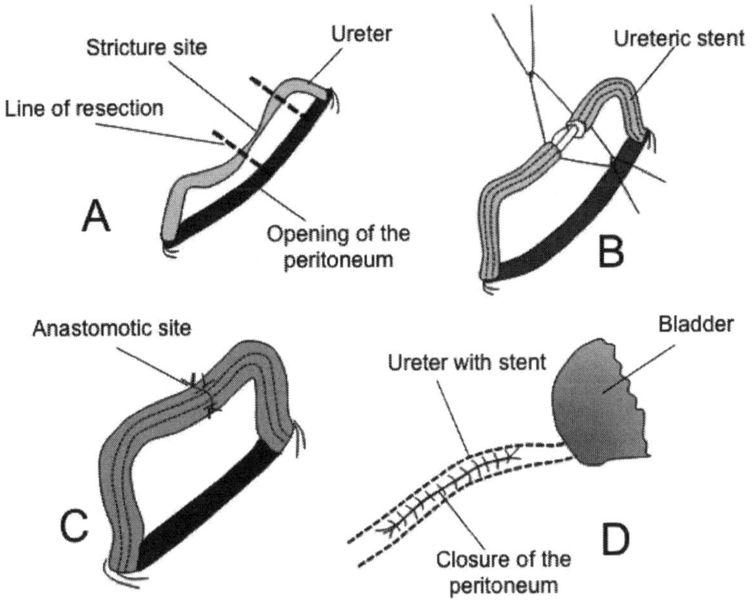

Figure 21.14 Resection and re-anastomosis of the ureter.

The bladder injury is the second most common type of urinary tract injury and with the increasing practice of laparoscopic surgery, the incidence of bladder injury has increased to 1–1.8%. Intraoperatively, bladder injury can be recognized by methylene blue test; instilling the methylene blue into the bladder via a urethral catheter and observe for any site of leakage. Bladder wall defect (muscular wall defect) is closed by continuous suturing using absorbable suture size 3/0 and if possible, avoid suturing the mucosa. Second layer of serosal suturing is advisable to ensure good integrity of the repair. Indwelling catheter is placed for 7–10 days.

Basic Surgical Techniques in Gynaecological Surgery

Fasting and Bowel Preparation

Traditionally, fasting should be at least 4–6 hours before surgery. However, based on current evidence, recently a patient can be allowed to take clear non-fizzy fluids up to 2 hours before surgery. The primary goals of bowel preparation are (a) reduction in the bacterial flora inhabiting the GIT and, therefore, reduction in the risk of bacteraemia and postoperative infection and (b) removal of solid faecal materials from the colon.

Following are the recommendations from British Consensus Guidelines on Intravenous Fluid Therapy for Adult Surgical Patient 2008, regarding bowel preparation:

(a) Routine use of preoperative mechanical bowel preparation is not beneficial and may complicate intra and postoperative management of fluid and electrolyte balance. Its use should therefore be avoided whenever possible.
(b) Where mechanical bowel preparation is used, fluid and electrolyte derangement commonly occurs and should be corrected by simultaneous intravenous fluid therapy with Hartmann's or lactate Ringer's solution.

Skin Preparation

It is advisable for the patients to shower or have a bath using soap on either the day before or the day of surgery. Avoid shaving if possible or shave as close to the time of surgery as possible. Studies have shown that 2% chlorhexidine gluconate was superior to 4% chlorhexidine or povidone iodine as a skin antiseptic prior to surgery in reducing microbial counts.

Skin Incision

The decision on the type of skin incision is very important because adequate exposure is one of the most important principles in any form of surgical treatment. Factors that would influence the type of incision include the nature of the pathology, type of surgery, the size of patients, history of previous surgery and size of the tissue to be removed.

There are three most important characteristics of appropriate skin incision:

(a) accessibility
(b) extensibility
(c) security

The most common type of skin incision in gynaecologic oncology surgery is the vertical and transverse skin incision. The types of skin incisions are shown in Table 21.4. Maylard's skin incision is the most common transverse incision performed in gynaecologic cancer surgery (Fig. 21.15). Paramedian skin incisions are no longer used and are only considered in a patient who had a previous similar incision. In Maylard's incision, the incision extends between anterior superior iliac spines, and it involves division of the rectus muscle and ligations of inferior epigastric vessels. This incision is suitable in the surgical treatment of cervical and uterine cancer. The advantages of this incision are cosmetically more acceptable and lower risk of incisional hernia. Midline incision is the method of choice for surgical treatment of ovarian cancer or in other cancers where upper abdominal exploration and surgery are anticipated. Midline incision will provide an excellent exposure and accessibility to the entire abdominal structures. The disadvantages of the midline incision (as compared to transverse incision) are higher risk of wound breakdown (1.7% versus 0.25%), incision hernia and postoperative pain.

Table 21.4 Type of abdominal skin incisions

1. **Vertical incision**: Midline incision, Paramedian incision
2. **Transverse and oblique incision**: Pfannensteil incision, Cheney's incision, Maylard's incision, Kocher's subcostal incision, McBurney's Grid iron
3. **Abdominothoracic incisions**

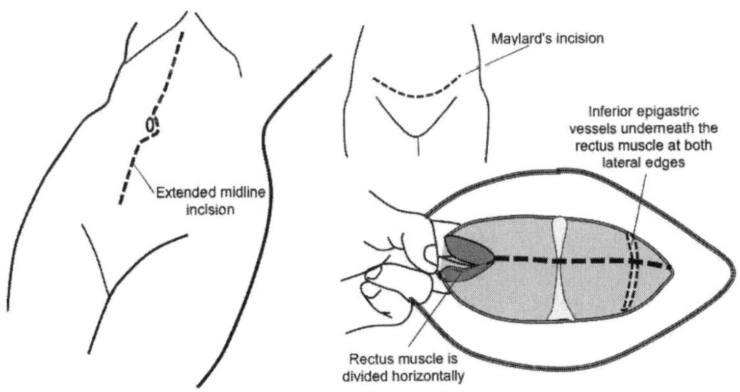

Figure 21.15 Most common skin incisions in gynaecologic cancer surgery (midline incision and Maylard's incision).

Surgical suture is used to hold tissues together after an injury or surgery. The ideal suture should have the following characteristics:

(a) high in vivo tensile strength during the critical wound-healing period
(b) rapid absorption rate once the critical period is over
(c) minimal tissue reactivity
(d) no memory (memory is a tendency of the suture to revert to its original form even after being twisted or bent)
(e) predictable performance
(f) easy suture handling and knot security

The size of the suture is defined by the diameter of the suture measured in tenths of a millimetre. It is described by a number plus or minus a 0 ranging from 5 (heavy braided suture for orthopaedics) to 11-0 (fine monofilament suture for ophthalmics). The surgical sutures are divided into two categories: (a) absorbable or non-absorbable sutures (either natural or synthetic) and (b) monofilament or multi-filament sutures (either natural or synthetic).

Surgical Drain

The routine use of surgical drain is controversial. The two most common aims of surgical drain are to prevent the accumulation of fluid (blood, pus and infected fluids) and to characterize the fluid in order to diagnose early surgical complication such as ongoing haemorrhage and anastomotic leak.

There are two categories of surgical drains:

(a) **Open or closed**: Open drains include corrugated rubber or plastic sheets that drain fluid onto a gauze pad or into a stoma bag. The disadvantage of this type of drain is they are likely to increase the risk of infection. Closed drains are formed by tubes draining into a bag or bottle, e.g. chest tube, portex drain, radivac drain, etc.
(b) **Active or passive**: Active drains are maintained under suction, while passive drains have no suction and work according to the differential pressure between body cavities and the exterior as well as gravity.

Basic Principles in Gynaecologic Oncology Surgery

Principle 1: Know the map of the pelvis

A detailed knowledge of the pelvic anatomy holds the key to a precise, neat and bloodless surgery.

The three important anatomical structures in order of importance to a surgeon are

(a) pelvic spaces
(b) pelvic vessels and nerves
(c) ureter

Here are the three simple steps you can do to get acquainted with your surgical field:

Step 1: Acquire theoretical knowledge on the following:

(a) pelvic spaces: their boundaries and contents
(b) ureter: its course and blood supply
(c) pelvic vessels: and their branches
(d) pelvic nerves: and their branches

Step 2: Get a visual understanding on what you have studied:

(a) to reinforce your knowledge
(b) pay attention to details like where the ureter will be found and where the vessels will be encountered

Step 3: Mental Exercise before each surgery

Go through the entire sequential steps of a procedure in your mind again and again before the surgery, e.g. steps to identify the ureter.

Principle 2: Traction and counter-traction

To comprehend the principle of traction and counter-traction one has to appreciate the following:

(a) Tissues and organs are separated and held together by loose connective tissues, which forms potential spaces (pelvic spaces).
(b) In some areas, the connective tissues condense to form ligaments (e.g. uterosacral ligament) and fascia (e.g. pre-sacral fascia).

(c) Blood vessels and nerves traverse through these soft connective tissues and spaces.
(d) By applying gentle opposing tractions between tissues, tissue planes will open up into spaces.
(e) This action separates the organs with ease and without bleeding.
(f) It also exposes the blood vessels and nerves clearly.

Dissection must be blunt and done in the direction parallel to the vessels and nerves, to avoid bleeding and nerve injury.

Principle 3: Optimal exposure

Achieving optimal exposure means you are

(a) able to clearly visualize the anatomy of the organ you wish to dissect
(b) able to dissect this organ in full comfort
(c) in a position to react to an unexpected complications (e.g. massive bleeding) quickly

It does not mean

(a) it has to be a laparotomy rather than a laparoscopy
(b) the incision has to be midline
(c) the incision has to be long

The ingredients for achieving an optimal exposure are as follows:

(a) choosing the appropriate approach (laparoscopy vs. laparotomy)
(b) using the appropriate incision (midline, Maylard's, Pfannensteil)
(c) applying an adequate retractor
(d) achieving good packing technique to displace the bowels away
(e) ensuring the abdominal muscle is fully relaxed.

Ten Guiding Thoughts and Principles

(1) Every good surgeon is a perpetual trainee at different phases, at different levels and in different fields of training.
(2) A bad laparoscopist would swear that laparotomy is superior, which is not the case.

(3) A good laparoscopist has a tendency to avoid laparotomy even when the indication is glaringly obvious to do so, and when things go awry, it confirms what a bad laparoscopist said is true.

(4) Master your pelvic dissection at laparotomy first; the skilful strokes will follow when you perform a laparoscopic dissection.

(5) Use a generous incision, midline if necessary, and graduating to smaller incision progressively and appropriately.

(6) Let logical medical indication prevail over cosmetic desire.

(7) Pay attention to setting up an optimal surgical field by applying good traction and pack away the bowels well.

(8) Provide feedback to your anaesthetist about the abdominal wall muscle tone to achieve optimal muscle relaxation.

(9) A good surgeon knows the operating tools well (sutures, instruments, equipment).

(10) A good surgeon has excellent basic surgical techniques (knotting, dissecting, clamping).

Chapter 22

Basic Principles of Radiotherapy

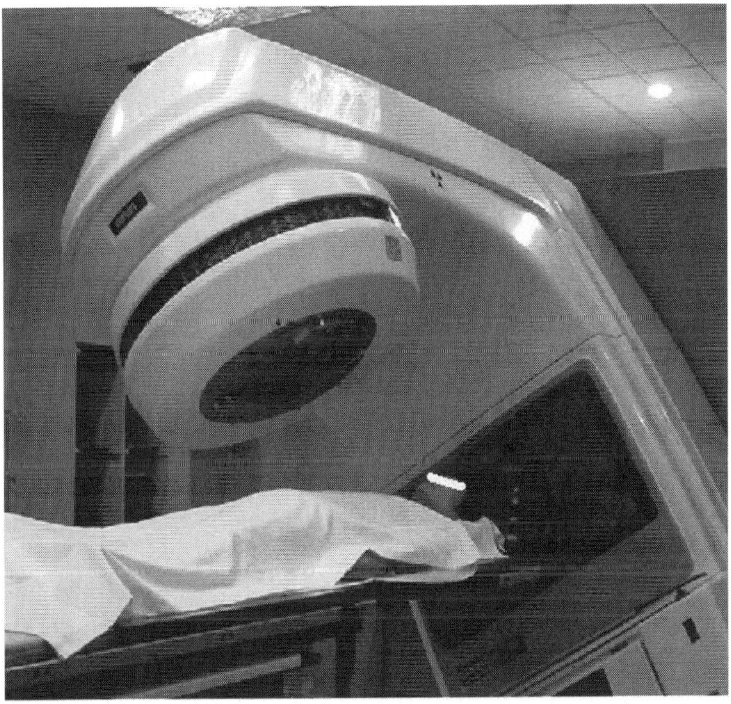

Gynaecologic Cancer: A Handbook for Students and Practitioners
Rushdan Noor, Eng Hseon Tay, and Jeffrey Low

ISBN 978-981-4463-06-5 (Hardcover), 978-981-4463-07-2 (eBook)
www.panstanford.com

Introduction

Historically, the first application of radiation for the therapeutic purpose was made in 1896 in Chicago by Grubbe for the treatment of breast cancer and the first case of the cure of malignant tumour by radiotherapy alone was reported on a patient with squamous carcinoma of the nose. Radiation therapy is defined as the use of high-energy radiation from X-ray, gamma rays, protons, neutrons, and other sources to kill cancer cells and shrink tumours. Radiation therapy is the most effective non-surgical treatment of cancer. Gynaecologic cancers were among the first malignancies treated with ionizing radiation more than 100 years ago. It remains an essential component of both as primary treatment and adjuvant post-operative treatment of selected gynaecological malignancies. Radiation therapy can also be palliative in metastatic disease and frequently used to alleviate the symptoms as a result of tumour invasion such as in bone, spine and brain metastases.

The most commonly used radiations in clinical practise are X-ray and gamma ray. These two types of radiations are a form of electromagnetic radiation with shorter wavelength than heat and light: also known as the high-energy photon. Both have similar properties but from different origins. Gamma ray originates from the nucleus emitted from a radioisotope, while X-ray originates from outside the nucleus, produced by bombardment of a target by high-speed electrons. Apart from high-energy photon, irradiation can also exist in particulate form (particle radiation) such as electron, proton, neutron and alpha particle. The most common form of radiation in clinical practice today is the high-energy photon (gamma-ray and X-ray). Deposition of energy by radiation exposure is called radiation-absorbed dose and is measured in rads. The SI unit of absorbed dose is the Gray (Gy); 1 Gy is equal to 100 rads or 1 joule/kg. The term ionizing radiation is used because it forms ions in the cells of the tissues it passes through as it displaces electrons from atoms.

External beam radiotherapy is commonly delivered by a linear accelerator utilizing high-voltage X-ray beam. This unit deposits the maximum dose beneath the surface; therefore, external beam radiotherapy is considered skin-sparing. External beam radiation therapy can also be delivered by Cobalt-60 unit; this unit provides relatively high-energy gamma rays, ideally suited for the treatment of head and neck cancers and other superficially located tumours such as breast cancers and soft tissue sarcomas of extremities. They are not adequate for the treatment of deep seated tumours. Linear accelerators have more advantages; for instance, high-energy beams can be created. The edges of the beams are sharper, can also treat superficial lesions and the dose rate can be adjusted much easier. Cobalt-60 units, however, are cheaper than a linear accelerator.

In brachytherapy, radioisotope is used to deliver radiation in the form of gamma rays. In the past, radium was the primary isotope used in brachytherapy; recently, because of its long half-life and high-energy output, radium has been replaced with caesium, gold and iridium, which have shorter half-life and lower energy (Fig. 22.1).

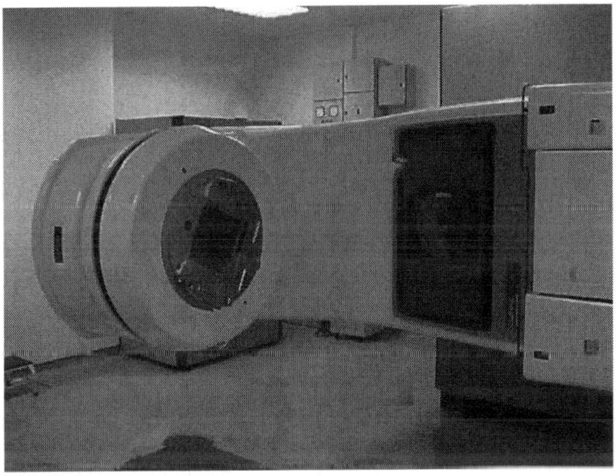

Figure 22.1 Linear accelerator delivers high-voltage X-rays for external beam radiotherapy.

Table 22.1 Physical characteristics of commonly used radioisotopes in radiotherapy

Isotope	Energy (MeV)	Half-life
Radium-226	0.830	1600 years
Caesium-137	0.662	30 years
Cobalt-60	1.250	5.26 years
Iridium-192	0.380	74.2 days
Gold-198	0.412	2.7 days

Biologic Effects of Radiation

The exact mechanism of cell death by radiation is still under extensive investigations. Neoplastic cells are usually more easily killed by radiation than are their parent cells in the surrounding normal tissues.

There are at least two mechanisms how radiation kills the cancer cells:

(a) **Molecular degradation** of large molecules, i.e. breaking into smaller units. Leading to severe alterations in morphology and biochemical properties of the molecules. These molecules can be proteins, enzymes, nucleic acids and certain lipids.

(b) **Cross-linking** of long molecules leading to dysfunction and insoluble in the system. Macromolecule will be held rigid.

The damage of cells can be lethal (the cell dies) or sub-lethal (the cell has an opportunity to repair itself). As results of irradiation, there will be morphologic and functional changes in irradiated cell. The therapeutic mechanism of irradiation is based on the intrinsic ability of cells to repair damage and the ability of the radiation oncologist to maximized radiation effect on tumour and minimized detrimental effect of radiation to normal tissues. Repeated small doses of radiation are less damaging to a sensitive cell than a single total dose. Cell nuclei are the major sites of radiation damage leading to cell death.

The tumour may be radioresistant or radiosensitive. Radiosensitivity is the relative susceptibility of cells, tissues, organ or organisms to the effect of the ionizing radiation. Generally rapidly dividing tumours are more radiosensitive to irradiation than slow growing tumour.

Radiocurability and Radiosensitivity

Radiocurability and radiosensitivity are common terminology used to measures the effectiveness of radiation therapy. Radiocurability is the ability of radiation therapy to eliminate or cure the tumour at either the primary site or metastatic site through direct effect of irradiation. Radiosensitivity is the response of the tumour to irradiation that can be measured by the extent and length of time of regression.

Radiosensitivity is not equal to radiocurability; a radiosensitive tumour may not be cured by radiation therapy if the disease has already metastasized. However, radioresistant tumour, if localized and accessible to high dose radiation therapy, can be cured, e.g. squamous cell carcinoma of the cervix.

Radiosensitivity of the tumour is depending on many factors, and the most important factors are:

(a) **Hypoxia**: Higher the hypoxic fraction of cells, less responsive the tumour to radiation. Exophytic friable cervical lesion with higher blood supply and better oxygenation respond better to radiation than endophytic/infiltrative cervical lesions. Hypoxic cells require 3× radiation dose needed by well-oxygenated cells. Surgical removal of the hypoxic cells decreases the radiation dose required and increases the probability of the local control.

(b) **Proportion of active proliferating cell**: More proportion of an active cell, more sensitive to radiation.

(c) **Type of tumour**: Dysgerminoma is more radiosensitive (requires 20–30 Gy) than cervical cancer (requires >70 Gy).

Tumour cells usually proliferate faster than the normal tissues. Shortening the time interval between surgery and radiation therapy reduces the repopulation of tumour cells, therefore long delay in the interval is best avoided.

Radiosensitivity of tumour can be predicted based on the following features:

(a) **Mitotic count**: High mitotic count and poor response;

(b) **Volume of tumour**: more volume, require higher dose;

(c) **A portion of tumour**: The central portion has less blood supply and, therefore, requires higher dose compared to the periphery with better oxygenation;

(d) **Cell cycle phase**: Cell in phase M is more sensitive to radiation than phase S (M and G2 are the most sensitive phase).

The other commonly used term in radiation therapy is the therapeutic ratio, which is defined as the relationship between the desired and unwanted effects of therapy. The aim of any radiotherapy is to achieve a high therapeutic ratio, which means good cancer control but fewer injuries to adjacent normal organs. One method to reduce the risk of normal tissue injury and increase the therapeutic ratio is dividing the treatment into 20–30 separate treatments and given daily over 4–6 weeks (fractionation).

Effects of Irradiation on Foetus

Moderately large doses of radiation (>200 cGy) delivered to the human embryo before 2–3-week gestation are not likely to produce severe abnormalities in most children born, although a considerable number of embryos may be resorbed or aborted (all or none phenomenon).

Irradiation between 4- and 11-week gestation leads to severe abnormality of many organs in most or all children. Irradiation between 11 and 16-week gestation may produce few eye, skeletal and genital organ abnormalities but stunted growth. Microcephaly and mental retardation are also frequently present. Irradiation between 16 to 30 weeks may lead to a mild degree of microcephaly, mental retardation and IUGR. Irradiation after 30 weeks is not likely to produce gross structural abnormalities.

General Concepts of Clinical Radiation Therapy

There are basically two modalities of radiation treatment:

(a) **External irradiation or external beam radiation therapy (EBRT)**: also known as teletherapy when the radiation source lies at a distance from the body.

(b) **Local irradiation (brachytherapy)**: sources are in direct proximity to the tumour. There are at least four types of brachytherapy:

   (a) intra-cavitary irradiation
   (b) interstitial irradiation
   (c) direct therapy
   (d) intra-peritoneal or intra-pleural

There are various machines or equipment for EBRT, such as linear accelerator (Fig. 12.1), Telecobalt Unit (Cobalt-60) and Telecaesium Unit. New equipment for EBRT comprises stereotactic radiotherapy and stereotactic radiosurgery (gamma knife). Linear accelerator is the most common EBRT machine, which is used to produce, X-rays of energy 6–20 MeV (Million electron volts).

Generally, there are four clinical uses of radiation therapy:

(a) **Radical radiotherapy** to produce a high rates of local tumour control (as primary treatment)
(b) **Adjuvant radiotherapy** to eradicate a loco-regional residual microscopic disease
(c) **Neoadjuvant radiotherapy** given prior to primary treatment usually surgery to increase operability by downstaging
(d) **Palliative radiotherapy** for pain (bone metastasis, visceral pain, etc.), bleeding, tumour obstruction of the hollow viscera (bronchus, rectum, etc.), superior vena cava obstruction, spinal cord compression, symptomatic nodal disease, etc.

Palliative radiotherapy is given over a shorter period of time with larger fraction sizes but a lower overall dose. Treatment may be given as a single fraction, e.g. 8–10 Gy or as a short fractionated course, e.g. 20 Gray in 5 fractions, 30 Gy in 10 fractions.

In Gynaecological cancer, standard pelvic radiotherapy (EBRT) is given to the following target volumes: (a) Primary tumour and (b) Pelvic lymph nodes up to the external iliac group. There are four boundaries (borders) in standard pelvic RT, i.e. upper border (L5-S1), inferior border (inferior border of obturator foramen), lateral border (1–2 cm from the edge of the pelvic brim/pelvic wall) and posterior border. Posterior border varies according to the site of primary tumour (mid-symphysis pubis anteriorly and middle of S2 posteriorly).

Each treatment session is called a fraction; for EBRT each fraction delivers 1.8–2.0 Gy and is given for 4–5 days in a week for 5–7 weeks (total dose ranging from 50–70 Gy). The lower the dose and the higher the fractionation, the better the normal tissue tolerance of the radiation given.

Brachytherapy is the treatment with radioactive material implanted or located very close to the tumour-bearing area (Fig. 22.2). Radioisotopes commonly used in brachytherapy are iridium, caesium, iodine and palladium. Current brachytherapy uses a remote afterloading unit where the delivery of radioisotope can be controlled from remote area to reduce the exposure to the staffs. There are two types of brachytherapy, i.e. low-dose-rate (LDR) brachytherapy and high-dose-rate (HDR) brachytherapy. Low dose rate requires admission to the hospital and lasts for 3 days with single or more insertion/fractions. High-dose-rate brachytherapy is delivered for a few minutes in each treatment session with a total of two to seven insertions within 1–2 weeks.

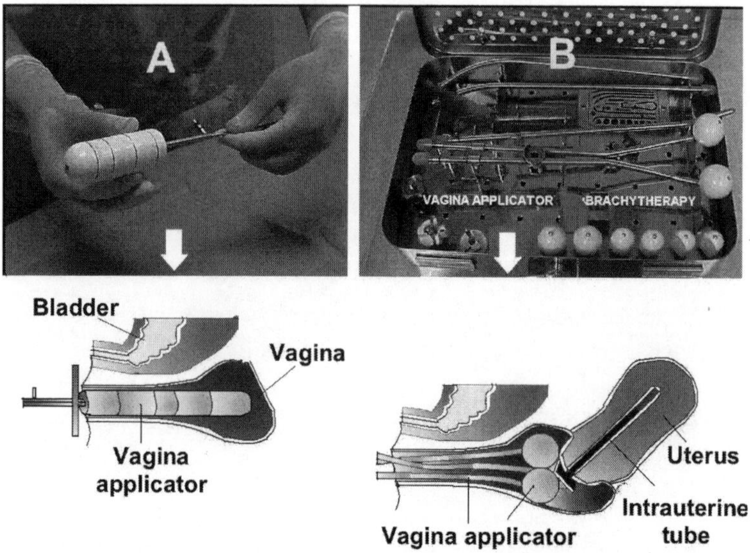

Figure 22.2 Brachytherapy; insertion of vaginal applicator. A: patient without the uterus and B: patient with uterus. The types of vagina applicator used in both patients are different.

Brachytherapy allows a high radiation dose to the tumour with low doses to the surrounding tissue; hence, it results in less toxicity to the surrounding normal tissues. Low-dose-rate brachytherapy delivers 0.4–2 Gy per hour radiation with a total of 30 Gy to point A (single dose for 24 hours). High-dose-rate brachytherapy delivers >12 Gy per hour, total 2–4 insertions/fractions; 1–2 insertions per week. Each insertion delivers 6 Gy within a few minutes. The most popular LDR source is caesium-137, while the most widely used HDR source is iridium-192.

Pelvic radiation delivered for a total dose of 5000 cGy given in five daily fractions each week for 5 weeks (total 25 fractions) is well tolerated in most instances. In gynaecological cancer, often both EBRT and BRT were given to a patient and BRT was initiated after the completion of EBRT.

The term **hyperfractionated irradiation** refers to the therapy given more than once daily, i.e. when the daily dose is divided into two treatment sessions, without changing the length of the treatment, while **accelerated irradiation** is when the total dose of radiation is given over a shorter period of time by giving the same dose of radiation more frequently (more than once a day).

Effects of Irradiation on Abdominal and Pelvic Normal Tissues

Similar to other treatment modalities, radiotherapy is not without risk. The tolerance of irradiated tissue depends on four factors:

(a) the fractionation technique
(b) total dose given
(c) dose rate
(d) volume irradiated

Cervix and uterus have very high tolerance to radiotherapy. Small bowel has better tolerance than large bowel because of its mobility, unless if it is immobile because of adhesion. Bladder tolerates more than sigmoid colon and rectum to radiotherapy.

According to a radiobiologist, in case of injury to normal tissues, only 5–20% of the damage is repairable. Therefore, repeat radiation at the same site is not recommended when the patient develops recurrence or new cancer. The risk of radiation toxicity to small bowel is less than large bowel because of the mobility of this organ. However, the risk will increase if the small bowel entrapped within the adhesion or adhered to the pelvis or abdominal wall. Attempt must be made to minimize adhesion formation during surgery to reduce the risk of radiation effect on bowels. Surgery like Wertheim's hysterectomy and lymph node sampling increased the risk of the radiation complications to large and small bowel. The retroperitoneal approach has decreased this complication rate and is the preferred method to evaluate the status of lymph node in cervical and endometrial cancer.

There are several other factors that contributing to the risk of radiation injuries:

(a) general and nutritional condition of the patient
(b) hygiene
(c) superimposed infection
(d) trauma (physical or chemical)

Potential Sites and Nature of Radiation Injuries in Gynaecologic Cancer Patients

- **Skin**: Acute effects are erythema (>20 Gy), desquamation, ulceration, necrosis (dose > 65 Gy). Late effects are atrophy of epidermis, loss of hair follicles, sebaceous gland and sweat glands, telangiectasia and hyperpigmentation.
- **Small and large intestines**: Acute: watery diarrhoea, intermittent abdominal pain (second to third week), absorption problem, rectal discomfort, tenesmus and mucus/blood in stool if the rectum included in the radiation. Ulceration and fibrosis leading to stenosis, perforation and fistula can occur (>60 Gy). *Doxorubicin and 5-FU enhance radiation effects in the intestine more than other cytotoxic agents.*
- **Liver**: Elevated liver enzyme (i.e. ALP), liver enlargement and acsites (dose > 30 Gy); with lower dose hepatitis can occur if concomitant chemotherapy.
- **Kidney**: Radiation nephritis (within 6 months of irradiation >20 Gy in 3–5 weeks) with symptoms of lassitude, headache, SOB, vomiting, nocturia and leg oedema. Signs are proteinuria, haematuria and hypertension. A late effect is chronic nephritis (after 18 months).
- **Bladder**: Radiation cystitis (acute) (>30 Gy)-self limiting condition in most cases. With a dose of >60 Gy to entire bladder, chronic cystitis and haematuria can occur. Other complications include fibrosis, decreased bladder capacity and vesicovaginal fistula.
- **Ovary**: In most of the radiation therapy to the abdomen, ovary will be exposed to about 1–2 Gy, transient effect to granulosa cell can occur leading to irregular menses and amenorrhoea. In a larger dose, the injury will be more severe, i.e. oocyte degeneration, follicles atrophy, etc. Permanent injury to the ovary is manifested as hypooestrogenaemia and elevated gonadotrophin hormones (single dose of 6.5–8 Gy or fractionated dose of 15–20 Gy exposure).
- **Vagina**: Radiation may lead to inflammation and thinning of the vaginal mucosa, scarring of the area may occur as it heals and can interfere with the ability of the vagina to stretch. Occasionally, ulceration, pain and post-coital bleeding can

occur. The radiation could shorten and narrow the vagina, which may interfere with sexual intercourse.

- **Bone marrow**: Acute effect normally observed after whole body radiation, i.e. reduction in lymphocytes then WBC (within hour). Granulocytopenia occurs after a day. Recovery occurs after 2–3 weeks. Thrombocytopenia occurs a bit later. More severe effect is permanent bone marrow damage.
- **Peripheral nerves**: Lumbosacral plexopathy—rare complication of pelvic irradiation.
- **Second cancer**: Theoretically, radiation can induce new cancer based on the knowledge about the link between radiation and cancer recognized among atomic bomb survivals. The incidence is unknown but very low, and it takes many years. Some cases of leukaemia are related to radiation exposure. Radiation to the chest has also been linked to the breast cancer and there was reported case of uterine cancer, bladder cancer and rectal cancer diagnosed many years after pelvic irradiation for cervical cancer. However, the radiation dose associated with the risk of second cancer was very high. For most cancers associated with radiation, risks were highest among long-term survivors and appeared concentrated among women irradiated at relatively younger ages (Boice et al.).

Combination of Irradiation with Other Therapeutic Modalities

Radiation therapy can be either alone or in combination with other modalities. It can be given pre-operatively, intra-operatively or post-operatively.

The rationales of pre-operative radiation therapy are

(a) to eradicate a subclinical disease beyond the margins of the surgical resection.
(b) to diminish tumour implantation by decreasing viable cell during operation.
(c) to sterilize lymph node metastases outside the operative field.
(d) to decrease potential for dissemination of clonogenic tumour cells that might metastases.

(e) to facilitate subsequent surgical treatment and increases the chances of optimal cytoreduction.

The main disadvantage of pre-operative radiation is it may interfere with normal healing of tissue affected by surgery.

Post-operative radiation therapy is the most common mode of radiation therapy in gynaecological cancers. The rationales of giving radiation therapy after surgery are

(a) destroying subclinical foci of tumour cells following surgery.
(b) eradicating adjacent subclinical foci, including LN.
(c) more effective in eradicating residual tumour due to smaller volume.

The potential disadvantage of post-operative radiation is that the initiation can only be started after wound healing and radiation effect may be affected by impairment of blood supply produced in tumour bed by surgery.

Radiation therapy can also be combined with chemotherapy either sequentially or concomitantly. Concomitant chemoradiation is currently the treatment of choice in many cancers, including cervical cancer. Combination of radiation therapy and other modalities of cancer treatment was found to be beneficial in many aspects. However, at the same time it also enhances normal tissue toxicity and should be administered with cautious and in selected patients.

Processes of Radiation Therapy

Radiation therapy is a complex process and involves many steps. Following is the step-by-step summary of radiotherapy processes (seven steps):

(1) **Pre-planning and counselling**: The patient is seen by radiation oncologist and complete information will be given to a patient regarding the reasons for therapy and technique involved. Ideally, the patient and family members should be seen by a team of specialists comprising surgical oncologist, radiation oncologist, oncology nurse, etc.

(2) **Treatment Planning**: Activities involved in the planning are a definition of the treatment volumes, prescription of the radiation dose and production of a treatment plan and the associated dataset needed for its implementation. The method of the patient's positioning and immobilization is also

determined to ensure that patient is going to be treated in the same position every day, comfortable than reproducible. Treatment planning is the most crucial part of the radiotherapy process (Fig. 22.4).

(3) **Choice of target volume**: The target volume must include gross tumour volume (gross tumour) and clinical target volume (predicted microscopic tumour around the gross tumour). Planning target volume (PTV) is an extended area from CTV and GTV taking into account for day-to-day variation due to patient and organ movement (Fig. 22.3).

(4) **Target volume localization and simulation**: Tumour localization is achieved with diagnostic imaging information such as X-ray, CT scan, and MRI and the use of a simulator. AcQSIM is an example of CT-based tumour localizer; AcQSIM software allows the radiologist/oncologist to rapidly visualize and localize a tumour and critical anatomy, then subsequently mark the patient's skin. Surface markings and tattoos are applied to help radiographers to produce the same field on each day of treatment.

(5) **Dosimetry**: Dosimetry is a calculation of the amount of radiation doses absorbed by the patient.

(6) **Treatment delivery**: The patient is positioned and beam parameters are set (gantry angles, beam collimation, etc.). Prescribed dose is then checked, and treatment is then delivered to a patient.

(7) **Verification**: To ensure the accuracy of the treatment through check-X-ray or using portal imaging systems that utilize computer software programs to produce images of the treated area.

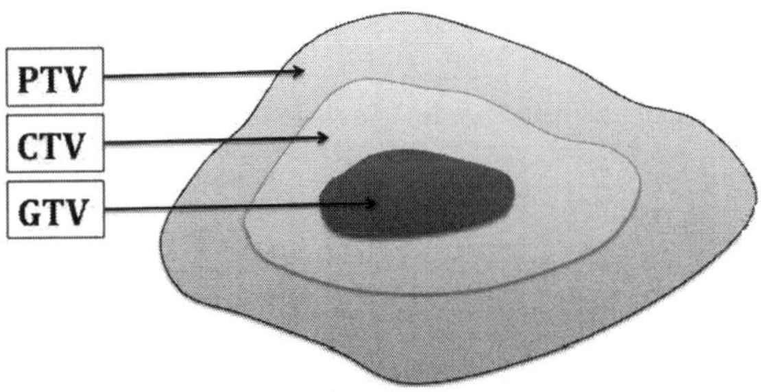

Figure 22.3 *Target volume. PTV:* planning target volume, *CTV: clinical target volume, GTV: gross tumour volume.*

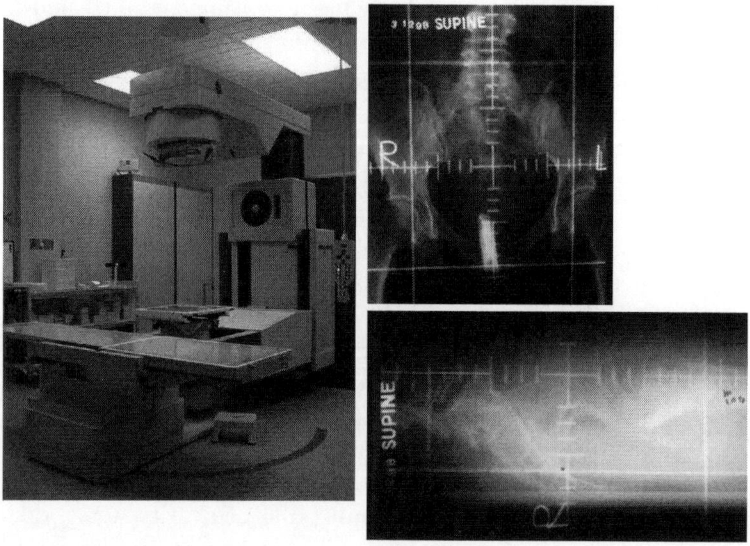

Figure 22.4 *One of the processes in planning of radiotherapy.*

Current Developments in Radiotherapy

The improvement of diagnostic imaging such as CT scans and MRI has been immensely helpful in radiation treatment planning. With these modalities together with sophisticated software, the accuracy and treatment planning has been improved and at the same time reduces the possibility of a "geographical miss".

Accurate localization of target volume can also reduce the volume of normal tissue irradiated by up to 50%. This is called "conformal" radiotherapy and one of the most important equipment to achieve this is via an apparatus known as a multi-leaf collimator which is located at the head of the linear accelerator (gantry comprising more than 40 pairs of tungsten bars. As compared to conventional shielding method using lead block, tungsten bars in the multi-leaf collimator can move independently to shape the treatment beam to irregular contours.

Intensified Modulated Radiation Therapy

Intensified modulated radiation therapy (IMRT) is a more advanced form of conformal radiotherapy. It is relatively a new technology and with this technology, target volume will receive radiation in precision and minimal effect on surrounding normal structure. Therefore, higher dose can be given to the primary tumour and improve the cure rate without increasing toxicity to adjacent normal organs. Intensified modulated radiation therapy is based on the concept of inverse treatment planning, which means than the clinician defines the treatment volume and surrounding normal tissue volumes and specifies certain dose restrictions on these volumes. The computer then calculates optimisation of beam parameters. With this information, the computer is then able to control the shape of the radiation beam and modify its intensity by moving multi-leaf collimators in and out of the treatment field. One of the main interests in gynaecological malignancy is radiotherapy for cervical cancer; IMRT may play an important role in the treatment of locally advanced cervical cancer to improve cure rate and significantly reduce gastrointestinal and genitourinary toxicity.

Image-Guided Radiation Therapy

In image-guided radiation therapy (IGRT), repeated imaging scan (CT, MRI or PET) are performed during treatment. These imaging scans are processed by computers to identify changes in a tumour's size and location due to treatment and to allow the adjustment of the patient's position and dose of radiation. This technique will allow reductions in the planned volume of tissue to be treated, thereby decreasing the total radiation dose to normal tissue. **Tomotherapy** is one of IGRT methods whereby the machine (with both treatment and imaging) can rotate completely around the patient similar to normal CT scanner.

Stereotactic Radiosurgery

Stereotactic radiosurgery is a 3D technique that delivers the radiation dose in one fraction by specially designed collimators attached to the linear accelerator. This technique will deliver a high dose of radiation to a small volume usually about 3 cm diameter. Stereotactic radiosurgery can be used in the treatment of arteriovenous malformation and brain tumour.

Other Types and Methods of Radiotherapy

Electron Radiation Therapy

Gamma-rays are delivered by radioisotope, while X-rays originate from outside the nucleus produced by bombardment of a target by high-speed electrons. Both gamma-rays and X-rays are also known as photons. The other type of radiation therapy is known as particle radiation therapy (electrons, protons, neutrons, alpha particles, and beta particles). **Electron radiation therapy** is delivered by the linear accelerator and used to irradiate superficial tumours such as skin cancer or tumour near the surface of the body. The other particles used for radiation are proton beams and neutron beams.

Proton Beams

Proton beams are a newer form of particle beam radiation; they cause little damage to tissues they pass through but are very good at killing cells at the end of their path. Proton beams differ from proton beams, mainly in the way they deposit energy in living tissue. Whereas protons deposit energy in small packets all along their path through tissue, protons deposit much of their energy at the end of their path (called the Bragg peak) and deposit less energy along the way. Proton beams may be able to deliver more radiation to the cancer while causing fewer side effects to normal tissues nearby. Proton beam radiation, however, requires highly specialized equipment and expertise.

Neutron Beam Therapy

Neutron beam therapy is another particle beam therapy often used to treat inoperable tumours or tumours that are radioresistant. Neutrons have a greater biologic impact on cells than other types of radiation. Neutron beam is effective even to hypoxic tissues/cells. The concern about neutron beams is toxicity. It has been applied for salivary tumour, prostate and some sarcomas.

Intra-Operative Radiation Therapy

Intra-operative radiation therapy (IORT) is another type of radiation where the patient, while undergoing a surgery, is put under a radiation machine or source and fine beam is being concentrated on the tumour bed. This is mainly helpful in areas, which are deep seated and difficult to treat with EBRT due to intervening normal tissues. The high-energy electron beams have been utilized in IORT. Some encouraging results with IORT have been reported in the treatment of various tumours of head and neck, paediatric soft tissue sarcomas, colorectal tumours, etc. Intra-operative radiation therapy can also be delivered in form of brachytherapy (IOHDR), especially in dealing with tumour in the pelvis, chest and skull base.

Hyperthermia and Radiotherapy

Hyperthermia and radiotherapy can be used either as a primary modality or as an adjunct to a cytotoxic drug or irradiation. This technique is still investigational and may be useful for the treatment of lesions that have previously failed to respond to other methods. The first notable use of hyperthermia in gynaecologic oncology is the use of interstitial hyperthermia for deep tumour of the pelvis. The tumour was exposed to a temperature of 43–44 degree for 30–40 minutes using radiofrequency heat followed by radiation 1–3 hours later.

Basic Equipment for Radiotherapy in Gynaecology Oncology

(1) High-dose-rate brachytherapy equipment (Fig. 22.5)

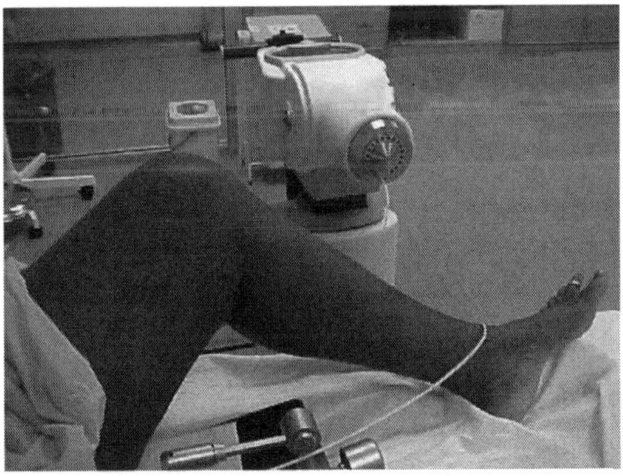

Figure 22.5 Nucleatron microselectron is the machine that delivers HDR brachytherapy. The radiation source is iridium (in pallets, delivered via long tubing that is connected to the vagina applicator).

Vaginal applicator for brachytherapy

(a) The patient with a uterus has two options: either three-channel (if their vagina is spacious) or one-channel applicator if the vaginal cavity is narrow or small (Fig. 22.6).

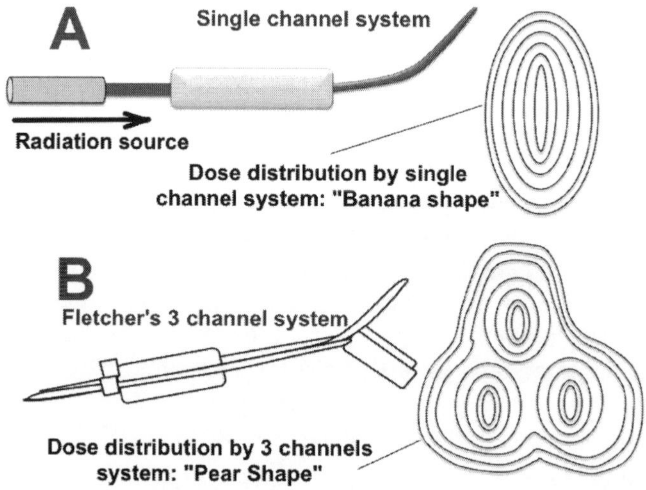

Figure 22.6 Brachytherapy in form of two- or three-channel system.

(b) Vaginal applicator for a patient without uterus is shown in Fig. 22.7.

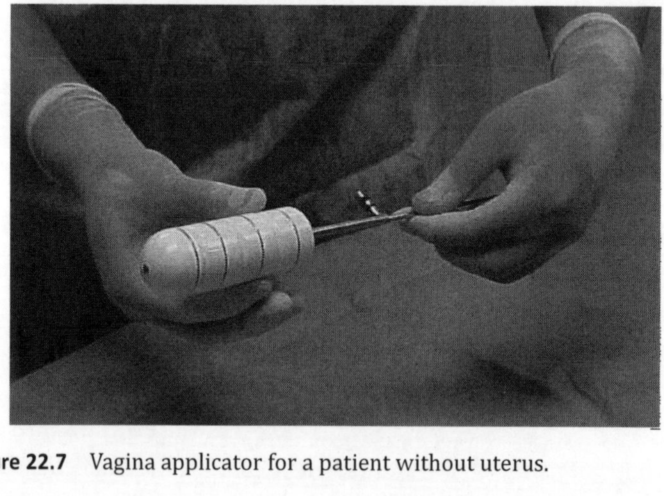

Figure 22.7 Vagina applicator for a patient without uterus.

(2) **Low-dose-rate brachytherapy unit** (Fig. 22.8)

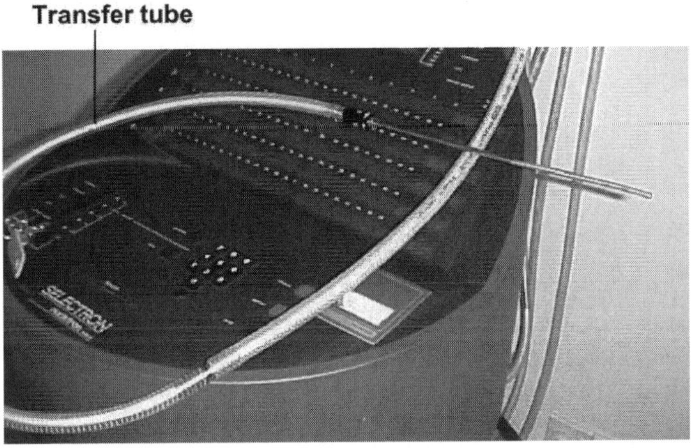

Figure 22.8 An example of the LDR brachytherapy unit. The patient has to be admitted, and the treatment lasts 24–30 hours.

(3) **External beam radiotherapy unit: linear accelerator** (Fig. 22.9)

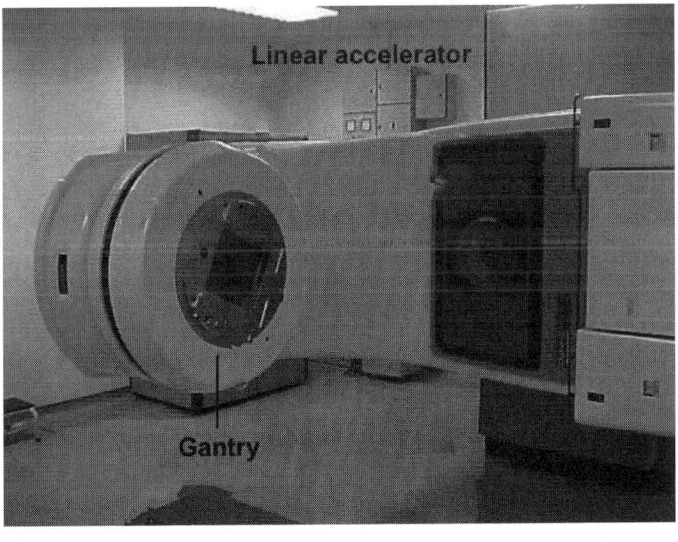

Figure 22.9 Linear accelerator machine. High-voltage X-ray beam is emitted from the gantry.

Shielding for EBRT

Shielding is the method used to provide protection for healthy tissue during radiotherapy of malignant tissue. In conventional method, shielding is provided by application of lead blocks and plate at the end of the gantry as shown in Fig. 22.10. There will be no radiation pass through the block/shield. Apart from shielding, wedge is also applied to filter the dose to ensure target volume received high dose, while the normal adjacent organ received minimal dose. The other new method of shielding is using multi-leaf collimator (MLC). Multi-leaf collimator is a device made up of individual "leaves" of a high atomic number material, usually tungsten (Fig. 22.11), that can move independently in and out of the path of a particle beam in order to block it. MLCs are used on linear accelerators to provide conformal shaping of radiotherapy treatment beams.

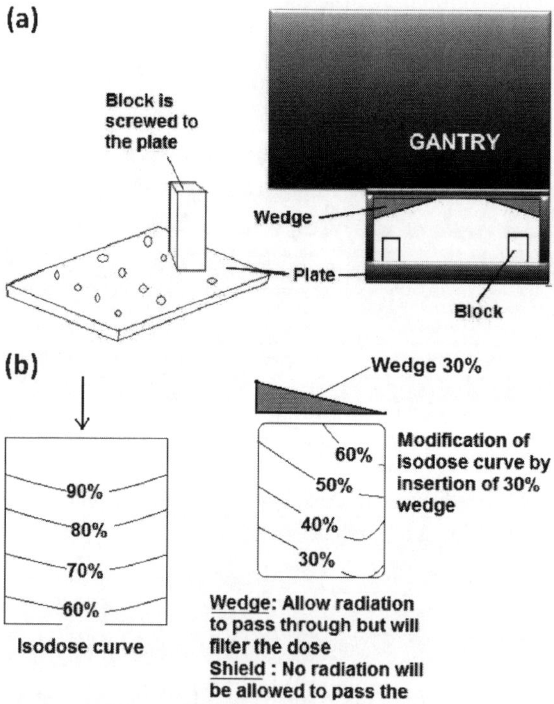

Figure 22.10 Shielding using conventional method with plate and block (a) and wedge is used to filter the dose (b).

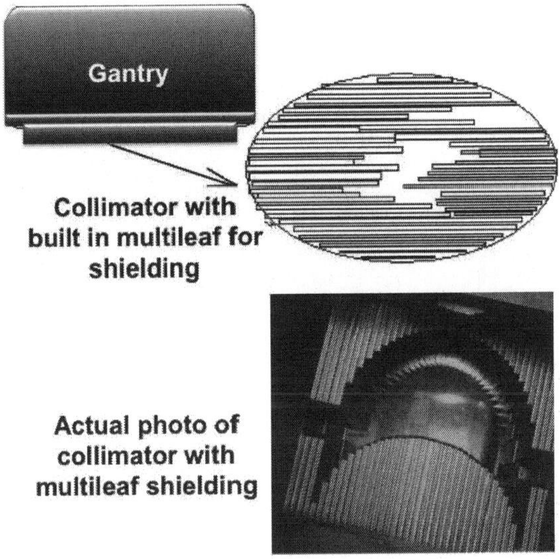

Figure 22.11 Collimator with built-in multileaf for shielding during EBRT.

References

American Cancer Society. Support and Treatment. Radiation therapy principles. Access at http://www.cancer.org/Treatment/Treatment-sandSideEffects/TreatmentTypes/Radiation/Radiation TherapyPrinciples, August 2010.

Boice JD, Engholm G, Kleinerman RA, et al. Radiation dose and second cancer risk in patients treated for cancer of the cervix. *Radiat Res* 1988; **116**: 3–55.

Kohler MF, Creasman WT. Radiation therapy in gynaecology. *eMed Obstet Gynaecol, updated*: July 22, 2008.

National Cancer Institute. Radiation Therapy for Cancer: Questions and Answers. Accessed at www.cancer.gov/cancertopics/factsheet/Therapy/radiation on June 29, 2009.

Rushdan MN. *Summary in Gynaecology Oncology*, 2nd, ed., 2009.

Schreiber GJ. Radiation therapy, general principles. *E-Medicine*, January 29, 2010.

Shafiq J, Barton M, Noble D, et al. Systematic Review. An international review of patient safety measures in radiotherapy practice. *Radiother Oncology* 2009; **92**: 15–21.

Sridhar T, Symonds RP. Principles of chemotherapy and radiotherapy. *Obstet, Gynaecol Rep Med* 2008; **19**(3): 61–67.

Symonds RP. Principles of gynaecological chemotherapy and radiotherapy. *Curr Obstet Gynaecol* 2003; **13**: 102–109.

Symonds RP, Foweraker K. Principles of chemotherapy and radiotherapy. *Curr Obstet Gynaecol* 2006; **16**: 100–106.

Chapter 23

Basic Principles of Chemotherapy

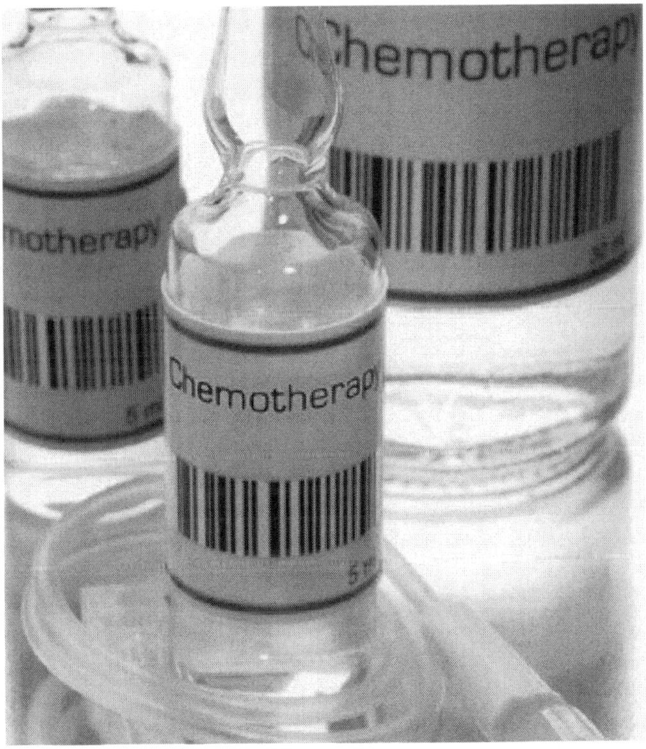

Gynaecologic Cancer: A Handbook for Students and Practitioners
Rushdan Noor, Eng Hseon Tay, and Jeffrey Low

ISBN 978-981-4463-06-5 (Hardcover), 978-981-4463-07-2 (eBook)
www.panstanford.com

Introduction

In cancer management, both surgery and radiotherapy are essentially local treatments directed at the primary tumour and any loco-regional disease. Chemotherapy is a systemic treatment and can treat distant metastases. In the majority of cancers, chemotherapy is used to improve the prognosis and curative only in minority of cancers. It is known that, chemotherapy is curative in lymphomas, leukaemias, testicular cancers and in choriocarcinoma.

The ideal anti-neoplastic drugs eradicate cancer cells without harming normal cells. However, current anti-neoplastic drugs have significant toxicity because it has difficulty distinguishing malignant from normal cells. To understand how anti-neoplastic drugs act on cancer cells, it is very important to understand the basic biology of normal and cancer cells (tumour biology).

In the early phases of growth, tumour cells appear to grow exponentially, but as tumour mass increases, the time that a particular tumour requires to double its volume appears to increase. The time taken to double their volume is called volume-doubling time. There are three main explanations why the volume-doubling time is prolonged: (a) increase in cell cycle time (mitosis to next mitosis), (b) decrease in the growth fraction (active cells) and (c) increase in cell loss (lack of nutrients).

The suitability of chemotherapy depends on the nature of neoplasm, extent of spread or stage and the patient's clinical condition or performance status. Not all cancers are chemosensitive. This depends on (a) how the drug distributed to the tumour, (b) drug transportation into the cell, (c) presence of drug-sensitive biochemical pathways in target cells and (d) relative rate of intra-cellular activation and inactivation of the drug.

Basic Cell Cycles

Stages of Cell Cycle

The cell cycle is an ordered set of events, culminating in cell growth and division into two daughter cells. Non-dividing cells are not considered to be in the cell cycle

- There are two phases in the cell cycle:
  (a) interphase
  (b) mitosis

Interphase

Interphase is further divided into the following stages (Fig. 23.1):

(a) **G1** (Gap 1): 46 chromatids
(b) **S** (synthesis): DNA replication occurs resulting in 46 pairs (92) of chromatids
(c) **G2** (Gap 2): 2 chromatids join at centromere (become chromosomes) and centrioles duplicate

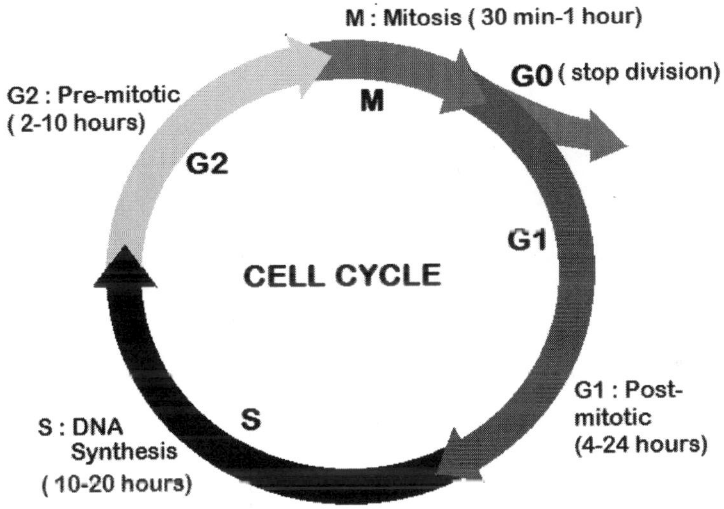

Figure 23.1 The cell cycle.

Mitosis

Stages of mitosis (Mnemonics: **PPMAT**)

- **Prophase** (Chromatin begins to condense, nucleolus disappears and centriols move to opposite ends)
- **Prometaphase** (Nuclear membrane dissolves, proteins attach to centromeres forming a kinetochores. Microtubules attach at kinetochores and chromosomes begin moving)

- **Metaphase** (chromosomes line up in the equatorial plane (middle) of the cells (Spindle fibres align the chromosomes along the middle of the cell nucleus)
- **Anaphase** (Chromosome migrates towards opposite poles, movement results from a combination of kinetochore movement along the spindle microtubules and physical interaction of polar microtubules)
- **Telophase** (Chromatids arrive at opposite poles, new membranes from around the daughter nuclei, cell wall begins to contract).

Gompertzian Growth Concepts

As a tumour mass increases in size, its mass-doubling time becomes progressively longer (see Fig. 23.2). A metastatic tumour is more sensitive to chemotherapy than primary tumour and it is more sensitive to cell cycle–specific agents.

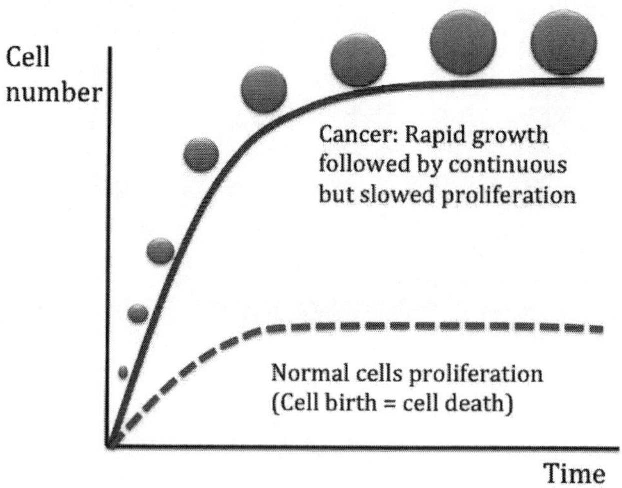

Figure 23.2 Gompertzian growth concepts.

Generation and Doubling Time

Generation time is the duration of time for cell to complete one cycle of growth. Lesser the blood supply, longer the generation time.

The **doubling time** for tumour depends on the generation time and the rate of cell death.

Tumours do not have faster generation times but have more cells in the active phases of replication than normal tissues. Normal tissues have a large number of cells in the Go phase.

The doubling time of the tumour is the time it takes for the mass to double its size.

(a) Embryonal tumour and lymphomas have shorter doubling time (20–40 days), while squamous cell and adenocarcinoma have longer doubling time (50–150 days).
(b) Metastatic tumour has generally shorter doubling time than primary tumour.
(c) One centimetre tumour mass may have undergone 30 doublings.
(d) In the late stages of tumour growth, small doublings will result in a very significant increase in tumour mass. Once the tumour becomes palpable, i.e. 1 cm, only three more doublings will produce a very large tumour mass (8 cm diameter).

One milligram of tumour usually consists of 1,000,000 cells. One cubic centimetre tumour consists of 1 billion cells but not all of these cells are viable, and it is the clonogenic cell component that must be destroyed. Two basic factors that regulate the speed of tumour growth are

(a) growth fraction (number of tumour cell that actively involved in cell divisions
(b) cell death

There are actually only small fractions of rapidly proliferating cells within a tumour mass. The majority of cells are often out of the cell cycle and resting. Anti-neoplastic agents appear to work by first-order kinetics, i.e. they kill a constant fraction of cells rather than a constant number.

Types of Anti-Neoplastic Agents Related to Cell Cycle

Most anti-neoplastic agents work by interfering with DNA synthesis or function. The anti-neoplastic drugs can be divided into two subgroups:

(a) **Cell cycle–specific agents** (effective during certain phases of the cell cycle)

(b) **Non-cell cycle–specific agents** (effective during all phases of the cell cycle)

The examples of a cell cycle–specific agents are (a) S-phase-specific agents (anti-metabolite (flourouracil, methotrexate [MTX]), topoisomerase I and II inhibitors, gemcitabine, etc.) and (b) G2-M phase-specific agents (bleomycin, vincristine, vinblastine, taxanes).

The examples of the non-cell cycle–specific agents are (a) alkylating agents (cyclophosphamide, ifosfamide, melphalan), (b) platinum (cisplatin, carboplatin), (c) bleomycin and (d) actinomycin D.

The rationale of sequential treatment of the non-cell cycle–specific agents and cell cycle–specific agents is that the first group will reduce the size of tumour mass, and once the tumour mass is reduced in size, there will be a higher percentage of metabolically active cells. These active cells will be tackling by subsequent cell cycle–specific agents, e.g. MTX.

At any given time, comparatively large numbers of cancer cells will be in the DNA synthesis phase (S), the only time during which cycle-dependent agents (those inhibiting DNS synthesis) can act. Thus, short-term high-dose cycle-dependent agents such as MTX are most effective in killing rapidly dividing tumour cells with relatively sparing of the normal bone marrow elements. Unfortunately, bone marrow cells, the epithelial cells lining the GIT and hair follicles all have generation times comparable to those of tumours and are therefore, vulnerable to compounds that inhibit DNA synthesis.

Tumour cell population grows more synchronously than cells in bone marrow, of which only small proportion is in S phase at a given time; hence, this explains the selectivity of phase-dependent compound.

Non-cycle–specific agents, e.g. akylating agents, are more effective against bulky and slow-growing tumour. Once the tumour mass is reduced, cells grow faster, i.e. more proportion of cell will be active; therefore, the cells are more sensitive to cell cycle–specific agents, e.g. MTX. This phenomenon during recovery after the effect of alkylating agents is the rationale of sequentially combining non-cycle–specific with cycle–specific agents in a new regime. Since, DNA is a main target site for these drugs, maximum cell killing is not possible when cells are in the S phase at the time of drug administration.

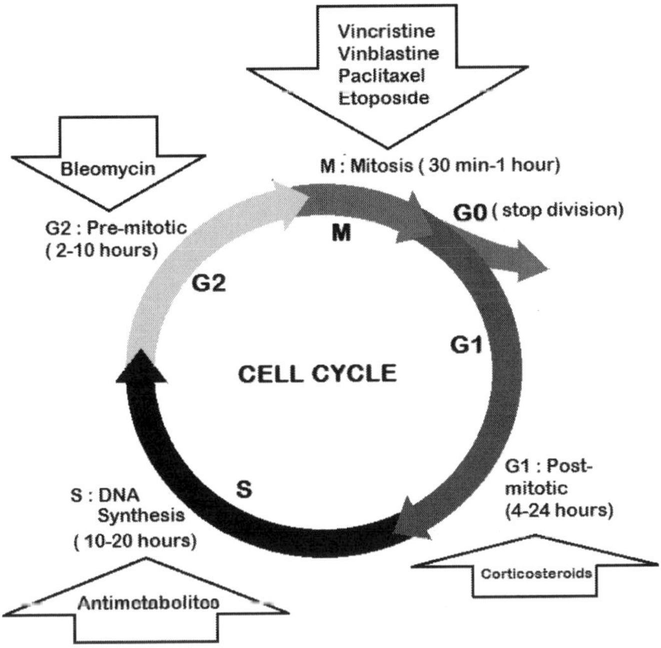

Figure 23.3 Cell cycle and anti-neoplastic drugs.

Drug Resistance

The effectiveness of any cancer treatment is limited by the development of acquired drug resistance. The actual mechanism of single drug resistance followed by multiple-drug resistance is unknown. Resistance to a single drug is usually associated with cross resistance to other drugs as well (including dissimilar drugs). This cross resistance is more commonly seen with drugs from natural products (i.e. doxorubicin, VP16 and vinca alkaloids).

"Goldie-Coldman" hypothesis: Most malignant cells begin with intrinsic sensitivity to chemotherapeutic agents but develop spontaneous resistance at variable rates (due to spontaneous mutation). Therefore, to minimize the emergence of drug resistance requires multiple effective drugs or therapies applied as early as possible throughout the patient's malignant disease process.

The discovery of a mechanism of drug resistance was mainly because of the extensive research carried out on MTX. Methotrexate is a folate antagonist which kills the cancer cells by inhibiting the enzyme dihydrofolate reductase (DHFR), thereby blocking the pathway of de novo DNA synthesis.

There are at least five major mechanisms of drug resistance in cancer cells:

(a) Altered transport of the drug (decreased influx, increase an efflux).
(b) Increase in the total amount of the target enzyme/protein (gene amplification), e.g. an increase in the amount of DHFR enzyme in MTX-resistant cells.
(c) Alteration in the target enzyme/protein (low-affinity enzyme). Mutation can lead to structural change in the target enzyme such as mutation of DHFR resulting in decreased binding affinity of MTX.
(d) Elevation of cellular glutathione (GSH). Glutathione is a tripeptide present in all mammalian cells to protect the cells by destroying the reactive oxygen compounds, free radicals and other toxic compounds either endogenous or exogenous. Drug-resistant tumour cells have been shown to contain much higher level of GSH.
(e) Inhibition of drug-induced apoptosis. Cell death caused by some cytotoxic drug is also dependent on the presence of factors that inhibit apoptosis. Any factor inhibiting apoptosis might lead to development of drug resistance in tumour. Examples of those factors are mutation or deletion of p53 gene products; increase expression of the bcl-2 gene, etc.

The other mechanisms of cytotoxic drug resistance are (a) overproduction of cytochrome P450 protein, (b) overexpression of ATP-binding cassette transporter breast cancer-resistant protein (BCRP), (c) overexpression of S-adenosoylmethionine synthetase and (d) Loss of functional retinoblastoma protein.

An understanding of the mechanism of cytotoxic drug resistance will provide the basis for the development of drugs that can specifically interact with the cause of resistance and restore its sensitivity against cancer cells (Fig. 23.1).

Possible Mechanisms Associated with Resistance to Some Commonly Used Anti-Cancer Drugs

Table 23.1 Mechanism of drug resistance in some commonly used anti-cancer drugs

Mechanism	Drugs
Increase in proficiency of repair of DNA	Alkylating agents, cisplatin
Decrease in cellular uptake or increase in efflux of drugs.	Cisplatin, doxorubicin, VP16, MTX, vinblastine, vincristine
Increased in GSH	Cisplatin
Increase in levels of "target" enzyme	MTX
Decrease in drug activation	Doxorubicin, 5FU
Increase in drug degradation	Bleomycin, cytosine arabinoside
Alternative biochemical pathways	Cytosine arabinoside
Inactivation of active metabolites by binding to sulfhydryl compounds	Alkylating agents, cisplatin, doxorubicin
Decrease activity of topoisomerase	Amsacrine, doxorubicin, etoposide
Alteration in 'target' enzyme	5FU, MTX
Inhibition of drug-induced apoptosis (mutation or deletion of p53)	Adramycin, cisplatin

Categories of Chemotherapeutic Drugs Used in the Treatment of Gynaecological Cancer

Most anti-cancer drugs cause DNA damage through various mechanisms, including disruption of cell cycle checkpoints, growth factors, growth factor receptors and signal transduction.

Alkylating Agents

- Alkylating agents are one of the earliest chemotherapy agents that started to be used in the early 1940s.
- Alkylating agents inhibit DNA replication by forming covalent bonds with DNA bases (cross-linking the DNA strands).

- Examples of alkylating agents are cyclophosphamide, ifosfamide, melphalan, procarbazine, busulfan, etc.
- Chlorambucil is the least toxic and can be given by mouth.
- Cyclophosphamide and ifosfamide can produce an acrolein metabolite which can cause haemorrhagic cystitis.
- Hydration and use of mesna has largely overcome the haemorrhagic cystitis. Mesna is rapidly excreted in the urine and inactivates the acrolein metabolites in the urine.
- Cyclophosphamide is not nephrotoxic and can be used in renal impairment. However, ifosfamide can cause cumulative renal tubular damage resulting in a Fanconi syndrome.

Platinum

- The first platinum-based chemotherapy drug is cisplatin, which was approved in 1978.
- Platinum is probably the most important cytotoxic drug in gynaecological cancer.
- Platinum compounds form DNA cross-links by an action similar to the alkylating agents.
- Cisplatin, carboplatin and recently oxaliplatin are platinum-based cytotoxic drugs.
- Cisplatin is more nephrotoxic and ototoxic than carboplatin.
- Carboplatin is a second-generation and oxaliplatin is the third-generation platinum-based cytotoxic agent.

Anti-Tumour Antibiotics and Anthracylines

- Anti-tumour antibiotics have various modes of action, including DNA cross-linking and topoisomerase inhibition. Some intercalates between base pairs of DNA and RNA inhibit RNA and DNA polymerase, generate oxygen-free radicals and alter cell membrane function.
- The most important members of this drug are doxorubicin (adriamycin) and epirubicin.
- Doxorubicin is isolated from mutated strain of streptomyces.
- Actinomycin D is also anti-tumour antibiotic (polypeptide antibiotic) isolated from the bacteria of the genus Streptomyces.

- Doxorubicin, epirubicin, idarubicin is also known as anthracycline drugs (anthracycline antibiotics).
- The short-term dose-limiting side effects of anthracycline drugs are myelosuppression and mucositis.
- Cardiomyopathy is also a dose-limiting side effect and can be prevented by controlling the total dose and the use of chemo-protectant cardioxane (dexrazoxane) prior to treatment.
- Liposomal doxorubicin is the modified form of doxorubicin to enhance efficacy and reduce the toxicity. The doxorubicin is encapsulated inside the liposome; liposome allows the doxorubicin to remain in the body for a longer duration. Encapsulated doxorubicin is also thought to reduce exposure of the active metabolite to myocardial tissue and therefore, reduces myocardial toxicity. Currently there are two types of liposomal doxorubicin available (differ in their lipid component), i.e. pegylated liposomal doxorubicin hydrochloride (**Caelyx/Doxil**) and **Myocet**. Myocet is indicated as a combination with cyclophosphamide in metastatic breast cancer.
- Bleomycin is also anti-tumour antibiotic, discovered in the 1960s. Bleomycin creates free oxygen radicals that break DNA strands, similar to anthracycline.
- They are commonly used in the treatment of breast cancer, uterine sarcoma and ovarian cancer.

Anti-Metabolites

- Anti-metabolites are cytotoxic agents that structurally resemble naturally occurring purines, pyrimidines and nucleic acids.
- Anti-metabolites can inhibit key enzymes involved in DNA synthesis.
- They can incorporate in the DNA or RNA of the cancer cells and interfere with the cell division process.
- Example of anti-metabolites is MTX, 5-fluorouracil, 6-mercaptopurine, gemcitabine, etc.
- Methotrexate is an anti-folate drug, which is structurally similar to folic acid and inhibits the activity of DHFR enzyme leading to inhibition of DNA and RNA synthesis.

- Gemcitabine is a deoxycytidine analogue, a pyrimidine anti-metabolite related to cytarabine. Gemcitabine is a pro-drug and metabolized intra-cellularly to the active forms known as dFdCDP and dFdCTP. Both active metabolites will incorporate into DNA and inhibit DNA synthesis resulting in apoptosis.

Vinca Alkaloids

- Vinca alkaloids are derived from the periwinkle plant, Vinca rosea (catharanthus roseus) which have been traditionally used by the natives of Madagascar to treat diabetes.
- Vinca alkaloids are also categorized under tubulin-binding drugs together with taxanes.
- Examples of vinca alkaloids are vincristine, vinblastine, vinorelbine and vindesine.
- Vinblastine and vincristine bind to tubulin dimers and prevent their assembly into microtubules.
- These drugs are highly vesicant. This drug should be injected into a central venous line or cannula where there is no resistance to injection and where blood can be freely drawn back.
- Vinorelbine is a synthetic vinca alkaloid that is available both intravenously and orally.

Topoisomerase Inhibitors

- Topoisomerase inhibitors (I and II) are a group of enzymes that allow unwinding and uncoiling of supercoiled DNA.
- Both Topoisomerase inhibitor I and II work by interfering with DNA transcription, replication and function to prevent DNA supercoiling.
- Topoisomerase I inhibitors are extracted from the bark and wood of the Camptotheca accuminata, they form a complex with topoisomerase DNA. Topotecan and Irinotecan are topoisomerase inhibitor I.
- Topoisomerase II inhibitors are extracted from the alkaloids found in the roots of May Apple plants. Topoisomerase II enzyme binds covalently to complementary strands of double-strand DNA, cleaving both strands. The inhibitors of this

enzyme will reseal these breaks. Example of toposimerase II inhibitors is Etoposide, teniposide and amsacrine. They are also classified under epipodophyllotoxins chemotherapy agents.

- The main side effect of topoisomerase inhibitors is haematological toxicity.
- They are excreted by the liver and renal tubules; therefore, dose adjustment may be necessary with renal and hepatic impairment.

Taxanes

- Taxanes are plant alkaloids that were first developed for therapeutic use in 1963.
- Taxanes are extracted from the yew tree.
- Paclitaxel is the first taxane discovered in 1971 and was made available for clinical use in 1993. Paclitaxel is isolated from the bark of the Western yew tree.
- Docetaxel is the second generation of taxanes derived from the needles of the European yew trees.
- Both paclitaxel and docetaxel work in the M-phase of the cell cycle and inhibit the function of microtubules by binding with them resulting in a sustained block in mitosis.

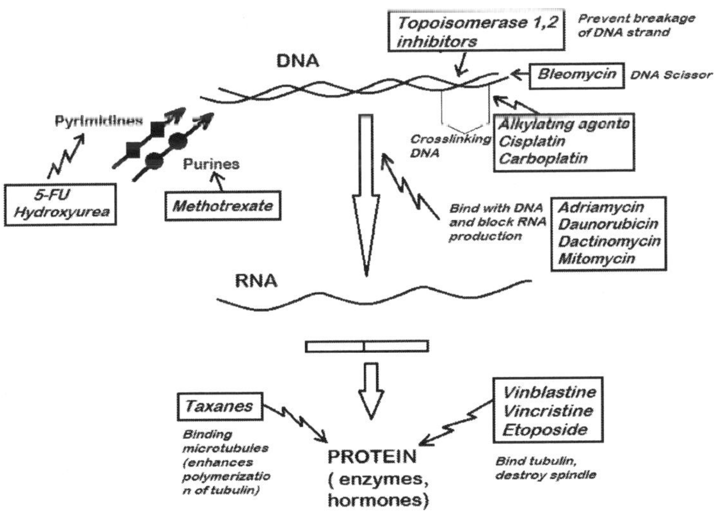

Figure 23.4 Mode of actions of commonly used anti-neoplastic drugs.

The summary of mode of actions of commonly used anti-neoplastic drugs in gynaecological cancers is shown in Fig. 23.4.

Chemotherapy and Toxicity

Chemotherapeutic agents must be used at doses that produce some degree of toxicity to normal tissue in order to be effective.

Haematologic Toxicity

- Most frequently seen side effect.
- Acute granulocytopenia occurs 6–12 days after administration.
- Recovery will occur in 2 weeks.
- Thrombocytopenia occurs a bit later.
- Mitomycin-C is famous in causing late myelosuppression, i.e. 28–42 days.
- Higher risk of infection if granulocytes count <500/mm 3 for 5 days.
- Risk of bleeding is real if platelet count <20,000; therefore platelet transfusion should be given.

Gastrointestinal Toxicity

- Concomitant granulocytopenia allows the injured mucosa to become infected by bacteria and fungal.
- Mucositis normally occurs 3–5 days before myelosuppression.
- Another GIT toxicity is necrotizing enterocolitis (abdominal pain, nausea, vomiting, fever, watery/bloody diarrhoea).

Skin Reactions

- Alopecia
- Allergic reaction
- Skin necrosis and sloughing strongly associated with adriamycin, actinomycin D, mitomycin C and vinca alkaloid
- Liposomal doxorubicin can cause palmar-plantar erythrodysesthesia (hand–foot syndrome)

Cardiac Toxicity

- Primarily with adriamycin
- Rarely with cyclophosphamide
- Cases report mitomycin C causing endocardial fibrosis and myocardial fibrosis

Genitourinary Toxicity

- Chronic haemorrhagic cystitis by cyclophosphamide (can be reduced by mesna (n-acetylcysteine)
- Renal tubular toxicity associated with azotemia and Mg wasting by cisplatinum
- Other agents: MTX and Mit-C

Neurologic Toxicity

- Most agents associated with mild neurologic side effects
- Vinca alkaloids: commonly associated with peripheral motor sensory and autonomic neuropathies. Loss of deep tendon reflexes, distal paraesthesias
- Most are reversible
- Cisplatinum cause ototoxicity and peripheral neuropathy (delayed type)
- 5-FU associated with cerebellar toxicity
- Ifosfamide has been associated with encephalopathy

Gonadal Dysfunction

- Alkylating agents can cause azoospermia and amenorrhea.
- In women older than 30 years, most chemotherapeutic regimes would be associated with a high incidence of premature ovarian failure.

Carcinogenicity

- Alkylating agents: Theoretical risk of acute leukaemia 5–10% after 10 years
- Most carcinogenic: melphalan and chlorambucil

Basic Practical Chemotherapy

Evaluation of New Agents

Before any chemotherapeutic drugs are allowed to be used in regular medical practice, they have to go through three trials:

Phase I trial: To evaluate toxicity and tolerance

Phase II trial: Determine the therapeutic dose and effectiveness and toxicity at that dose

Phase III trial: To compare the new chemotherapeutic drugs with currently used drug ("gold standard")

Important Considerations before Using Chemotherapeutic Drugs

- **Natural history of the malignancy**: Histology must be confirmed, primary site and extent of disease must be identified.
- **Patient characteristics**: Age, nutritional status, co-morbid conditions, performance status, vital organ function, extent of previous treatment, support from family and community, financial status.
- **Availability of adequate facilities** to evaluate, monitor and treat potential drug toxicities.
- **Availability of parameter and methods to monitor objective response to treatment.**
- **Probability of achieving a useful response**: curative, improved survival. For example, a patient with choriocarcinoma and germ cell tumour should be treated aggressively due to its chemosensitivity and curability. Advanced epithelial ovarian cancer has 75% chances of response to first-line chemotherapy; the patient should receive a full dose during initial treatment. Advanced endometrial and cervical cancer have lower response rates to chemotherapy, i.e. 30%. Change quickly to other modalities if the tumour progresses. In leiomyosarcoma, chemotherapy play a restricted role.

  Important message: *The decision to embark on chemotherapeutic drugs therapy is very complex. Optimal patient care demands a careful review of the multiple factors affecting therapy to maximize the possibilities for improving survival and quality of life.*

Performance Status

Performance status is an easy scoring system to assess the status of a patient in terms of their functional capability and physical fitness. Performance status can be an important determinant of patient fitness, response and outcome in cancer treatment.

Many scoring systems are available and one of the most commonly used is the Eastern Cooperative Oncology Group (ECOG) scale (or WHO scale: Zubrod); see Table 23.2. The other common performance status scale is called Karnofsky performance status as shown in Table 23.3.

Table 23.2 The Eastern Cooperative Oncology Group performance status scale (Zubroid)

Score	Performance status
0	Fully active; able to carry on all pre-disease activities without restriction
1	Restricted in physically strenuous activity but ambulatory and able to carry out work of a light or sedentary nature, e.g. light housework or office work
2	Ambulatory and capable of all self-care, but unable to carry out work activities; active in more than 50% of waking hours
3	Capable of only limited self-care; confined to bed or chair 50% or more of waking hours
4	Completely disabled; cannot carry out any self-care; totally confined to bed or chair

Table 23.3 Karnofsky performance index

Score	Definition
100	Normal; no complaints; no evidence of disease
90	Able to carry on normal activity; minor signs or symptoms of disease
80	Normal activity with an effort; some signs or symptoms of disease
70	Cares for self; unable to carry on normal activity or to do active work
60	Requires occasional assistance but is able to care for most needs
50	Requires considerable assistance and frequent medical care

Types of Chemotherapy

- **Primary therapy:** chemotherapy as a primary therapy, e.g. MTX in treatment of choriocarcinoma.
- **Adjuvant therapy**: use of systemic chemotherapy after surgery and/or radiotherapy with curative intent if the subsequent risk of recurrence is high.
- **Concurrent chemoradiation**: use of chemotherapy to sensitize the tumour to radiation with curative intent. Given concomitantly and the dose of chemotherapy drug is less than usual to reduce toxicity.
- **Neoadjuvant chemotherapy**: use of chemotherapy in the management of locally advanced disease that will facilitate subsequent definitive/curative treatment.
- **Induction chemotherapy**: initial systemic chemotherapy for patients with disseminated disease for which regional therapy (i.e. surgical resection or radiotherapy) is incomplete or not indicated.
- **Salvage chemotherapy**: chemotherapy given for recurrence after initial chemotherapy or second-line chemotherapy fails to respond to initial induction therapy. Generally, the goal is palliation not cure.
- **Consolidation chemotherapy**: extended chemotherapy more than the usual regimen, chemotherapy may be extended to a total of 10–12 cycles.
- **Palliative chemotherapy**: chemotherapy for relief in the symptoms in incurable cancer.

Definitions of Response (WHO Guidelines)

- **Complete Response (CR)**: Complete resolution of all evidence of disease lasting at least 1 month.
  (a) Complete clinical response (CCR)
  (b) Complete Pathologic Response: It surgically documented (CPR)
- **Partial Response (PR)**: A decrease of ≥50% in the product of the diameters (maximal and minimal) of all measurable lesions lasting at least 1 month without the development of new lesions.

(a) Partial clinical response (PCR)
(b) Partial pathologic response: It surgically documented (PPR)

- **Stable Disease (SD)**: A decrease of <50% or an increase of <25% in the product of the diameters of all measurable disease.
- **Progression**: An increase of ≥25% in the measurable lesions as described above or the identification of new lesions.

Response Evaluation Criteria in Solid Tumours (RECIST)

The WHO definition of response above has gained wide acceptance in clinical practice. However, the National Cancer Institute (NCI) has proposed and implemented newer standard response criteria called Response Evaluation Criteria in Solid Tumours (RECIST). The differences between these guidelines are outlined in Table 23.4.

Table 23.4 Comparison between RECIST and WHO guidelines of the definition of response

Response	RECIST	WHO
Objective response (OR)	Target lesions change in sum of the longest diameter. Maximum 5 per organ up to 10 (more than one organ)	Measurable disease change in the sum of the products of longest diameter and greatest perpendicular diameters, no maximum number of lesions specified
Complete response (CR)	Disappearance of all target lesions, confirmed at ≥ four-week disappearances	Disappearance of all known disease, confirmed at ≥ 4 weeks
Partial response (PR)	≥ 30% decrease from baseline, confirmed at ≥ 4 weeks	≥ 50% decrease from baseline, confirmed at ≥ 4 weeks
Progressive disease (PD)	≥ 20% increase over smallest sum observed or appearance of new lesions	≥ 25% increase in one or more lesions or appearance of new lesions
Stable disease (SD)	Neither PR nor PD criteria met	Neither PR nor PD criteria met (no change)

Calculation of Dosage

- **Body surface area (BSA)** versus weight. BSA is preferred because body surface area is relatively unchanged or less likely to be altered during therapy, and variation in the total dose between an obese and thin patient is also minimized.

  BSA (Mostellar equation) (m^2) = $(W \times H)^{1/2} \times 1/60$ or
  BSA (DuBois formula) (m^2) = $(0.425W \times 0.725H) \times 0.007184$
  W: Patient's weight in kilogram
  H: Patient's height in inches

- **Creatinine clearance** (for anti-cancer drug that eliminated via kidney)

Methods	Calculation of creatinine clearance (CrCl)
Jelliffe Method	CrCl (mL/min/1.73 m^2) = $\frac{98 - 0.8\,(\text{Age} - 20)}{\text{Serum creatinine}}$
Cockroft–Gault Method	CrCl = $\frac{(140 - \text{Age})(\text{Weight in kg})}{27 \times \text{Serum creatinine (gm/100 mL)}}$

- **Calvert formula** is used to calculate the dose of cytotoxic drug based on the value of creatinine clearance (GFR) and AUC
  - (a) There is evidence showing that there is an inverse linear correlation between the GFR and the area under the curve (AUC) of drugs such as carboplatin. In order to obtain the desire AUC, the dose not only must be decreased in patients with low renal function, but it should be higher than standard doses in patients with high renal clearance values.
  - (b) Calvert formula = AUC × (GFR + 25)
  - (c) Carboplatin dose (mg) = target AUC × (GFR + 25)
  - (d) Recommended individualized dosing of Carboplatin

    AUC 5: Untreated patients, when used in combination chemotherapy

    AUC 5: In previously treated patients

    AUC 7: In previously untreated patients, single agent.

Important Tips in Chemotherapy

Management of Recurrent Disease

- Patients with recurrent disease after chemotherapy usually do poorly to subsequent chemotherapy because of the following reasons:
  - (a) Development of chemo drug resistance.
  - (b) General status of a patient has been compromised by disease and previous drugs.
- Therefore, the aim of therapy is palliative.
- Single agent is preferable unless if the patient is platinum-sensitive.
- In the absence of excessive toxicity, without further disease progression, the patient may remain on therapy for prolonged periods of time with acceptable quality of life.

Principle of combination chemotherapy

- Each component should have activity against the target tumour as a single agent.
- Each component should have a different mechanism of actions, ideally with a biochemical basis for additive or synergistic effects without evidence of antagonistic interaction.
- Optimal sequences of drug administration should be determined from pre-clinical data and early clinical trials to maximize the tumour cell kill.
- Distinct mechanisms of resistance are desirable to minimize the emergence of drug-resistant phenotypes.
- Minimal overlap of non-haematologic toxicity is desirable to safely maintain full therapeutic doses of each component.

Supportive and Preventive Care for Chemotherapy-Induced Myelosuppression

- This can be achieved by administering haematopoietic growth factors.
- Aims of administering the haematopoietic growth factors are:

(1) amelioration of therapy related myelosuppression
(2) modulation of disease related myelosuppression
(3) enhanced host defence to infection

The characteristic of haematopoietic growth factors (cytokines family) is shown in Table 23.5.

Table 23.5 Characteristic of haematopoietic growth factors (cytokines family)

Factors	Source	Function
1. GM-CSF	T cells, endothelial cells, stroma cells	Stimulates haematopoiesis of granulocytes and macrophage, activates granulocytes and macrophages
2. G-CSF	Endothelial cells, monocytes, stroma cells	Stimulates haematopoiesis of granulocytes lineage, activate granulocytes.
3. Erythropoietin	KIDNEY	Stimulates erythroid growth and development.
4. IL-1	Monocytes/ macrophages, B and T cells, endothelial cells.	Co-stimulates early stages of haematopoiesis, T&B cell activation
5. IL-3	T-cells	Stimulates early stages of haematopoiesis
6. IL-6	T cells. Monocytes/ Macrophage, fibroblast	Co-stimulates early stages of haematopoiesis, T&B cells activation.

Note: GM-CSF, granulocytes-macrophage colony-stimulating factors; G-CSF, granulocytes colony-stimulating factors; IL, interleukin.

GM-CSF and G-CSF

- These two agents can induce large numbers of haemopoietic stem and progenitor cells to leave their normal havens within the inter-medullary compartment of the bone marrow and to circulate in the peripheral blood.
  (a) Subcutaneous administration is better than intravenous infusion.

(b) Recommended dose is 250 ug/m^2.
(c) In some instances, smaller dose is more stimulating than a higher dose.
(d) It may enhance neutrophil function, i.e. adherence, phagocytic, and chemotaxis.
(e) Administration of both would indirectly reduce the incidence of fever, antibiotic usage and days in the hospital.
(f) Routine use of these drugs may not be cost-effective.

- Adverse effects of GM-CSF and G-CSF are

  (a) cutaneous eruption of macules and papules
  (b) exacerbation of underlying autoimmune disease
  (c) stomach distension and on rare occasion rupture
  (d) anaphylaxis: rare
  (e) thrombosis
  (f) theoretical possibility of exacerbation of the underlying malignancy

Erythropoietin

- Produced through gene cloning.
- Kidney is the main site for endogenous erythropoietin production.
- Endogenous production is stimulated by anaemia and hypoxia.
- However, a patient who undergoes chemotherapy less responsive to such stimulant.

Overcoming Nausea and Vomiting during Chemotherapy

Nausea and vomiting are the most commmon and important side-effects encountered by cancer patients while receiving chemotherapy. Overcoming chemotherapy-induced nausea and vomiting is extremely important to ensure good quality of life and better compliance. Therefore, there will be minimal interruption of the progress of chemotherapy. The category of anti-neoplastic drugs according to their emetogenic potential is shown in Table 23.6.

Table 23.6 Category of anti-neoplastic drugs according to their emetogenic potential

Level	Frequency of emesis	Agent	
1	<10%	Bevacizumab Bleomycin Busulfan Chlorambucil Fludarabine 5-Fluorouracil (500 mg/m^2)	Hydroxyurea Methotrexate (<50 mg/m^2) Rituximab Vinblastine Vincristine Vinorelbine
2	10–30%	Bortezomib Capecitabine Cetuximab Cytarabine <1000 mg/m^2 Doxetaxel Etoposide 5-Fluorouracil (500–1000 mg/m^2)	Gemcitabine Methotrexate Mitomycin Mitoxantrone Paclitaxel Pemetrexed Topotecan Trastuzumab
3	30–90%	Busulphan > 4 mg/day Carboplatin Cisplatin <50 mg/m^2 Cyclophosphamide (<1500 mg/m^2) Cyclophosphamide (oral) Cytarabine ≤ 1 g/m^2 Dactinomycin	Daunorubicin Doxorubicin Epirubicin < 90 mg/m^2 Idarubicin Ifosfamide Irinotecan Oxaliplatin Procarbazine
4	>90%	AC/EC combination Carmustine < 250 mg/m^2 Cisplatinum > 50 mg/m^2 Cyclophosphamide > 1500 mg/m^2 Cytarabine > 1 gm/m^2 Dacarbazine Methotrexate > 1000 mg/m^2	

General Principles

- Patients should be counselled about nausea and vomiting following chemotherapy.
- Anti-emetics should be given routinely to all patients receiving moderate or highly emetogenic chemotherapy.
- Intravenous route is preferred though oral anti-emetics can be as effective.

Type of Chemotherapy-Induced Nausea and Vomiting

- **Delayed emesis:** vomiting occurs more than 24 hours after chemotherapy. It can last for 6–7 days. Common drugs are cisplatin, carboplatin, cyclophosphamide and doxorubicin.
- **Anticipatory nausea/vomiting:** Nausea or vomiting occurs before chemotherapy due to previous experience of vomiting while on chemotherapy.
- **Breakthrough vomiting**: It occurs despite treatment to prevent it; this type of vomiting requires more anti-nausea and vomiting treatment.
- **Refractory vomiting:** persistent vomiting despite treatment

Table 23.7 Guidelines for anti-emetic prescription with chemotherapy based on emetogenic levels

Ematogenic level	With chemotherapy D1	Take home (oral) D2–3	Options
4	5-HT3 A AND Dexamethasone	Dexamethasone ±metoclopramide	Aprepitant D1–3 Lorazepam
3	5-HT3 A AND Dexamethasone	Dexamethasone ±metoclopramide	Aprepitant D1–3
2	Dexamethasone and/or metoclopramide	Dexamethasone ±metoclopramide	—
1	Nil or Metoclopramide	Nil or metoclopramide	—

Table 23.8 Anti-emetic drugs and dosages

Drug	Dose	Route	Frequency
Granisetron	1 mg 0.01 mg/kg 2 mg	IV IV PO	Daily
Ondansetron	8 mg 24 mg	IV PO	Daily
Tropisetron	5 mg	IV/PO	Daily
Dexamethasone	12 mg 8 mg	IV PO	Stat daily
Metoclopramide	10–20 mg	IV OR PO	tds
Lorazepam	0.5–2 mg	PO	tds or qid
Prochlorperazine	10 mg	PO or IV	Tds or qid
Haloperidol	1–2 mg 1–3 mg	PO IV	tds or qid
Aprepitant	1 pack (125 mg 80 mg)	 PO PO	 Day 1 Days 2 and 3

The guidelines for anti-emetic prescription of chemotherapy based on emetogenic levels is shown in Table 23.7. Table 23.8 showed the most commonly used anti-emetic drugs and the dosages.

Dose Modification Guidelines[1]

To reduce treatment-related morbidity and treatment cancellation, dose modification is important in patients who developed significant drug toxicity. The decision on dose modification must be individualized and should be discussed with the consultant oncologist.

---

[1]Adapted from Malaysian MOH Systemic Therapy of Cancer, 2nd edition.

General Principle of Dose Modification

Haematological toxicity	Actions
Inadequate blood counts on day of treatment	Delay 1 week; use same dose
Inadequate counts after 1 week delay	Delay 1 more week; dose reduction by 25%
Inadequate counts after 2 weeks	Review regime/plan
Non-haematological toxicity	Actions
Grade 3	Consider for dose reduction; dose reduction by 25% from previous dose
Grade 4	MUST reduce the dose and review the regime; use 50–75% of previous dose
Renal toxicity Creatinine clearance GFR > 60 mL/min = 100% cisplatin dose GFR 40 to 60 mL/min = 50% cisplatin dose GFR < 40 mL/min = omit cisplatin	Cisplatin dose 100% 50% Omit
Neuropathy including ototoxicity (platinum, vince, taxane) Grade 2 Grade 3–4	 Dose reduction by 25% Omit
Cystitis (cyclophosphamide, ifosfamide) Grade 2	Increase fluid intake > 2L per day; add or increase mesna dose

References

English MW. Principle of chemotherapy. *Paediatr Child Health* 2009; **20**(3): 123–128.

Fujiwara T, Grimm EA, Mukhopadhyay T, Zhang WW. Induction of chemosensitivity in human lung cancer cells in vivo by adenovirus-mediated transfer of the wild-type p53 gene. *Cancer Res* 1994; **54**: 2287–2291.

Garattini S. Pharmacokinetics in cancer chemotherapy. *Eur J Cancer* 2007; **43**: 271–282.

Iqbal MP. Review Article. Mechanism of drug resistance in cancer cells. *Pak J Med Sci* 2003; **19**(2): 118–127.

Lowe SW, Bodis S, McClatchey A, et al. p53 status and the efficacy of cancer therapy in vivo. *Science* 1994; **266**: 807–810.

McFadyen MC, Mcleod HL, Jackson FC, Melvin WT, Doehmer J, Murray GI. Cytochrome P450 CYP1B1 protein expressions: a novel mechanism of anticancer drug resistance. *Biochem Pharmacol* 2001; **62**: 207–212.

Parnell C, Woll PJ. Principles of cancer chemotherapy. Safe Prescribing (Foundation years 1: 2) 2005: 18–22.

Schweitzer BI, Dicker AP, Bertino JR. Dihydrofolate reductase as a therapeutic target. *FASEB J* 1990; **4**: 2441–2452.

Sridhar T, Symonds RP. Principles of chemotherapy and radiotherapy. *Obstet, Gynaecol Reprod Med* 2008; **19**(3): 61–67.

Symonds RP. Principles of gynaecological chemotherapy and radiotherapy. *Curr Obstet Gynaecol* 2003; **13**: 102–109.

Symonds RP, Foweraker K. Principles of chemotherapy and radiotherapy. *Curr Obstet Gynaecol* 2006; **16**: 100–106.

William FM, Flintoff WF. Isolation of a human cDNA that complements a mutant hamster cell defective in methotrexate uptake. *J Biol Chem* 1995; **270**: 2987–2992.

Zubrod CG, Schneiderman M, Frei E, et al. Appraisal of methods for the study of chemotherapy of cancer in man: comparative therapeutic trial of nitrogen mustard and triethylene thiophosphoramide. *J Chron Dis* 1960; **11**: 7–33.

Chapter 24

Modulating Agents, Biologic Response Modifiers and Targeted Therapy in Gynaecological Cancer

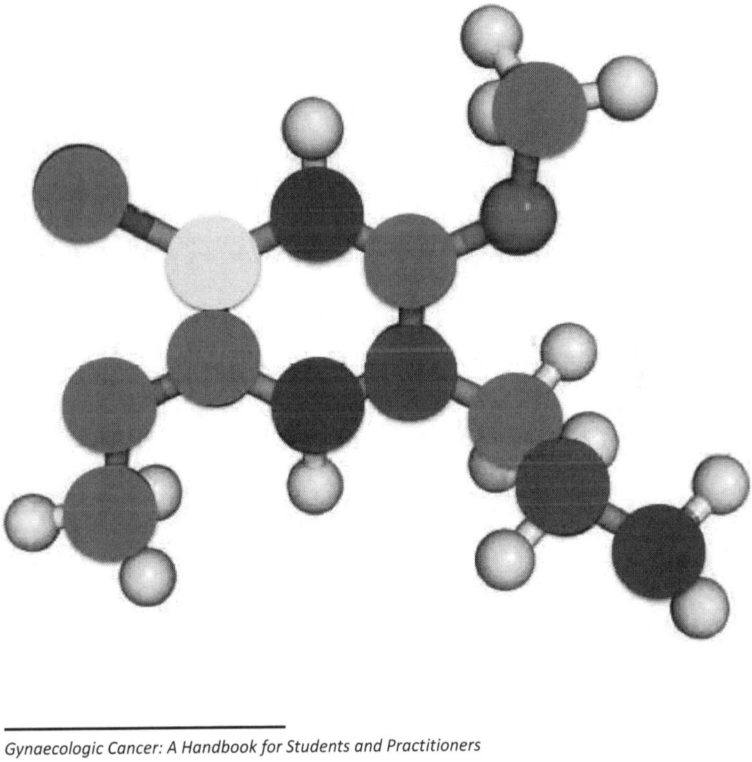

Gynaecologic Cancer: A Handbook for Students and Practitioners
Rushdan Noor, Eng Hseon Tay, and Jeffrey Low

ISBN 978-981-4463-06-5 (Hardcover), 978-981-4463-07-2 (eBook)
www.panstanford.com

Modulating Agents in Cancer

There are two main limiting factors for successful chemotherapy, namely (a) development of chemo-resistance and (b) toxic effects of chemo drugs to normal tissues.

Modulating agents are used to improve the therapeutic index of chemotherapy. They can be divided into three main classes:

(a) agents that protect host tissue from a toxic effect of chemo drugs
(b) agents that potentiate anti-cancer drugs
(c) agents that reverse acquired drug resistance

Modulating Agents

Folinic Acid (e.g. Leucovorin)

Folinic acid is the reduced form of folic acid. It can readily be converted to tetrahydrofolate, which does not require an action of dihydrofolate reductase. Tetrahydrofolate has vitamin activity equivalent to folic acid. Methotrexate (MTX) inhibits dihydrofolate reductase.

The objective of folinic acid administration is to overcome high-dose MTX-induced toxicity to bone marrow and lining of gastrointestinal tract ("rescue bone marrow and GIT"). It can rescue cells by replenishing the intra-cellular reduced-folate pool and preventing (MTX) toxicity via blockage of thymidine synthesis. It acts in a dose- and time-dependent fashion (given within 48 hours). Folinic acid is normally started 24 hours after MTX is given. This delay gives the MTX a chance to exert its anti-cancer effects.

Folinic acid can also potentiate anti-tumour activity of 5-fluorouracil by enhancing the binding of 5-FU with a specific enzyme in cancer cell. Combination of folinic acid and 5-FU is given in colorectal cancer.

Therefore, folinic acid can either enhance chemotherapy effectiveness or acting as a chemoprotector. Folinic acid is also used to treat a patient who has accidentally received an overdose of MTX. The route of administration of folinic acid is oral, intravenous and intra-muscular injection.

Dexrazoxane (Zinecard)

Anthracyclines, alkylating agents, 5-fluorouracil and paclitaxel are chemotherapeutic agents most often associated with cardiac toxicity. Doxorubicin has been the most widely studied cardiotoxic agent in adult and paediatric patients. Dexrazoxane is chemoprotective agents to reduce cardiotoxicity of doxorubicin and approved by the FDA to be used in a breast cancer patients.

The indication of dexrazoxane is to reduce the incidence and severity of cardiomyopathy associated with doxorubicin administration in women with advanced breast cancer who have received a cumulative doxorubicin dose of 300 mg/m^2. A phase III trial evaluating cardioprotective potential of dexrazoxane has shown that dexrazoxane arm yielded significantly fewer cardiac events (13% vs. 39%). It is not recommended for use with the initiation of doxorubicin therapy and with chemotherapy regimens that do not contain an anthracycline.

Dexrazoxane is given via intravenous injection (250/500 mg vial) and the dosage is slow infusion (15 minutes), 500 mg/m^2 with 50 mg/m^2 doxorubicin (dosage ratio of 10:1) given prior to doxorubicin administration (within 30 minutes). Dexrazoxane should be given no less than 30 minutes before adriamycin.

The protective mechanism is through chelation of free and iron bound within anthracycline complexes, thereby preventing the formation of cardiotoxic reactive oxygen radicals. Dexrazoxane can also enhance the effects of cisplatin in both drug-sensitive and drug-resistant human ovarian cell lines. Unfortunately, dexrazoxane administration may add to the myelosuppression caused by chemotherapeutic agents.

Thiol-Based Chemoprotectors

Glutathione

Glutathione (GSH) is a tripeptide with a gamma peptide linkage between the amine group of cysteine and the carboxyl group of the glutamate side-chain. It is an anti-oxidant, preventing damage to important cellular components caused by reactive oxygen species such as free radicals and peroxides. Glutathione is not an essential nutrient since it can be synthesized in the body. Glutathione protects against platinum and alkylating agents. However, this drug is still being investigated.

Amifostine (Ethyol)

Amifostine is an organic thiophosphate and most extensively developed cytoprotective agent. It is protective to both chemotherapy and radiation therapy. Amifostine is taken into a normal cell but not into a cancer cell. The mechanism of actions is scavenging oxygen-free radical, detoxification of active chemo agents (alkylating and platinum), induction of hypoxia, etc. Amifostine also stimulates bone marrow progenitor cells and increased sensitivity of cancer cell to cytotoxic drugs, e.g. paclitaxel and carboplatin. Therefore, amifostine has dual action, i.e. protective and potentiator. It has been approved by the FDA to reduce renal toxicity by cisplatin.

Amifostine has been shown in the clinical trial to reduce nephrotoxicity and neurotoxicity of cisplatin and haematotoxicity of cyclophosphamide: 26% versus 10% with amifostine.

Amifostine can alter the pharmacokinetics of carboplatin and increase its efficacy. This effect is minimal in cisplatin.

A controlled study using amifostine (910 mg/m^2) in advanced ovarian cancer showed that an addition of amifostine in a cyclophosphamide and cisplatin regimen decreased renal toxicity (5% vs. 15%).

Interestingly, amifostine is also radioprotector. Phase 3 multi-centre randomized control trial had shown intravenous infusion (3 minutes) of amifostine administered at a dose of 200 mg/m^2 given 15–30 minutes before radiotherapy significantly reduced the incidence of grade 2 and more xerostomia (51% versus 78%) in patients with head and neck cancer as compared to radiotherapy alone. Amifostine was also found to increase the patient's tolerability to a higher dose of radiotherapy.

To date, there is no strong evidence to show that amifostine has neuroprotective property.

Sodium Thiosulphate

Sodium thiosulphate is a reactive thiol agent often used as an antidote to cyanide and nitroprusside poisoning. It was later found to have chemoprotector properties. Sodium thiosulphate acts as a modulator in cisplatin-induced toxicity (ototoxicity, neurotoxicity and nephrotoxicity) and it can reduce nephrotoxicity by cisplatin. The FDA has approved this drug.

The clinical utility of sodium thiosulphate as a chemoprotectant when used with high-dose cisplatin would appear to be confined to use in intra-peritoneal therapy and other regional therapy. It is also potential protector for cisplatin-induced hearing loss (ototoxicity). Sodium thiosulphate is given after the administration of cisplatin or carboplatin. The possible mechanism of actions are direct binding and inactivation of platinum agents, displacing platinum from cellular bound targets, decreasing DNA damage, increasing cellular glutathione levels, or scavenging platinum-induced free radicals.

Mesna

Mesna is one of the oldest known cytoprotectants. It is clinically used for protection against bladder toxicity (haemorrhagic cystitis) from alkylating agents. It is known that the risk of haemorrhagic cystitis without mesna is 18–40%. Mesna inactivates active metabolites of alkylating agents known as acrolein, which accumulated in bladder and responsible in urotoxicity (causing oedema, ulceration, neovascularization, haemorrhage dan necrosis). Sulphhydryl group present in mesna binds to acrolein within the urinary tract and acts as a neutralizing agent.

Mesna has also been found to prevent or reduced cytotoxicity effect of cisplatin when given simultaneously. Therefore, mesna should not be given simultaneously with cisplatin.

Intravenous mesna is given as a bolus dose (20% of ifosfamide dose) prior to ifosfamide followed by another two doses 4 and 8 hours later. Mesna can also be given orally and subcutaneously.

Glutamine

Glutamine is the most prevalent amino acid in the human body. It is given as an oral medication 10 gm three times a day or 0.5 gm/kg/day. Studies on cytoprotective effects of glutamine have produced conflicting results. The studies were mainly looking into protective effect of glutamine against mucositis and gastrointestinal ulceration induced by anthracycline-based chemotherapy. A randomized control double blind crossover study shows patients with breast cancer receiving oral glutamine together with anthracycline-based chemotherapy had a lower incidence of WHO grade 2 and more oral mucositis (38.7% vs. 49.7%) and significantly lower incidence of grade 3 and above oral mucositis (1% vs. 7%).

Fibroblast Growth Factors

Fibroblast growth factors (FGFs) are naturally occurring human amino acid proteins attributing to regulation and early development of organogenesis. One of the subfamilies of FGFs is keratinocyte growth factor (KGF). Keratinocyte growth factor stimulates the proliferation and differentiation of epithelial cells. Some studies have shown that systemic administration of recombinant human KGF (rHuKGF) also known as palifermin provides cytoprotection against mucositis in patients with haematologic, head and neck and colorectal cancer. Palifermin was given prior to chemotherapy or in patients with haematologic malignancies receiving myelotoxic therapy requiring haemopoietic stem cell transplantation. In the later group of patients, palifermin was given before and after myelotoxic therapy. There was also evidence that palifermin has a protective effect against cyclophosphamide-induced ulcerative haemorrhagic cystitis and chemotherapy/radiation induced mucositis. A double blind phase III study in non-Hodgkin's lymphoma patients undergoing bone marrow transplantation showed that an addition of palifermin before and after radiotherapy had significantly reduced grade 3–4 oral mucositis than those who received placebo (63% vs. 98%).

Recombinant Human Erythropoetin (rhEPO)

Erythropoetin (EPO) is a glycoprotein stimulating production and maturation of red blood cells. EPO is synthesized predominantly by interstitial kidney (80%) and liver cells (20%) in response to tissue hypoxia. EPO can also be synthesized in vitro. Recombinant human erythropoietin (rhEPO) is produced by DNA recombinant technology. There are at least three types of (rhEPO), rhEPO alpha, beta and darbapoetin. Few meta-analysis had revealed a positive and negative effect of rhEPO on overall survival, risk of death and thromboembolism. The American Society of Clinical Oncology and American Society of Hematology published joint recommendation (2005) regarding rhEPO. These recommendations advise the use of epoetins only in patients with anaemia related to chemotherapy. The European Organization for Research and Treatment of Cancer (EORTC) guidelines 2007 had recommended epoetins only be given in anaemic cancer patients who are symptomatic and not based on fixed haemoglobin concentration.

Granulocyte-Colony Stimulating Factor (G-CSF) and Granulocyte Macrophage-Colony Stimulating Factor (GM-CSF)

Granulocyte-colony stimulating factor (G-CSF) is a cytokine (substances that are secreted by specific cells of the immune system). It stimulates maturation and growth of neutrophil progenitors into mature cells. Granulocyte-colony stimulating factor is produced by endothelial cells, fibroblasts, keratinocytes and macrophages. It promotes the release of premature neutrocytes from the bone marrow and activates their phagocytic activity.

Second type of colony stimulating factors (CSFs) is granulocyte macrophage-colony stimulating factor or GM-CSF. Granulocyte macrophage-colony stimulating factor stimulates neutrophils but also macrophages, dendritic cells, basophils and eosinophils. Newer CSFs available recently is pegfilgrastim.

Generally there are three main indications of the colony stimulating factors: (1) primary prophylaxis of febrile neutropenia, (2) secondary prophylaxis of febrile neutropenia and (3) treatment of afebrile and febrile neutropenia. According to American Society of Clinical Oncology, febrile neutropenia is designated as a body temperature of approximately 38.5°C or higher, sustained for more than 1 hour and developing concurrently with absolute neutropenia of less than 500 cells/mm^3. CSFs are indicated for primary prophylaxis against febrile neutropenia if the risk of febrile neutropenia is >20% (American Society of Clinical Oncology [ASCO], EORTC and National Comprehensive Cancer Network [NCCN] 2006 guidelines). Patient-related risk factors for developing febrile neutropenia are age more than 65 years, poor performance status, advanced cancer, bone marrow infiltration, previous episode of neutropenia, anaemia, poor nutritional status, severe comorbidities etc. Secondary prophylaxis is CSFs administration in patients who developed febrile neutropenia in previous chemotherapy and did not receive primary prophylaxis. In general, CSFs is not recommended for afebrile neutropenia.

In febrile neutropenia, ASCO guidelines state that the use of CSFs should be considered in patients with febrile neutropenia that are at high risk of infection-associated complications or who have prognostic factors that are predictive of a poor clinical outcome (e.g. prolong pyrexia > 10 days, profound neutropenia (ANC < 100/ mm^3), age > 65 years, hypotension, multi-organ dysfunction, etc.). To date, meta-analysis and randomized controlled trials assessing the role of CSFs in afebrile and febrile neutropenia did not show any advantage in terms of overall survival.

Biologic Response Modifiers

Biologic response modifiers (BRM) are agents and approaches to the treatment of cancer with a mechanism of action that involves modulation of the individual's own biologic responses. In addition, they also can be used to lessen certain side effects that may be caused by some cancer treatments.

Inflammation and Tumour

Chronic inflammation resulting from low-grade, persistent chemical, bacterial, viral agents predisposes the formation of the pre-neoplastic foci and subsequently promotes tumour development. Following are some facts about the link between inflammation and neoplastic transformation:

- link between ulcerative colitis and colon cancer
- chronic pancreatitis and pancreatic cancer
- HPV and cervical cancer
- hepatitis C and hepatocellular cancer
- *Helicobacter pylori* and gastric cancer
- schistosoma infection and bladder cancer

- free radical and nitrogen species linked with mutation
- inflammations induced by chronic exposure to ultraviolet and other environmental chemical, e.g. asbestos were linked with melanoma, skin cancer and mesothelioma
- nitrates in food processing chemical transformed to nitrosamine and can lead to pre-malignant condition of the stomach

Cytokines and Tumour Growth

Cytokines are a large group of a polypeptide secreted by living cells that act non-enzymatically to regulate cellular functions (regulation of immune cell activity, haematopoiesis and regulation of proliferation). They are signalling molecules that are key mediators of inflammation or an immune response. They have a wide variety of cellular functions and are stimulated when tissue homeostasis is altered.

Cytokines can be classified into two main groups:

(a) pro-inflammatory (e.g. interleukin 1, 6, 15, 17, 23 and Tumour Necrosis Factor α (TNFα)

(b) anti-inflammatory (e.g. interleukin 4, 10, 13, transforming growth factor (TGFβ) and interferon α)

Their net effect will be either pro- or anti-tumourigenic depending on the balance of these two groups. Pro-inflammatory cytokines (e.g. TNFα) are pro-tumourigenic and anti-inflammatory cytokines are anti-tumourigenic. Cytokines will bind to membrane receptors and activate a very complex signal transduction pathway that leads to apoptosis, cell proliferation, angiogenesis and cellular senescence. In an animal model, the moderate amount of TNFα can increase tumour growth, stimulate angiogenesis, cause DNA damage and increase the metastatic potential of tumours. Inhibition of TNFα by anti-TNFα antibodies reduce the tumour burden and metastasis. Treatment with anti-inflammatory cytokines, e.g. IL10, TGFβ to animal model with *Helicobacter hepaticus* infection was found to prevent chronic inflammation and adenocarcinoma of colon.

Chemokines and Tumour Growth

As mentioned above, inflammatory insults will lead to up-regulation of non-specific pro-inflammatory cytokines such as IL-1α/β, IL-6, interferon (IFN)-α, and tumour necrosis factor (TNF)-α. These cytokines subsequently induce the expression of pro-inflammatory chemokines. Chemokines are soluble, small molecular weight (8–14 kDa) proteins that bind to their cognate G-protein coupled receptors (GPCRs) to elicit a cellular response, usually directional migration or chemotaxis (migration and recruitment of leukocytes). Chemokines are important in many biological events such as embryogenesis, wound healing, angiogenesis, Th1/Th2 Th1/Th2 development, leukocyte homeostasis and lymphoid organ development, inflammatory diseases, pro and anti-tumour responses. In addition to a role in chronic inflammation associated with tumour progression, chemokines are involved in tumour angiogenesis and in homing of tumour cells to the sentinel lymph nodes, metastasis to specific organs, as well as metastasis of the metastatic lesions.

Chemokines are classified into four main groups, namely, CXC, CC, CX3C and C chemokine. Studies are still being carried out to determine the role of each chemokine in cancers such as colorectal cancer, small cell lung cancer, ovarian cancer, multiple myeloma, prostatic cancer, etc. In future, anti-cancer drug targeting specific chemokines can be developed to eradicate pre-cancerous state or cancer at a very early stage.

Cyclooxygenase and Tumour

Cyclooxygenases (COX) are enzymes that convert fatty acids to prostaglandins. Prostaglandins, mainly PGE2, are key mediators of inflammation and inflammation-associated cancer. There are two types of COX: (1) COX-1 and (2) COX-2. Cyclooxygenases-2 is primarily responsible for the increased cyclooxygenase activity due to chronic inflammation. Cyclooxygenases-2 has now been found to be highly expressed in nearly every tumour type examined, including in the pre-cancerous state, suggesting that COX-2 has an important role in tumour initiation and maintenance. The use of NSAIDs that inhibit COX-2 activity is associated with reduced risk of malignancies such as colorectal, oesophageal, stomach, lung, breast and ovarian cancers.

Biologic Response Modifiers in Current Clinical Practices

Interferons

Interferon is the family of glycoprotein produced by several different cell types. Interferons are types of cytokines that occur naturally in the body. They were the first cytokines produced in the laboratory for use as biologic response modifiers. The greatest therapeutic usefulness of interferon is in the treatment of hairy cell leukaemia.

There are two types of interferons:

(a) **Type 1 (alpha and beta)**: produced by induced leukocytes and fibroblasts
(b) **Type 2 (gamma)**: produced by lymphocytes and monocytes.

The modes of actions of interferon are as follows:

(a) Interferon has anti-viral properties.
(b) It has an effect on the immune system (enhances antibody production and lymphocytes blastogenesis, enhances macrophage phagocytosis, NK activity, etc.)

Interferon alpha is the type most widely used in cancer treatment. The FDA has approved the use of interferon alpha for the treatment of certain types of cancer, including hairy cell leukaemia, melanoma, chronic myeloid leukaemia and AIDS-related Kaposi's sarcoma. Researchers are exploring combinations of interferon alpha and other BRMs or chemotherapy in clinical trials to treat many cancers.

Interleukins (IL-1, 2, 3, 4)

Interleukin is a polypeptide produced by lymphocytes and macrophage. It is also a cytokine that occurs naturally in the body and can be prepared in the laboratory. Many interleukins have been discovered; interleukin-2 (IL-2) is the most widely studied in cancer treatment. It stimulates proliferation, differentiation, and function of T lymphocytes, B lymphocyte, etc. The FDA has approved IL-2 for the treatment of certain cancers such as metastatic renal cancer and metastatic melanoma. The role of IL-2 was also evaluated for other cancers such as leukaemia, lymphoma, colorectal, ovarian, breast and prostate cancers.

Tumour Necrosis Factor

Tumour necrosis factors (TNFs) are a group of cytokines that can cause cell death or apoptosis. There are two types of TNF: Alpha (TNFα) and Beta (TNFβ). Tumour necrosis factors are produced by activated monocytes (TNFα) and lymphocytes (TNFβ). They can also be produced in vitro by recombinant DNA technology. So far, only TNFα being evaluated in clinical. Tumour necrosis factors are able to induce haemorrhagic necrosis and tumour regression in animal. Responsive tumour includes melanoma, colon cancer, breast cancer, cervical cancer, ovarian cancer, lung cancer and astrocytoma.

Retinoids

The retinoids are a class of chemical compounds that are related chemically to vitamin A. In medicine, retinoids are useful due to their ability to regulate epithelial cell growth. Epithelial system needs vitamin A for display of a proper morphology and function. Vitamin A is protective to epithelial tumour and Retinoid acid is also used for some dermatological condition such as actinokeratosis, pre-cancerous and Basal cell carcinoma.

Modulators of Resistance to Chemotherapy

One of the main concerns about chemotherapy is the emergence of chemo-resistant malignant cells. Resistant tumours express a resistant phenotype due to their inherited genotype. Tumour resistance can also be acquired following sub-lethal exposure to anti-cancer drugs. The mechanism of tumour resistance is complex and multi-factorial. The multi-factorial mechanisms of drug resistance have led to the use of combined chemotherapy. Strategies are being designed to reverse or modulate the development of tumour resistance to cytotoxic drugs. Some of the examples of such agents that have been evaluated are buthionine sulphoximine, glutathione-S-transferase inhibitors, lonidamine, aphidicolin, azidothymidine and novobiocin.

Modulators of P-Glycoprotein

Two multi-drug resistant (MDR) genes have been identified: (a) P-glycoprotein (P-gp) gene and (b) MDR-associated protein (MRP) gene. The expression of these proteins in tumour is associated with reduced drug accumulation leading to resistance to a broad spectrum of anti-cancer drugs. Substances that can interfere with function of these proteins can increase the sensitivity of tumour to anti-cancer drugs.

P-glycoprotein (P-gp) modulators that are being studied are

(a) **Cyclosporin A analogs**
Cyclosporin A analogs are potential potent reversing agent of P-gp-mediated drug resistance. However, phase II trial in ovarian cancer for cisplatin resistance did not show encouraging results.

(b) Verapamil and quinine
This combination results in additive or synergistic chemo-sensitization through their effect on blocking P-gp-mediated MDR.

Targeted Therapy in Cancer

The traditional cytotoxic therapy remains the treatment of choice in many cancers. These cytotoxic drugs work primarily through the inhibition of cell division. Targeted cancer therapies are drugs or other substances that block the growth and spread of cancer by interfering with specific molecules involved in tumour growth and progression. Targeted therapy blocks the proliferation of cancer cells by interfering with specific molecules required for tumour development and growth. Some of these molecules may be present in normal tissue, but they are often mutated or overexpressed in tumour.

Targeted therapies are approved as one of the important component of treatment in many cancers, including breast, lung, colorectal, pancreatic and haematological cancers. The number of new targeted therapies approved by the FDA has exceeded the number of traditional chemotherapeutic drugs. Since 2000, the FDA has approved 15 targeted therapies. However, currently the cost of targeted therapies is very expensive.

The most common molecular pathways targeted in solid tumours are (a) epidermal growth factor receptors (EGFR), also known as HER1, (b) vascular endothelial growth factors (VEGF) and (c) HER-2/neu.

The following pathways can be inhibited at many levels:

(a) binding and neutralizing ligands
(b) occupying receptor-binding sites
(c) blocking receptor signalling within the cancer cell
(d) interfering with downstream intra-cellular molecules

There are two types of targeted agents:

(a) Monoclonal antibody with larger molecules (**large-molecule inhibitors**): It targets extra-cellular component such as ligand and receptor. The route of administration of this group is intravenous. The examples of large-molecule inhibitors are bevacizumab, trastuzumab, alemtuzumab, cetuximab, gemtuzumab ozogamicin, panitumumab and rituximab.
(b) **Small-molecule inhibitors**: They can enter cells, thereby blocking receptor signalling (mainly tyrosine kinase) and interfering with downstream intra-cellular molecules.Tyrosine kinase signalling initiates a molecular cascade that leads to cell growth, proliferation, migration and angiogenesis in normal and malignant tissues. As compared to large-molecule inhibitors, small-molecule inhibitors are commonly administered in oral form and are cheaper than large-molecule inhibitors. The examples of small-molecule inhibitors are bortezomib, dasatinib, erlotinib, gefitinib and others such as imatinib, lapatinib, sorafenib and sunitinib.

Epidermal growth factor receptors are also present in normal cells; therefore, EGFR inhibitors can cause a dermatologic complications such as a skin rashes and gastrointestinal complication such as diarrhoea and abdominal pain.

Anti-VEGF is also known as anti-angiogenesis; without new vessel formation, the tumour cannot grow. Due to better blood supply in the remaining tumour, the delivery of anti-cancer drugs will be more efficient. However, anti-VEGF will also affect normal blood vessels leading to bleeding, thrombosis and proteinuria due to alteration in glomerular infiltration, bowel perforation and hypertension.

Only patients who have overexpression of VEGF or EGFR will respond to anti-VEGF/EGFR. Example in breast cancer, 25% of patients will have HER 2/neu (target molecule related to EGFR) positive, therefore, only 25% of patients will respond to anti-HER2/neo, i.e. trastuzumab (herceptin).

Until recently, targeted therapies have been approved by the FDA mainly in non-gynaecological cancer such as breast cancer, leukaemia, non-small cell lung cancer, lymphoma, renal cell cancer, colo-rectal cancer, etc. The role of targeted therapy in gynaecologic cancer is still investigational.

References

Bokemeyer C, Aapro MS, Courdi A, et al. For the European organization for research and treatment of cancer (EORTC) taskforce for the elderly. EORTC guidelines for the use of erythropoietic proteins in anaemic patients with cancer: 2006 update. *Eur J Cancer* 2007; **43**: 258–270.

Brizel DM, Wasserman TH, Henke M, et al. Phase III randomized trial of amifostine as a radioprotector in head and neck cancer. *J Clin Oncol* 2000; **18**: 3339–3345.

Cuzick, J, et al. Aspirin and non-steroidal anti-inflammatory drugs for cancer prevention: an international consensus statement. *Lancet Oncol* 2009; **10**: 501–507.

Gerber DE. Targeted Therapies: a new generation of cancer treatments. *Am Fam Physician* 2008; **77**(3): 311–319.

Gridelli C, Aapro MS, Barni S, et al. Role of colony stimulating factors (CSFs) in solid tumours: results of an expert panel. *Clin Rev Oncol/Hematol* 2007; **63**: 53–64.

Harned TM, Kalous O, Neuwelt A, et al. Sodium Thiosulfate administrated six hours after cisplatin does not compromise antineuroblastoma activity. *Clin Cancer Res* 2008; **14**(2): 533–540.

Kemp G, Rose P, Lurain J, et al. Amifostine pretreatment for protection against cyclophosphamide and cisplatin-induced toxicities: results of a randomized controlled trial in patients with advanced ovarian cancer. *J Clin Oncol* 1996; **14**: 2101–2112.

Lima MV, Ferreira FV, Macedo FY, et al. Histologic changes in bladders of patients submitted to ifosfamide chemotherapy even with mesna prophylaxls. *Cancer Chemother Pharmacol* 2007; **59**: 643–650.

Marty M, Espie M, Llombart A, et al. A phase III study to investigate the cardioprotective potential of dexrazoxane in advanced/metastatic breast cancer patients undergoing anthracycline-based chemotherapy (abstr/poster 50520. 27th Breast Cancer Symposium; 2004 (December): San Antonio, TX.

Peterson DE, Petit RG. Oral mucositis incidence and severity reduced with AES-14: results of a phase III pivotal trial in patients with breast cancer (poster). Presented at 1st Annual Chicago Supportive Oncology Conference (CSOC); 2005, October: Chicago, IL.

Raman D, Baugher PJ, Thu YM, Richmond A. Role of chemokines in tumour growth. *Cancer Lett* 2007; **256**: 137–165.

Schetter AJ, Heegaard NHH, Harris CC. Inflammation and cancer: interweaving microRNA, free radical, cytokine and p53 pathways. *Carcinogenesis* 2010; **31**(1): 37–49.

Spielberger R, Stiff P, Bensinger W, et al. Palifermin for oral mucositis after intensive therapy for hematologic cancers. *N Engl J Med* 2004; **351**: 2590–2598.

Willam P, Hogle. Cytoprotective agents used in the treatment of patient with cancer. *Semin Oncol Nurs* 2007; **23**(3): 213–224.

Winczura P, Jassem J. Combined treatment with cytoprotective agents and radiotherapy. Cancer Treatment Review. 2009 (December), Article in Press.

Chapter 25

Immunotherapy and Hormonal Therapy in Gynaecological Cancer

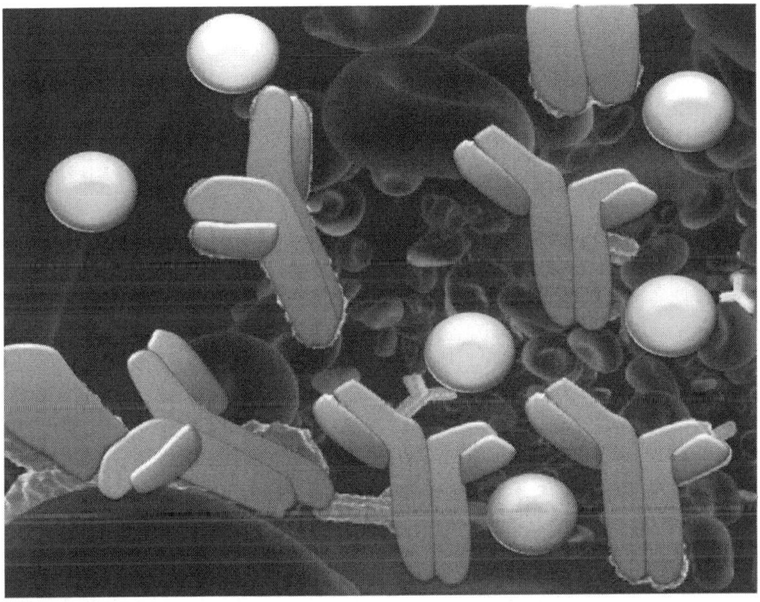

Gynaecologic Cancer: A Handbook for Students and Practitioners
Rushdan Noor, Eng Hseon Tay, and Jeffrey Low

ISBN 978-981-4463-06-5 (Hardcover), 978-981-4463-07-2 (eBook)
www.panstanford.com

Tumour Immunology and Immunotherapy

The tumour microenvironment is an important aspect of cancer biology that contributes to tumour initiation, tumour progression and responses to therapy. Cells and molecules of the immune system are a fundamental component of the tumour microenvironment. Tumour cells express most of the same cell surface antigens (e.g. HLA antigen) as in normal cells. Many tumour cells express specific antigens not found in similar normal cells. This is term as tumour-associated antigens **(TAAs)**. See Fig. 25.1.

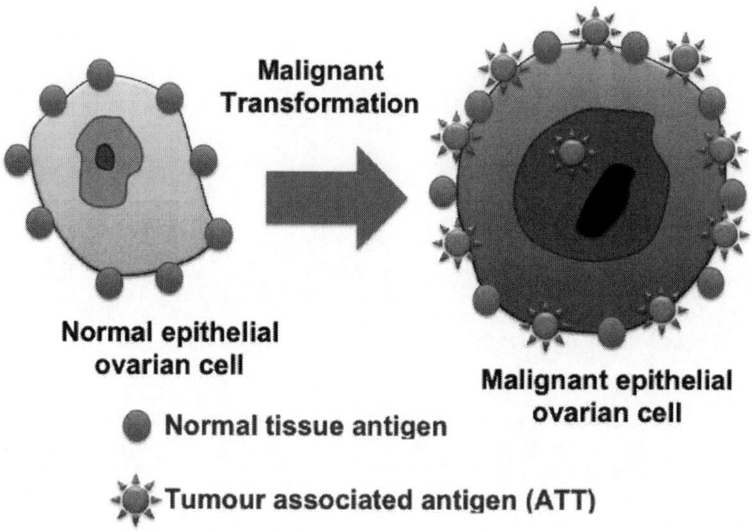

Figure 25.1 Tumour-associated antigens are additionally expressed on the tumour cell surface.

Tumours vary widely in their immunogenicity. In general, neoplasms induced experimentally in vivo with chemical or viral agents are highly immunogenic, while tumour arising spontaneously in vivo (e.g. human malignancies) are poorly immunogenic. There are also antigens that can only be found in the foetus but re-expressed in cancer cells. This oncofoetal antigen is more common than tumour-associated antigens. The example of oncofoetal antigens are carcinoembryonic antigen (CEA) and alpha foetoprotein (AFP). T cells are said to be key effector cells in anti-tumour immunity.

Antigen recognition by T cells involves binding of the T cell receptor to specific major histocompatibility complex (MHC)-peptide combination. By analyzing the T cells that recognize tumours, many TAAs have now been identified. Tumour-associated antigens can be classified into five broad groups: (1) mutated antigens (unique to cancer cells, e.g. mutated beta-catenin, caspase, k-ras, etc., in CML, (2) cancer testis antigens (restricted to testis germ cells, ovary and trophoblast, e.g. MAGE, BAGE, etc.), (3) overexpressed antigen (can be found in normal cell, e.g. p53, Her2/neu), (4) differentiation antigens (only expressed on particular tissue types, e.g. prostate-specific antigen, tyrosinase, etc.), (5) oncogenic viral products (in virally induced cancers, e.g. Epstein–Barr virus antigens in lymphomas, HPV virus antigens E6, E7 in anogenital cancers, etc.).

The immune system may prevent tumours in three main ways: (1) resolving inflammation, (2) eliminating oncogenic viral infections and (3) immunosurveillance.

Following are the arguable evidences that humans have tumour-limiting factors (immunosurveillance):

(1) Spontaneous regression (very rare) has been reported in cancers such as melanoma, renal cancer and neuroblastoma. Many have observed that this tumour regression was preceded by surgical intervention (e.g. biopsy, partial resection), infections, administration of bacterial vaccines, transfusion reaction, etc.).
(2) Self-healing melanomas.
(3) Regression of metastases after resection of primary neoplasms.
(4) Regression of tumour after non-cytotoxic doses of chemotherapy.
(5) Reappearance of metastases after a long latent period.
(6) Frequent failure of circulating tumour cells to form metastases.
(7) Infiltration of tumours by mononuclear cells.
(8) Higher incidence of tumours after clinical immunosuppression.
(9) High incidence of tumour in immune deficiency diseases.
(10) Increased incidence of malignancy with aging.

Following are the evidences to show that tumour-limiting factors may be attributed to an immune system:

(1) Transplant patients are more prone to develop cancer, especially virus-induced cancer, e.g. Herpes virus 8 (Kaposi's sarcoma), HPV (cervical cancer), Epstein–Barr virus (lymphoma) and hepatitis B and C (hepatoma).
(2) Two- to five-fold increase incidence of colon, lung and prostate cancer in kidney transplant recipients.
(3) Patients with Chediak Higashi syndrome (impaired NK cells cytotoxicity) have 200-fold increased risk of malignancy.
(4) Correlation between the presence of TILs (tumour-infiltrating lymphocytes) and prognosis. Presence of TILs correlates with better prognosis.

Despite the ability of the immune system to eliminate the tumour growth, in many instances, tumours can still evade the immune system.

Following are the postulated mechanisms by which foreign or mutant cells (including cancer cells) might avoid an interaction with potentially damaging immune systems:

(1) Lower tumour antigenicity (antigenic modulation): Loss of antigenicity or change in the antigenic markers by which tumour cells may avoid immunologic destruction.
(2) Sneaking through.
(3) Immunoresistance: Similar to antibiotic resistance, cancer cells may developed diminished sensitivity to immune rejection and becomes resistant cancer.
(4) Vascularization (neoplasm keeps proliferate with their antigens locked away behind a wall of new blood vessels, which is recognized as self).
(5) Immunosuppression: Some degree of immunosuppression has been found in almost all cancer patients studied.
(6) Blocking factors, e.g. blocking antibodies, Ag–Ab complexes, etc.
(7) Tumour secreting a range of soluble immunosuppressive mediators, e.g. nitric oxide, transforming growth factor-β and IL-10.

(8) The immune system does not recognize the tumour cells as foreign (through a complex mechanism involving T cells and dendritic cells (DC) instead the immune system treat the tumour as "self".

Principles of Immunotherapy

The first report of successful immunotherapy was in 1881 by William Coley, who treat sarcomas by administrating bacterial toxins. The ultimate goal of immunotherapy is the complete destruction of all neoplastic cells. Immunotherapy has shown more effectiveness in neoplasms that are highly antigenic, such as Burkitt's lymphoma, malignant melanoma and neuroblastoma.

Tumour has the ability to vary their antigenic profile and suppress the immune response. It is well established that tumours down-regulate many of the molecules involved in processing and presentation of peptide on MHC class I, and that changes occur in the antigenic profile of tumours as they progress and metastasize.

The tumour microenvironment is also known to be immunosuppressive due to hypoxia, induction and recruitment of suppressor cells, oxidative stress, etc. This reason is part of explanations why many immunotherapies failed.

Single agent immunotherapy is ineffective. They may be combined with radiotherapy or chemotherapy. Cancer vaccine is currently the most promising immunotherapy. However, there are three main challenges: (1) to identify the "right antigen" that is different from normal cell to minimize self-destruction, (2) to find right adjuvant to enhance an immune response (at present only two adjuvants, aluminium-based salt and squalene oil–water–emulsion (MF56)); other potential adjuvants are cytokines, bacterial products, heat-shock protein, viral-like particles, etc., and (3) to induce the right immune response, which is effective in eradicating tumour cells, sustainable and excellent immune memory. The ultimate goal of vaccine-based cancer immunotherapy is to elicit a potent immune response that will cause the eradication of the tumour as well as generate a long-term memory response that will guarantee complete remission and keep the cancer in check. Immunotherapy is still investigational and so far the results are disappointing.

Immunotherapeutic Approaches

There are two main approaches in immunotherapy: (a) **active Immunotherapy** and (b) **passive Immunotherapy**.

Active Immunotherapy

Active immunotherapy induces in the host a state of immune responsiveness to tumour. There are two types of active immunotherapy: (a) ***non-specific:*** (biologically immunostimulant, e.g. BCG, MER, etc.; chemical immunostimulants, e.g. cimetidine, levamisole, etc.; chemotherapeuutic agents, e.g. cyclophosphamide, doxorubicin, cinca alkaloid, cisplatin; cytokines, e.g. interferon, IL-2, TNF) and (b) ***specific***: Inactivated tumour vaccines.

Passive Immunotherapy

In passive immunotherapy, the host immunologically active substances are transferred directly to the tumour. There are two types of passive immunotherapy: (a) **non-specific** (LAK cells (IL-2), activated macrophages—interferon, cytostatic or cytotoxic cytokines) and (b) **specific** (monoclonal antibodies, radiotherapeutic coupled to alpha- or beta-emitting radionuclides, chemotherapeutic (adriamycin, MTX, etc.), allogeniec bone marrow transplant with ablative chemotherapy or radiation therapy, etc.).

The example of non-specific passive immunotherapy is using lymphokine-activated killer (LAK) cells. Lymphocytes from a patient were removed using leukopheresis machine. These lymphocytes were then treated with a lymphokine called Interleukin-2 (IL-2). This converted lymphocytes into lymphokine-activated killer (LAK) cells that were capable of destroying cancer cells but not normal cells. These LAK cells were infused along with IL-2 back into the patient. The IL-2 induced the LAK cells to multiply for a short time in the body, thus enhancing their ability to destroy cancer cells. This method has been shown to mediate regression of established pulmonary and hepatic metastases in a variety of human neoplasm. Cancers that had been evaluated are renal cell carcinoma, melanoma, colorectal cancer and non-Hodgkin's lymphoma in very advanced stage.

In specific passive immunotherapy, antisera produced from an animal or other cancer patients are injected into the patient. Using the technology of monoclonal antibody, immunizing an animal with antigen and fusing it spleen cell with the long-lived malignant B cell line, antibodies is then produced by this B cell. Monoclonal antibodies could be of benefit in clearing tumours cells from the blood and in diminishing the amount of circulating tumour antigens that could have a blocking effect on subsequent immunotherapy.

Potential Approaches for Cancer Vaccination Strategy

Anti-Idiotypic Antibody-Based Vaccine (Using Monoclonal Antibody Technology)

The most important advantage of this vaccination strategy is that it allows effective vaccination against non-protein antigens, such as tumour specific sugars or lipids, against which it is otherwise difficult to elicit T cell responses.

Dendritic Cell-Based Vaccines

Dendritic cells, the sentinels of the immune system, play a crucial role in activation of antigen-specific immune responses. Since they are the most powerful activators of naïve T cells, DC are being used in vaccines to induce the appropriate antigen-specific immunity.

DNA and RNA Vaccines

The use of naked DNA or RNA encoding the tumour antigen instead of the antigen itself as a vaccine is of great interest because of their expected ease of production. These vaccines elicit immune responses only to the encoded antigens, compared to other types of nucleic acid-based vaccines that depend on tumour antigen expression by various viral vectors.

Viral Vector-Based Vaccines

Naked DNA and RNA can be made more immunogenic by incorporating them into viral vectors. Live recombinant viral vaccines have been tested in cancer for the past 10 years. Viral vectors are an attractive choice for antigen delivery because they mimic a natural infection.

Particle-Based Vaccines

Particulate carriers of antigens, such as microparticles, emulsions, immune stimulating complexes, liposomes, virsomes and virus-like-particles (VLPs) are increasingly being used in vaccine formulations as vehicles to deliver the desired antigen to APC and increase its immunogenicity.

Hormonal Interactions and Hormonal Therapy in Cancer

Hormones

Hormones are chemical messengers that are synthesized and secreted by specific cell type into the circulatory system to target cells. It released continuously or in short bursts. Hormones are inactivated by the liver and excreted by the kidneys. They will bind to the receptor in target cells.

Types of Hormones

There are at least five types of hormones:

(1) **steroids,** e.g. sex hormones, corticosteroid, calcitriol
(2) **eicosanoids** (derived from arachidonic acid), e.g. prostaglandin, leukotrienes
(3) **amines** (derived from tyrosine or tryptophan), e.g. dopamine, epinephrine, melatonin
(4) **peptides** (all hypothalamic, anterior pituitary and digestive hormones)
(5) **nitric oxide**

Receptors

In cell biology, receptor is a structure on the surface of a cell (or inside a cell) that selectively receives and binds a specific substance. Receptors have following properties: (a) protein, (b) specific and high affinity to particular hormones, (c) saturable and (d) binding will result in biologic response. Receptors can be in the cell membranes, cytoplasma or in the nucleus. Hormones bind to the receptors and hormones-receptor complexes will be translocated into the nucleus resulting in specific RNA transcription.

The quality and concentration of receptors can be measured using monoclonal antibody test or immunohistochemical assays. Monoclonal antibody test and immunohistochemical assays in frozen or paraffin-embedded tissue sections are used to qualitatively estimate the distribution and localization of receptors. Determination of oestrogen receptors and progesterone receptors status has been shown to be of clinical value in the management of patients with some cancers arising in hormonally responsive tissue.

Hormonal Interactions in Breast Cancer

Endogenous Sex Steroid and Breast Cancer

The longer duration of endogenous sex steroid exposure would increase breast cancer risk. Multiple studies have linked an increased risk of breast cancer with post-menopausal obesity (relative risk of 1.27 for women with BI > 33 kg/m^2) and weight gain (45% higher risk in women who gained at least 25 kg since age 18).

Exogenous Sex Steroid and Breast Cancer

Women's Health Initiative (WHI), a large multi-centre trial in the United States, involved 16,608 post-menopausal women randomized into two groups, placebo versus combined HRT (conjugated equine oestrogen 0.625 mg and medroxyprogesterone acetate 2.5 mg). After 5.2 years of the WHI study, there was 24% increase in the risk of invasive breast cancer, abnormal mammogram and increased breast density with HRT usage compared to placebo.

In women with breast cancer, HABITS trial from Stockholm involving 447 breast cancer survivors, HRT group was found to have over twice the risk of breast cancer recurrence compared to controls. Results were similar regardless of oestrogen receptor status and tamoxifen use.

HRT used in above studies was found to be more strongly associated with hormone-receptor-positive cancers than negative.

Oestrogen and Anti-Oestrogen in Breast Cancer

Although the WHI study did not see an association between unopposed oestrogen alone and breast cancer risk (average follow-up of 7.1 years), the longer-term effect of this hormone is still unknown. Oestrogen receptor positive breast cancer responds better to hormonal manipulation, while receptor negative tumour is more aggressive. Oestrogen receptor can be quantified, the more the receptor the better the response. Studies have shown that oestrogen receptor positive tumour has a longer disease-free interval and longer survival with adjuvant endocrine therapy compared with receptor negative.

Tamoxifen is a selective oestrogen receptor modulator used as an adjuvant treatment for ER positive early-stage breast cancer and metastatic disease. Tamoxifen (10–20 mg daily) therapy in advanced breast cancer in the post-menopausal patients has been associated with longer disease-free interval and survival and reduced recurrence rate (in ER-positive patient). Anti-tumour effect of Tamoxifen is mediated by anti-oestrogenic activity. The net result is slowing of cell proliferation and even regression. It also may directly influence apoptosis. Tamoxifen also has modest oestrogenic activity on the endometrium. It has been reported that 10% of tamoxifen-treated women will develop endometrial pathology within 5 years. The risk of endometrial cancer in a patient treated with Tamoxifen is RR 2.53 (CI 1.35–4.97). A study showed almost seven-fold increased risk of endometrial cancer. Duration of tamoxifen use is an important determinant, i.e. two-fold increased risk after 2 years, and five-fold after 5 years). Tamoxifen-induced endometrial cancer was found to be more of prognostically unfavorable histotype. The annual risk of endometrial cancer in a patient on tamoxifen is approximately 2–3 per 1000. Routine endometrial sampling in asymptomatic women is not cost effective. No survival advantage if Tamoxifen continued for more than 5 years in women with node negative and receptor positive. Longer used of tamoxifen was also found to be associated with other uterine pathology, i.e. polyps, adenomyosis, fibroids, endometrial hyperplasia. The other future hormones that may be useful in breast cancer are toremifene, raloxifene and other SERMs.

Aromatase inhibitor (AI) is an alternative to tamoxifen as an adjuvant treatment for post-menopausal early-stage ER positive breast cancer. AI suppresses oestrogen synthesis by inhibiting aromatase (blocking the conversion of androgen to oestrogen). Anastrazole is an example of aromatase inhibitor. It has been proven to be effective in preventing breast cancer recurrences and safer than tamoxifen in terms of endometrial pathology. A study showed anastrazole could reverse the tamoxifen-induced endometrial lesions.

Progestogen and Breast Cancer

In WHI trial, progestogen component in HRT was found to be responsible in the breast cancer risk and not oestrogen component. It is hypothesized that progesterone may increase cell division and thereby lead to the accumulation of DNA damage.

Hormonal Therapy in Endometrial Adenocarcinoma

General

Endometrium contains high-affinity, steroid-specific receptors for both oestrogens and progesterone. Maximum oestrogen receptors (ER) and progesterone receptor (PR) concentration occur in mid to late proliferative phase. Progesterone produced by corpus luteum results in downregulation of both ER and PR in the endometrium. Progesterone also inhibits proliferation of endometrial cells. The concentration of ER in endometrial neoplasia is in the same range with ER concentration in late proliferative phase of the normal endometrium. Almost all endometrial carcinomas are ER positive. PR is comparable with those found in secretory phase of the normal menstrual cycle. Progesterone receptor concentration varied with the degree of differentiation of tumour. An aggressive endometrial cancer has lower PR and ER.

The correlation between PR positivity and response to progesterone treatment is still being evaluated. Many studies suggested, although a significantly higher response rate is observed in a patient with PR-positive tumour, a variable response is found in both the receptor positive and negative. There is more than one factor involved.

Progestogen Therapy in Endometrial Neoplasia

Endometrial Hyperplasia

Adenomatous and atypical hyperplasias are more resistant to progestogen therapy than simple hyperplasia with response rate of 80% and 50%, respectively. Intra-uterine levonorgestrel gives better response rate than oral progestogen (100% vs. 60%, respectively).

Endometrial Carcinomas

Progesterone was shown to have an anti-oestrogenic effect on the endometrium. It acts as anti-oestrogen by reducing oestrogen receptor content and increasing oestradiol dehydrogenase. Progestogen can also reverse well-differentiated endometrial adenocarcinoma in young women desirous of childbearing. The regression rate following high-dose progestogen therapy in early-stage and grade 1 endometrial cancer is 60–70%. The recurrence rates of as high as 24–46% was reported at the median follow-up of 40 months.

The other indications for hormonal therapy are as follows: (a) In recurrent endometrial cancer, the response rate is poor, i.e. 15–25%. (b) In metastatic endometrial carcinoma, the common dosage of Provera is 50 mg tds. A study comparing progestogen dose of 1000 mg versus 200 mg per day showed no additional benefit to doses greater than 200 mg/day. The route of administration does not affect the outcome and PR positive tumour has slightly better response rate (37% vs. 8% in GOG81) compared to PR negative.

Other Potential Hormonal Treatment for Endometrial Carcinoma

(1) **GnRH analogues**: Minig et al. (2011) evaluate the efficacy of combined therapy of levonorgestrel-release intrauterine

device (LNG-IUD) and GnRH analogue in patients with atypical endometrial hyperplasia and stage 1A, well differentiated endometrial cancer who would like to preserve their fertility. The treatment consisted of the insertion of LNG-IUD for 1 year plus GnRH analogue for 6 months. Complete response rate was observed in 95% of patients with atypical endometrial hyperplasia and 57.1% of patients with endometrial cancer. However, the samples involved in this study were small.

(2) **tamoxifen** (response rate of 10% in advanced and recurrent disease): A study showed better response rate with a combination of progestogen and tamoxifen (up to 22%)

(3) **Aromatase inhibitors** (study very limited, response rate 9–15% in recurrent endometrial cancer).

Steroid Receptors and Predictive Tests for Endometrial Cancer

Are there any predictive tests or factors to determine progestogen responsiveness? At present, no accurate test is available. The detection and measurement of steroid receptors have been proposed but the problem is to isolate tumour cell from normal epithelial. The epithelial lining makes up 50% of the normal endometrium. The presence of small proportion of normal epithelial will affect the tumour receptor status. Measurement of steroid receptors in breast cancer is easier because of much smaller proportion of normal epithelium in the whole breast tissue. Recently, with the emergence of Monoclonal antibodies test with immunohistochemical technology, receptor status in endometrial tumour could be measured more accurately; however the clinical usage of this information is still controversial.

Endometrial Stromal Sarcoma

Low-grade endometrial stromal sarcoma may respond to hormonal therapy due to their steroid receptor concentration. A response rate of 50% had been reported in recurrent low-grade endometrial stromal sarcoma (ESS). A small study on GnRH (Leuprolide) given to shrink the tumour size has been reported.

Hormonal Therapy and Receptors in Ovarian Carcinoma

Steroid receptor status in normal ovary and ovarian tumour is not completely known. A study on ER and PR in carcinoma of ovary and relation with tumour grade, histology grade and prognosis are conflicting. Trial has been done to evaluate the activity of tamoxifen in patients refractory to cytotoxic chemotherapy. In GOG protocol, Tamoxifen 20 mg bd was given in a patient with stage 3 and 4 ovarian epithelial carcinoma with persistent or recurrence after first line therapy: complete response was observed in 10–15% and 89% of these patients had elevated oestrogen receptor. The highest response to tamoxifen is seen in endometroid histology.

Review of 18 trials on hormonal therapy in advanced ovarian cancer showed 13% overall response rate (majority uses tamoxifen). Recent meta-analysis, specifically on tamoxifen involving 14 studies showed overall response rate of 9.6% and stable disease in 31.9%.

Progestogen (50 mg tds) has also been use but complete response rate less than 5%. Overall response rate was only 8% in the Northern California Oncology Group study using high-dose megestrol. The other potential hormonal treatments in recurrent ovarian cancer are aromatase inhibitors (letrozole and anastrozole) and GnRH analogue (response rate between 9% and 12%).

HRT in Patients Treated for Gynae Malignancy

Oestrogen replacement can be given to patients with cervical cancer. A study demonstrates a reduction in long-term radiation complications to rectum, vagina and bladder were less if given oestrogen. Combined HRT should be given, as not all endometrial linings will be completely irradiated.

In endometrial cancer, the benefit of HRT outweighs the risk of stimulating occult tumour growth. Caution must be taken in using HRT in patients with high-risk prognostic factor, e.g. myometrial invasion, high grade, etc. Data are still limited but available data so far show no increased in recurrence rate among endometrial cancer patients who were on oestrogen replacement therapy following primary treatment.

All uterine sarcoma except low-grade endometrial stromal sarcoma are non-hormonal dependent tumour. A small case series studying women treated for ESS showed HRT to adversely affect the course of disease.

Two meta-analyses with conflicting results on the impact of HRT on epithelial ovarian cancer (EOC) development have been published—the first suggesting no increase in relative risk of EOC in post-menopausal women taking HRT and a second showing a small, but significant, increase of risk after a prolonged use for more than 10 years. Endometroid EOC is oestrogen sensitive tumour. However, studies have failed to show an association between HRT use and the development of EC or the course of disease after treatment. Ovarian granulosa cell tumour is known to secrete steroid hormones and commonly present with symptoms of hyperoestrogenism.

Squamous carcinoma of cervix is not hormonal-sensitive tumour and therefore there is no contraindication of HRT in cervical cancer survival. In adenocarcinoma of the cervix, epidemiological data have shown an increased risk association of adenocarcinoma of the cervix with the prolonged use of oral contraceptive (OC) pills, more so in human papilloma virus (HPV) positive women. The mechanism of an increased cervical cancer (adenocarcinoma) risk in HPV-positive patients taking OC pills may be related to an oestrogen metabolite—16-alpha-hydroxyestrone, which acts as a cofactor together with oncogenic HPV to promote cell proliferation.

Conclusion: Based on the biological knowledge and published clinical information, SCCs of the uterine cervix, vulva carcinoma, vagina carcinoma, ovarian carcinoma, endometrial serous carcinomas and most uterine sarcomas are not oestrogen dependent (except endometrial stromal sarcoma) and therefore, HRT can be given safely.

OCP and Prevention of Ovarian and Endometrial Cancer

A meta-analysis demonstrated a significant reduction in risk of ovarian epithelial cancer with the use of OCP: 50% reduction in risk if used more than 5 years duration. Ten years of OCP usage in women with strong family history of ovarian cancer reduced their risk of developing ovarian cancer lower than women without family history and who never used OCP. OCP also protects those who have a mutation BRCA1 and BRCA2, i.e. 60% reduction in women taking OCP for 6 years. OCP also reduced the risk of endometrial cancer even only for 1-year usage, i.e. 50% reduction.

References

Anderson GL, Limacher M, Assaf AR, et al. Effects of conjugated equine oestrogen in postmenopausal women with hysterectomy: the women's health initiative randomized controlled trial. *J Am Med Assoc* 2004; **291**(14): 1701–1712.

Barakat RR, Brundy BN, Spirtos NM, Bell J, Mannel RS. Randomized double-blind trial of estrogen replacement therapy versus placebo in stage I or II Endometrial cancer: a gynaecologic oncology group study. *J Clin Oncol* 2006; **24**: 587–592.

Bergman L, Beelen M, Gallee M, et al. The Comprehensive Cancer Centres ALERT Group. Risk and prognosis of endometrial cancer after tamoxifen for breast cancer. *Lancet* 2000; **356**: 881–887.

Chen WY. Exogenous and endogenous hormones and breast cancer. *Best Pract Res Clin Endocrinol Metab* 2008; **22**(4): 573–585.

Copier J, Dalgleish AG, Britten CM, et al. Improving the efficacy of cancer immunotherapy. *Eur J Cancer* 2009; **45**: 1424–1431.

Coughlin SS, Giustozzi A, Smith SJ, Lee NC. A meta-analysis of estrogen replacement therapy and risk of epithelial ovarian cancer. *J Clin Epidemiol* 2000; **53**: 367–375.

Clemente CG, Mihm MC Jr, Bufalino R, et al. Prognostic value of tumour infiltrating lymphocytes in the vertical growth phase of primary cutaneous melanoma. *Cancer* 1996; **77**: 1303–1310.

Eliassen AH, Colditz GA, Rosner B, et al. Adult weight change and risk of postmenopausal breast cancer. *J Am Med Assoc* 2006; **296**(2): 193–201.

Ferguson SE, Soslow RA, Amsterdam A, Barakat RR. Comparison of uterine malignancies that develop during and following tamoxifen therapy. *Gynecol Oncol* 2006; **101**: 322–326.

Ferguson G, Herzog T. Current research on the use of hormonal therapy in the treatment of advanced or recurrent endometrial cancer. *Women's Oncol Rev* 2004; **4**: 175–180.

Gaddy SP, Finn OJ. Cancer Vaccines: Accomplishment and Challenges. *Crit Rev Oncol/Hematol* 2008; **67**: 93–102.

Garrett A, Quinn MA. Hormonal therapies and gynaecological cancers. *Best Pract Res Clin Obstet Gynaecol* 2008; **22**(2): 407–421.

Garuti G, Cellani F, Centinaio G, et al. Prospective endometrial assessment of breast cancer patients treated with third generation aromatase inhibitors. *Gynecol Oncol* 2006; **103**: 599–603.

Gottschalk S, Edwards OL, Sili U, et al. Generating CTLs against the subdominant Epstein–Barr virus LMP1 antigen for the adoptive immunotherapy of EBV-associated malignancies. *Blood* 2003; **101**: 1905–1912.

Holmberg L, Iversen OE, Rudenstam CM, et al. Increased risk of recurrence after hormone replacement therapy in breast cancer survivors. *J Natl Cancer Inst* 2008; **100**: 475–482.

Lai C, Huang H. The role of hormones for the treatment of endometrial hyperplasia and endometrial cancer. *Curr Opin Obstet Gynecol* 2006; **18**: 29–34.

Mascarenhas C, Lambe M, Bellocco R, et al. Use of hormone replacement therapy before and after ovarian cancer diagnosis and ovarian cancer survival. *Int J Cancer* 2006; **119**: 2907–2915.

Menada MV, Costantini S, Moioli M, et al. Evaluation of endometrial thickness in hormone receptor positive early stage breast cancer postmenopausal women switching from adjuvant tamoxifen treatment to anastrozole. *Breast* 2008; **17**: 631–636.

Minig L, Franchi D, Boveri S, et al. Progestin intrauterine device and GnRH analogue for uterus-sparing treatment of endometrial precancers and well-differentiated early endometrial carcinoma in young women. *Ann Oncol* 2011; **22**(3): 643–649.

Ostrand-Rosenberg S. Animal models of tumour immunity, immunotherapy and cancer vaccines. *Curr Opin Immunol* 2004; **16**: 143–150.

Prestwich RJ, Errington F, Hatfield P, Merrick AE, Ilett J, Selby PJ, Melcher AA. Overview: the immune system-is it relevant to cancer development, progression and treatment? *Clin Oncol* 2008; **20**: 101–112.

Rosenberg SA. Progress in human tumour immunology and immunotherapy. *Nature* 2001; **411**: 380–384.

Rossouw JE, Anderson GL, Prentice RL, et al. Writing group for the Women's Health Initiative investigators. risks and benefits of estrogen plus progestin in healthy postmenopausal women. *JAMA* 2002; **288**: 321–333.

Sheil AG, Disney AP, Mathew TH, Livingston BE, Keogh AM. Lymphoma incidence, cyclosporine, and the evolution and major impact of malignancy following organ transplantation. *Transplant Proc* 1997; **29**: 825–827.

Singh P, Oehler MK. Review: Hormone replacement after gynaecological cancer. *Maturitas* 2010; **65**: 190–197.

Smith JS, Green J, Berrington de Gonzalez A, et al. Cervical cancer and use of hormonal contraceptives: a systematic review. *Lancet* 2003; **361**: 1159–67.

Sousa Antonio MR, Makuch DS. The immune system as key to cancer treatment: Triggering its activity with microbial agents. *Bioscience* 2009; **2**: 388–392.

William C, Simera I. Tamoxifen for relapse of ovarian cancer. *Cochrane Database Syst Rev* 2001; I: CD001034.

Chapter 26

Management of Long-Term Side Effects of Gynaecologic Cancer Treatment

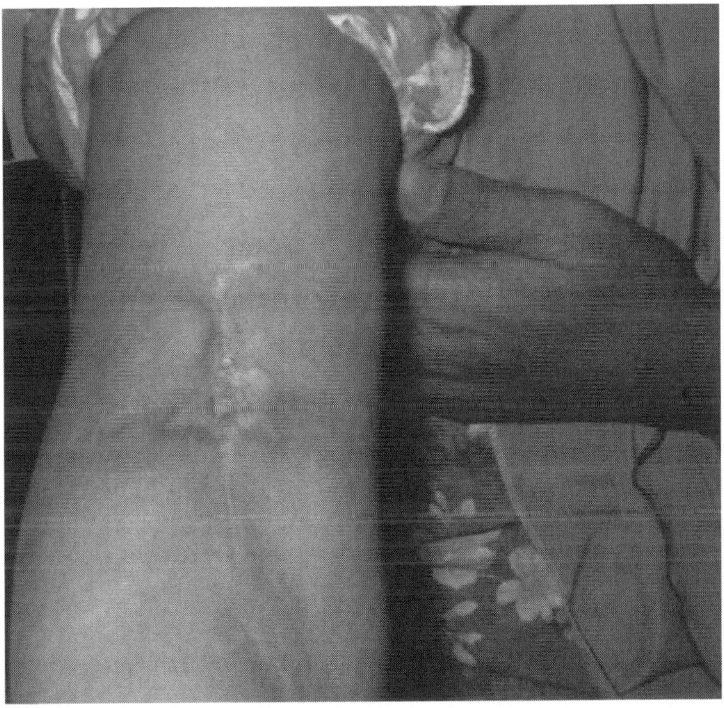

Gynaecologic Cancer: A Handbook for Students and Practitioners
Rushdan Noor, Eng Hseon Tay, and Jeffrey Low

ISBN 978-981-4463-06-5 (Hardcover), 978-981-4463-07-2 (eBook)
www.panstanford.com

Introduction

Treatment for patients with gynaecological cancer comprises surgery, chemotherapy and radiotherapy in the form of either single or combined modalities. Each treatment modality carries potential side effects either locally or systemically. Long-term side effects are those developed several months after the initiation of treatment. This chapter highlights the prevention and management of long-term side effects of gynaecological cancer treatment.

Side Effects of Chemotherapy

Mucositis

Mucositis is commonly associated with anthracyclines, methotrexate, alkylating agents and 5-FU.

Therapeutic measures for mucositis are

(a) Nystatin syrup if associated with fungal infection
(b) Sucking ice chips
(c) Gargle with sodium bicarbonate, chlorhexidine, thymol, etc.
(d) Lignocaine gel for symptomatic

Alopecia

Majority of cytotoxic drugs will cause some degree of alopecia. Alopecia is most commonly associated with anthracyclines, taxanes and etoposide. The hair will grow back 2–3 months following chemotherapy.

Following are some suggestions for patients to minimize alopecia:

(a) Use a gentle shampoo and a soft brush.
(b) Avoid dyeing, perms, bleaches and hair sprays.
(c) Protect the scalp from sun exposure.
(d) The use of a scalp tourniquet is controversial.

Myelodysplastic Syndrome and Acute Non-Lymphocytic Leukaemia

This is the most feared long-term complication of cancer treatment. Alkylating agents if given for a long duration increase the risk of acute non-lymphocytic leukaemia by 10-fold. The peak incidence of myelodysplastic syndrome and acute non-lymphocytic leukaemia is after 4–5 years of chemotherapy. The risk still persists up to 8 years after the cessation of chemotherapy. Data regarding cisplatin and acute leukaemia are conflicting. The benefits of cisplatin were found to outweigh the risk of leukaemia. The use of etoposide has also been recently found to increase the risk of acute leukaemia.

Cardiac Toxicity

Doxorubicin can cause acute cardiac toxicity, i.e. arrhythmias, pericarditis or, more commonly, chronic heart failure. Cardiotoxicity is rare if a total dose of doxorubicin is less than 350 mg. The risk of cardiac toxicity is 1–10% if a cumulative dose is more than 550 mg/m^2. The risk of cardiotoxicity is increased if the cardiotoxic drug is combined with Paclitaxel. Patients who had cardiac irradiation have an increased risk of developing chemotherapy-induced cardiac toxicity.

The dose of doxorubicin must be reduced if patients are known to have (a) hypertension and pre-existing cardiac disease, (b) diabetes, (c) prior mediastinal irradiation and (d) age more than 70 years.

Following are measures to reduce the risk of cardiotoxicity by doxorubicin:

(a) Slow continuous intravenous infusion for several days instead of bolus dose.
(b) Chemoprotector agent, i.e. dexrazoxane, which reduces the anthracycline-induced cardiac injury.
(c) Liposososmal doxorubicin is less cardiotoxic.

Pulmonary Toxicity

The most serious pulmonary toxicity by bleomycin is subacute and chronic interstitial pneumonitis. Pneumonitis can lead to fibrosis. Early symptoms of pneumonitis are cough and dyspnoea. The risk of pulmonary toxicity is 5% if cumulative dose of bleomycin is less than 450 mg. The other risk factors that increase the risk of pulmonary toxicity are (a) age more than 70 years, (b) prior chest irradiation, (c) pre-existing emphysema and (d) single dose of more than 25 mg/m^2. The pathogenesis of bleomycin-induced pulmonary toxicity is unknown. Slow infusion of bleomycin is known to reduce the risk or pulmonary toxicity and bleomycin has to be discontinued if the pulmonary function test shows the reduction of more than 15%. Mitomycin C is another drug that has a similar effect if the cumulative dose is more than 20 mg/m^2.

Neurotoxicity

Peripheral neuropathy is associated with platinum, vinca alkaloids and taxanes. Vinca alkaloids can also cause autonomic neuropathy. Platinum, ifosfamide and 5-FU had been linked with a rare complication of encephalopathy. Neuropathy and ototoxicity are dose-limiting side effects of cisplatin.

Among neurologic side effects of cisplatin are

(a) peripheral sensory neuropathy (most common)
(b) ototoxicity leading to high-frequency hearing loss, tinnitus
(c) retinal toxicity
(d) seizures
(e) autonomic dysfunction

In some cases, the initial symptoms of neurotoxicities are only manifested after months of initiating the treatment. The incidence is 15% if a cumulative cisplatin dose is more than 300 mg/m^2 and the incidence increases to 85% if a cumulative dose is more than 300 mg/m^2. The neurotoxicity improves a few months after the cessation of treatment. The exact aetiology of neurotoxicity is unknown; it may be due to low magnesium levels and interaction of cisplatin with vitamin B12. Besides cisplatin, paclitaxel also has a similar side effect. The combination paclitaxel and cisplatin can increase the incidence of severe peripheral neuropathy to as high as 20–25%. The treatment options for neurotoxicity are (a) amitriptylline, (b) carbamazepine and (c) gabapentin.

Renal Insufficiency

Renal insufficiency is most commonly associated with cisplatin. The renal damage is reversible in the majority of cases and the damage often involves the renal tubules system. Hypomagnesaemia is one of the manifestations of chemotherapy-induced renal insufficiency. The other cytotoxic drug that has been associated with renal insufficiency or nephrotoxicity is Mitomycin.

Nephrotoxicity can be minimized by selection of less nephrotoxic cytotoxic drugs, appropriate pre-chemotherapy hydration before administration of nephrotoxic drug, close monitoring of renal function and the use of chemoprotector such as amifostine. Amifostine can reduce the harmful effect of cisplatin to renal tubules. It is given as slow intravenous infusion 30 minutes prior to chemotherapy. It is readily taken up by cells, where it binds to and detoxifies reactive metabolites of platinum and alkylating agents as well as scavenges free radicals.

Infertility and Mutagenic Potential

Chemotherapy-induced amenorrhoea is more common in older age group. In patients younger than 24 years, the incidence of amenorrhoea is 28%. The data regarding the incidence of infertility are limited. There is no increase risk in foetal congenital anomalies and neuro-developmental impairment if exposure occurs before conception.

Neutropenic Sepsis

Patients on chemotherapy are prone to developing infection. Infection can be life threatening and patients must be counselled about fever following chemotherapy and the need to seek medical attention. Fever is common if the patient develops neutropenia.

The definitions of febrile neutropenia are

(a) **Fever**: Single oral temperature of 38.3°C and above or persistent temperature of 38.0°C for more than 1 hour
(b) **Neutropenia**: Neutrophil count < 500 cells/mm^3, or a count of <1000 cells/mm^3 with a predicted decrease to <500 cells/mm^3
(c) **Febrile neutropenia**: Presence of both fever and neutropenia

Bacterial infections occurring during episodes of febrile neutropenia are caused predominantly by aerobic Gram-negative bacilli (especially *Escherichia coli, Klebsiella pneumonia* and *Pseudomonas aeruginosa*) and Gram-positive cocci have become more prominent in recent years with the increasing use of indwelling intravenous catheters. The other organisms responsible in neutropenic sepsis are fungus and viruses.

Patients with neutropenic sepsis should be admitted, and septic work-up should be done. Empirical antibiotics must be started as either monotherapy or dual therapy. Combination antibiotics may be preferred in cases with severe neutropenia.

Colony-stimulating factors such as G-CSFs should be considered in patients with febrile neutropenia with the following high-risk features:

(a) age more than 65 year old
(b) expected prolonged (more than 10 days) and profound neutropenia ($<0.1 \times 10^9$/L)
(c) altered sensorium
(d) uncontrolled medical disease
(e) hypotension and multi-organ dysfunction
(f) possible hospital-acquired infection
(g) as secondary prophylaxis for patients who experienced febrile neutropenia from a previous cycle of chemotherapy.

G-CSF should be given 24–72 hours after the administration of myelotoxic chemotherapy and continue until the absolute neutrophil count $\geq 1 \times 10^9$/L. The recommended doses of CSF are 5 μg/kg/day for G-CSF and 250 μg/m^2/day for GM-CSF given subcutaneously.

Central Nervous System Adverse Effects Induced by Chemotherapy

Various chemotherapy-induced CNS toxicities have been reported in the literature. Chemotherapy-induced CNS toxicity can be acute or delayed. Headache and seizures have been reported in many chemotherapeutic drugs, including platinum and vinca alkaloids. The causes of seizures include direct toxic effects and indirect metabolic derangement during chemotherapy. Vincristine has been known to cause inappropriate anti-diuretic hormone secretion with encephalopathy. Ifosfamide can cause an encephalopathy leading to confusion or even a coma; this is usually reversible. Cerebellar syndrome was reported to occur following administration of 5-fluorouracil and high dose cytarabine. Mitomycin can trigger thrombotic microangiopathy, and anti-VEGF drugs can cause cerebral haemorrhage and arterial infarction. Intrathecal chemotherapy (methotrexate, cytarabine) can produce aseptic meningitis and very rarely, transverse myelopathy, which can generally be prevented with concomitant corticosteroids. Central nervous system chemotherapy-induced side effects are more common in a patient treated for brain tumour when they received intrathecal chemotherapy.

Most chemotherapeutic agents do not efficiently cross the blood–brain barrier but animal studies have shown that some chemotherapeutic agents such as cisplatin, fluorouracil and carmustine given intravenously can increase blood–brain barrier permeability, which could raise CNS toxicity. Combination chemotherapy is more commonly associated with CNS toxicity as compared to single agent chemotherapy. The exact mechanism of CNS toxicity in chemotherapy is unknown.

Side Effects of Radiation Therapy

In gynaecological malignancy, radiation injuries occur mainly to the bladder, ureter, rectosigmoid and small bowel. A late complication to bowel and urinary tract occur 6–24 months after completion of therapy. Radiation can also leads to bladder complications such as haemorrhage, vesicovaginal fistula and contracted bladder.

The other complication of radiation therapy is gastrointestinal toxicity such as proctitis, sigmoiditis, stricture, obstruction and fistula.

Barillot et al. have reported that the 5-year actuarial rates of late radiation toxicity in more than 600 patients with cervical cancer were 42% for grade 1, 23.5% for grade 2, 10% for grade 3 and 3% for grade 4. The majority were related to reproductive organ (31%) and rectum (21.5%). Generally, the risk of developing late grade 3 and 4 toxicity associated with radiotherapy is in between 3–9.3% (Perez et al., 1999; Eifel et al., 1995).

A major radiation complication requiring admission occurs in 12% of cases, and among the complications are ureteric stricture (risk 0.7%) mainly at the uretero-vesical junction and large bowel injury such as fistula, which occurs after 6–18 months. The risk of ureteric stricture is significantly increased with combination of radical surgery and radiotherapy.

Femoral head fracture and necrosis can occur after radiation therapy. In a study, the cumulative actuarial incidence of femoral neck fracture was found to be 2% at 5 years and 15% at 10 years.

Predisposing Factors to Radiation-Related Complications

The predisposing factors to radiation-related complications can be divided into host factors, disease-related and treatment-related factors.

Host Factors

(a) Poor tissue oxygenation, i.e. hypoxia due to anaemia
(b) Poor nutritional status

Disease-Related Predisposing Factors

(a) Medical disorders that reduce tissue oxygenation, i.e. hypertension, diabetes, etc.
(b) Pre-existing pelvic pathology, e.g. PID, diverticulitis, previous surgery
(c) Locally advanced cancer can indirectly produce poor tissue oxygenation and distorted of normal anatomy and this lead to altered distribution of radiation dose.

Treatment-Related Predisposing Factors

(a) External beam irradiation: Predisposing factors is related to dose per-fraction, total dose (10% risk of total dose 45–50 Gy), Beam energy and number of treatment field.
(b) Intra-cavitary irradiation; Predisposing factors is related to placement and type of applicator, dose rate (high dose rate, 2–3 Gy/min is associated with the risk of cystitis and proctitis).

Gastrointestinal Radiation Toxicity

The risk of gastrointestinal toxicity in patients following radiotherapy varies depending on the type and dose of radiotherapy, concomitant chemotherapy, general condition of patients, surgical treatment prior to radiotherapy, etc. With current development of better radiotherapy technique, the risk of gastrointestinal toxicity is expected to be lower than before. The risk of grade 3 and 4 gastrointestinal toxicity is ranging from 9–23%. Chen et al. reported 13.4% of patients developed RTOG grade 2 and greater gastrointestinal toxicity with median latency of 18 months following radiotherapy for cervical cancer. Late gastrointestinal toxicity is especially attributed to vascular insufficiency (chronic ischaemia) and fibrosis. Intestinal radiation injuries occur mainly in cervical cancer due to exposure to higher dose of radiation. About 74% of intestinal radiation injuries developed within 2 years of therapy. Late radiation effects on the small bowel can result in ulceration and inflammation causing malabsorption and bacterial overgrowth. The most common site is the ileum because small intestines are more sensitive than colon. Rectosigmoid and caecum are second most common sites.

In radiation-induced gastrointestinal toxicities, the most common indications for surgery are obstruction and fistula. Small bowel obstruction was observed in 3.9–5.3% and can occur up to 20 years after treatment.

The most common large bowel complications are haemorrhage, rectal ulceration, proctitis and fistula with the average latency period of 6–18 months. Radiation fistula to the rectosigmoid is difficult to manage (incidence is 3% at 20 years). Recurrent tumour has to be excluded. Fistula repair is done after faecal diversion procedure. Opening site has to be closed by tissue with blood supply. These tissues can be bulbocavernosus fat pad, gracilis and rectus muscle and folded piece of normal colon as patch (Bricker's technique) (see Fig. 26.1).

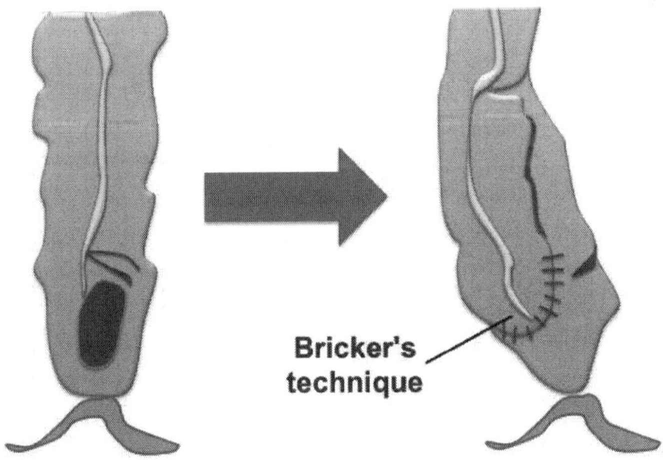

Figure 26.1 Surgical treatment for radiation fistula with Bricker's technique.

Pathogenesis of Acute and Late Radiation Toxicity

One of the most important radiation toxicity is related to gastrointestinal tract (GIT). GIT epithelial has short cell cycle time (12–15 hours) and therefore, sensitive to radiation. Radiation cause damage of epithelial leading to thinning of the mucosa and later denuding. Acute inflammatory reaction causes malabsorption and fluid/electrolytes loss. A late complication has different pathogenesis. Late effects are due to vascular endothelial damage, i.e. capillary endarteritis and fibrosis leading to tissue hypoxia. Tissue hypoxia leads to ulceration, fibrosis, perforation and fistula. There is no correlation between an early and late effect in terms of risk and severity. It is advisable to avoid biopsy to radiation ulcer because it can be predisposed to fistula formation. The risk of radiation-induced fistula is approximately 1–2%.

Urinary Tract Radiation Injury

Urinary tract radiation injury is a serious complication but less common than a bowel complications. Ureteral and bladder radiation injuries manifested 1–3 years after radiotherapy. One-third of patients presented within 1 year of radiotherapy. Late bladder toxicity appears to be the result of damage to the vascular endothelial cells.

Ureteric Radiation Injury

Ureteric injury occurs in 0.6–1.7% of radical hysterectomies. The risk of ureteric stricture is 1% and the most common site to radiation ureteric stricture is 4–6 cm above the uretero-vesical junction at the point ureter passes parametrium. Unilateral ureteric stricture occurs in 60% of cases. Before any surgical repair, tumour recurrence has to be first excluded. If the ureter has to be resected, uretero-neocystostomy may be difficult as the bladder also may be abnormal due to radiation. Lateral dome of bladder usually receives lesser dose of radiation and, therefore, is the preferred site of ureteric re-implantation.

If the bladder has been severely affected by radiation, segment of the intestine can be used to cover the implantation site in bladder.

Transuretero-ureterostomy is an alternative if the opposite ureter is normal. If both ureters are abnormal, urinary diversion is the only option.

Bladder Radiation Injuries

Radiation can cause cystitis, haematuria, contracture, necrosis and fistula formation. Anti-cholinergic drug can be used to increased bladder capacity and reduced frequency in a patient with radiation cystitis. Irrigation of bladder with the corticosteroid solution may be helpful in some patients. Uncontrolled bleeding is often treated with electrocoagulation using diathermy cystoscopically.

Intra-vesical instillation of 1% formalin may be useful in severe chronic haematuria (exclude ureteric reflux before proceed, formalin is toxic to upper tract and kidney).

Fistula is most commonly occurring between the anterior vaginal wall and posterior bladder wall. The risk of radiation vesico-vaginal fistula is 1–2%. Simple closure in radiation vesico-vaginal fistula is often unsuccessful. Fistula closure is done using well-vascularized tissue such as gracilis muscle, omentum and bulbocavernosus muscle. Permanent urinary diversion may be necessary.

Sexual Function

Sexual dysfunction has been reported approximately in 50% of patients following radiation therapy for cervical cancer. Reported complications related to sexual function are deterioration in sexual interest (49%), frequency of intercourse (47%), lubrication problem (46%), failed to achieve orgasm (49%) and dyspareunia (36%). Vaginal stenosis was reported in 30% of patients.

Secondary Malignancies

Breast, bone marrow and thyroid gland are the most sensitive organ that can develop secondary malignancies after exposure to radiation. An increased risk of solid cancer usually does not appear until 10 years or more following radiation exposure. Endometrial cancer is a potential secondary malignant tumour developed following pelvic irradiation. The estimated incidence is less than 1% and the risk of uterine sarcoma was found to be 5.4 times higher than non-radiated population.

Surgical Complications in Gynaeoncologic Surgery

Urinary Tract Injuries

Intra-operative urinary tract injuries

Bladder injuries occur in 1–2% of radical hysterectomy, while ureteric injury occurs in 1% of radical hysterectomy. The causes of ureteric injuries are (a) Crushing injury by clamp or ligature and (b) Laceration and transaction. In crushing injury, if the blood supply is not impaired, it can be managed conservatively with ureteric stenting. Severe crushing injury requires resection of the damaged site and followed by end-to-end anastomosis or re-implantation of ureter into the bladder (uretero-neocystostomy). Injuries below the pelvic brim generally require re-implantation of the ureter. Permanent suture materials should never be used in repairing uroendothelium. Urinary diversion is indicated if there is no possibility of ureteric repair. There are two types of urinary diversion: (a) continent type and (b) incontinent type.

Post-operative urinary tract injuries

The incidence of uretero-vaginal fistula is 1–2% in radical hysterectomy and it may will only apparent on 5th to 14th day post-operatively. The treatment for uretero-vaginal fistula is either conservative or surgical repair. If the conservative approach is adopted, the patient is given antibiotics, undergoes ureteric stenting and awaits spontaneous resolution in 6–8 weeks. Surgical treatment is indicated if there is significant intra-abdominal urine leak and repair should be done immediately. Surgery is also indicated if failed conservative approach. As compared to uretero-vesical fistula, vesico-vaginal fistula is less common but often closed by itself if the defect is small. Vesicovaginal fistula occurs after both irradiation and radical surgery invariably required surgical correction.

One of the most common urinary tract complications following radical hysterectomy is bladder dysfunction. Bladder dysfunction after radical hysterectomy is due to disruption of nerve supply and 2–3% of patients develop severe form of bladder dysfunction.

Intestinal Injuries

Surgery for gynaecological cancer particularly for advanced ovarian cancer has lead to various intestinal complications. Intestinal injuries can be divided into (a) intra-operative intestinal injuries and (b) post-operative intestinal injuries.

Intra-operative Injuries

The predisposing factors for intra-operative intestinal injuries are (a) previous surgery, (b) prior irradiation, (c) inflammatory bowel disease and (d) intra-peritoneal chemotherapy. The types of intestinal injuries include serosal injuries, laceration, transected and impairment of blood supply. Small intestines can be repaired by continuous suturing because of high blood supply. Large intestines should be repaired by interrupted suture to minimize vascular impairment. The most common suture material used to repair the intestines is vicryl/silk size 3/0. Bowel preparation is important prior to surgery to reduce the risk of bowel injury and minimized its complications.

Post-operative Injuries

Intestinal obstruction can occur due to adhesion, most resolved spontaneously after conservative management. Anastomotic leak was reported in 1–6% of cases, while the risk of post-anastomotic stricture was reported in 3%. Intestinal leak can also occur spontaneously due to ischaemic necrosis and unrepaired intestinal wall tear. Enterocutaneous fistula and mild leak can be managed conservatively: (a) nil by mouth, (b) intravenous drip and total parenteral nutrition, (c) gastric suction and (d) somatostatin to reduce intestinal secretion. Paralytic ileus is common post-operative complication gynaecological oncology surgery and it often resolved after conservative treatment. Small bowel obstruction can be treated conservatively. However, large bowel complete obstruction has to deal surgically to avoid caecal perforation (if caecum acutely dilated > 10 cm).

Appendix

Common Toxicity Criteria (Simplified CTC Ver. 3.0)

- Common toxicity criteria are a standardized classification of side effects used in order to determine the severity of treatment-related side effects.
- The latest version of Common Terminology Criteria for Adverse Event (CTCAE) is version 4 released by US Department of Health and Human Services in May 2009. It is endorsed by US National Institutes of Health and National Cancer Institute.
- Grade 5 is death and, therefore, is not stated in the following table.

Blood/Bone Marrow

Adverse event	Grade 1	Grade 2	Grade 3	Grade 4
Haemoglobin (g/dl)	<LLN–10.0	8.0–10.0	6.5–8.0	<6.5
Leukocytes (mm^3)	<LLN–3000	2000–3000	1000–2000	<1000
Neutrophil (mm^3)	1500–2000	1000–1500	500–1000	<500
Platelets (000/mm^3)	<LLN–75	50–75	10–50	<10

Febrile Neutropenia

ANC < 1000, fever >38.5°C	—	—	Present	Life-threatening sepsis

Constitutional Symptoms

Fatigue	**Increased fatigue, normal activity**	**Difficulty in performing some activities**	**Severe or loss of ability to perform some activities**	**Bedridden or disabling**
Fever, AGC >1000	38.0–39.0c	39.1–40c	>40.0 for <24 hours	>40.0 for >24 hours
Weight gain/loss	5–10%	10–20%	≥20%	—

Lymphatics

Adverse event	Grade 1	Grade 2	Grade 3	Grade 4
Lympoedema	Mild	Moderate, requires compression	Severe, limiting function	Severe, limiting function, ulcer

Neurology

Adverse event	Grade 1	Grade 2	Grade 3	Grade 4
Neuropathy	Paresthesias or loss of deep reflexes	Interfering with function	Interfering with daily activities	Permanent sensory loss

Gastrointestinal

Adverse event	Grade 1	Grade 2	Grade 3	Grade 4
Anorexia	Loss of appetite	Significantly reduced oral intake.	Requiring IV fluids	Requiring NGT or IV nutrition
Constipation	Requires stool softener/ change of diet	Requiring laxatives	Enema or manual evacuation	Obstruction/toxic megacolon
Dehydration	Dry mucosa, skin turgor diminished	Brief fluid replacement	Sustained fluid replacement	Haemodynamic collapse, requires intensive care
Diarrhoea, no colostomy	Increased to <4 stools/ day	4–6 stools/day, nocturnal stool	≥stools/day, incontinence, dehydration	Hemodynamic collapse, requires intensive care
Diarrhoea with colostomy	Mild increase, loose, watery colostomy o/p	Moderate increase, normal activity	Severe increase, interfering with normal activity	Hemodynamic collapse, requires intensive care
Oesophagitis, odynophagia, dysphagia ± due to radiation	Mild dysphagia, can eat regular diet	Requiring soft or liquid diet	Requiring IV hydration or NGT feeding	Complete obstruction, perforation or ulceration with bleeding
Mouth dryness	Mild	Moderate	—	—
Mucositis due to radiation	Erythema of mucosa	Patchy <1.5 cm pseudo-membranous reaction	Confluent pseudo-membranous reaction	Necrosis/deep ulcer ± bleed
Nausea	Able to eat	Decreased oral intake	Requiring IV fluids	—

(*Continued*)

(*Continued*)

Adverse event	Grade 1	Grade 2	Grade 3	Grade 4
Proctitis	Increase frequency, blood streaked stool, rectal discomfort, no medication required	As grade 1 but requiring medication, anal fissure	Req. IV fluids, transfusion or persistent discharge requiring pads (mucus)	Perforation, necrosis or bleeding requiring surgical intervention
Salivary gland changes	Slightly thick saliva, altered taste	Thick, ropy sticky saliva, markedly altered taste	—	Acute gland necrosis
Taste disturbance	Slightly altered	Markedly altered	—	—
Vomiting	1 in 24 hours	2–5 in 24 hours	≥6 in 24 hours, IV fluids	Hemodynamic collapse

Dermatology/Skin

Adverse event	Grade 1	Grade 2	Grade 3	Grade 4
Alopecia	Mild hair loss	Pronounced hair loss	—	—
Hand-foot skin reaction	Skin changes without pain	Painful skin changes, normal function	Painful skin changes, interfering function	—
Injection site	Pain, itchy, erythema	Pain/swelling with phlebitis	Severe/ prolonged ulcer/necrosis or requiring op	—
Nail changes	Discoloration, ridging/ pitting	Loss of nail or painful nail bed	—	—
Pigmentation	Localized	Generalized	—	—
Radiation dermatitis	Faint erythema, dry desquamation	Moderate-brisk erythema or oedema or desquamation confined to skin fold or creases	Confluent moist desquamation ≥1.5 cm, not confined to skin fold, pitting oedema	Necrosis or ulceration of full thickness dermis,–/+ spontaneous bleeding

Pain

Adverse event	Grade 1	Grade 2	Grade 3	Grade 4
Pain due to radiation Or bone pain	Mild, not Interfering with function	Pain/analgesics interfering with function	Interfering with Daily activities	disabling

Pulmonary

Adverse event	Grade 1	Grade 2	Grade 3	Grade 4
Cough	Mild	Req. narcotic Anti-tussive	Severe, poorly Controlled by treatment	—
Pneumonitis or Pulmonary fibrosis	Radiographic changes ± mild symptoms	Requiring steroid or diuretics	Requiring oxygen	Requiring assisted ventilation

Renal/Genitourinary

Adverse event	Grade 1	Grade 2	Grade 3	Grade 4
Dysuria	Mild, requiring no intervention	Symptoms relieved with therapy	Symptoms not relieved with therapy	—
Urinary frequency/ urgency	Nocturia, frequency up to 2 × normal	Frequency > 2 × normal but < hourly	≥ hourly with urgency or requiring catheter	—
Hematuria	Microscopic	Intermittent gross bleeding	Persistent gross bleeding, clots	Necrosis, deep ulcer, surgery

Non-Haematological Toxicities

- Anything requiring medication is often grade 2.
- Reactions needing admission and/or support is usually ≥grade 3.
- Life-threatening reactions are invariably grade 4 but not all grade 4 are life threatening.
- Whenever unsure, mild, moderate and severe corresponds to grades 1, 2 and 3, respectively.

References

Barillot I, Horiot JC, Maingon P, et al. Impact on treatment outcome and late effects of customized treatment planning in cervix carcinoma: baseline results to compare new strategies. *Int J Radiat Oncol Biol Phys* 2000; **4**: 189–200.

Bruner DW, Lanciano R, Keegan M, Corn B, Martin E, Hanks GE. Vaginal stenosis and sexual function following intracavitary radiation for the treatment of cervical and endometrial carcinoma. *Int J Radiat Oncol Biol Phys* 1993; **27**: 825–830.

Coia LR, Myerson RJ, Tepper JE. Late effects of radiation therapy on the gastrointestinal tract. *Int J Radiat Oncol Biol Phys* 1995; **31**: 1213–1236.

Czesnin K, Wronkowski Z. Second malignancies of the irradiated area in patients treated for uterine cervix cancer. *Gynecol Oncol* 1978; **6**: 309–315.

Dreyer G. Operative management of cervical cancer. *Best Pract Res Clin Obstet Gynaecol* 2005; **19**(4): 563–576.

Eifel PJ, Levenback C, Wharton JT, Oswald MJ. Time course and incidence of late complications in patients treated with radiation therapy for FIGO stage 1B carcinoma of the uterine cervix. *Int J Radiat Oncol Biol Phys* 1995; **32**: 1289–1300.

Holland CM, Shafi MI. Radical Hysterectomy. *Best Pract Res Clin Obstet Gynaecol* 2005; **19**(3): 387–401.

Hoskin WJ, Perez CA, Young RC. *Principles and Practise of Gynecologic Oncology*, 4th ed., Lippincott William & Wilkins.

Landoni F, Maneo A, Cormio G, et al. Class II versus Class III radical hysterectomy in stage 1B-2A cervical cancer: a prospective randomized study. *Gynecol Oncol* 2001; **80**: 3–12.

Maduro JH, Pras E, Willemse PHB, de Vries EGE. Acute and long-term toxicity following radiotherapy alone or in combination with chemotherapy for locally advanced cervical cancer. *Cancer Treat Rev* 2003; **29**: 471–488.

Moreno A, Clemente J, Crespo C, et al. Pelvic insufficiency fractures in patients with pelvic irradiation. *Int J Radiat Oncol Biol Phys* 1999; **44**: 61–66.

Pearcey R, Brundage M, Drouin P, et al. Phase III trial comparing radical radiotherapy with and without cisplatin chemotherapy in patients with advanced squamous cell carcinoma of the cervix. *J Clin Oncol* 2002; **20**: 966–972.

Perez CA, Grigsby PW, Lockett MA, Chao KSC, Williamson J. Radiation therapy morbidity in carcinoma of the uterine cervix: dosimetric and clinical correlation. *Int J Radiat Oncol Biol Phys* 1999; **44**: 855–866.

Pikaart DP, Holloway RW, Ahmad S, et al. Clinical-pathologic and morbidity analyses of Type 2 and 3 abdominal radical hysterectomy for cervical cancer *Gynecol Oncol* 2007; **107**(2): 205–210.

Soussain C, Ricard D, Fike JR, et al. CNS complications of radiotherapy and chemotherapy. *Lancet* 2009; **374**: 1639–1651.

Sridhar T, Symonds RP. Principles of chemotherapy and radiotherapy. *Obstet, Gynaecol Reprod Med* 2008; **19**(3): 61–67.

Saibishkumar SP, Patel FD, Sharma SC. Original Article. Evaluation of late toxicities of patients with carcinoma of the cervix treated with radical radiotherapy: An audit from India. *Clin Oncol* 2006; **18**: 30–37.

Symonds RP. Principles of gynaecological chemotherapy and radiotherapy. *Curr Obstet Gynaecol* 2003; **13**: 102–109.

Symonds RP, Foweraker K. Principles of chemotherapy and radiotherapy. *Curr Obstet Gynaecol* 2006; **16**: 100–106.

Chapter 27

Nutritional Support for Gynaecologic cancer Patients

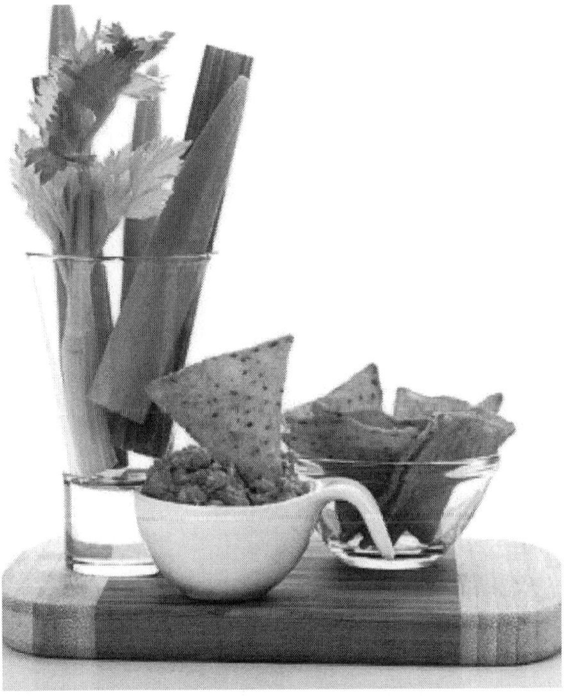

Gynaecologic Cancer: A Handbook for Students and Practitioners
Rushdan Noor, Eng Hseon Tay, and Jeffrey Low

ISBN 978-981-4463-06-5 (Hardcover), 978-981-4463-07-2 (eBook)
www.panstanford.com

The relationship between nutrition and cancer is not yet fully understood, but researchers do know that well-nourished patients have a better prognosis. In patients with potentially curable or stable disease, nutritional support, when indicated, is an important and often critical part of the overall treatment plan. Before the advent of enteral and parenteral nutrition, the inability to receive nutrients through oral intake inevitably led to wasting and death. Many of the cancer patients actually died because of dehydration and starvation.

Nutritional status before treatment is one of the independent prognostic factor for cancer. Malnourished patients undergoing major surgery have higher morbidity and mortality. Finding and treating nutrition problems early may help the patient gain or maintain weight, improve the patient's response to therapy, and reduce complications of treatment.

Table 27.1 Metabolic abnormalities in cancer patients

	Metabolic abnormalities
Carbohydrate	• Increased gluconeogenesis from amino acid, lactate and glycerol
	• Increased glucose disappearance and recycling
	• Insulin resistance
Lipid	• increased lipolysis
	• increased glycerol and fatty acid turnover
	• lipid oxidation non-inhibited by glucose
	• decreased lipogenesis and lipoprotein lipase activity
	• non-constant increase in plasma levels of NEFA and lipid
Protein	• increased muscle protein catabolism
	• increased whole-body protein turnover
	• increased liver protein synthesis and decreased muscle protein synthesis

Malnutrition is a complex, multi-factorial phenomenon that leads to progressive weight loss and deficiency of specific nutrients. Cancer and its various therapeutic modalities contribute to malnutrition. In a multi-centre cooperative study of more than 3000 cancer patients, DeWys et al. reported substantial weight loss in more than 50% of patients. The highest frequency and severity of weight loss occurred in patients with gastrointestinal malignancies (including pancreas and stomach). The most common form of malnutrition in a cancer patient is protein-calorie malnutrition. Specific nutrient deficiency such as Mg and vitamin B12 deficiency can also occur. Malnutrition is mostly seen in advanced ovarian cancer with intra-abdominal metastases leading to impaired GIT function. Table 27.1 shows metabolic abnormalities in cancer patients.

Nutritional Assessment

Ability to tolerate treatment is better for the well-nourished patient. Screening and assessment of nutritional status are done before beginning of anti-cancer therapy. Assessment determines the complete nutritional status of the patient and identifies if nutrition therapy is needed.

Methods of Nutritional Assessment

There are at least two methods of nutritional assessment: (a) antropometric and biochemical markers and (b) subjective global assessment (SGA).

Anthropometric and Biochemical Markers

Measuring weight, skinfold thickness, mid-arm muscle circumference and creatinine/height index are common antropometric nutritional assessment. However, it has many limitations, e.g. weight can be affected by ascites. Serum creatinine, serum protein, transferrin and others are biochemical markers for nutritional assessment. Biochemical markers alone also has few limitations, e.g. creatinine measurement can be affected by renal impairment due to chemotherapy and serum protein and transferrin can also be misleading of nutritional status because they are not specific. Combined parameter may be more beneficial, e.g. Prognostic Nutritional Index (PNI), which uses serum albumin, transferrin, triceps skin folds and delayed cutaneous hypersensitivity (immunology).

Subjective Global Assessment

Subjective global assessment (SGA) provides a simple, reproducible and accurate method to identify malnourished patients who need nutritional support. It is based on complete history and physical examination. In SGA, special emphasis is given to six areas: changes in weight, dietary intake, GIT symptoms, functional capacity, physiologic stress and physical signs of nutritional deficiencies. Patients are then categorized as Group A (normal), B (mild) and C (severe malnutrition).

Aetiology of Malnutrition

The aetiology of malnutrition is multi-factorial. It can be broadly divided into three causes: (a) decreased food intake, (b) malabsorption and (c) metabolic derangement.

Decreased Food Intake

Tumour itself and therapy (chemotherapy and radiotherapy) can reduce food intake through direct GIT involvement or systemic effects leading to anorexia. Tumour can also cause anorexia; mechanism of action is unknown probably through cytokines. Furthermore, depression that is commonly inflicted on cancer patients can reduce appetite and food intake.

Malabsorption

Malabsorption can be due to direct effect of tumour or therapy or both. Gastrointestinal tract tumour can cause intra-luminal obstruction. Extensive resections of the small bowel can lead to malabsorption of fluids and nutrients. Chemotherapy can cause mucositis, ileus and malabsorption.

Metabolic Derangement

Even with normal nutrient intake, cancer patients can become malnourished due to inefficient nutrient utilization and wasteful metabolic pathways. It is known that cancer patients have an increase in basal energy expenditure and are often associated with glucose intolerance and peripheral insulin resistance. Cancer can also lead to lipid metabolism abnormalities, including increase in lipolysis with high serum triglycerides. Studies have found that cancer patients have high protein body turnover leading to depletion in muscle mass, and this could be mediated through cytokines.

Nutritional Therapies

There are two main objectives of nutritional support in cancer patients: (a) provision of nutrition during anti-cancer therapy to improve an outcome and (b) permanent support for a patient with GIT failure.

There are four types of nutritional therapies:

(a) enteral nutrition
(b) oral dietary therapy
(c) drug therapy to increased appetite and food intake
(d) parenteral nutrition

Goals of Nutritional Therapy

Following are the main goals of nutritional therapy in cancer patients:

(1) Prevent or correct malnutrition.
(2) Prevent wasting of muscle, bone, blood, organs, and other lean body mass.
(3) Help the patient tolerate treatment.
(4) Reduce nutrition-related side effects and complications.
(5) Maintain strength and energy.
(6) Protect the ability to fight infection.
(7) Help recovery and healing.
(8) Maintain or improve the quality of life.

Enteral Nutrition

Enteral feeding is defined as delivery of liquid nutrient formula into the GIT through tubes or catheters placed into the stomach or small intestine. Enteral feeding is preferred to parenteral feeding because it preserves the gastrointestinal architecture and prevents bacterial translocation from the gut. Enteral feeding has fewer complications and cheaper than total parenteral nutrition.

Compared to oral feeding, enteral nutrition has several advantages, i.e. ability to deliver nutrients beyond obstructed areas and nutrients can be delivered at a slow, continuous rate thereby permitting a longer period for nutritional absorbency in patients with limited absorptive capacity, e.g. extensive small bowel resection and extensive mucosal injury due to chemotherapy or radiotherapy.

The prerequisite for enteral nutrition is adequately functioning small intestinal mucosa for absorption of nutrients. If the intestines have limited capacity due to radiation enteritis, short bowel syndrome (remaining bowel 3–4 feet with good function) or partial obstruction, enteral feeding can be given by slow continuous infusion to maximize absorption.

There are two routes of administration of nutrient formula:

(1) nasogastric or nasoenteric tubes if GIT access to be obtained for short term < 2 weeks (some nutritionists recommend 4 weeks)
(2) gastrostomy and jejunostomy for those who require longer nutritional supports.

Gastrostomy and jejunostomy tubes have more advantages such as the following: (a) Calibre is larger and less likely to be obstructed, (b) Risk of aspiration is less and (c) They are more comfortable and aesthetically pleasing.

Gastrostomy and jejunostomy enable the patients to receive 90% of prescribed feeding compared to 55% in NGT feeding (due to frequent dislodging of the tube). The method of choice of gastrostomy is percutaneous gastrostomy tube inserted endoscopically due to ease and safety, and it can be performed as outpatient procedures. The nutrients should be administered distal to the ligament of Treitz to avoid aspiration pneumonia and gastric ileus.

There are four basic types of nutrient formulae (more than 100 types of nutrient formulae available commercially):

(a) complete nutrition
(b) single nutrients
(c) fluid and electrolytes
(d) disease-specific enteral formula for diabetes, renal impairment, hepatic and pulmonary dysfunction.

Complete nutrition formula normally provides 1500–2000 kcal/day.

Types of Administration of Enteral Feeding

There are two types of administration of enteral feeding: (a) bolus feeding and (b) continuous infusion.

Bolus Feeding

(a) tip of catheter in the intact stomach
(b) up to 500 mL can be infused within 10–15 minutes
(c) gravity or by syringe

Continuous Infusion

(a) tip of catheter distal to pylorus
(b) to avoid abdominal distension and diarrhoea
(c) rate of infusion up to 150 mL/hour

Efficacy of Enteral Feeding

Studies have failed to demonstrate any clear benefit of enteral feeding as adjuvant therapy for cancer. Routine use of enteral nutrition support in patients receiving chemotherapy or undergoing an operation for cancer cannot be justified. A large study of the Italian Society for Parenteral and Enteral Nutrition randomizing malnourished patients to early post-operative standard enteral nutrition or TPN demonstrated that patients receiving enteral nutrition had a significantly decrease in post-operative complications and duration of post-operative stay (Bozzetti et al.).

Indications for Enteral Nutrition in Cancer Patients

The indications for enteral nutrition in cancer patients are (a) obstruction of upper GIT and not a candidate for an operation, (b) chronic malnutrition due to inadequate oral intake and (c) peri-operative support of a malnourished patient.

Complications of Enteral Nutrition

Following are the potential complications of enteral nutrition:

(a) **Aspiration** (1–32%): most serious, can be minimized by upright position during bolus feeding and use of jejunal feeding.
(b) **Diarrhoea** (5–30%): due to medication given (e.g. antacid, antibiotics, etc.) and underlying bowel problem.
(c) **Metabolic complications**: dehydration, azotaemia, hyperglycaemia and hyperkalaemia.

Measures that can reduce or avoid complications of enteral nutrition are as follows:

(a) choosing an appropriate formula
(b) infusion into an appropriate portion of GIT
(c) correct infusion method
(d) providing clinical and metabolic monitoring

Not all patients are suitable for enteral nutrition. Enteral nutrition is not appropriate for the following patients:

(1) patients who had major surgery or resection of stomach and intestines
(2) patients with bowel obstruction
(3) patients who have severe nausea, vomiting, and/or diarrhoea
(4) patients with coagulation disorder such as thrombocytopenia
(5) uncooperative patients

Home Enteral Nutrition

The main purpose of home enteral nutrition (HEN) is to provide nutrients and fluids outside the hospital. It was found to be safe with complication rate of 0.4%. An overall survival rate for a cancer patient on HEN is 30% and in gynaecological malignancies, HEN is useful for a patient with upper GIT obstruction, who cannot be treated surgically.

Oral Dietary Therapy

The indications of oral dietary therapy in cancer patients are as follows:

(a) able to eat but impaired GIT, e.g. partial small bowel obstruction, chronic radiation enteritis and short bowel syndrome
(b) patients with a special metabolic requirement

Diet is modified based on the pathophysiologic changes induced by underlying disorder. Usually oral dietary therapy is given for a short period of time due to taste fatigue.

Following are the recommendations of the types of diets in three categories of patients:

(1) Patients with partial small bowel obstruction, diet should be
  (a) frequently small amounts
  (b) high calories
  (c) low fibre
(2) Patients with radiation enteritis, diet should be
  (a) low fat
  (b) low fibre
  (c) lactose-free
(3) Patients with short bowel syndrome:
  (a) frequent small amount
  (b) low fibre
  (c) low lactose, simple sugar
  (d) taking fluid separately from meals
  (e) mineral and vitamins supplementation, e.g. calcium, zinc, magnesium and vitamin B12.

With the above recommendation, a study found that it reduces the incidence of diarrhoea and increases the ability of the body to cope with the situation.

Pharmacologic Agents

In a human clinical trial, these agents provided a modest gain in weight but no improvement in the quality of life and no other benefits.

Appetite Stimulants

Steroid such as prednisolone or dexamethasone may improve nutritional parameters and appetite but the risks probably outweigh the benefits. Muscle wasting is a recognized side effect.

Progestational agents such as megestrol acetate (approved by the FDA) can improve appetite and reduce weight loss (dose used in a study was 160–1200 mg/day, effect only seen after 8 weeks). Cochrane Reviews concluded that megestrol acetate improved appetite and weight gain, but there was no impact on the quality of life.

Combination of megestrol acetate and ibuprofen (or indomethacin) has been recommended as an appetite stimulant. Megestrol stimulates appetite and ibuprofen reduces systemic inflammation (one of the attributing factors to cancer cachexia), and both thereby attenuate the metabolic abnormalities underlying cachexia.

Cytokine Inhibitors

Studies have shown that monoclonal antibodies against TNF improve appetite and reduce protein loss. Monoclonal antibodies against IL-1, IL-6 also reduced protein loss in an animal study. Thalidomide and pentoxyfylline have been shown to inhibit TNF. Only thalidomide reduced weight loss associated with tuberculosis and AIDS.

Other Agents and Modality to Increase Weight

Anabolic androgenic steroid stimulates muscle protein synthesis, resulting in muscle mass. Testosterone, nandrolone decanoate and exandrolone have been tested positive in a number of catabolic states but their potential in cancer cachexia is still unknown.

Oral nutritional supplements such as eicosapentaeoic acid (EPA) derived from fish oil may attenuate the metabolic abnormalities associated with cachexia. Randomized trials have shown improvement in food intake and increased physical activity among patients who consume nutritional supplement and EPA. However, this nutritional supplement has no benefit in terms of lean body mass and cancer survival.

Combinations of oral nutritional supplements/EPA/anti-inflammatory (indomethacin) are being evaluated, but the outcomes are still unknown.

Total Parenteral Nutrition

Total parenteral nutrition (TPN) delivers nutrients directly into the circulation, avoiding the problems with poor oral intake and gastrointestinal dysfunction seen in patients with cancer-induced cachexia. Total parenteral nutrition is indicated in patients unsuitable for oral or enteral nutritional support and it can be life-saving. In cancer patients, TPN can be used during chemotherapy and/or radiotherapy. It can overcome major causes of cancer cachexia, i.e. decreased food intake and dysfunction of GIT. Total parenteral nutrition, however, does not alter the metabolic derangement.

Routine TPN is not justifiable and not all patients are suitable; it has to be very selective. Improvement in nutritional parameters afforded by TPN in patients receiving chemotherapy is not necessarily translated into improved clinical outcomes (Statement NIH, American Society for Parenteral and Enteral Nutrition and Clinical Nutrition).

Indications of Total Parenteral Nutrition

Following are the indications of TPN:

(a) prevention of the effect of starvation in a patient who is predicted to be unable to tolerate oral or enteral feeding for >7 days
(b) maximization of performance status in a malnourished patient prior to chemotherapy or surgery
(c) malnourished patient undergoing bone marrow transplant

Roles of Total Parenteral Nutrition in Cancer Patients

The role of TPN in the survival and its effect on the efficacy of cancer treatment is still unclear. A study has shown that chemotherapy is more toxic in weight-losing patients limiting the total dose of cytotoxic drugs and consequently, the response to treatment and perhaps survival.

Generally patients require 30 kcal/kg non-protein calories (dextrose or lipid), 1 g/kg amino acid and 2 L fluid.

Total parenteral nutrition is not without risks. The risks of TPN are:

(a) central line and catheter site infection (11%)
(b) fluid overload (2%)
(c) metabolic complications (hyperglycaemia, hypokalaemia, hypophosphataemia) (13%)
(d) fatty liver

Total parenteral nutrition does not appear to benefit well-nourished or mildly malnourished patients undergoing chemotherapy, radiotherapy or surgery. Studies have shown that patients with mild and moderate malnutrition given TPN and on chemotherapy have increased risk of infection. This finding is reverse in severe malnutrition.

Patients with massive intestinal resection, entero-cutaneous fistula, bone marrow transplant recipients and severe radiation enteritis and in whom cancer has been cured can benefit from long-term TPN at home. In advanced, incurable and ill patients, long-term TPN can only do more harm than good.

Indications for TPN in Hospitalized Patients with Gynaecologic Cancers

The therapeutic goals for TPN in cancer patients are to improve the function and outcome of patient by:

(a) preventing and treating undernutrition/cachexia
(b) enhancing compliance with anti-cancer treatments
(c) controlling some adverse effects on anti-cancer treatments
(d) improving the quality of life

The peri-operative indications of TPN are:

(a) seven to ten days pre-operatively in a severely malnourished patient (who cannot be fed enterally)
(b) post-operative complications that prevent oral or enteral intake for more than 7–10 days
(c) patient with entero-cutaneous fistula

The indications of TPN during radiation therapy or chemotherapy are:

(a) maximization of performance status prior to therapy in a malnourished patient who cannot be fed enterally

(b) severe persistent (>7–10 days) mucositis, diarrhoea, ileus or emesis

In general, TPN is indicated after 7–10 days of inability to tolerate oral or enteral feeding due to any cause.

Ethical Consideration of Nutritional Support in Terminally Ill Patients

The role of nutritional support for the terminally ill patient is a subject filled with ethical and legal dilemmas. Patients have their autonomy and may refuse any nutritional support. Relative may, on the other hand, request the continuation of TPN in terminally ill and their request is in line with medical futility.

Regarding the issue of patient's autonomy, a report from the President's Commission for the Study of Ethical Problems in Medicine and Biomedical and Behavioral Research states: "*The voluntary choice of a competent and informed patient should determine whether or not life sustaining therapy will be undertaken, while healthcare institutions and professionals should try to enhance patient's abilities to make decisions on their own and to promote understanding of the available options*".

As for treatment (chemotherapy, radiation therapy etc), Physician's recommendations may form the sole basis for the patient's decision because patient's knowledge and experiences are too limited to decide. This is, however do not apply to nutritional support. Therefore, the autonomy and medical futility as well as religious beliefs should govern decisions for both initiation and withdrawal of an ongoing therapy in terminally ill patients unresponsive to all treatments available.

Referring to President's Commission statement, a justification that is adequate for not commencing treatment is also sufficient for ceasing it. Moreover, establishing a higher requirement for cessation might unjustifiably discourage vigorous initial attempts to treat seriously ill patients that sometimes succeed.

The provision of food and water by enteral or parenteral routes is often failed to improve comfort and in fact, may add to discomfort and uneasiness. The TPN can only be considered if it will enhance the quality of life of a patient who is not at imminent risk of dying in spite of widely metastasized disease (life expectancy > 2 months). Even when this situation exists, we still have to weigh between risks and benefits before considering TPN.

References

American College of Physicians. Parenteral nutrition in patients receiving cancer chemotherapy. *Ann Int Med* 1989; **110**: 734–736.

Berenstein EG, Ortiz Z. Megestrol acetate for the treatment of anorexia-cachexia syndrome. *Cochrane Database Syst Rev* 2005; **2**: CD004310.

Bozzetti F, Braga M, Gianotti L, Gavazzi C, Mariani L. Postoperative enteral versus parenteral nutrition in malnourished patients with gastrointestinal cancer: a randomised multicentre trial. *Lancet* 2001; **358**: 1487.

Bozzetti F. Basics in Clinical Nutrition: nutritional support in cancer. e-SPEN, the European e-Journal of Clinical Nutrition and Metabolism (2009), doi: 10.1016/j.eclnm. 2009.06.018.

Bozzetti F, Arends J, Lundholm K, Micklewright A, Zurcher G, Muscaritoli M. ESPEN Guidelines on Parenteral Nutrition: non-surgical oncology. *Clin Nutr* 2009; **28**(4): 445–454.

Buzby GP, Mullen JL, Mathews DC, et al. Prognostic nutritional index in gastrointestinal surgery. *Am J Surg* 1980; **139**: 160–167.

DeWys WD, Begg C, Lavin PT, et al. Prognostic effect of weight loss prior to chemotherapy in cancer patients. Eastern Cooperative Oncology Group. *Am J Med* 1980; **69**: 491–497.

Fearon KC, von Meyenfeldt M, Moses AGW, et al. An energy and protein dense, high n-3 fatty acid oral supplement promotes weight gain in cancer cachexia: a randomised double blind trial. *Gut* 2003; **52**: 1479–1486.

Fearon KCH. Cancer cachexia Developing multimodal therapy for a multidimensional problem. *Eur J Cancer* 2008; **44**(8): 1124–1132.

Klein S, Koretz RL. Nutritional support in patients with cancer: What do the data really show? *Nutr Clin Pract* 1994; **9**: 91–100.

Koretz RL, Lipman TO, Klein S, American Gastroenterological Association. AGA technical review on parenteral nutrition. *Gastroenterology* 2001; **121**: 970.

McKinlay AW. Nutritional support in patients with advanced cancer: permission to fall out? *Proc Nutr Soc* 2004; **63**: 431–435.

Moses AW, Slater C, Preston T, et al. Reduced total energy expenditure and physical activity in cachectic patients with pancreatic cancer can be modulated by an energy and proteindense oral supplement enriched with n-3 fatty acids. *Br J Cancer* 2004; **90**: 996–1002.

Rivadeneira D, Evoy D, Fahey TJ, Lieberman MD, Daly JM. Nutritional support of the cancer patient. *CA Cancer J Clin* 1998; **48**: 69–80.

Schattner M. Enteral nutritional support of the patient with cancer: route and role. *J Clin Gastroenterol* 2003; **36**: 297–302.

Chapter 28

Basic Surgical Procedures in Gynaecologic Oncology

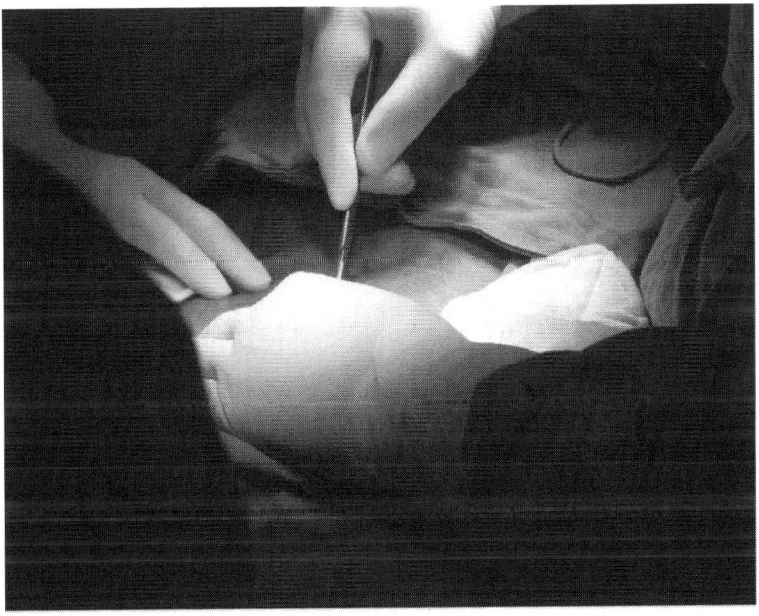

Gynaecologic Cancer: A Handbook for Students and Practitioners
Rushdan Noor, Eng Hseon Tay, and Jeffrey Low

ISBN 978-981-4463-06-5 (Hardcover), 978-981-4463-07-2 (eBook)
www.panstanford.com

Urethral Catheterization

Urethral catheterization is one of the most common gynaecological procedures. The ability to insert a urinary catheter is an essential skill. Catheters are sized in units called French, where one French equals 1/3 mm. Catheters vary from 12 FR (4 mm) to 48 FR (16 mm) in size.

Step-by-step urethral catheterization (10 steps)

(1) Drape the patient with towels.
(2) Wear sterile gloves and perform swabbing:
  (a) Use the left hand to part the labia to expose the introitus.
  (b) Use the right hand to swab down 6× using one swab for each stroke, swabbing downwards from the introitus to the (do a gentle swabbing)
    - swab centrally from clitoris to vagina
    - swab left labium majora
    - swab right labia majora
    - swab left labia minora
    - swab right labia minora
    - swab urethral meatus
(3) Discard the gloves and put on another pair of sterile gloves.
(4) Place the kidney dish below the introitus, part the labia with the left hand to expose the urethral meatus.
(5) Lubricate a Foley's catheter tip with a sterile solution, and with the right hand insert the catheter for about 7 cm. We do not need to change the glove if we inserted the catheter with a forcep.
(6) Leave open end of catheter inside the kidney dish to allow urine to drain.
(7) Inflate retaining balloon with 10 mL of sterile water.
(8) Withdraw the catheter until resistance is felt.
(9) Clean open end of catheter with sterile gauze and connect to drainage bag.
(10) Remove the gloves.

Pleurocentesis

Pleural effusion is an abnormal collection of fluid in the pleural space resulting from fluid production or decreased absorption.

Normal pleural fluid volume is 0.13 mL/kg body weight serves as a lubricant to facilitate movement of the pleural surfaces against each other during respiration. This volume is keeping consistent by the balance of hydrostatic and oncotic pressure as well as lymphatic drainage. Disturbance of any one of these components will lead to pathology, including pleural effusion. Pleurocentesis/thoracocentesis is removal of pleural fluid.

Characteristics of Normal Pleural Fluid

- Clear colour
- Protein less than 2%
- pH 7.60–7.64
- Glucose content similar with plasma
- Sodium, potassium and concentration similar with interstitial fluid

Causes of Pleural Effusion

- hypoalbuminaemia
- malignancy
- inflammation
- infection
- pulmonary embolism
- congestive heart failure
- trauma
- uraemia
- liver disease
- systemic lupus erythematosus
- Meig's syndrome

Symptoms

- dyspnoea
- chest pain
- symptoms associated with underlying disease process

Purpose of Pleurocentesis

- for diagnostic purpose
- symptomatic relief

Contraindications

- uncooperative patient
- top of the rib below the puncture site cannot be felt
- coagulopathy
- patient with known bullous lung disease
- patient with only one lung
- patient on peep
- patient with markedly raised left hemidiaphragm

Techniques of Pleurocentesis

(1) Pre-medicate with analgesia (morphine can be used as analgesia and also cough suppression).
(2) Position the patient sitting up and supporting herself on a bedside table.
(3) Identify the site for needle insertion, usually one or two interspaces below the highest point of effusion, but NOT LOWER than the eighth intercostal space.
(4) Make a mark on the posterior axillary line of the chosen interspace over the superior aspect of the lower rib.
(5) Clean and drape with sterile materials.
(6) Infiltrate with local analgesia the skin and deeper soft tissues and down to the pleura.
(7) The intercostal artery on the inferior aspect of the upper rib must be avoided at all times.
(8) A 14 G needle with the outer cannula is attached to a syringe and advanced over the superior aspect of the lower rib, maintaining gentle negative pressure.
(9) When the pleural space is entered, identified by withdrawal of fluid, the patient is asked to hold her breath in expiration, the needle withdrawn as the cannula is advanced.
(10) A three-way tap and 60 mL syringe are attached to the cannula before the patient is told to start breathing again.
(11) An infusion tubing connected to a drainage bag is attached to the three-way tap and aspiration commenced.
(12) If an indwelling catheter is required, a 16 G catheter connected to a three-way tap is inserted into the 14 G needle. The needle is advanced slowly, and once the pleural space is entered

the catheter is pushed gently into the pleural space, and the needle removed.

(13) Never pull back on the catheter with the needle in place as the catheter tip may shear off.

(14) Removal of 400–500 mL of pleural fluid is often sufficient to alleviate shortness of breath. The recommended limit is 1000–1500 mL in a single pleurocentesis.

(15) After completion of the pleurocentesis, the cannula or catheter is removed and pressure applied over the puncture site for 2–3 minutes.

(16) Apply a sterile dressing

(17) An expiratory chest-X-ray is done to exclude a pneumothorax.

Potential Complications of Pleurocentesis

- pneumothorax
- infection
- cough
- haemothorax
- air embolism

Chest Tube Insertion

Chest tube insertion or tube thoracostomy is the insertion of the tube into the pleural cavity to drain air, blood, bile, pus or other fluids.

Indications

- pneumothorax
- haemothorax
- drainage of pleural effusion
- chylothorax
- empyaema

Contraindications

- coagulopathy
- pulmonary bullae

- pulmonary, pleural or thoracic adhesions
- loculated pleural effusion or empyaema
- skin infection over the chest tube insertion site

Equipment

- iodine and alcohol swabs for skin prep
- sterile drapes and gloves
- #11 scalpel blade and handle
- Mayo clamp
- Kelly clamp
- silk suture (size 0)
- needle holder
- sterile gauze
- vaseline gauze
- tape
- suction apparatus
- chest tube (size 28 to 32 Fr, depending on clinical setting)
- 1% lidocaine with epinephrine, 10 cc syringe, 25 G and 22 G needles

Techniques of Chest Tube Insertion

(1) Obtain informed consent.

(2) Position the patient with affected side up. Identify the insertion site, which is generally at the anterior axillary line just behind the lateral edge of the pectoralis major at the level of the nipple. Prep and drape the insertion site. Generously anesthetize the insertion site along the insertion tract to the pleura. Appropriate position can be checked by aspirating through the needle used for instilling the local anaesthetic. The patient should be positioned supine or at a 45° angle.

(3) With aseptic techniques, infiltrate 5 mL of local anaesthesia to a wide area of subcutaneous tissue superior to the expected initial incision. Inject another 10 mL of LA into the periosteum, intercostals muscle and the pleural.

(4) The skin incision is made in between the midaxillary lines over a rib that is below the intercostals level selected for chest tube insertion. Skin incision should be in the same direction as the rib itself.

(5) The skin should be incised directly over the body of the rib, the incision length being 3–4 cm long overlying the rib that is below the desired intercostals levels of entry.

(6) The Kelly or Mayo clamp is then used to bluntly dissect superiorly over the superior margin of the next higher rib. The Mayo clamp is then pushed through the parietal pleura with tips closed and with slow steady pressure.

(7) Once the pleura has been penetrated, the clamps are opened wide to enlarge the insertion tract and removed. Operator's index finger can also be inserted along the tract to further enlarge the opening if needed.

(8) The chest tube is grasped near the end to be inserted with the Mayo clamp (jaws of the clamp parallel to the length of the tube), and advanced into the pleural space.

(9) Once the tube is inserted so that all drainage ports are inside the thoracic cavity, the tube is connected to suction and sutured in place with silk suture by closing the skin edges of the incision around the tube and tying the suture ends up around the tube. The area should be dressed with vaseline gauze and sterile gauze sponges. Make sure to provide enough padding between the chest tube and the chest wall.

(10) Chest X-ray should be obtained to ensure correct placement of the chest tube.

Complications of Chest Tube Insertion

- haemorrhage at the site of insertion
- infection
- haematoma
- lung laceration
- laceration of intra-abdominal organs if tube is inadvertently inserted into the abdominal cavity
- tube dislodgment

Pleurodesis

Pleurodesis (or pleural sclerosis) is the procedure performed to produce an adhesion or obliteration of the pleural spaces. Pleurodesis is indicated to prevent a recurrent pneumothorax or pleural effusion.

In cancer, pleurodesis is often performed to control malignant pleural effusion in order to palliate the symptoms. Pleurodesis is unsuitable for patients with poor performance status, life expectancy less than 3 months, patients with trapped lung, i.e. the lung cannot expand because of tumour or scarring, etc.

A chemical known as a sclerosant is used to induce chemical inflammation and subsequently adhesions between parietal and visceral pleural to obliterate the pleural spaces. Despite high success rate, recurrence rate of pleural effusion is common.

Commonly used sclerosants in pleurodesis and success rate are as follows:

- talc (90–96%)
- doxycyline (90%)
- bleomycin (84%)
- quinacrine (70–90%)
- nitrogen mustard (52%)

The sclerosant can be injected or instilled into the pleural cavity through chest tube insertion or thoracoscopy. In thoracoscopy, thoracoscope is used to visualize the pleural space and sclerosant can be placed under direct visualization. Thoracoscopy, however, has to be done in the operation theatre and usually under general anaesthesia.

Pleurodesis (using bleomycin) through chest tube: Techniques

(1) It can be done as a bedside procedure.

(2) Under local anaesthesia, the chest tube is inserted at the lower part of the chest and connected to the bottle as mentioned above.

(3) Leave the chest tube to drain pleural fluid until dry. Usually it takes 2–5 days for the pleural fluid to be drained completely.

(4) Before pleurodesis, give analgesic to the patient. Local anaesthetic agent such as lignocaine (200 mg) or lidocaine

can be instilled into the pleural spaces either separately of together with sclerosant.

(5) If instillation of lignocaine is done separately, the patient should be turned in six different positions after 10 minutes.

(6) Bleomycin solution (maximum 40 mg) in 50 mL normal saline is then injected into the pleural spaces (via chest tube) followed by another 50 mL of normal saline flushing.

(7) Clamp the chest tube for 2 hours.

(8) The patient is turned to six different positions (every 15 minutes for 2 hours) to ensure the bleomycin is well distributed throughout the pleural spaces.

(9) Monitor vital signs and any evidence of allergic reactions.

(10) After 2 hours, reconnect the chest tube to underwater seal or Pleur-e-vac.

(11) The chest tube is then removed when the drainage becomes minimal (< 50 mL) usually after at least 24 hours.

Potential Risks of Pleurodesis

- infection
- pain
- bleeding at the chest tube site
- pneumothorax
- rarely related to the type of sclerosant used (fever, pain, nausea, low blood pressure, etc.)

Abdominal Paracentesis for Ascites

Ascites is an accumulation of an abnormal amount of fluid in the peritoneal cavity. Healthy men have little or no intra-peritoneal fluid, but women may normally have as much as 20 mL, depending on the phase of their menstrual cycle.

Causes of Ascites

(a) normal peritoneum
- portal hypertension
- hypoalbuminaemia

- miscellaneous conditions, e.g. chylous ascites, bile ascites, nephrogenic ascites, urinary ascites, ovarian hyperstimulation syndrome, Meig's syndrome

(b) diseased peritoneum
- infection (bacterial peritonitis, TB peritonitis, fungal peritonitis, etc.)
- malignancy
- others (vasculitis, eosinophilic peritonitis, granulomatous peritonitis, etc.)

Ascites can be either transudate or exudate. The serum-ascites albumin gradient (SAAG) is the best single test for classifying ascites into a portal hypertensive (SAAG >1.1 g/dl) and non–portal hypertensive (SAAG <1.1 g/dl) causes. Calculated by subtracting the ascitic fluid albumin value from the serum albumin value, it correlates directly with portal pressure. The specimens should be obtained relatively simultaneously. The accuracy of the SAAG results is approximately 97% in classifying ascites. The terms high-albumin gradient and low-albumin gradient should replace the terms transudative and exudative in the description of ascites.

Abdominal paracentesis is a procedure in which a needle or catheter is inserted into the peritoneal cavity to remove an ascitic fluid. Paracentesis can either be diagnostic, therapeutic or both.

Contraindications of Paracentesis

- acute abdomen
- cellulitis of abdominal wall
- severe coagulopathy
- distended bowel
- extensive intra-peritoneal adhesions

Techniques of Abdominal Paracentesis

(1) Explain to a patient and obtain informed consent.
(2) Empty the urinary bladder either voluntarily or with a catheter.
(3) Identify the site for insertion of the cannula. Ultrasound guidance can be useful in choosing the best site for paracentesis.

(4) Two recommended sites for paracentesis are (a) Two centimetre below the umbilicus in the midline or (b) Five centimetre superior and medial to the anterior superior iliac spines on either side.
(5) Clean and drape in a sterile manner.
(6) Infiltrate with LA (lignocaine/lidocaine 1%) the skin and full thickness of the proposed site of paracentesis with 5 mL syringe and 25 G needle.
(7) Switch to the longer 20 G needle and administer 4–5 mL of LA along the catheter/needle insertion tract. Anaesthetize all the way down to the peritoneum, alternating injection and intermittent aspiration until into the peritoneal cavity.
(8) Insert a 14 G needle (with three-way tap connected to a 50/60 mL syringe) into the abdominal cavity.
(9) Continuously apply negative pressure to the syringe as the needle is advanced.
(10) Withdraw the needle when free flow of fluid is aspirated and advance the cannula.
(11) For dependent drainage, attach an infusion tubing to the cannula.
(12) An alternative to 14 G needle is a catheter, size 8 F over 18 G, 7.5 inch needle with three-way stopcock. With this needle, a small skin nick using size 11 scalpel has to be made prior to insertion. Insertion techniques are similar.
(13) During the procedure, the patient can be placed in different positions to facilitate drainage.
(14) To minimize the risk of a persistent leak from the puncture site, use a small gauge needle or take a "Z" track during insertion of the needle.

Additional Facts

- Dietary sodium restriction and diuretics do not often provide symptomatic relief of refractory ascites in patients with advanced stages of cancer.
- Although paracentesis does effectively drain ascitic fluid, the ascites invariably will recur, and repeated procedures are necessary.

- A total of >20 L of ascitic fluid can be removed safely but each removal should not be more than 5 L.
- Up to 5 L of ascitic fluid can be removed in each paracentesis.
- Removal of 5 L and more ascitic fluid is considered as large volume paracentesis and albumin transfusion is given after the procedures.
- Volume expander using normal saline is sufficient if the volume of ascitic fluid removed is less than 5 L.

Potential Complications of Paracentesis

- Wound infection
- Persistent leaking from the puncture site
- Abdominal wall haematoma
- Bowel injury
- Laceration of major blood vessels (aorta, mesenteric artery, etc.)
- Catheter loss in the abdominal cavity
- Dilutional hyponatraemia
- Post-paracentesis hypotension (delayed complication occur after 12 hours of procedure if a large volume of ascitic fluid removed)
- A rare complication of spontaneous haemoperitoneum due to mesenteric variceal bleeding after removal of a large amount of ascitic fluid (>5 L)

Bladder Retraining and Care of Suprapubic Urinary Catheter

A patient who underwent radical hysterectomy often has bladder dysfunction. Some gynaecologic oncologist will insert a suprapubic catheter at the end of the surgery.

The suprapubic catheter is a tube used to drain urine from your bladder. This flexible tube is inserted into the bladder through an incision in suprapubic region. The catheter will be left unclamped for few days (3–7 days) to rest the bladder before a bladder retraining is initiated.

Bladder Retraining (Instruction to Patient)

(1) Go to the bathroom at least every 3 hours. You should not worry if it takes some time to retrain your bladder.
(2) Try to pass your urine normally into a container.
(3) Measure the amount of urine in the container.
(4) Unclamp your catheter.
(5) Drain your urine from your catheter.
(6) Measure the amount of urine.
(7) Clamp your catheter.
(8) Write the amounts of urine that you passed normally and the amount from your catheter on the record form (see Table 28.1).
(9) Add the two amounts together and record the total.
(10) Catheter should not be left clamped for more than 4 hours. If after 4 hours, you do not have an urge to pass your urine, the catheter should be unclamped and urine output is measured. This will avoid overdistended bladder.
    - Good sign of bladder recovery is increasing volume of urination and decreasing volume of urine removed from the catheter.
    - When the amount of urine removed from the catheter consistently less than 50 mL for at least 24 hours, catheter can now be removed.

Table 28.1 Example of urinary chart

Date	Time	Amount urinated	Amount of urine from catheter	Total
25.2.10	8.30 AM	90	50	140
	11.45 PM	100	80	180
Total				

Care of Suprapubic Catheter (Instruction to Patient)

Some patients are allowed to go home with their suprapubic catheter, and they are instructed to perform bladder training at home. Taking care of the suprapubic catheter is very important to ensure lower risk of infection, especially at the site of the catheter. Infection can spread down to subcutaneous tissue and bladder. Infection can also delay wound healing following removal of catheter.

Materials

- Tape
- Povidone–iodine ointment
- Q-tip
- Waste basket/plastic bag
- Povidone–iodine swabsticks (or cotton balls and povidone–iodine solution)
- Dressing sponges (4 × 4) split half way into the middle

Care of your suprapubic catheter (instruction to patient)

(1) Gather the supplies.

(2) If you are using a dressing, take off the old dressing. Be careful not to pull on the tube. Check the dressing for any unusual or foul drainage. Place the dressing in a plastic bag and throw away in the wastebasket.

(3) Wash your hands with soap and water.

(4) Look carefully at where the catheter leaves the skin (exit site). Check for any unusual or foul drainage, swelling, bleeding, skin irritation, or tract formation. A tract occurs around a tube if there is too much pressure from the tube on the skin. A tract looks like an open sore next to the exit site. Take swab for culture and sensitivity if you suspect local infection.

(5) Wash around the shield gently with soap and water. You may take a shower with the tube. It will not hurt it to get wet.

(6) Using one povidone–iodine swabstick, clean under the shield and clean around the exit site of the catheter. Start at the exit site and clean outward 3–4 inches in a circular motion. Never clean back towards the tube. Throw away the used swabstick and do it again with a new one. Let the area dry. An alternative to povidone is hibitane solution (Fig. 28.1).

(7) Put a thin layer of povidone–iodine ointment around the catheter with a Q-tip.

(8) Place a split 4 × 4 around the catheter. Tape it in place.

(9) Tape the catheter to your abdomen.

(10) Change this dressing every day. If the dressing falls off, becomes dirty or for any other reason, such as foul drainage or urine leakage, needs to be changed, change the dressing using the above steps.

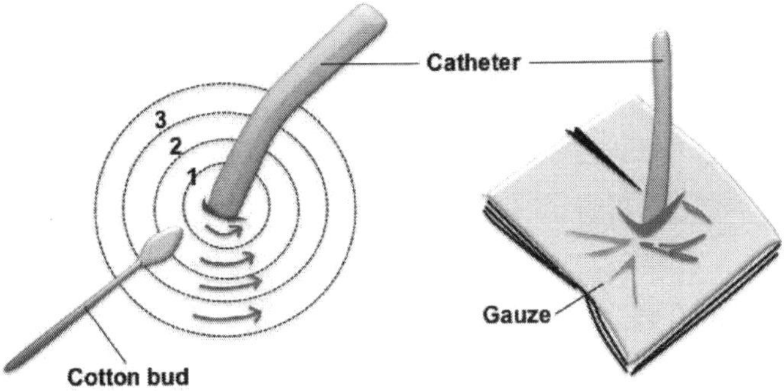

Figure 28.1 Care of suprapubic catheter site.

Chemoport

Chemoport is an implantable vascular access device to provide repeated access to the vascular system for the delivery of medications, intravenous fluids, parenteral nutrition solutions and blood products.

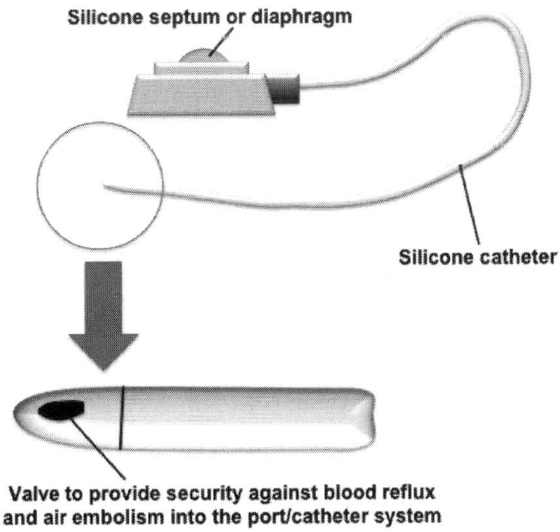

Figure 28.2 Basic components of chemoport.

There are two components (Fig. 28.2):

- injection port with a self-sealing silicone septum
- radiopaque silicone catheter

All material is biocompatible and can be used with virtually all injectable solutions.

Indications for Use of Chemoport

- patients requiring repeated vascular access for therapy
- infusion of fluid, TPN, blood product
- blood withdrawal

Contraindications

- presence of device related infection
- patient's body size unable to accommodate the device
- allergic to material
- severe chronic obstructive lung disease
- previous episodes of venous thrombosis or vascular surgical procedures at the prospective placement site.

Possible Complications

- air embolism
- bleeding
- brachial plexus injury
- cardiac arrhythmia
- cardiac temponade
- hydrothorax
- local tissue reaction, inflammation, etc.
- catheter or port erosion through the skin
- catheter embolism
- pneumothorax
- endocarditis

Implantation Instructions (Fig. 28.3)

(1) Aseptic technique.

(2) Site of port implantation, i.e. infraclavicular region, avoid pinch-off area (area where the first rib is overlapping the clavicle).
(3) Flush the catheter with normal saline before insertion.
(4) Cutaneous tissue thickness over the port should be appropriate, i.e. 0.5 to 2 cm.
(5) Vein (external jugular, internal jugular, subclavian vein).
(6) Patient in Trendelenburg position with head turned away.
(7) Incision over the intended vein.
(8) Expose the vein.
(9) Use the right angle to pick the thread around the vessel 2× to occlude the vessel during incision.
(10) Skin incision is made over the port site and creat a subcutaneous tract using artery forcep to the first incision.
(11) Using the silk to tight at the tip of catheter and pull the catheter toward the vein.
(12) Incise the vein and slide the catheter tip into the vein.
(13) Catheter tip should be at the junction of the superior vena cava and the atriam.

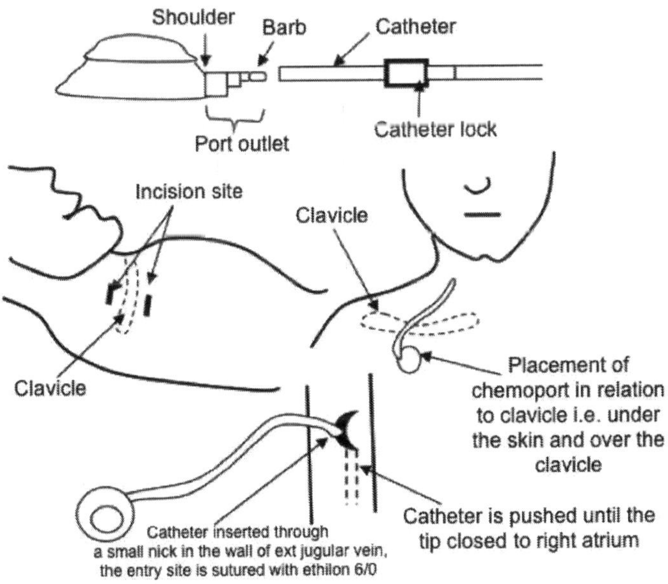

Figure 28.3 Single lumen chemoport and technique of insertion.

Accessing Implanted Port

Equipment: (1) non-coring needle and (2) syringe, at least 10 mL
Procedures:

(1) Locate the port septum/diaphragm by palpation.
   (a) Locate the base of the port with the non-dominant hand.
   (b) Triangulate the port between the thumb and the first fingers of the non-dominant hand. Aim for the centre point of these three fingers.

(2) Insert the needle perpendicular to the port diaphragm. Advance the needle through the skin and the diaphragm until reaching the bottom of the reservoir.

(3) Verify the correct needle placement by blood aspiration.

(4) Always flush the port following injection.

(5) Perform the saline lock procedure.

Saline lock procedure: It is meant to prevent clot formation and catheter blockage. Saline is filled after each use and if no injection is given for long time. Saline lock should be replaced every 4 weeks. Flushing volume is between 10 and 20 mL.

Chapter 29

Laparoscopic and Robotic Surgery in Gynaecologic Oncology

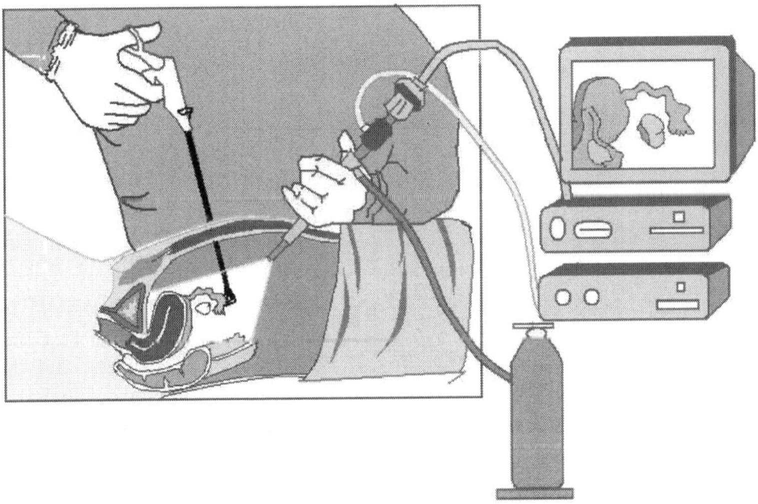

Gynaecologic Cancer: A Handbook for Students and Practitioners
Rushdan Noor, Eng Hseon Tay, and Jeffrey Low

ISBN 978-981-4463-06-5 (Hardcover), 978-981-4463-07-2 (eBook)
www.panstanford.com

Introduction

Developments in laparoscopic equipment in the past two decades have made minimally invasive surgery feasible in the modern management of gynaecologic cancers. It is associated with decreased blood loss, lower transfusion rates, decreased analgesic requirements, shorter lengths of hospital stay, improved cosmesis and faster return to normal daily activities. Adjuvant radiation or chemotherapy can be initiated earlier, and radiation complications from bowel adhesions are minimized. Robotic surgery is now considered the most advanced platform of minimally invasive surgery and is being increasingly used to perform surgery in patients with a number of gynaecologic malignancies.

Endometrial Cancer

Laparoscopy has been used for endometrial cancer in three conditions:

(a) primary staging in the form of hysterectomy, bilateral salpingo-oophorectomy, lymphadenectomy and washings
(b) re-staging of patients who have not been staged
(c) evaluation and management of recurrences

Total laparoscopic hysterectomy (TLH) and laparoscopy-assisted vaginal hysterectomy (LAVH) are the two basic surgical approaches. Data indicate significantly more pelvic lymph nodes removed, smaller changes in post-operative blood counts, lower pain medication requirements, shorter hospital stay, earlier return to full activity and work and a higher level of satisfaction with their treatment.

A GOG Study known as LAP2 was published in *Journal of Clinical Oncology*. The objective of this study was to compare laparoscopy versus laparotomy for comprehensive surgical staging of uterine cancer. Patients with clinical stage I to IIA uterine cancer were randomly assigned to laparoscopy (n = 1696) or open laparotomy (n = 920), including hysterectomy, salpingo-oophorectomy, pelvic cytology and pelvic and para-aortic lymphadenectomy. The main study end points were 6-week morbidity and mortality, hospital length of stay, conversion from laparoscopy to laparotomy, recurrence-free survival, site of recurrence and patient-reported quality-of-life outcomes. Laparoscopy was initiated in 1682 patients and completed without conversion in 1248 patients (74.2%). Conversion from laparoscopy to laparotomy was secondary to poor visibility in 246 patients (14.6%), metastatic cancer in 69 patients (4.1%), bleeding in 49 patients (2.9%) and other cause in 70 patients (4.2%). Laparoscopy had fewer moderate to severe post-operative adverse events than laparotomy (14% vs. 21%, respectively; $P < 0.0001$) but similar rates of intra-operative complications, despite having a significantly longer operative time (median, 204 vs. 130 minutes, respectively; $P < 0.001$). Hospitalization of more than 2 days was significantly lower in laparoscopy versus laparotomy patients (52% vs. 94%, respectively; $P < 0.0001$). Pelvic and para-aortic nodes were not removed in 8% of laparoscopy patients and 4% of laparotomy patients ($P < 0.0001$). No difference in overall detection of advanced stage (stage IIIA, IIIC or IVB) was seen (17% of laparoscopy patients vs. 17% of laparotomy patients; $P < 0.841$). This study indicates that comprehensive surgical staging of endometrial cancer can be performed using laparoscopy without increased intra-operative injuries, with fewer post-operative complications and with shorter hospital stay (Walker et al., 2009).

Ovarian Cancer

Role of Laparoscopy in the Evaluation of Adnexal Mass

Following are important facts about the roles of laparoscopy in the evaluation of an adnexal mass with suspicious features on ultrasound:

(1) Complete pre-operative workup is essential.
(2) Thorough initial assessment of the abdominal cavity should be performed as in a laparotomy.
(3) Aspiration of cysts should be avoided.
(4) Endobags should be used to prevent spillage of the cyst fluid content into the abdominal cavity.
(5) The prognosis associated with intra-operative rupture is poorly understood. Perhaps it is not the rupture of the cyst at the time of laparoscopy but rather the delay in the patient receiving treatment that results in the poor outcomes. If rupture occurs,

then vigorous irrigation should be undertaken. There should be pre-operative consent for and the capabilities to proceed with a full staging procedure if a malignancy is encountered. If the patient cannot be staged immediately, then planned re-staging should be undertaken as soon as possible.

Role of Laparoscopy in the Staging and Re-Staging

Laparoscopy has roles in the staging or re-staging of apparently early ovarian cancer. Laparoscopic detection of abdominal and lymphatic metastases may be equivalent to historical controls for staging by laparotomy, with acceptable complication rates, shorter hospital stay and upstaging in up to 26.6% of patients. Shorter recuperation is an advantage in the event that adjuvant treatment is required. Laparoscopy is also suitable when fertility-sparing unilateral oophorectomy and surgical staging are indicated. Feasibility of laparoscopic re-staging in patients with incompletely staged ovarian, fallopian tube, endometrial and primary peritoneal cancers was demonstrated in GOG 9302 and 9402. Fifty-eight patients underwent complete laparoscopic staging, confirmed with photographic documentation. Nine patients were incompletely staged laparoscopically due to the lack of peritoneal biopsies, cytology or bilateral lymph nodes. Seventeen patients underwent laparotomy. In comparing patients who were managed laparoscopically with those managed with laparotomy, the laparoscopic group demonstrated significantly less blood loss, hospital stay and comparable nodal yields.

Role of Laparoscopy in Advanced Ovarian Cancer

There are three potential applications of laparoscopy in advanced ovarian cancer, namely (a) triage for resectability—96% accuracy and 100% negative predictive value, (b) second look evaluation—within a research protocol and (c) selected cases of primary or secondary cytoreduction, sometimes done in conjunction with hand-assisted laparoscopic surgery (HALS). However, data are limited and more long-term studies are needed.

Neoadjuvant chemotherapy and downstaging may allow for laparoscopic interval debulking to optimal status as demonstrated in one small series, but long-term survival data for such an approach are lacking. Laparoscopic second look surgery may have a role in a research setting.

Cervical Cancer

Primary Surgical Treatment for Early-Stage Disease

There is increasing evidence that radical hysterectomy may be performed laparoscopically, with lower blood loss, equivalent operating duration, clear surgical margins, reduced wound infection, decreased post-operative pain, shorter median length of stay and earlier return to full activity and similar recurrence and mortality rates. Dargent first performed laparoscopic pelvic lymphadenectomy followed by a Schauta radical vaginal hysterectomy. Hatch et al. then reported 37 patients treated by laparoscopic pelvic and para-aortic lymphadenectomy followed by radical vaginal hysterectomy. Subsequent series have shown that the complication rates go down as the operator's experience increases. There are now increasing reports of laparoscopic radical hysterectomy. Puntambekar reported on 248 patients with early-stage cervical cancer, noting a median operative time of 292 minutes, median number of resected pelvic lymph nodes of 18, median blood loss of 165 mL and a median length of stay of 3 days. Every report on laparoscopic lymphadenectomy and radical hysterectomy has noted a significant decrease in blood loss and transfusion rates, with decreased hospital stay and rapid return to normal function. GOG 206 is now under way to investigate the sensitivity of the sentinel lymph node in predicting lymph node metastasis in patients with invasive cervical carcinoma by using laparoscopy or laparotomy.

Locally Advanced Cervical Cancer

Pre-treatment laparoscopic nodal staging may offer valuable information for individualized treatment planning with minimal morbidity. There was demonstrable improvement in accuracy of nodal assessment over CT and MRI. In younger patients, ovarian function can be preserved by laparoscopic ovarian transposition before the initiation of radiation therapy.

Radical Trachelectomy with Laparoscopic Lymphadenectomy

The indications for radical trachelectomy and laparoscopic lymphadenectomy are

(1) desire for future childbearing.
(2) stage 1A1 disease with extensive lymph-vascular space invasion
(3) stage IA2 disease
(4) stage IB1 ≤2 cm diameter with no involvement of the upper endocervix on MRI or intra-operative frozen section

The histology is squamous cell carcinoma, adenocarcinoma or adenosquamous and there should be no metastases to regional lymph nodes or lymphovascular space invasion. The risk factors for recurrence include lesion size greater than 2 cm, depth of invasion greater than 1 cm and lymph-vascular space invasion.

Some authors suggest that conservative fertility-sparing surgery may be appropriate for select patients with larger lesions that are clearly exophytic.

Milliken and Shepherd reported that a total of 709 patients had radical vaginal trachelectomy between 1994 and 2008. There have been 29 cases of recurrence (4%) and 16 reported deaths from recurrence (2%). In the last few years, there have been case reports for total laparoscopic-assisted trachelectomies or robotic-assisted trachelectomies, but it is not a routinely performed procedure.

Other Roles of Laparoscopy in Cervical Cancer

Laparoscopy can be used as method of assessment before pelvic exenteration. The other role of laparoscopy is to verify and guide for the interstitial radiation needle implant placement to decrease treatment-related morbidity.

Robotic Surgery

The potential technical drawbacks of conventional laparoscopy include limited range of motion intra-abdominally (only four degrees of freedom), counter-intuitive movements, amplification of tremors in prolonged cases because of the length and rigidity of the instrumentation, reduced depth perception secondary to a two-dimensional view, thick abdominal wall resistance against instrument movement and poor surgeon ergonomics.

The da Vinci surgical system (Intuitive Surgical, Sunnyvale CA) is currently the only commercially available robotic surgical system that is FDA approved for gynaecologic and other surgical procedures.

Following are the components of the da Vinci system:

(1) The surgeon console is a remote unit that allows the seated surgeon to manipulate the robotic instruments while viewing a 3-D operative field.
(2) Patient-side cart, which provides three or four robotic arms, which in turn control the endoscope and instrument arms.
(3) EndoWrist instrumentation, which provides seven degrees of motion, mimicking the full range of motion of a surgeon's hand and wrist.
(4) In-vision system, which allows for three-dimensional imaging. The Vision System incorporates a high-resolution three-dimensional endoscope, which provides 3-D vision when the surgeon utilizes the stereoscopic viewer. An additional vision tower provides operative field visualization for the rest of the surgical team, although images are two-dimensional.

The advantages of the robotic system include three-dimensional high-definition vision, tremor reduction, seven degrees of intra-abdominal articulation, motion scaling and surgeon comfort. The use of the da Vinci robotic-assisted laparoscopic radical prostatectomy (RALP) was pivotal in bringing about the subsequent widespread use of the tool in gynaecology. It is an ideal tool for teaching since it allows expert surgeons to instruct novice surgeons from distant sites, a practice known as telementoring with the use of dual consoles and telestration. In addition, robotic surgery allows for telepresence, whereby a surgeon may operate on a patient from a distant site. At present, the key roles of robotic surgery in gynaecological cancer are (a) endometrial cancer staging, (b) radical hysterectomy for early cervical cancer and (c) radical trachelectomy.

The disadvantages of robotic surgery are the high initial cost, limited instrumentation and increased operation theatre space needed for robotic surgical cart and surgical console.

Following are the standard port placements for gynaecologic robot-assisted surgery (Fig. 29.1):

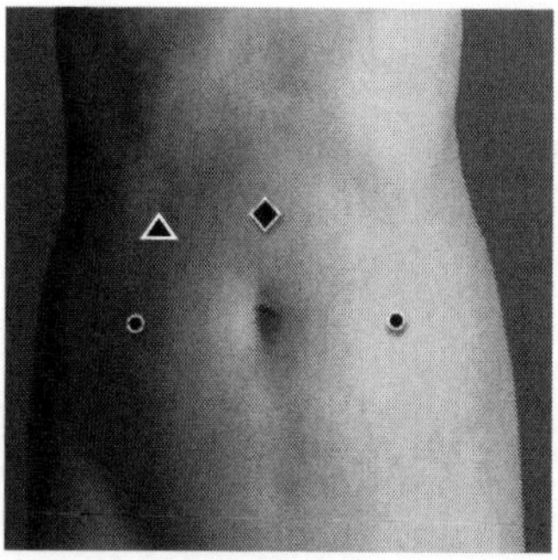

Key:

- ◆ 12 mm robotic camera port
- ● 8 mm robotic instrument ports
- ▲ 5 mm laparoscopic assistant port

Figure 29.1 Standard port placement for gynaecologic robot-assisted surgery (© 2010 GRACES Singapore).

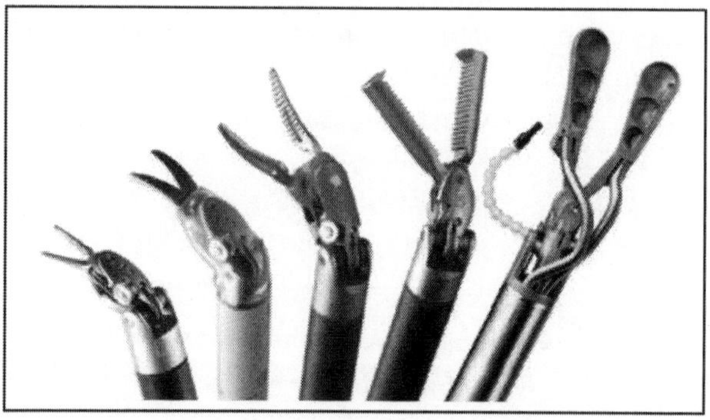

Figure 29.2 Da Vinci instruments, © 2011, Intuitive Surgical, Inc.

(a) 12 mm camera port is placed in the midline.
(b) Two 8 mm instrument ports are placed in the same horizontal line drawn through the umbilicus.
(c) Port positions describe a rough arc, which is more suited to the shorter xipho-pubic distance in the Asian population.

Complications of Laparoscopy

Key Factors Related to Complications Laparoscopy

Surgeon training and surgical expertise are important key factors to determine the success of the laparoscopic surgery. Studies have shown that as the surgeons perform more cases by laparoscopy their level of skill will improve and the complication rate will decrease.

Patient factors include weight—patients who are overweight or obese have a higher complication rate due to difficulty with exposure during the surgery. In addition, these patients also may pose difficulty with ventilation during the surgery leading to pulmonary complications. Patients who are obese and with multiple medical co-morbidities often benefit from laparoscopic surgery because of the fact that patients undergoing laparoscopic surgery have a much faster return to normal activities and full recovery. The other patient factor is prior surgical history: A patient with history of abdominal surgery has higher risk of complications during laparoscopic surgery because of an increased risk of adhesion (scar tissue) formation from their previous surgeries. A patient with medical co-morbidities is known to have higher risk of laparoscopic complications related to anaesthesia and post-operative recovery.

The other important factors that contributed to the risk of laparoscopic complications are the quality and the selection of the instrumentation.

The specific complications of laparoscopic surgery include vascular injury, gastrointestinal injury, urinary injury, incisional hernias and thermal injuries. Less common complications include port-site recurrences and gas embolism.

Vascular Injuries

Vascular injuries can occur during initial entry into abdominal cavity, during dissection of tissue lying in close proximity to major vessels, or by excessive traction on tissue. It can be prevented by controlled insertion of initial trocar, proper anatomical orientation and localization of the major blood vessels, or by avoiding use of insufflating needles for abdominal infusion of insufflation gas. In the event of a major vascular injury, the surgeon should consider immediate conversion to laparotomy, along with adequate patient stabilization and judicious use of vascular surgeon consultant.

Gastrointestinal Injuries

Laparoscopic surgery can lead to gastrointestinal injuries and potentially carries a significant morbidity, particularly if unrecognized. It can occur from insufflation needle, trocar insertion or operative dissection. The management depends on the extent of the injury, the site of the bowel affected and the overall status of the patient at the time of presentation.

Urinary Injuries

Urinary injuries usually occur because of trocar insertion, particularly in patients with previous pelvic surgery or multiple caesarean sections, or by pelvic dissection with poor exposure due to a large pelvic mass or enlarged uterus. Ureteral injuries can occur through narrowing, partial transaction (cutting), suture occlusion, thermal injury or complete transection. Repair is aimed based on the location and extent of the injury.

Incisional Hernias

The risk factors for incisional hernias include the use of multiple ancillary ports, procedures where a large mass is removed through the small incision made for trocar placement, instruments requiring 10–12 mms ports, increased operating room time, use of port-anchoring devices, failure to close large fascial (layer of support of the anterior abdominal wall) defects and history of prior incisional hernias. The majority of patients present with pain at the incisional site, fever, nausea and vomiting. The average time to presentation is 10 days post-operatively. Approximately 20% of patients will require a bowel resection as a result of the incisional hernia.

Port-Site Metastases

The rate of incisional metastases is the same in laparoscopic surgery as it is in laparotomy. The factors contributing to the occurrence of port-site metastases include wound contamination, effects of pressure to create abdominal distention, aerosolization of tumour cells, local immune response and surgical technique—more common in patients with widely disseminated disease, while factors which may decrease the risk include minimizing tissue trauma, retrieving the specimen in an endoscopic bag to prevent spread of malignant cells to the incision, suturing the fascial defect and deflating the abdomen with trocars in place.

Gas Embolism

Gas embolism is an extremely rare complication of laparoscopic surgery. It occurs when a sufficient quantity of gas is forced into open veins and into the circulation. After the gas collects in the heart, no blood could be effectively pumped into the heart or brain and the patient may die acutely.

References

Amara DP, Nezhat C, Teng NN, et al. Operative laparoscopy in the management of ovarian cancer. *Surg Laparosc Endosc* 1996; **6**: 38–45.

Boggess JF, Gehrig PA, Cantrell L, et al. A comparative study of 3 surgical methods for hysterectomy with staging for endometrial cancer:robotic assistance, laparoscopy, laparotomy. *Am J Obstet Gynecol* 2008; **199**: 360.e1–360.e9.

Chi DS, Abu-Rustum NR, Sonoda Y, et al. The safety and efficacy of laparoscopic surgical staging of apparent stage I ovarian and fallopian tube cancers. *Am J Obstet Gynecol* 2005; **192**: 1614–1619.

Childers JM, Hatch KD, Tran AN, et al. Laparoscopic para-aortic lymphadenectomy in gynecologic malignancies. *Obstet Gynecol* 1993; **82**: 741–747.

Childers JM, Spirtos NM, Brainard P, et al. Laparoscopic staging of the patient with incompletely staged early adenocarcinoma of the endometrium. *Obstet Gynecol* 1994; **83**: 597–600.

Chen Y, Xu H, Zhang Q, Li Y, Wang D, Liang Z. A fertility preserving option in early cervical carcinoma: laparoscopy-assisted vaginal radical trachelectomy and pelvic lymphadenectomy. *Eur J Obstet Gynecol Reprod Biol* 2008; **136**: 90–93.

Dargent D. A new future for Schauta's operation through a presurgical retroperitoneal pelviscopy. *Eur J Gynaecol Oncol* 1987; **8**: 292–296.

Fagotti A, Fanfani F, Ludovisi M, et al. Role of laparoscopy to assess the chance of optimal cytoreductive surgery in advanced ovarian cancer: a pilot study. *Gynecol Oncol* 2005; **96**: 729–735.

Hatch KD, Hallum AV III, Nour M. New surgical approaches to treatment of cervical cancer. *J Natl Cancer Inst Monogr* 1996; **21**: 71–75.

Kornblith AB, Huang HQ, Walker JL, et al. Quality of life of patients with endometrial cancer undergoing laparoscopic international federation of gynecology and obstetrics staging compared with laparotomy: a gynecologic oncology group study. *J Clin Oncol* 2009; **27**: 5337–5342.

Magrina JF, Kho RM, Weaver AL, et al. Robotic radical hysterectomy: comparison with laparoscopy and laparotomy. *Gynecol Oncol* 2008; **109**: 86–91.

Milliken DA, Shepherd JH. Fertility preserving surgery for carcinoma of the cervix. *Curr Opin Oncol* 2008; **20**: 575–580.

Morice P, Camatte S, Larregain-Fournier D, et al. Port-site implantation after laparoscopic treatment of borderline ovarian tumors. *Obstet Gynecol* 2004; **104**: 1167–1170.

Littell RD, Hallonquist H, Matulonis U, et al. Negative laparoscopy is highly predictive of negative second-look laparotomy following chemotherapy for ovarian, tubal and primary peritoneal carcinoma. *Gynecol Oncol* 2006; **103**: 570–574.

Nezhat FR, Datta MS, Liu C, et al. Robotic radical hysterectomy versus total laparoscopic radical hysterectomy with pelvic lymphadenectomy for treatment of early cervical cancer. *JSLS* 2008; **12**: 227–237.

Nezhat FR, Datta MS, Lal N, et al. Laparoscopic cytoreduction for primary advanced or recurrent ovarian, fallopian tube, and peritoneal malignancies. *Gynecol Oncol* 2008; **108**: S60.

Nezhat F, Yadav J, Rahaman J, et al. Analysis of survival after laparoscopic management of endometrial cancer. *JMIG* 2008; **15**: 181–187.

Nezhat F, Ezzati M, Rahaman J, et al. Laparoscopic management of early ovarian and fallopian tube cancers: surgical and survival outcome. *Am J Obstet Gynecol* 2009; 200: **83**.e1–83.e6.

Pahisa J, Martínez-Román S, Martínez-Zamora MA, et al. Laparoscopic ovarian transposition in patients with early cervical cancer. *Int J Gynecol Cancer* 2008; **18**: 584–589.

Plante M, Renaud MC, Tetu B, et al. Laparoscopic sentinel node mapping in early-stage cervical cancer. *Gynecol Oncol* 2003; **91**: 494–503.

Plantae M. Fertility preservation in the management of cervical cancer. *CME J Gynecol Oncol* 2003; **8**: 128–138.

Puntambekar SP, Palep RJ, Puntambekar S, et al. Laparoscopic total radical hysterectomy by the Pune technique: our experience of 248 cases. *J Minim Invasive Gynecol* 2007; **14**: 682–689.

Ramirez PT, Wolf JK, Leveback C. Laparoscopic port-site metastases: etiology and prevention. *Gynecol Oncol* 2003; **91**: 179–189.

Reich H, McGlyn F, Wilkie W. Laparoscopic management of stage I ovarian caner: a case report. *J Reprod Med* **35**: 601–604.

Seamon LG, Cohn DE, Henretta MS, et al. Minimally invasive comprehensive surgical staging for endometrial cancer: robotics or laparoscopy? *Gynecol Oncol* 2009; **113**: 36–41.

Sjövall K, Nilsson B, Einhorn N. Different types of rupture of the tumor capsule and the impact on survival in early ovarian carcinoma. *Int J Gynecol Cancer* 1994; **4**: 333–336.

Spirtos NM, Eisekop SM, Boike G, et al. Laparoscopic staging in patients with incompletely staged cancers of the uterus, ovary, fallopian tube, and primary peritoneum: a Gynecologic Oncology Group (GOG) study. *Am J Obstet Gyencol* 2005; **193**: 1645–1649.

Tillmanns T, Lowe MP. Safety, feasibility, and costs of outpatient laparoscopic extraperitoneal aortic nodal dissection for locally advanced cervical carcinoma. *Gynecol Oncol* 2007; **106**: 370–374.

Tozzi R, Malur S, Koehler C, et al. Laparoscopy versus laparotomy in endometrial cancer: first analysis of survival of a randomized prospective study. *JMIG* 2005; **12**: 130–136.

Vergote I, De Wever I, Tjalma W, et al. Neoadjuvant chemotherapy or primary debulking surgery in advanced ovarian carcinoma: a retrospective analysis of 285 patients. *Gynecol Oncol* 1998; **71**: 431–436.

Vergote I, De Brabanter J, Fyles A, et al. Prognostic importance of degree of differentiation and cyst rupture in stage I invasive epithelial ovarian carcinoma. *Lancet* 2001; **357**: 176–182.

Walker JL, Piedmonte MR, Spirtos NM, et al. Laparoscopy compared with laparotomy for comprehensive surgical staging of uterine cancer: gynecologic oncology group study LAP2. *J Clin Oncol* 2009; **27**: 5331–5336.

Index